Atlas of Cranial Base Surgery

Special Contributing Editors:

NEUROANATOMY:

JOHANNES LANG, M.D.

Professor of Anatomy Emeritus
Anatomical Institute
Würzburg, Germany

NEURORADIOLOGY:

JOHN BENTSON, M.D.

Professor of Neuroradiology
UCLA Department of Radiology
Los Angeles, California

NEUROPATHOLOGY:

G. F. WALTER, M.D.

Professor and Chairman of Neuropathology
Medical School Hannover
Hannover, Germany

Atlas of Cranial Base Surgery

UCLA and Hannover Experience

MADJID SAMII, M.D., Ph.D.
Professor and Neurosurgical Chair
Medical School Hannover
Chairman of the Neurosurgical Clinic
Nordstadt Hospital
Hannover, Germany

MELVIN L. CHEATHAM, M.D.
Clinical Professor
UCLA Division of Neurosurgery
Director, Cranial Base Surgery Laboratory
UCLA School of Medicine
Los Angeles, California

DONALD P. BECKER, M.D.
Professor and Chief
UCLA Division of Neurosurgery
Director, Cranial Base Surgery Program
UCLA School of Medicine
Los Angeles, California

Illustrated by Joseph I. Bloch, CMI

W.B. SAUNDERS COMPANY
A Division of Harcourt Brace & Company
PHILADELPHIA, LONDON, TORONTO, MONTREAL, SYDNEY, TOKYO

W.B. SAUNDERS COMPANY
A Division of Harcourt Brace & Company

The Curtis Center
Independence Square West
Philadelphia, PA 19106

Library of Congress Cataloging-in-Publication Data

Atlas of cranial base surgery / [edited by] Madjid Samii, Melvin L. Cheatham, Donald P. Becker.
p. cm.
ISBN 0-7216-3882-1
1. Skull base—Tumors—Surgery—Atlases. I. Samii, Madjid.
II. Cheatham, Melvin L. III. Becker, Donald P.
[DNLM: 1. Skull—surgery—atlases. WE 17 A8797 1994]
RD662.5.A85 1995
617.4′8—dc20
DNLM/DLC 94-4811

ATLAS OF CRANIAL BASE SURGERY ISBN 0-7216-3882-1

Printed in the United States of America.

Last digit is the print number: 9 8 7 6 5 4 3 2 1

CONTRIBUTORS

MARIO AMMIRATI, M.D.

Assistant Professor, Division of Neurosurgery, UCLA Medical Center. Attending Neurosurgeon, UCLA Medical Center; Chief, Division of Neurosurgery, Olive View/UCLA Medical Center, Los Angeles, California.

Pre-sigmoid Sinus Approach

JAMES C. ANDREWS, M.D.

Associate Professor, Division of Head and Neck Surgery, UCLA School of Medicine. Attending Head and Neck Surgeon, UCLA Medical Center, Los Angeles, California.

Translabyrinthine Approach; Transcochlear (Transotic) Approach; Middle Cranial Fossa Approach

KEITH BLACK, M.D.

Professor, Division of Neurosurgery, UCLA School of Medicine. Co-Director, Brain Tumor Program; Co-Director, Cranial Base Surgery Program, UCLA Medical Center, Los Angeles, California.

JOSEPH I. BLOCH, CMI

Medical Illustrator; Active Member, Association of Medical Illustrators. Department of Neurosurgery, Allegheny General Hospital, Pittsburgh, Pennsylvania.

RINALDO F. CANALIS, M.D.

Professor, Division of Head and Neck Surgery, UCLA School of Medicine. Chief, Division of Head and Neck Surgery (Otolaryngology), Harbor UCLA Medical Center; Vice Chief, Division of Head and Neck Surgery, UCLA Medical Center, Los Angeles, California.

Translabyrinthine Approach; Transcochlear (Transotic) Approach; Orbitotomy: Caudal Approach

MELVIN L. CHEATHAM, M.D.

Clinical Professor, Division of Neurosurgery, UCLA School of Medicine. Administrative Director, Cranial Base Surgery Laboratory, UCLA Medical Center, Los Angeles, California.

GARY DUCKWILER, M.D.

Assistant Professor, Department of Radiology, UCLA School of Medicine. Director, Neuroradiology Fellowship Program, UCLA Medical Center, Los Angeles, California.

Endovascular Therapy

ROBERT ALAN GOLDBERG, M.D.

Assistant Professor of Ophthalmology, Department of Ophthalmology, UCLA School of Medicine. Chief, Division of Orbital and Ophthalmic Plastic Surgery, Jules Stein Eye Institute; Director, UCLA Orbital Disease Center, Los Angeles, California.

Orbitotomy: Medial Approach (Paranasal-Ethmoidal); Orbitotomy: Lateral Approach; Orbitotomy: Cranial Approach (Frontal-Orbital); Orbitotomy: Caudal Approach; Panoramic Orbitotomy; Transsphenoidal Optic Canal Decompression; Optic Glioma

J. PATRICK JOHNSON, M.D.

Assistant Professor, Division of Neurosurgery, UCLA School of Medicine. Co-Director, UCLA Comprehensive Spine Center, UCLA Medical Center, Los Angeles, California.

Transoral Approach to the Clivus and C1–C2

WESLEY A. KING, M.D.

Assistant Professor, Division of Neurosurgery, UCLA School of Medicine. Co-Director, Pituitary Program, UCLA Medical Center, Los Angeles, California.

Transsphenoidal Approach; Pituitary Tumors

HOWARD R. KRAUSS, M.D.

Assistant Clinical Professor, Department of Ophthalmology and Division of Neurosurgery, UCLA School of Medicine. Attending Surgeon, UCLA Medical Center; Jules Stein Eye Institute; Los Angeles; St. John's Hospital, Santa Monica, California.

Orbitotomy: Medial Approach (Paranasal-Ethmoidal); Orbitotomy: Lateral Approach; Orbitotomy: Cranial Approach (Frontal-Orbital); Orbitotomy: Caudal Approach; Panoramic Orbitotomy; Transsphenoidal Optic Canal Depression; Optic Glioma

NEIL A. MARTIN, M.D.

Associate Professor, Division of Neurosurgery, UCLA School of Medicine. Head, Neurovascular Surgery, UCLA Medical Center, Los Angeles, California.

Subtemporal Transtentorial Approach; Vascular Lesions (Aneurysms and Skull Base Arterial Bypasses)

MADJID SAMII, M.D.

Professor of Neurosurgery, Medical School Hannover. Visiting Professor of Neurosurgery in Continuum, UCLA Division of Neurosurgery. Chairman of the Neurosurgical Clinic, Nordstadt Hospital, Hannover, Germany.

MARCOS TATAGIBA, M.D.

Assistant Professor, Department of Neurosurgery, Neurosurgical Clinic, Nordstadt Hospital, Hannover, Germany.

FERNANDO VINUELA, M.D.

Professor of Radiology, Department of Radiology, UCLA School of Medicine. Director, Endovascular Therapy Service, UCLA Medical Center, Los Angeles, California.

Endovascular Therapy

PHILLIP A. WACKYM, M.D.

Assistant Professor, Section of Otology, Neuro-otology and Skull Base Surgery, Division of Head and Neck Surgery, UCLA School of Medicine. Attending Head and Neck Surgeon, UCLA Medical Center, Los Angeles, California.

Translabyrinthine Approach; Transcochlear (Transotic) Approach; Middle Cranial Fossa Approach

ACKNOWLEDGMENTS

We extend thanks to Mr. Edwin Best and Mrs. Thelma Best Komasa for their very generous financial support of the UCLA Cranial Base Surgery Program through a Unitrust. This offered the inspiration that led to the writing of this atlas.

Appreciation is also extended to Jianya Ma, M.D., and Zhongtao Mei, M.D., who contributed to the microneurosurgery laboratory work on this atlas during their time as Fellows in the UCLA Division of Neurosurgery.

Special thanks are also given to Miss Ina Malo for her secretarial help and to Mr. Stefen Brinkmann and Mrs. Gena Behnke for their photographic assistance.

PREFACE

Tumors and other lesions at the skull base have historically been largely inoperable or attended by high risk of morbidity or mortality when surgically approached. During recent years, with the advent of CT and MRI coupled with development of microsurgical techniques, the exciting new field of cranial base surgery has risen to its present high level of expertise. Also responsible for these exciting new advances have been the contributions from the areas of neuroanatomy, neuroradiology, and neuropathology.

In developing the field of skull base surgery, neurosurgeons have been joined by specialists in ENT, ophthalmology, and plastic surgery and further aided by the expertise of interventional neuroradiologists. This team effort by an interdisciplinary group has made previously inoperable tumors now operable.

This ATLAS of CRANIAL BASE SURGERY has not been written simply to bring forth another textbook in this field. It is intended to be an ATLAS dealing with the anatomical, pathological, and surgical aspects of the very complex area of the cranial base in a clear, concise, simple, and practical manner. We have tried to avoid that which is theoretical or experimental and to present those principles that are basic and essential in performing surgery at the skull base.

Contained within the pages of this ATLAS are key anatomical illustrations depicting structures that can be studied through cadaver dissections in the laboratory. Also presented in a concise, serial manner are the various surgical approach techniques. In Section One, the Conventional Approaches are demonstrated and Section Two presents the Special Approaches to the cranial base.

Section Three of this ATLAS deals with Specific Problems that are encountered in cranial base surgery. In it the reader will find text and illustrations showing the location, the extension, and the behavior of different types of pathology in this area. It then presents the method of surgical approach and technique for surgical excision of these lesions.

In addition to striving to be concise in preparation of text, and as clear and helpful as possible in presenting illustrations, we have attempted to be as informative as possible in defining key points and "pearls of wisdom," based upon long collective experience. Perhaps the hallmark of excellence in communication is to present difficult, complicated subject matter in a concise manner and with optimal logic of thought and clarity. This we have attempted in creating this ATLAS.

Special thanks are given to our neurosurgery colleagues, and skull base specialists from allied disciplines, who work with us as the UCLA Cranial Base Surgery Team, and whose contributions to this ATLAS have been so valuable.

MADJID SAMII, M.D.
MELVIN CHEATHAM, M.D.
DONALD BECKER, M.D.

CONTENTS

I. CONVENTIONAL SURGICAL TECHNIQUES OF CRANIOTOMY —APPROACHES TO THE CRANIAL BASE

1
Subfrontal Approach (Unilateral, Bilateral). 3

2
Frontotemporal (Pterional) Approach. 6

3
Subtemporal Approach. 9

4
Suboccipital Lateral Retrosigmoid Approach. 12

5
Suboccipital Medial Approach. 16

6
Translabyrinthine Approach. 18
James C. Andrews, Phillip A. Wackym, and Rinaldo F. Canalis

7
Transcochlear (Transotic) Approach. 24
James C. Andrews, Phillip A. Wackym, and Rinaldo F. Canalis

8
Middle Cranial Fossa Approach. 26
Phillip A. Wackym and James C. Andrews

9
Transsphenoidal Approach. 32
Wesley A. King

II. SPECIAL SURGICAL APPROACHES TO THE CRANIAL BASE

1. Temporo-Occipital-Petrosal Approaches

10
Subtemporal-Transzygomatic Approach. 40

11
Lateral Approach to Middle Skull Base (Temporal-Infratemporal Fossa, Carotid Artery, and Jugular Foramen). 43

12
Lateral Approach to the Craniocervical Junction. 54

13
Pre-sigmoid Sinus Approach. 62
Mario Ammirati

14
Subtemporal Transtentorial Approach. 67
Neil A. Martin

2. Frontal Approaches

15
Transfrontal-Basal Approach. 75

16
Bifrontal Orbital Approach. 79

17
Frontal-Temporal-Orbital Approach (With Approaches to Cavernous Sinus). 82

3. FACIAL APPROACHES

18
Sublabial Transnasal Transmaxillary Sphenoidal Approach to the Sella and Clivus (Modified Midface Degloving). 86

19
Ethmoidal Sphenoidal Approach to the Sella and Clivus. 93

20
Transoral Approach to the Clivus and C1–C2. 95
J. Patrick Johnson

21
Orbitotomy: Medial Approach (Paranasal-Ethmoidal). 98
Howard R. Krauss and Robert Alan Goldberg

22
Orbitotomy: Lateral Approach. 102
Howard R. Krauss and Robert Alan Goldberg

23
Orbitotomy: Cranial Approach (Frontal-Orbital). 105
Howard R. Krauss and Robert Alan Goldberg

24
Orbitotomy: Caudal Approach. 107
Robert Alan Goldberg and Rinaldo F. Canalis

25
Panoramic Orbitotomy. 109
Robert Alan Goldberg and Howard R. Krauss

26
Transsphenoidal Optic Canal Decompression. 112
Robert Alan Goldberg and Howard R. Krauss

III. SPECIFIC CRANIAL BASE PATHOLOGY: PRINCIPLES OF SURGICAL APPROACHES

27
Meningiomas. 117

28
Acoustic Neurinomas. 152

29
Epidermoids and Dermoids. 170

30
Craniopharyngiomas. 176

31
Chordomas, Chondromas, and Chondrosarcomas. 186

32
Chemodectomas (Paraganglioma). 190

33
Cholesterol Granuloma. 197

34
Vascular Lesions (Aneurysms and Skull Base Arterial Bypasses)...... 201
Neil A. Martin

35
Pituitary Tumors.. 212
Wesley A. King

36
Optic Glioma.. 224
Robert Alan Goldberg and Howard R. Krauss

37
Esthesioneuroblastoma... 226

38
Juvenile Nasopharyngeal Angiofibroma.......................... 233

IV. INTERVENTIONAL SKULL BASE NEURORADIOLOGY

39
Endovascular Therapy.. 241
Fernando Vinuela and Gary Duckwiler

INDEX... 257

I

CONVENTIONAL SURGICAL TECHNIQUES OF CRANIOTOMY— APPROACHES TO THE CRANIAL BASE

Subfrontal Approach (Unilateral, Bilateral) 1

INDICATIONS

The subfrontal approaches are indicated for surgery of tumors or other lesions of the anterior cranial fossa as well as the suprasellar area.

POSITION

The patient is positioned supine with slight flexion of the trunk and knees. All pressure points are well padded. The head is placed in a three-point fixation headholder and elevated above the heart for venous drainage. The vertex is tilted down with slight extension of the neck to allow the frontal lobes to fall away without retraction (Figure 1). This arrangement provides a comfortable working position for the surgeon and offers exposure of the entire frontal fossa floor.

INCISION

A bicoronal incision extending from 1 cm anterior to the tragus over the root of the zygoma to the vertex at the bregma and to the opposite side is used for the subfrontal craniotomy (see Figure 1).

The flap is retracted with multiple fish hooks. Unilateral subfrontal exposure requires that the incision extend from the ipsilateral tragus to the contralateral superior temporal line. The scalp flap, including the pericranium, is sharply dissected from the bone. The pericranium should be protected with a moistened sponge and preserved in case it is needed later as a vascularized, pedicled flap for dural repair and frontal sinus closure.

The temporalis muscle is split vertically and retracted as needed for placement of the lateral burr hole.

CRANIOTOMY

A free bone flap is elevated for either unilateral or bilateral exposure. Unilateral craniotomy requires a burr hole placed just posterior to the origin of the zygomatic process of the frontal bone, about 1 cm above the frontozygomatic suture line (Figure 2A). With this location of the keyhole burr hole, the surgeon avoids entering the orbit. If the burr hole is not low enough, the dura can be elevated to identify the location of the anterior fossa floor and additional bone can be removed. The importance of this burr hole is to reach the level of the lateral anterior fossa. This is the position of the keyhole burr hole as it usually is described in this atlas; it is higher than the classic keyhole described by MacCarty. The position of the MacCarty keyhole is lower by about 1 cm and is just behind the zygomatic process and overlying the frontosphenoidal suture line (Figure 2B). Properly placed, the MacCarty burr hole offers entry into the anterior fossa above and the orbit below, with the orbital roof visible in the midportion of the burr hole.

Another burr hole is placed at the midline, as low as possible (Figure 3A). The pediatric burr is used to create a small opening over the frontal sinus. For a unilateral frontal craniotomy, a third burr hole is placed halfway between the first two burr holes and 5 cm above the orbital ridge (Figure 4).

For bilateral frontal craniotomy, burr hole placement at both keyhole sites and low in the midline at the glabella are necessary. Single or paired burr holes are placed over or adjacent to the sagittal sinus at a point 5 cm above the glabella (see Figure 3A and B). The dura is then separated in preparation for elevating the bone flap. Care is exercised in separating the dura in the midline overlying the sagittal sinus.

The craniotome is used to elevate the bone flap (see Figure 3A). As long as the orbital contents are not involved, it is unnecessary to remove the orbital roof. It is essential to extend the frontal craniotomy as low as possible to avoid a bony balcony along the supraorbital area, which reduces the surgical window.

DURAL OPENING

For a unilateral dural opening, a low transverse dural incision is made and curved slightly at the lateral end in a posterior direction (Figure 5). This opening preserves the frontal lobe veins that are draining into the superior sagittal sinus and provides adequate exposure to the anterior cranial fossa.

If a bilateral subfrontal approach is made (Figure 6), the dura is incised on both sides. Double ligation and division of the proximal superior sagittal sinus is done. The falcine dura is detached from the crista galli and the frontal lobes are gradually retracted. The basilar cisterns are opened to allow drainage of cerebrospinal fluid.

CLOSURE

Closure of the subfrontal craniotomy focuses on reapproximation of the superior sagittal sinus and watertight closure of the dura. This is achieved by the initial placement of several dural sutures to help with anatomical alignment, followed by closure with a running interlocking suture of 4-0 nylon. Additional dural defects are reconstructed with pericranium, if needed.

If the frontal sinus has been opened and part of the mucosa has been removed, the sinus has to be treated to achieve good nasal drainage and to avoid the development of a mucocele. We use a vascularized pedicle of pericranium to assure closure of the sinus and closure of the dural defect in the anterior fossa as far as the sphenoid wings and planum sphenoidale.

The bone flap is replaced and held secure with several nonabsorbable sutures. The burr holes are filled with bone dust or methyl methacrylate. A two-layer scalp closure is done with 3-0 Vicryl in the galea and 3-0 nylon or skin staples in the scalp.

RECOMMENDED READING

Kempe, L.: Operative Neurosurgery. Vol. 1. New York, Springer-Verlag, 1968.

MacCarty, C., Brown, D.: Orbital tumors in children. Clin. Neurosurg. 11:76–88, 1964.

Poppen, J.: Operative techniques for removal of olfactory groove and suprasellar meningiomas. Clin. Neurosurg. 11:1–7, 1964.

Samii, M., Draf, W.: Surgery of the Skull Base: An Interdisciplinary Approach. New York, Springer-Verlag, 1989.

Schramm, V., Myers, E., Maroon, J.: Anterior skull base surgery for benign and malignant disease. Laryngoscope 89:1077–1091, 1979.

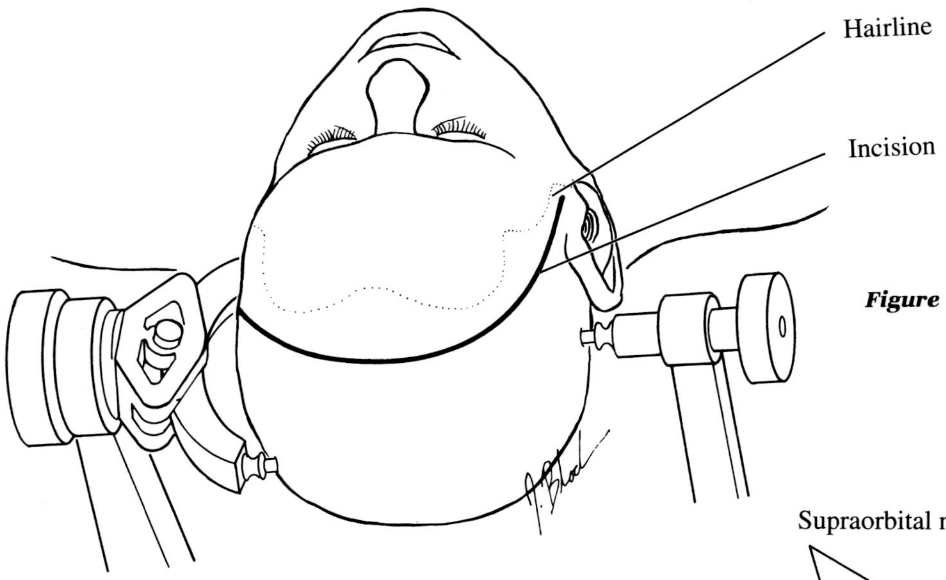

Figure 1. Patient position. Bicoronal scalp incision.

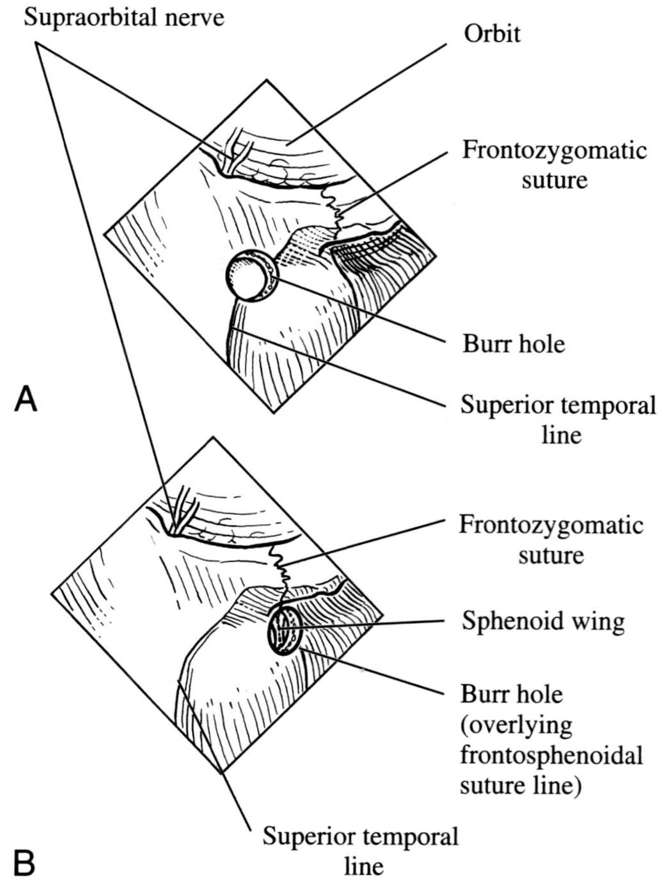

Figure 2. *A*, Placement of keyhole burr hole for the subfrontal approach. *B*, Position of MacCarty burr hole.

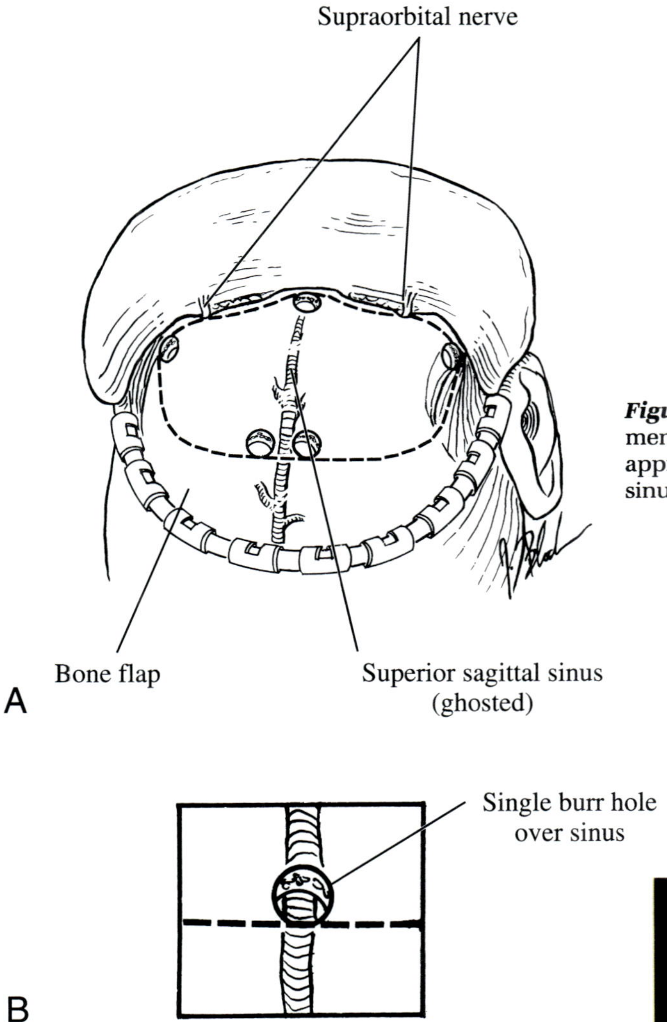

Figure 3. *A*, Low midline burr hole placement. Bilateral burr hole placement adjacent to sagittal sinus. Outline for elevation of bone flap, bilateral approach *(dotted line)*. *B*, Single burr hole placement over the sagittal sinus.

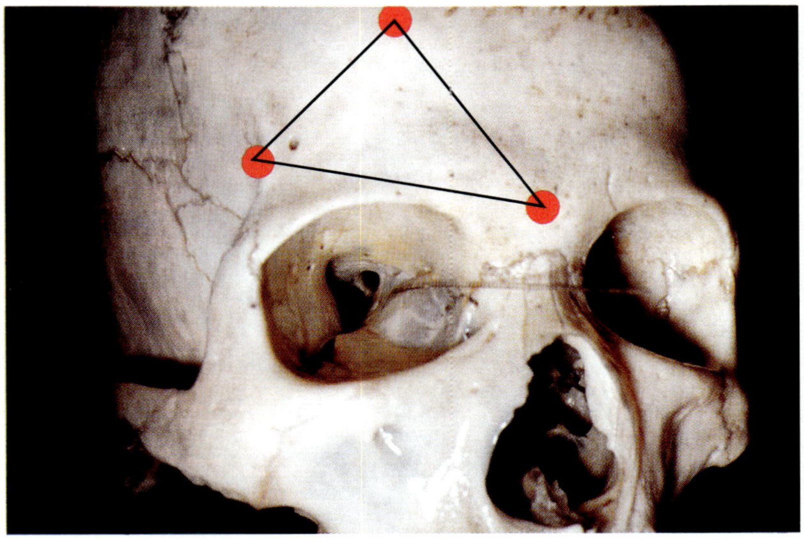

Figure 4. Placement of burr holes for unilateral subfrontal craniotomy.

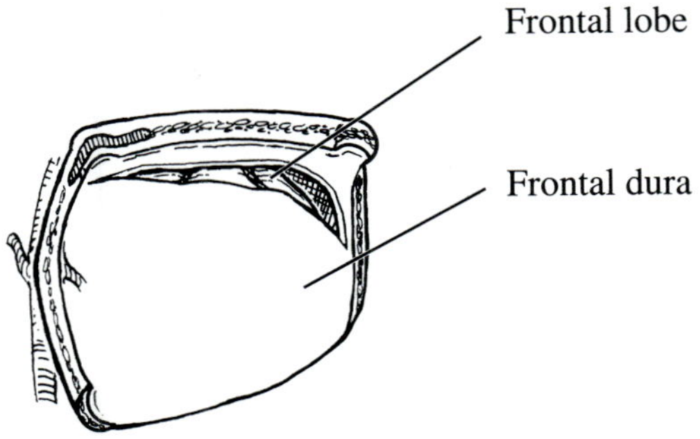

Figure 5. Unilateral frontal bone flap. Dural opening.

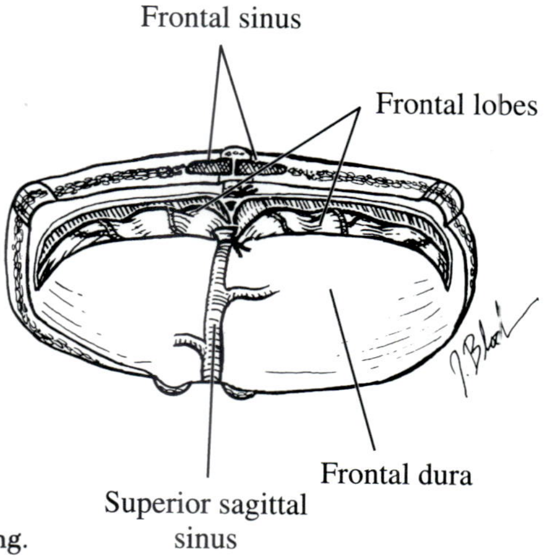

Figure 6. Bilateral frontal bone flap. Dural opening.

2 Frontotemporal (Pterional) Approach

INDICATIONS

The frontotemporal craniotomy is the most common and versatile exposure to the anterior and middle fossae for a wide variety of pathologies.

POSITION

The patient is placed in a supine position with the trunk and knees slightly flexed. The shoulder and hip on the side of the craniotomy are elevated to minimize rotation of the head when placed in the headholder in three-point fixation (Figure 1). A radiolucent headholder is used when intraoperative angiography is planned for aneurysm and arteriovenous malformation surgery.

The optimal position of comfort for the surgeon can be achieved by rotating the patient's head 30 to 60 degrees from vertical, depending on the location of the lesion. Thirty degrees of rotation provides transsylvian exposure of the basilar apex and many tentorial and perimesencephalic lesions.

The head is rotated to 45 degrees for exposure of the carotid-optic, suprasellar, and parasellar regions. Sixty degrees of rotation provides exposure of the frontal fossa floor as well as the anterior cerebral circulation to the proximal A2, sphenoid wing, anterior middle fossa, and subtemporal region.

The head is elevated above the heart to enhance venous drainage and the vertex is tilted down, allowing the frontal lobe to fall away with gravity.

INCISION

The skin incision and temporalis muscle dissection vary, depending on the pathology. The standard pterional incision we use provides excellent exposure of the frontal fossa and sylvian fissure for lesions of the lateral frontal fossa; sphenoid wing; superior orbital fissure; parasellar, suprasellar, and carotid-optic regions; optic nerves; chiasm; and many anterior circulation aneurysms.

The incision extends from 1 cm anterior to the tragus and gently curves on the forehead. For cosmetic reasons, it is carried behind the hairline, if possible (see Figure 1, incision A). The temporal lobe and middle fossa floor can be fully exposed with extension of the incision into a question-mark shape low over the ear (see Figure 1, incision B).

The temporalis fascia and muscle are then incised vertically. A cuff of fascia along the superior temporal line is left for later closure (Figure 2). The scalp and galea are elevated and dissection of the temporalis muscle is completed. The cutaneous flap and temporalis muscle are retracted with multiple fish hooks. The temporalis muscle and fascia along the posterior 1 cm of the zygoma can be partially incised for further anterior retraction of the muscle (Figure 3).

CRANIOTOMY

A free-flap craniotomy is preferred. Two burr holes are placed: the first in the frontal zygomatic keyhole position (see Figure 2) and the second low in the squamous portion of the temporal bone above the root of the zygoma (see Figure 3). The craniotomy flap is then elevated.

The saw cuts are directed low in the frontal and temporal fossae and toward the sphenoid wing to leave maximum bone on the flap and minimize the cosmetic defect. A well-planned craniotomy fractures the lateral sphenoid wing off with the bone flap to begin bone removal from the skull base. Routine epidural bone removal includes the entire lateral sphenoid wing to the superior orbital fissure. Further extradural bone removal of the anterior clinoid process, optic foramen, and superior orbital fissure can be performed as needed, depending on the pathology.

DURAL OPENING

The dura usually is opened circumferentially around the sphenoid wing from the floor of the frontal fossa to the tip of the temporal lobe (Figure 4). The dura is tacked up tautly with 4-0 nylon sutures for maximal exposure and hemostasis. The dura overlying the temporal lobe can be incised inferiorly for further exposure of the middle fossa.

The sphenoid ridge, anterior clinoid process, arteries of the anterior circle of Willis, and optic nerves and chiasm can be well exposed by this pterional approach (Figure 5).

CLOSURE

The dura is closed primarily in a watertight manner with 4-0 nylon in a running lock stitch. Peripheral 4-0 nylon tack-up sutures are placed to prevent epidural hematoma. The bone flap is secured in position with 0 nylon sutures and central tack-up sutures with 4-0 nylon. The temporalis muscle and fascia and the galea are closed anatomically with 3-0 Vicryl suture. Monofilament nylon or staples are used for scalp closure.

RECOMMENDED READING

George, B., Clemenceau, S., Cophignon, J., et al.: Anterior skull base tumor. The choice between cranial and facial approaches, single and combined procedure. From a series of 78 cases. Acta Neurochir. Suppl. (Wien) 53:7–13, 1991.

Hassler, W., Zentner, J.: Pterional approach for surgical treatment of olfactory groove meningiomas. Neurosurgery 25(6):942–945; discussion, 945–947, 1989.

McDermott, M., Durity, F., Rootman, J., Woodhurst, W.: Combined frontotemporal-orbitozygomatic approach for tumors of the sphenoid wing and orbit. Neurosurgery 26(1):107–116, 1990.

Samii, M., Ammirati, M., Mahran, A., et al.: Surgery of petroclival meningiomas; report of 24 cases. Neurosurgery 24(1):12–17, 1989.

Smith, P., Grubb, R., Kletzker, G., Leonetti, J.: Combined pterional-anterolateral approaches to cranial base tumors. Otolaryngol. Head Neck Surg. 103(3):357–363, 1990.

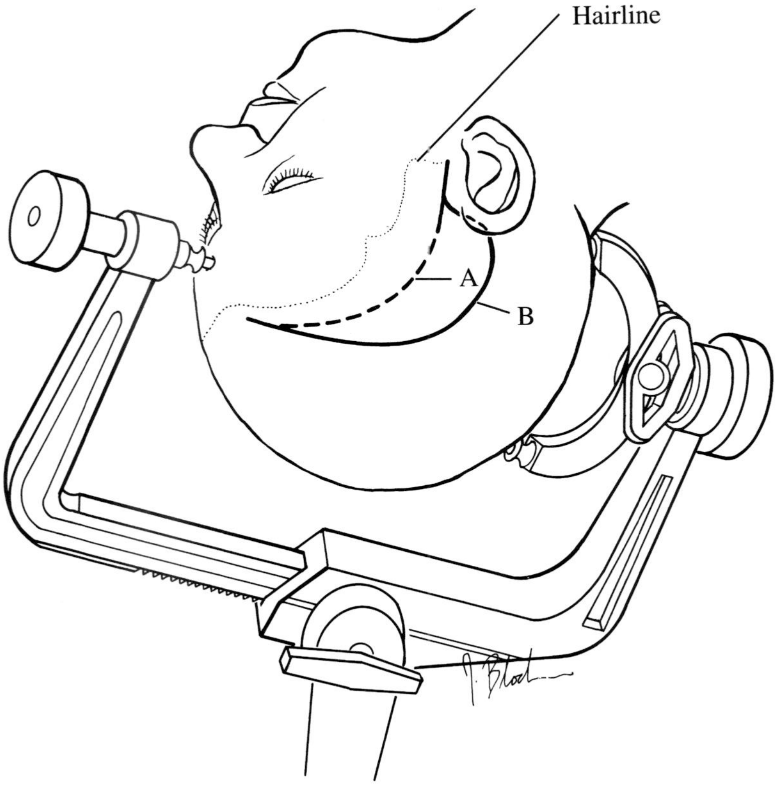

Figure 1. Patient position showing incision options A and B.

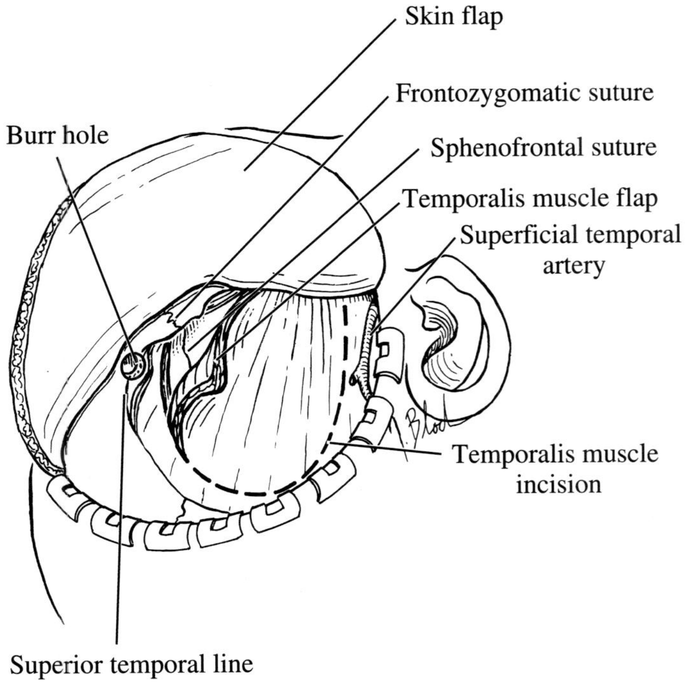

Figure 2. Scalp flap elevated showing placement of keyhole burr hole.

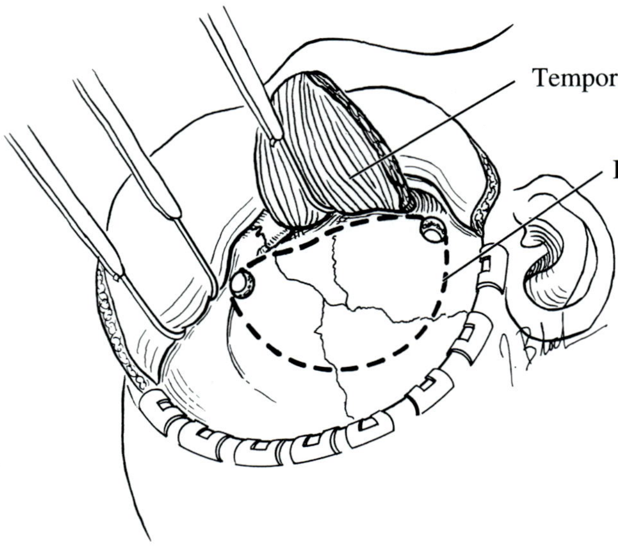

Figure 3. Burr hole placement and plan for craniotomy flap.

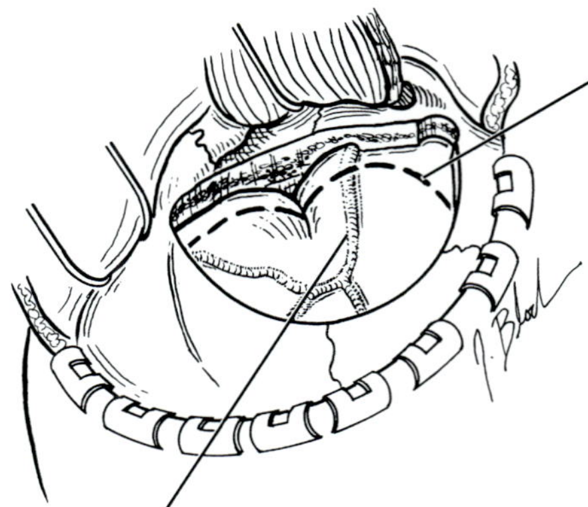

Figure 4. Dural opening for pterional approach (incision A).

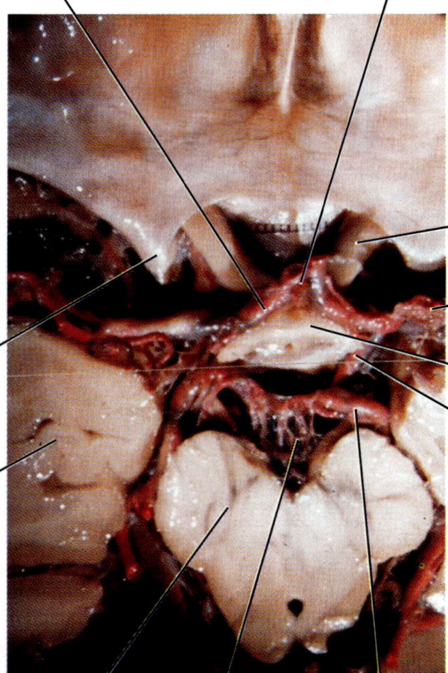

Figure 5. Cadaver dissection showing anatomical structures that may easily be exposed by a pterional approach.

Subtemporal Approach 3

POSITION

The patient is placed in the park bench, or lateral, position. The head is immobilized in three-point fixation positioned parallel to the floor and elevated 15 degrees above the level of the heart.

INCISION

Depending on the position and extent of the desired operative exposure, a choice of three skin incisions is made. For a small, limited subtemporal exposure, a 6-cm vertical incision is made in the temporal area 1 cm anterior to the tragus. The inferior limit of this incision is the zygomatic arch (Figure 1). If a larger, more posterior subtemporal exposure is needed, a 6 × 8-cm inferiorly based U-shaped incision is made (Figure 2). For a more extensive subtemporal exposure, including exposure of the sphenoid ridge, a preauricular incision extending from the zygomatic arch 1 cm anterior to the tragus is carried upward and curved first posteriorly above the ear and then anteriorly toward the midpupillary line (Figure 3). The posterior extent of this exposure is described in detail in Chapter 2.

CRANIOTOMY

For a small, limited subtemporal exposure (as may be needed for trauma or for approaching the internal auditory canal), the temporalis muscle is incised vertically in a manner similar to that for the scalp incision. A temporal craniotomy performed as a free bone flap may be done using one or more burr holes connected by the craniotome with beveling of the cut (Figure 4). The initial burr hole is placed low in the temporal area just above the zygomatic arch. After removal of the free bone plate, additional temporal bone is ronguered away inferiorly to allow easy access to the middle fossa floor, thus avoiding undue temporal lobe retraction.

For the more posterior subtemporal approach, the temporalis muscle may be incised vertically and separated more extensively, or it may be incised in a U-shaped manner, stripped away from the temporal bone, and reflected inferiorly. A 5-mm cuff of temporalis muscle is left superiorly to allow for later closure.

The more anterior subtemporal exposure involves curving the temporalis muscle incision anteriorly, as far as the orbital rim if needed.

DURAL OPENING

For some subtemporal operations, the dissection is extradural and the dura is not opened. For procedures that require an intradural dissection, the dural opening depends on the position and extent of the craniotomy as well as the pathology.

An example of the type of tumor that can be removed through a subtemporal approach is the trigeminal neuroma shown in the magnetic resonance imaging scans in Figure 5. In Figure 6, the tumor along the medial floor of the middle fossa is exposed by gentle elevation of the temporal lobe after opening of the dura. The tumor is shown during removal in Figure 7.

CLOSURE

Watertight dural closure is completed with 4-0 nylon, using a running lock stitch. Dural-to-pericranium tack-up sutures are placed along each bone edge. The free bone flap is secured in place at three points with 0 silk sutures passed through drill holes in the cranium and the bone plate.

The temporalis muscle and fascia are closed with absorbable 3-0 suture. The galea is closed with the same suture, and scalp closure is completed using monofilament 3-0 nylon or skin staples.

RECOMMENDED READING

Dautheribes, M., Migueis, A., Vital, J., Guerin, J.: Anatomical basis of the extended subtemporal approach to the cerebellopontine angle: Its value and limitations. Surg. Radiol. Anat. 11(3):187–195, 1989.

Harsh, G., Sekhar, L.: The subtemporal, transcavernous, anterior transpetrosal approach to the upper brain stem and clivus. J. Neurosurg. 77(5):709–717, 1992.

Knosp, E., Tschabitscher, M., Matula, C., Koos, W.: Modifications of temporal approaches: Anatomical aspects of a microneurosurgical approach. Acta Neurochir. Suppl. (Wein) 53:159–165, 1991.

Labbe, D., Hubert, P., Rigot-Jolivet, M., Madjidi, A.: Subperiosteal subtemporal approach: Technique and applications. Neurosurgery 30(5):744–747, 1992.

Sen, C., Sekhar, L.: The subtemporal and preauricular infratemporal approach to intradural structures ventral to the brain stem. J. Neurosurg. 73(3):345–354, 1990.

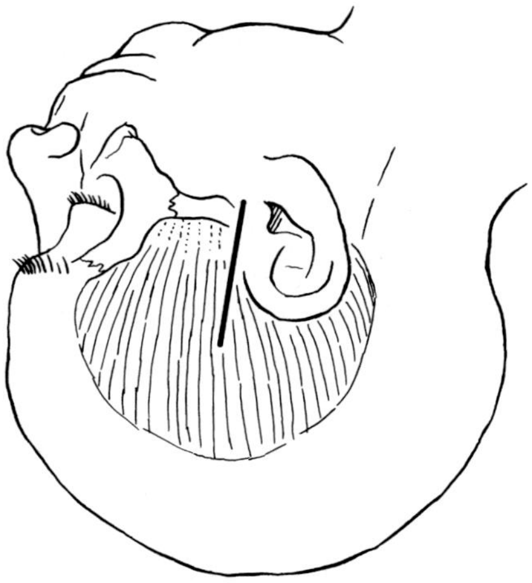

A

Figure 1. Vertical incision of subtemporal approach.

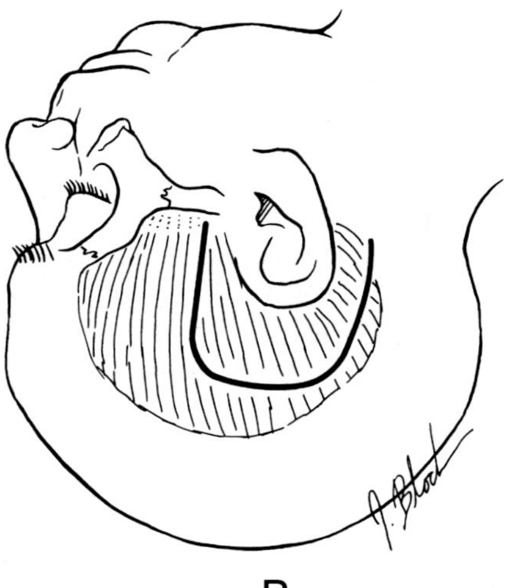

B

Figure 2. U-shaped incision for subtemporal approach.

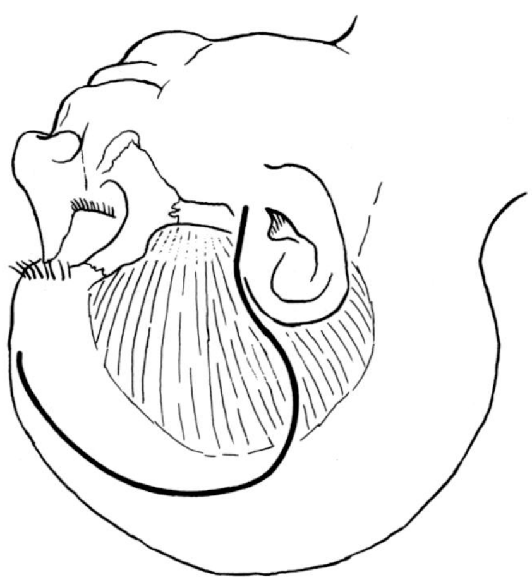

C

Figure 3. Curved incision for subtemporal approach.

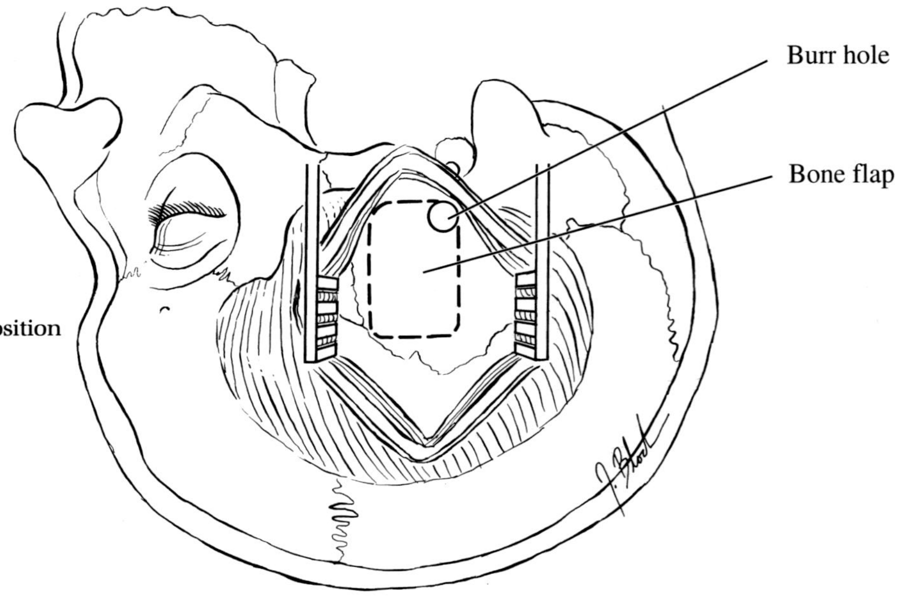

Figure 4. Temporal craniotomy bone flap position with use of single burr hole.

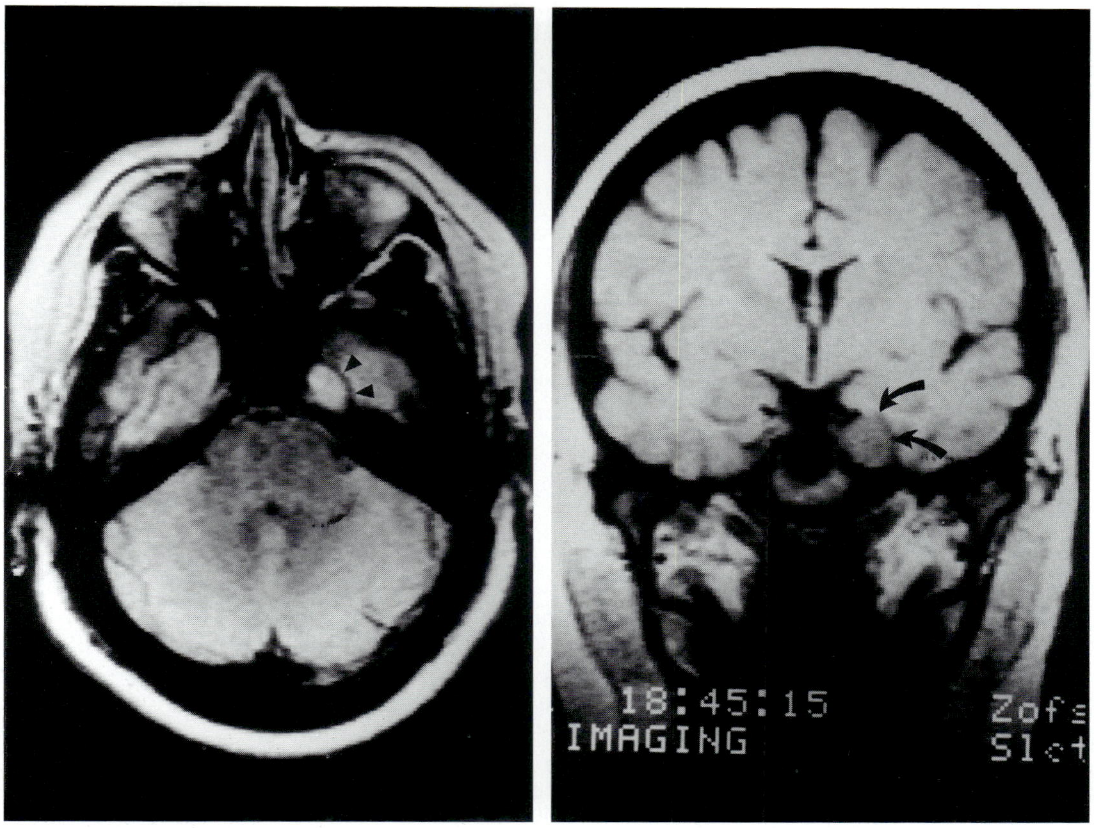

Figure 5. Magnetic resonance imaging scan showing a tumor *(arrows)* in Meckel's cave.

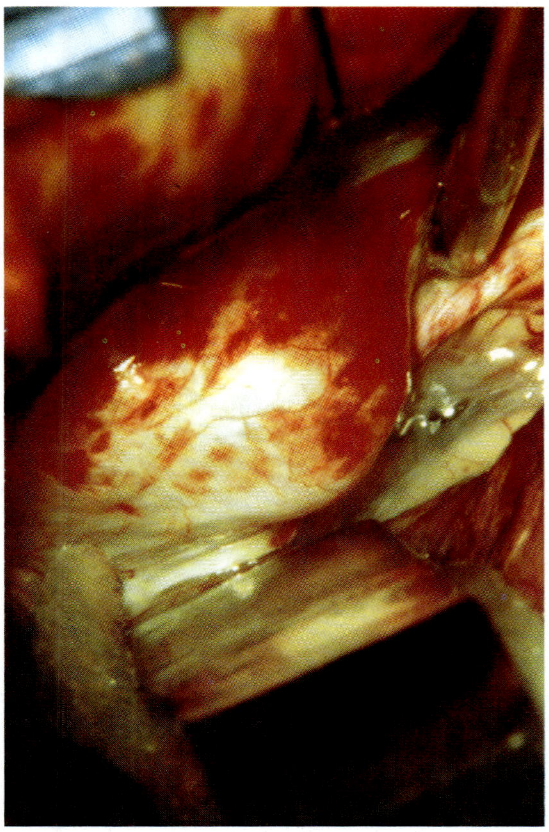

Figure 6. Exposure of trigeminal neuroma shown in Figure 5 after dural opening.

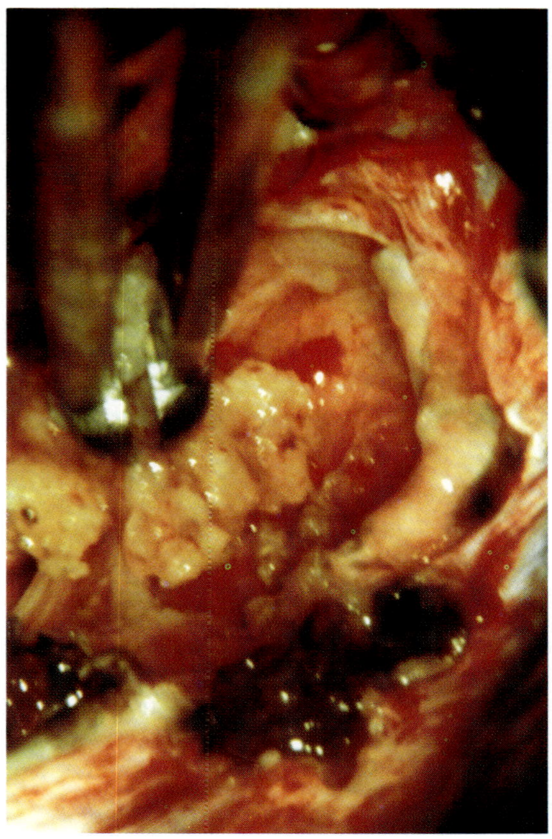

Figure 7. Partial removal of tumor shown in Figure 5.

4 Suboccipital Lateral Retrosigmoid Approach

INDICATIONS

The suboccipital lateral retrosigmoid approach is the standard procedure for entry to the cerebellopontine angle and the lateral posterior skull base.

POSITION

The suboccipital lateral retrosigmoid approach can be performed with the patient in a semisitting position (Figure 1), lateral position (Figure 2), three-quarters prone (park bench) position (Figure 3), or prone position (Figure 4). We prefer the semisitting and lateral positions for exposure of the cerebellopontine angle in most cases.

For the semisitting position, the patient is padded at all pressure points and the back of the operating table is elevated to 30 degrees. The head is secured in three-point fixation in a headholder, turned 30 degrees to the side of the craniotomy, and slightly flexed (Figure 1). The head and neck are in a natural anatomical position without unnecessary strain or compromise of cervical venous drainage.

For the lateral position, the patient is supported and padded in a beanbag with the legs flexed. The head is positioned neutral with the neck slightly flexed (Figure 2). The head of the operating table is slightly elevated for venous drainage.

For the park bench position, the patient is positioned similar to that for the lateral but with the head turned downward an additional 15 degrees. For the prone position, the patient is placed on bolsters and the head is immobilized in three-point fixation with 15 degrees of flexion. In each of these positions, the head is elevated 15 degrees above the level of the heart.

For the semisitting position, arterial blood pressure is monitored intraoperatively. A central venous catheter is placed in the right atrium, and a precordial Doppler is used to monitor for signs of air embolism. An end-tidal carbon dioxide sensor is used.

INCISION

A linear, slightly curved incision is placed behind the ear (Figure 5) 4.5 cm (in women) or 5 cm (in men) behind the external auditory canal. The incision extends from just above the superior nuchal line to the level of C1. The occipital artery and greater occipital nerve are preserved. A self-retaining retractor is used to maintain exposure.

The trapezius and splenius capitis muscles are detached from the superior nuchal line, and the remaining muscles at the skull base can be detached hemostatically with the bipolar cautery. The arch of C1 and the vertebral artery can be palpated below the foramen magnum, but they do not need to be exposed. The foramen magnum is not opened. Care is taken to avoid injury to the vertebral artery as it courses along the superior surface of the arch of C1.

CRANIECTOMY

An important bony landmark is the external occipital protuberance that overlies the confluence of the sinus. The superior nuchal line is a reliable landmark overlying the transverse sinus.

A single burr hole is placed over the cerebellar hemisphere as described by Lang and Samii (see Figure 5). This is just below the Frankfurt horizontal line and 4.5 to 5 cm behind the external auditory canal. The dense occipital bone is thinned with a high-speed drill. The dura is separated, and bone is removed with ronguers to enlarge the craniectomy to 4 to 5 cm square, exposing the edge of the transverse and sigmoid sinuses superiorly and laterally (Figure 6). Mastoid sinus air cells are packed with muscle. The foramen magnum is maintained intact with a ledge of inferior occipital bone preserved.

DURAL OPENING

There are many variations for dural opening, but the technique we often use is to open the dura along the sigmoid and transverse sinuses. The dura is laid on the cerebellar hemisphere with an overlying cottonoid to keep it moist and to protect the cerebellum. The dural edges along the sinus are retracted with tack-up sutures. A wide retractor blade supports the cerebellar hemisphere for exposure of the cerebellopontine angle (Figure 7).

The cerebellopontine angle cistern is opened to allow drainage of cerebrospinal fluid and improve exposure. In Figure 8, a cadaver dissection photograph shows the anatomical structures seen through this lateral suboccipital (retrosigmoid) approach.

CLOSURE

Before closure, the anesthesiologist is asked to give several periods of jugular compression to help identify unnoticed venous bleeding points. It is important to achieve careful hemostasis.

The dura is closed in a watertight manner with 4-0 nylon, using a continuous locking stitch. A lyophilized dura graft or fascia lata is used if there is a dural defect. Fibrin glue can be used for additional sealing along the suture line. Muscle and fascia are closed in several layers with interrupted 0 Vicryl suture. Subcutaneous closure is performed with interrupted 3-0 Vicryl suture. The skin is closed with monofilament nylon or staples.

RECOMMENDED READING

Ebersold, M., Harner, S., Beatty, C., et al.: Current results of the retrosigmoid approach to acoustic neurinoma. J. Neurosurg. 76:901–909, 1992.

Harner, S., Beatty, C., Ebersold, M.: Retrosigmoid removal of acoustic neuroma: Experience 1978–1988. Otolaryngol. Head Neck Surg. 103(1):40–45, 1990.

Lang, J., Samii, A.: Retrosigmoid approach to the posterior cranial fossa. An anatomical study. Acta Neurochir. (Wien) 111:147–153, 1991.

Rhoton, A.: Microsurgical anatomy of the brainstem surface facing an acoustic neuroma. Surg. Neurol. 25:326–339, 1986.

Samii, M., Draf, W.: Surgery of the Skull Base: An Interdisciplinary Approach. New York, Springer-Verlag, 1989.

Smith, M., Lagger, R.: Hearing conservation in acoustic neurilemmoma surgery via the retrosigmoid approach. Otolaryngol. Head Neck Surg. 92:168–175, 1984.

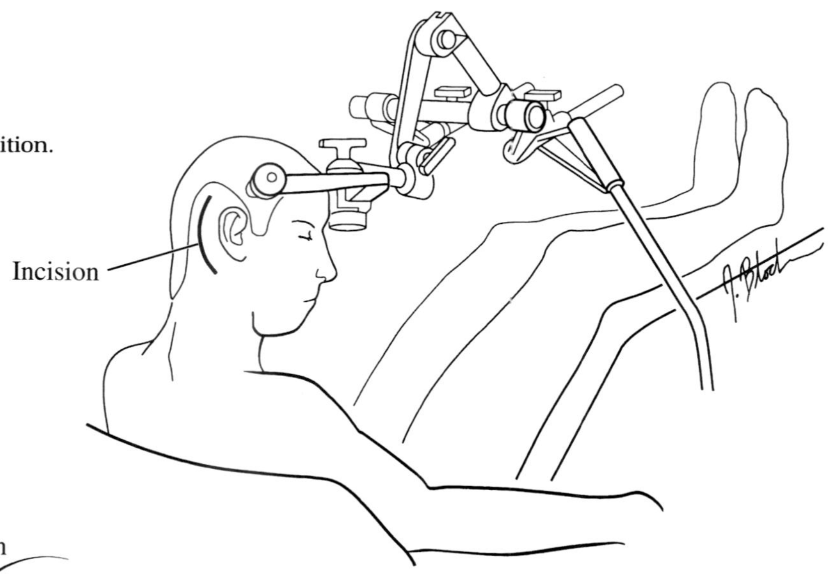

Figure 1. Semisitting position.

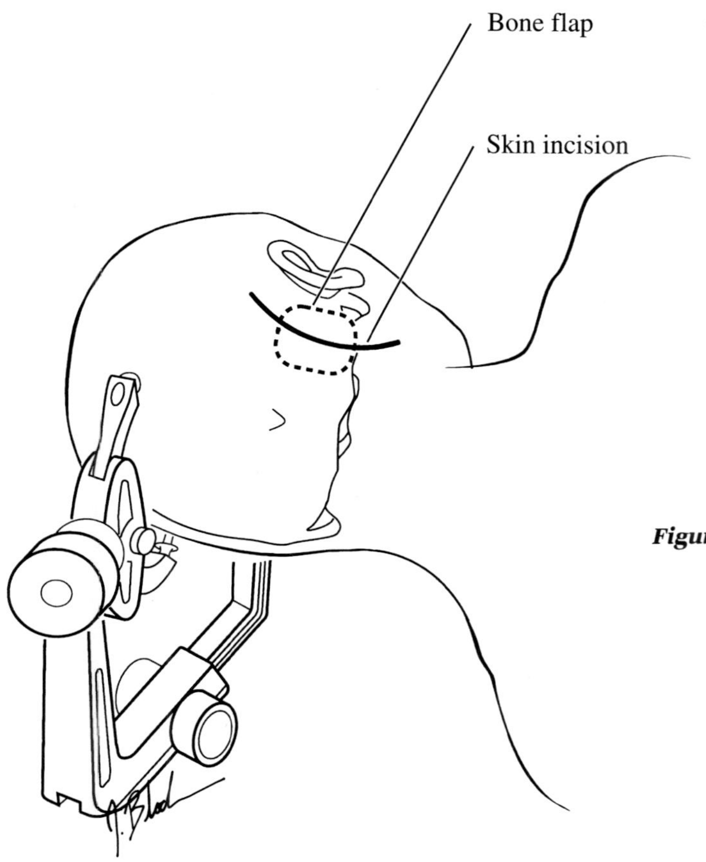

Figure 2. Lateral position.

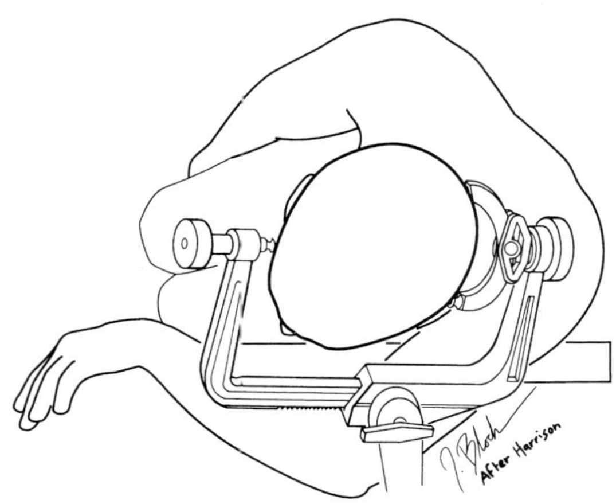

Figure 3. Three-quarters prone (park bench) position.

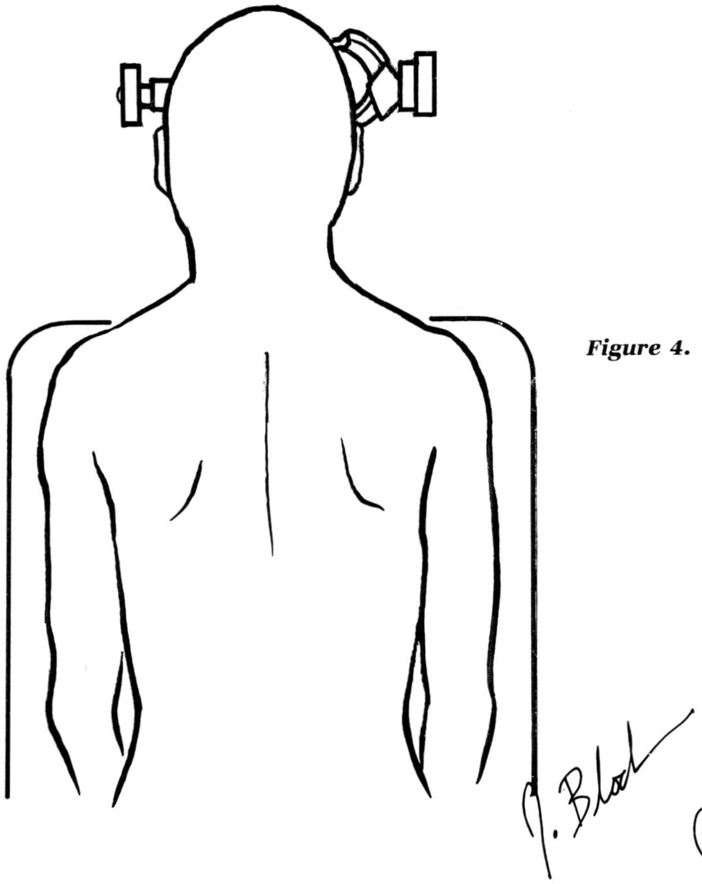

Figure 4. Prone position.

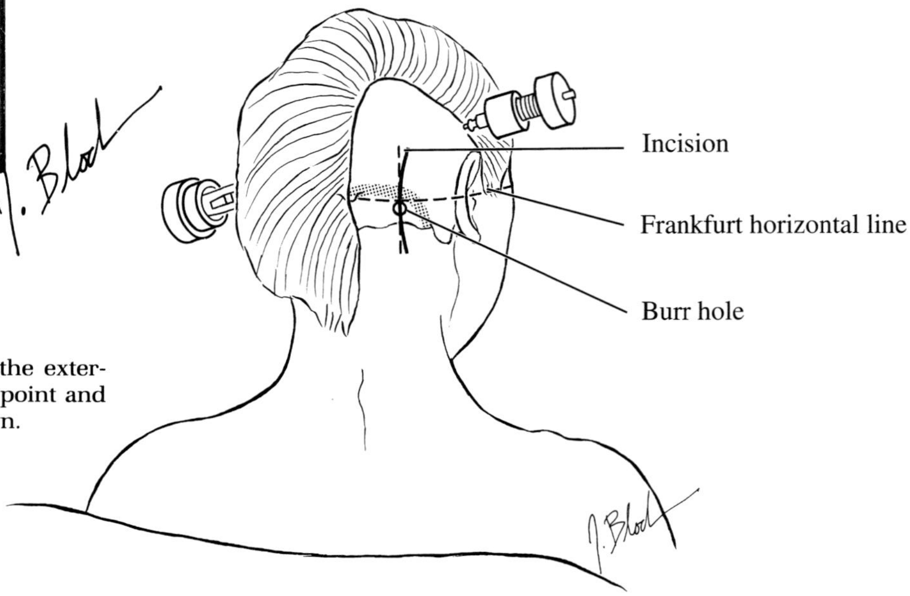

Figure 5. Linear incision 4.5 to 5 cm behind the external auditory canal. Burr hole placement at this point and just below the Frankfurt horizontal line is shown.

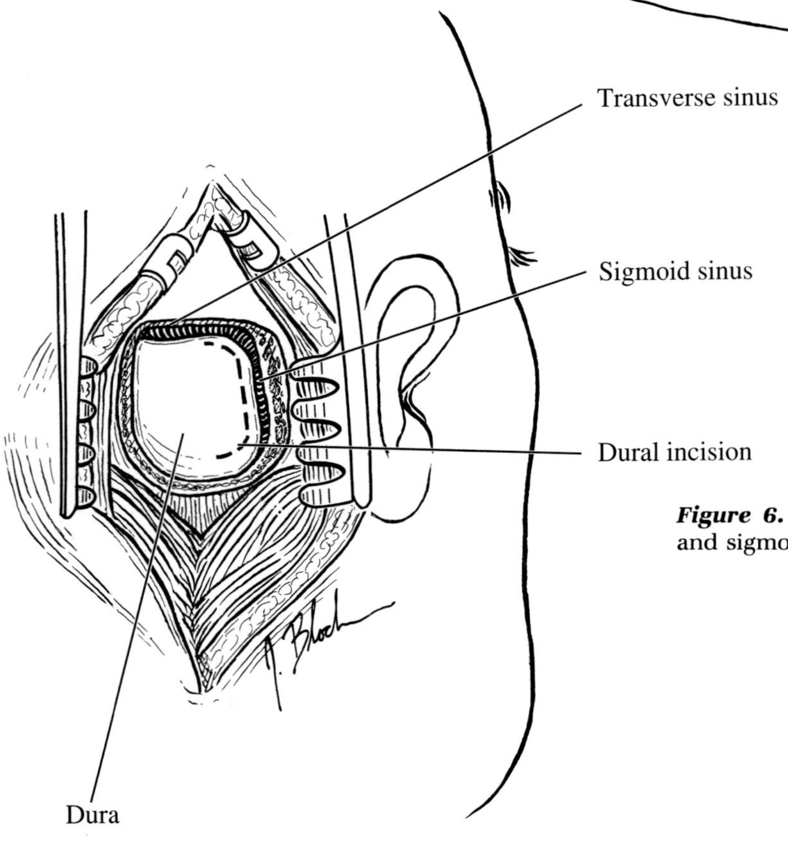

Figure 6. Occipital craniectomy 4 to 5 cm square with transverse and sigmoid sinuses exposed.

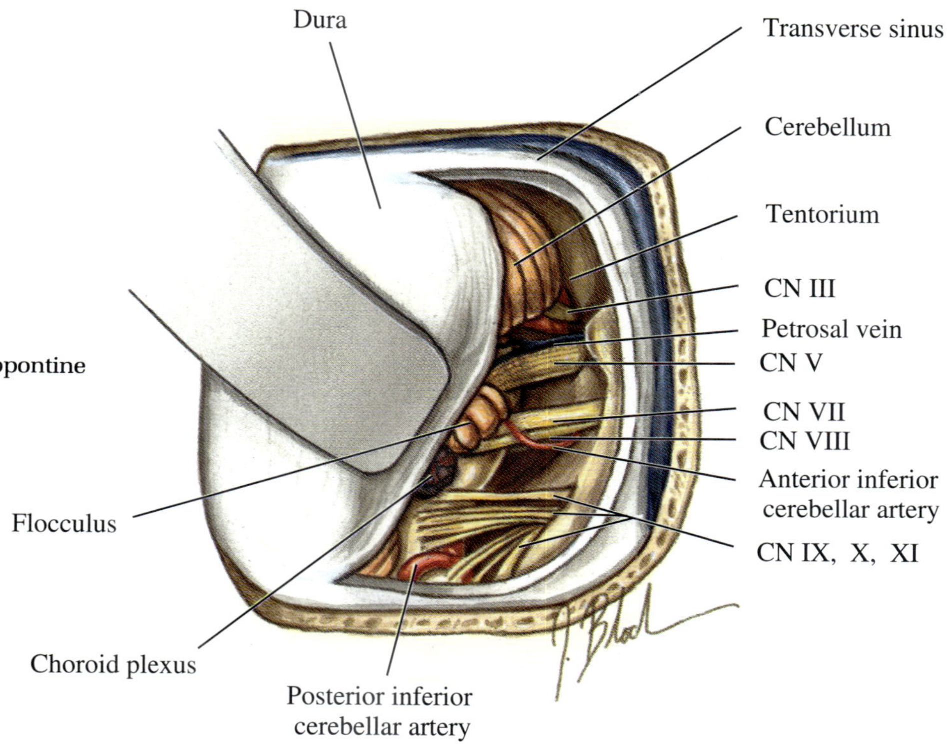

Figure 7. Dura opened and cerebellopontine angle exposed.

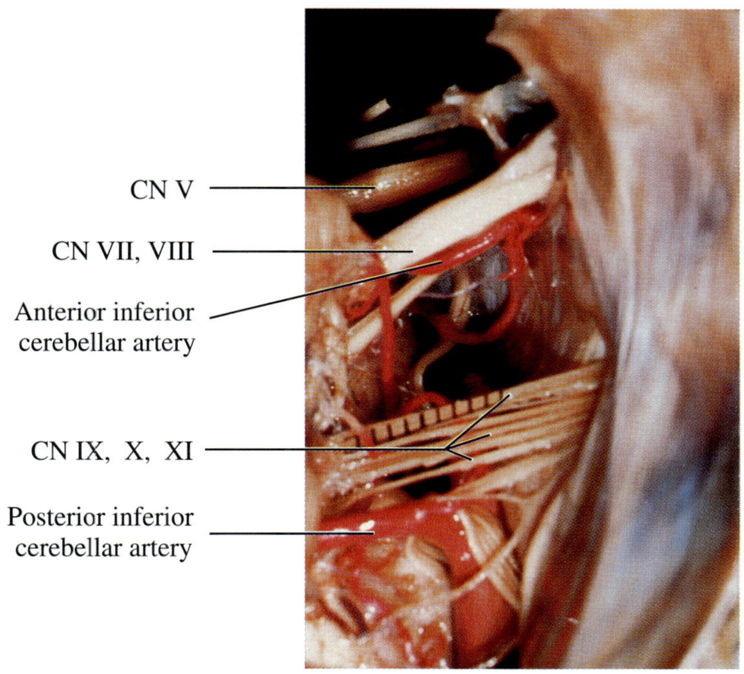

Figure 8. Anatomical exposure of the cerebellopontine angle structures as seen in cadaver dissection through a lateral suboccipital (retrosigmoid) approach.

5 Suboccipital Medial Approach

INDICATIONS

The suboccipital medial approach is indicated for many processes at the craniocervical junction that are located primarily in the midline posterior to the medulla oblongata and upper cervical spinal cord.

POSITION

The midline suboccipital craniotomy can be carried out in the prone, park bench, or semisitting position (see Chapter 4, Figures 1 through 4), depending on the location of the pathology and the surgeon's preference. The three-point headholder is used to fix the head for these positions.

INCISION

A midline incision is made extending from above the external occipital protuberance downward to C2. Cautery is used to expose the occipital bone, the arch of C1, and the spinous process of C2 in the midline raphae, and a self-retaining retractor is placed for soft tissue exposure (Figure 1).

CRANIOTOMY

Burr holes are placed bilaterally in the occipital bone, the dura is separated, and a suboccipital craniectomy is completed using a large rongeur. The inferior edge of the transverse sinus is exposed, and the posterior rim of the foramen magnum is removed. Removal of the posterior arch of C1 can provide exposure of the craniocervical junction and the upper cervical spinal cord (Figure 2).

DURAL OPENING

The dura is opened in a Y-shaped configuration extending from just below the transverse sinus bilaterally and is carried inferiorly in the midline to a point below the foramen magnum, exposing the cervicomedullary junction (see Figure 2). If bleeding occurs, the occipital sinus is ligated with 4-0 nylon. The superior part of the dura is elevated with temporary sutures, exposing the cerebellum. The arachnoid is incised in the midline, and the cisterna magna is opened (Figure 3). Figure 4 shows the anatomical structures that are exposed through the medial suboccipital approach.

CLOSURE

The dura is initially approximated with a few single sutures to ensure excellent anatomical alignment and then is completely closed in a watertight manner using a 4-0 nylon running lock stitch. With a careful dural opening, the surgeon can almost always achieve a complete dural closure. In case of a dural defect, a lyophilized dura graft or fascia lata is used.

The muscle and fascia are closed with interrupted 0 absorbable sutures in anatomical layers. The dermal layer is closed with inverted 3-0 absorbable sutures, and the skin is closed with 3-0 monofilament nylon sutures.

RECOMMENDED READING

De Oliveira, E., Rhoton, A., Peace, D.: Microsurgical anatomy of the region of the foramen magnum. Surg. Neurol. 24:293–352, 1985.

Hammon, W., Kempe, L.: The posterior fossa approach to aneurysms of the vertebral and basilar arteries. J. Neurosurg. 37:339–347, 1972.

Kempe, L.: Operative Neurosurgery. Vol. 2. New York, Springer-Verlag, 1970.

Rand, R., Jannetta, P.: Micro-neurosurgery for aneurysms of the vertebral-basilar artery system. J. Neurosurg. 27:330–335, 1967.

Yasargil, M.: Microneurosurgery. Vol. 1. New York, Georg Thieme Verlag, 1984.

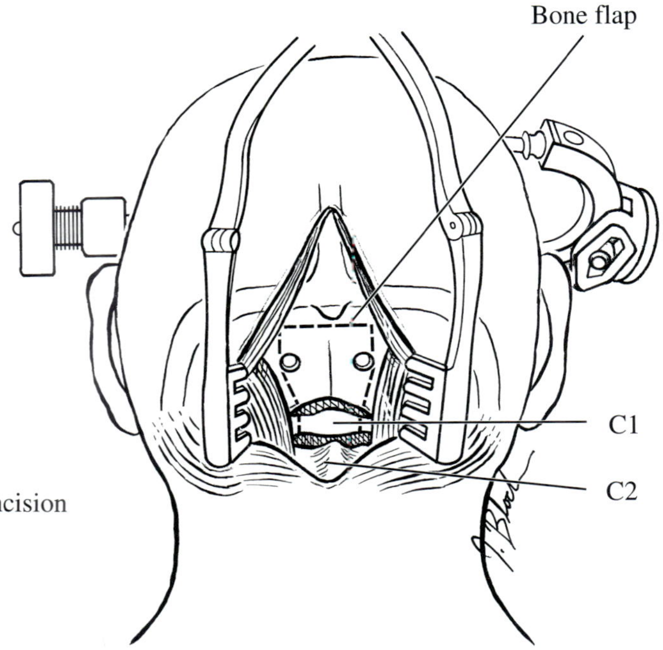

Figure 1. Midline occipital incision from external occipital protuberance downward to C2.

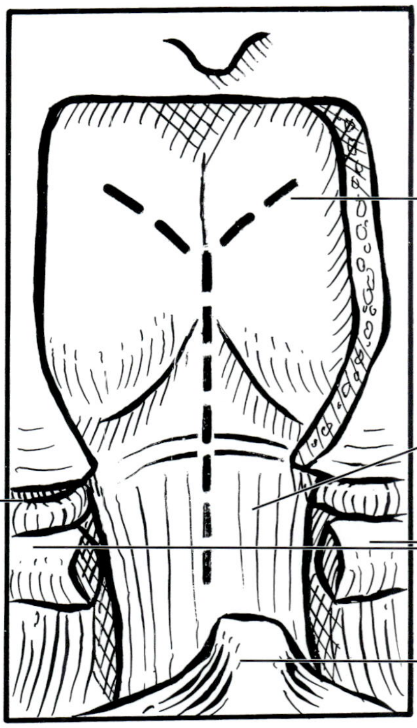

Figure 2. Suboccipital craniectomy completed and arch of C1 removed. Line of dural incision is shown with dotted line.

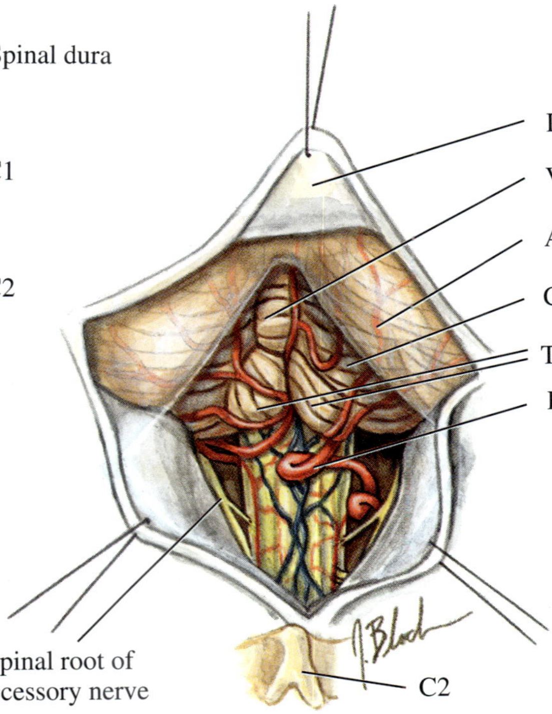

Figure 3. Exposure of cisterna magna with cervicomedullary junction and posterior inferior cerebellar artery in view.

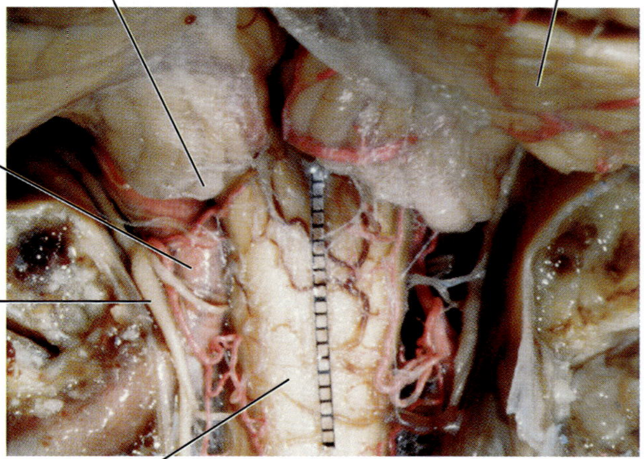

Figure 4. Cadaver dissection showing the anatomical structures as seen through a medial suboccipital approach.

6 Translabyrinthine Approach

James C. Andrews, Phillip A. Wackym, *and* Rinaldo Canalis

INDICATIONS

The translabyrinthine and transcochlear (transotic) approaches provide the most direct access with the shortest working distance to the internal auditory canal and most regions of the cerebellopontine angle without cerebellar retraction. A primary advantage of these approaches lies in the consistency in the anatomy of the region with the reliability of finding all the crucial structures of the temporal bone, including the facial nerve, cochlear and vestibular nerves, carotid artery, sigmoid and petrosal sinuses, and jugular vein. The disadvantage of the translabyrinthine and transotic approaches is the destruction of the cochlear and vestibular end organs with the inherent ipsilateral loss of hearing and balance. In many lesions of the internal auditory canal and cerebellopontine angle, the pathophysiology of the underlying disorder has resulted in preoperative cochlear and vestibular losses, making this only a relative consideration. With a normal contralateral ear, the benefit of preserving a malfunctioning inner ear is minimal at best. General guidelines have been established as to hearing that is considered worthy of preserving in the face of a normal opposite ear. These guidelines commonly are referred to as the rule of 50s. An ear with average hearing thresholds worse than 50 dB, a speech reception threshold less than 50 dB, or speech discrimination less than 50 per cent yet with normal contralateral hearing is not considered useful. This rule is relative and should not be used with potential disorders that may affect both ears, such as Meniere's disease. Experience has shown that the possibility of preserving hearing in the case of acoustic neuromas and other processes in the cerebellopontine angle is increasing with the use of middle cranial fossa and retrosigmoid approaches. Every attempt should be made to preserve hearing at any level.

No guides have been established for the preservation of vestibular function. Even minimal vestibular dysfunction, if uncompensated, may be problematic for a patient. With complete ipsilateral vestibular destruction, central compensation using vestibular afferent input from the normal contralateral ear is sufficient to provide functionally normal balance.

Indications for these procedures include vestibular nerve section, acoustic neuroma, and other lesions of the cerebellopontine angle. Contraindications include an approach to the cerebellopontine angle in which there is a need to preserve hearing and excessively large tumors (greater than 3.5 cm in diameter).

POSITION

The patient is placed in the supine position with the head turned away from the surgeon. Head-holding devices are not usually utilized in the translabyrinthine approach. A doughnut ring can be useful in supporting the head and maintaining its position.

INCISION

A wide C-shaped postauricular incision is made about 3 to 4 cm posterior to the helical rim (Figure 1). The incision is carried to the temporalis fascia superiorly and to the periosteum of the temporal bone inferiorly. A skin flap in the subgaleal plane is elevated forward to the external auditory canal with care taken to keep the cartilagenous canal intact. An anteriorly based rectangular periosteal flap is incised and pedicled over the region of the external auditory canal. From the posterior corners of the flap, 45-degree diagonal incisions superiorly and inferiorly are made in the periosteum to facilitate soft tissue elevation from the surface of the temporal bone. All soft tissue is retracted and preserved for a layered closure at the conclusion of the procedure.

CRANIOTOMY

A complete mastoidectomy is performed as follows (see Figure 1). Using a large cutting burr, drilling is begun over the mastoid antrum. The tegmen tympani and external canal are preserved as the mastoid is entered. Drilling is continued posteriorly to the sigmoid sinus, which is skeletonized, leaving a thin layer of bone residing over the structure. Bone over the sinodural angle is completely removed. The sigmoid sinus is followed inferiorly to the region of the jugular bulb. The cells of the mastoid tip are completely opened. The digastric ridge is located posteriorly and followed anteriorly to the region of the stylomastoid foramen. Further drilling is performed parallel to the stylomastoid foramen until the periosteum of the foramen is identified. A medium-sized diamond burr is then used as drilling extends closer to the facial nerve, which eventually is identified. Alternatively, the facial nerve can be identified anterior and inferior to the horizontal semicircular canal. The facial nerve is then followed superiorly to the region of the horizontal semicircular canal. Care is taken to completely visualize the facial nerve throughout its entire vertical and the beginning of its horizontal course within the temporal bone to prevent iatrogenic injury because further drilling is deep to the facial nerve. Intraoperative facial nerve electromyographic monitoring is useful throughout this dissection.

The retrofacial mastoid air cells are opened, and bone over the jugular bulb is removed. Drilling is performed into the labyrinthine portion of the temporal bone. The lateral semicircular canal is carefully drilled away with exposure of the second genu of the facial nerve in this region. Further drilling is then deep to the horizontal and vertical course of the facial nerve. The openings of the lateral semicircular canal are followed into the labyrinth. The posterior semicircular canal is identified and opened (Figures 2A, 3, and 4). At the crus communis, the junction of the nonampullary aspect of the superior and posterior semicircular canals, the vestibule of the labyrinth is entered. The superior semicircular canal is opened, and bone in and around this region is removed. The subarcuate artery lies in the center of the arc of the superior semicircular canal and may serve as a landmark to further direct drilling into the petrous tip (see Figure 2*B*).

Special consideration must again be given to the facial nerve as it loops back proximally from the geniculate ganglion into the labyrinthine portion, the most narrow and tenuous aspect of the intratemporal facial nerve, just lateral to the internal auditory canal. The labyrinthine portion of the facial nerve lies about 2 mm anterior and 2 mm superior to the ampulla of the superior semicircular canal.

The blue line of the internal auditory canal is identified next as drilling is extended further into the petrous tip. Bone should be drilled to an eggshell thinness superiorly, posteriorly, and inferiorly along the extent of the internal auditory canal and including the posterior lip of the porus (see Figure 2*C*). This shell of bone can then be removed using a Fisch microraspatory and a small right-angle hook. At the fundus of the internal auditory canal, the free nerve endings of the superior and inferior vestibular nerves (because the end organs have been removed) are found. These are divided by a transverse crest of bone within the canal (Figures 5 and 6; see also Figure 2*D*). Anteriorly and superiorly the facial nerve can be identified, separated from the vestibular nerve by a vertical crest of bone within the internal auditory canal. Intraoperative electrophysiologic monitoring and bipolar electrostimulation of the facial nerve are useful in precisely locating the nerve.

In the course of this procedure, it can be useful to maintain an island of bone over the sigmoid sinus (Bill's island) to prevent injury to the sinus from the shank of the burr because the surgeon's attention is directed toward the petrous tip (see Figure 2*A*). The need to completely remove the surrounding residual temporal bone, including the tegmen tympani over the middle fossa dura and the bone overlying the posterior fossa dura, depends largely on the procedure performed. A translabyrinthine vestibular neurectomy does not require additional bone removal. Once the internal canal is widely opened and the vestibular nerve identified and separated from the other structures within the canal, transection can be made proximal to Scarpa's ganglion. For an acoustic tumor, it is necessary to remove all bone over the middle and posterior fossa dura, internal auditory canal, and jugular bulb. The increased working space is necessary to safely approach and open the cerebellopontine angle.

CLOSURE

The facial recess is opened by drilling between the facial nerve and the chorda tympani. Through this exposure, the incudostapedial joint can be separated. Then by rotating the incus posteriorly toward the surgeon, the incudomalleal joint will separate, and this ossicle can be removed. Using a heavy Mayo scissors, the long process of the incus is cut from the ossicle and discarded, leaving the short process of the incus. The patient is now rotated away from the surgeon such that looking into the opening provided by the facial recess dissection will allow visualization directly into the eustachian tube. Bone wax is placed into the eustachian tube followed by the short process of the incus and then fibrin glue to effectively seal this structure and to prevent future cerebrospinal fluid leakage into the nasopharynx. After removal of the tumor from the internal auditory canal or the cerebellopontine angle, the defect of the dura may be large. The defect should be repaired by laying a rectus abdominis fascia graft in it. Abdominal fat cut into small strips is then used to fill the petrous tip and mastoid cavity. The temporalis muscle is then tightly reapproximated over the fat using 3–0 Vicryl. If necessary for tight closure, an anteriorly based temporalis muscle flap can be created and rotated over the surgical site. Fibrin glue is again applied. The skin is tightly closed using interrupted 3–0 nylon or skin staples. A mastoid dressing is applied.

RECOMMENDED READING

Brackmann, D., Green, J.: Translabyrinthine approach for acoustic tumor removal. Otolaryngol. Clin. North Am. 25(2):311–329, 1992.

Giannotta, S.: Translabyrinthine approach for removal of medium and large tumors of the cerebellopontine angle. Clin. Neurosurg. 38:589–602, 1992.

Hardy, D., Macfarlane, R., Baguley, D., Moffat, D.: Surgery for acoustic neurinoma. An analysis of 100 translabyrinthine operations. J. Neurosurg. 71(6):799–804, 1989.

House, W.: Evolution of trans-temporal bone removal of acoustic tumors. Arch. Otolaryngol. 80:731–741, 1964.

Tos, M., Thomsen, J.: The translabyrinthine approach for the removal of large acoustic neuromas. Arch. Otorhinolaryngol. Suppl. 246(5):292–296, 1989.

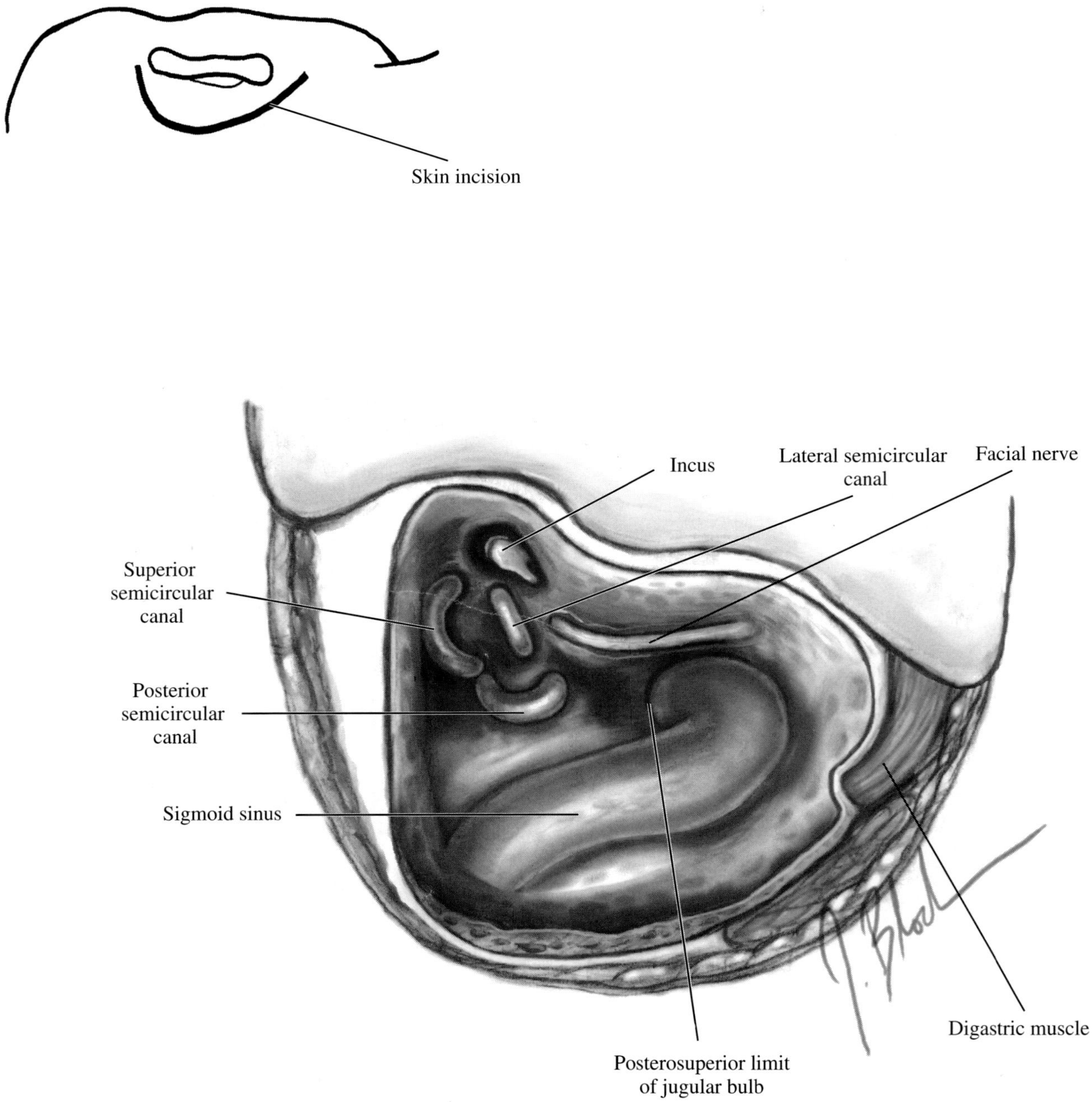

Figure 1. *Top left:* For the right translabyrinthine approach to the internal auditory canal, the patient is positioned supine with the head on a doughnut headrest and turned to the left. Post-auricular C-shaped incision is shown by bold line. *Bottom:* Retrosigmoid craniectomy and complete mastoidectomy with bone-covered sigmoid sinus, vertical segment of the facial nerve, and intact semicircular canals.

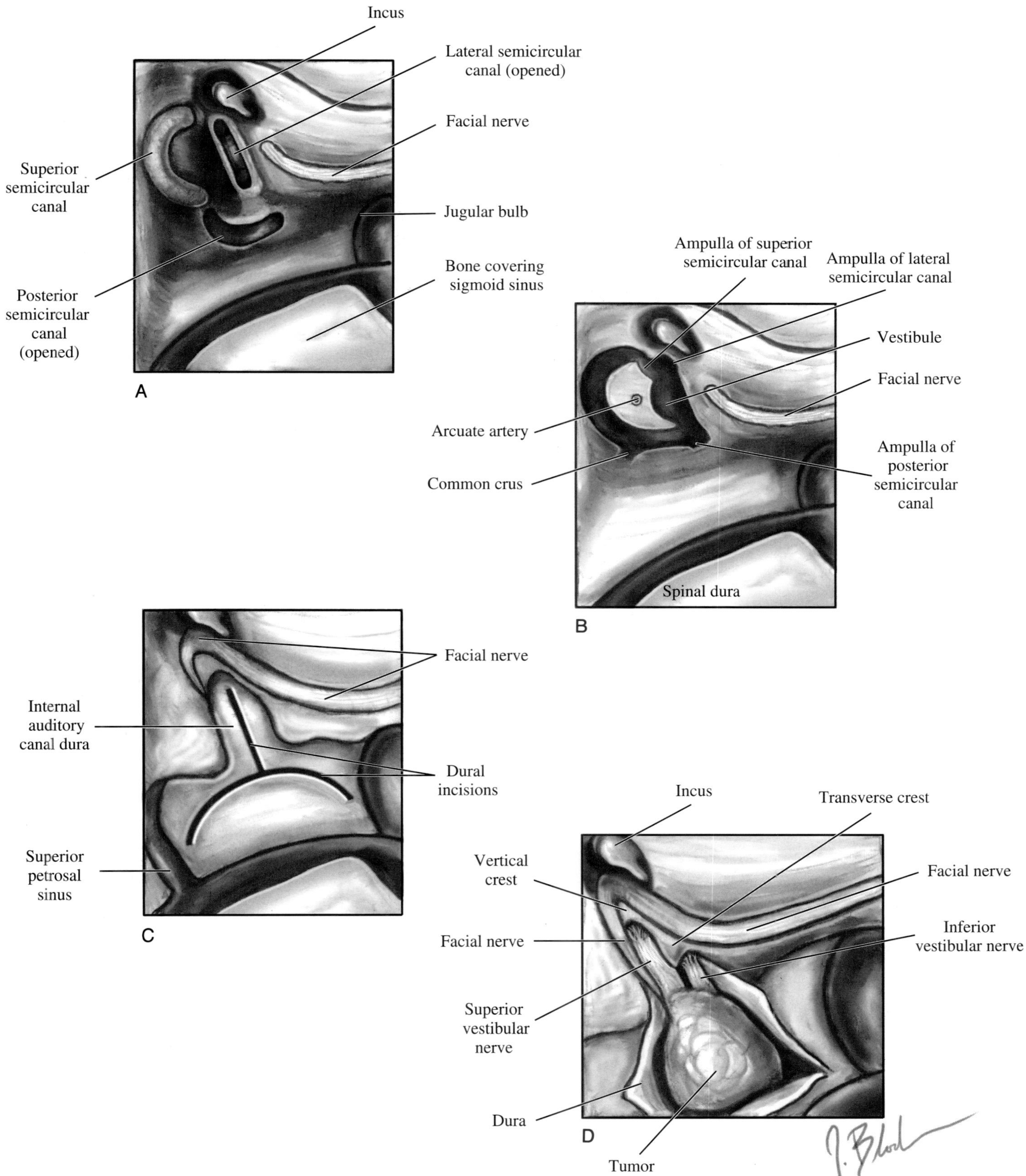

Figure 2. *A,* Controlled fenestration of the semicircular canals and creation of Bill's island of bone over the sigmoid sinus. *B,* Dissection of otic capsule is followed to the vestibule. Subarcuate artery is a constant landmark during this portion of the procedure. *C,* All bone between the superior petrosal sinus, sigmoid sinus, and beginning of the jugular bulb is removed. Presigmoid and internal auditory canal dural incisions. *D,* Medium-sized acoustic neuroma arising from the superior vestibular nerve. Note the relation between the facial nerve, superior vestibular nerve, and tumor. The facial nerve is identified distal to the tumor and separated from the capsule in a lateral-to-medial direction.

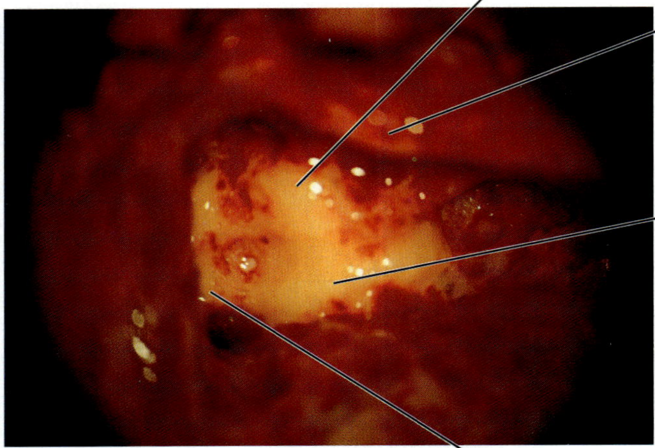

Figure 3. Intraoperative photograph of semicircular canals after complete mastoidectomy. Translabyrinthine approach for right acoustic neuroma.

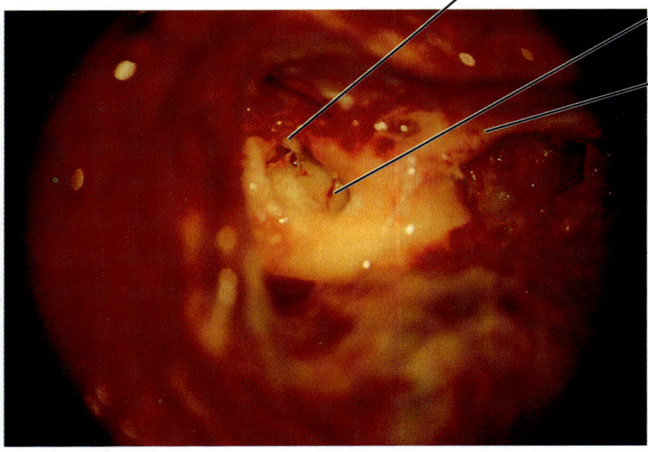

Figure 4. Otic capsule dissection into vestibule.

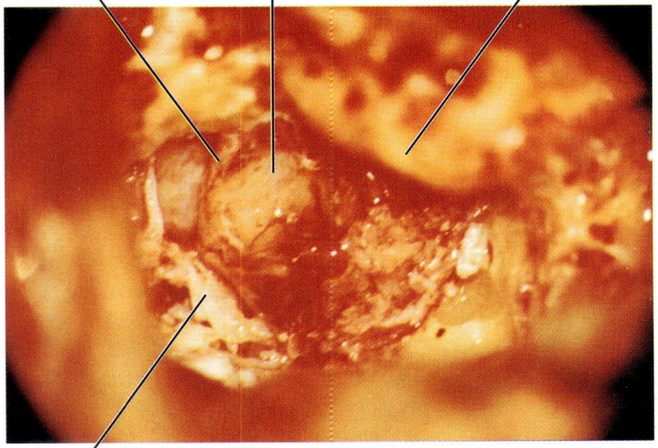

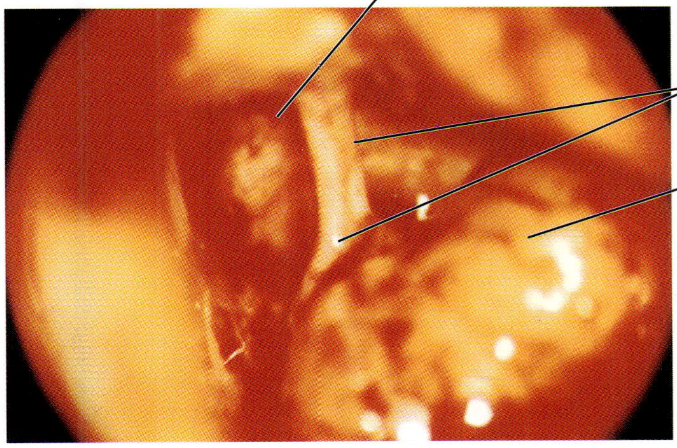

Figure 5. *A,* Exposure of acoustic neuroma within the internal auditory canal and cerebellopontine angle. *B,* Relation of normal facial nerve distal to the acoustic neuroma within the internal auditory canal.

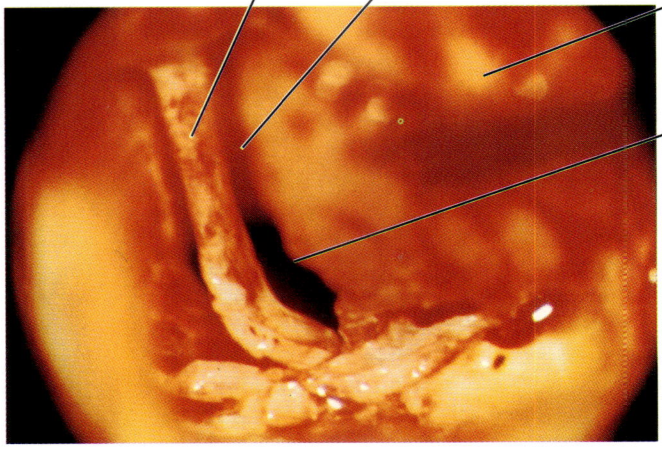

Figure 6. Intact facial nerve after complete resection of acoustic neuroma. Course of the facial nerve seen through the internal auditory canal and cerebellopontine angle.

7 Transcochlear (Transotic) Approach

James C. Andrews, Phillip A. Wackym, *and* Rinaldo Canalis

The transcotic approach to the internal auditory canal and cerebellopontine angle is an extension of the translabyrinthine approach that provides a much wider exposure of the cerebellopontine angle. This is accomplished by removing the cochlea in addition to the vestibular labyrinth. Through the transotic approach, an opening to the cerebellopontine angle can be provided from the petrous portion of the internal carotid artery anteriorly to the sigmoid sinus posteriorly and from the tegmen tympani and mastoideum of the middle cranial fossa superiorly to the jugular bulb inferiorly.

POSITION

The patient is placed in the supine position with the head turned away from the surgeon. Head-holding devices are not usually utilized in the transcochlear (transotic) approach. A doughnut ring can be useful in supporting the head and maintaining its position.

INCISION

A large C-shaped incision is made 4 cm posterior to the helical rim. A subgaleal skin flap is raised above the temporalis fascia superiorly and the mastoid periosteum inferiorly until the cartilagenous external auditory canal is reached. An anteriorly based rectangular flap centered over the region of the cartilagenous external auditory canal is created in the temporalis muscle and periosteum over the temporal bone. Superiorly and inferiorly directed diagonal incisions are created from the posterior corners of the incised flap and the soft tissue elevated off the temporal bone. The posterior aspect of the external canal skin is incised at a point medial to the junction of the body and cartilagenous external auditory canal to open the canal. Using a hemostat, dissection is performed between the parotid tissue and the anterior canal skin. The external auditory canal wall incision is then completed, allowing further elevation of the external ear and periauricular skin from the temporal bone. Using curved Iris scissors, the external canal skin of the auricle is dissected laterally for 1 to 1.5 cm from the surrounding canal wall cartilage of the auricle. A cuff of conchal cartilage is resected to facilitate eversion of the external auditory canal skin. A suture is placed in the medial aspect of the superior and inferior canal skin and then passed through the canal to allow the canal skin to be everted. Interrupted 4-0 Vicryl is then used to close the external canal skin as a blind sac. On the medial aspect of the auricular skin flap, the previously created rectangular flap of temporalis and periosteal soft tissue is transposed anteriorly and used as a second-layer closure for the external canal (Figure 1).

The skin lining the bony external canal is resected, and the tympanic membrane is elevated with the annulus from the bony annular sulcus. A malleus nipper is used to divide the manubrium from the head of the malleus. After incising the tensor tympani muscle and the chordae tympani nerve, the entire tympanic membrane and bony external canal wall skin can be removed. Failure to completely remove all squamous tissue from the temporal bone can result in the formation of a cholesteatoma.

CRANIOTOMY

A translabyrinthine bony dissection is completed as described previously. Before bone removal is completed over the internal auditory canal, the dissection is extended to the external canal, middle ear, and cochlea. The bony external canal is removed down to the level of the facial nerve. Drilling along the tegmen tympani of the middle fossa dura is extended from the mastoid region anteriorly to the middle ear region. The remainder of the ossicles are then removed (see Figure 1). Using a medium-sized diamond burr, drilling is begun in the eustachian tube so as to identify the internal carotid artery just deep to the medial wall of the eustachian tube. After the carotid artery is identified, this vessel is followed superiorly until it starts to bend anteriorly at the petrous apex and further anteriorly and superiorly, if needed.

Drilling is resumed below the vertical segment of the facial nerve and extended anteriorly toward the middle ear and cochlea (Figure 2). Drilling is continued along and below the facial nerve as it extends anteriorly beyond the second genu through the middle ear and toward the geniculate ganglion. The jugular bulb is followed below the facial nerve and into the region medial to the middle ear and below the cochlea. The remainder of the cochlea is removed by drilling over and below the facial nerve. When the bony dissection has been completed, the facial nerve passes through the center of the operative field as an isolated structure with a thin layer of bone surrounding it. The internal auditory canal can be isolated about 270 degrees around from the superior region where the labyrinthine segment of the facial nerve joins the cochleovestibular nerve.

CLOSURE

Closure is similar to that for the translabyrinthine approach. To prevent cerebrospinal fluid leakage, the eustachian tube anterior to the internal carotid artery is packed with fascia followed by the body of the incus to obstruct this structure. Fibrin glue is then applied. The dural defect needs to be reinforced with fascia. The freestanding facial nerve can be used as a structure under which a fat graft can be tucked to help maintain the position of the underlying fascial repair of the dura. Removal of the mastoid tip can facilitate reduction in the size of the mastoid cavity.

RECOMMENDED READING

Fisch, U., Mattox, D.: Microsurgery of the Skull Base. New York: Thieme Medical Publishers, 1988.

Horn, K.L., Hankinson, H.L., Erasmus, M.D., Beauparalant, P.A.: The modified transcochlear approach to the cerebellopontine angle. Otolaryngol. Head Neck Surg. 104(1):37–41, 1991.

House, W., Hitselberger, W.: The transcochlear approach to the skull base. Arch. Otolaryngol. 102:334–342, 1976.

House, W.F., Luetje, C.M.: Acoustic Tumors. Baltimore: University Park Press, 1979.

Tos, M., Thomsen, J.: Translabyrinthine Acoustic Neuroma Surgery: A Surgical Manual. New York: Thieme Medical Publishers, 1991.

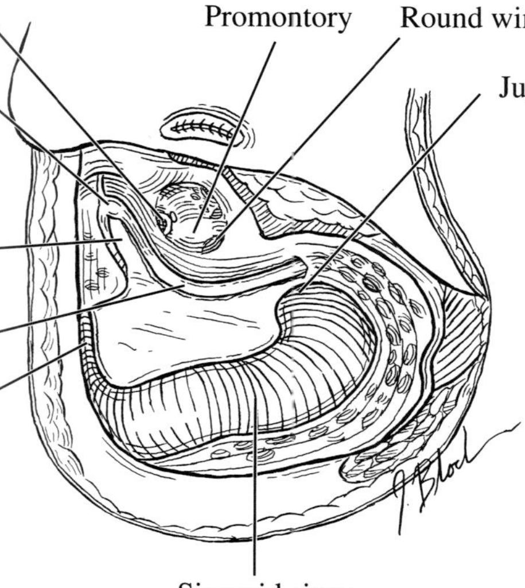

Figure 1. Anterior extension of the dissection after the translabyrinthine exposure. The cartilaginous external auditory canal skin is everted and oversewn. The bony external auditory canal is removed down to the bone-covered facial nerve. The tympanic membrane, malleus, and incus are removed.

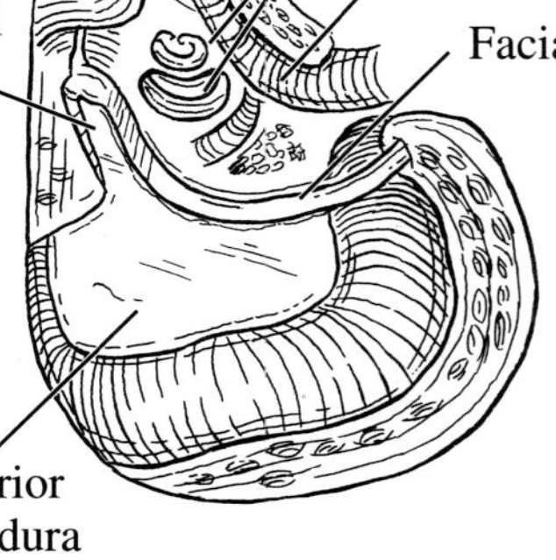

Figure 2. The cochlea is opened, and the infralabyrinthine bone is removed. The internal carotid artery is exposed anteromedially.

8 Middle Cranial Fossa Approach

Phillip A. Wackym *and* James C. Andrews

INDICATIONS

The middle cranial fossa approach is used as an alternative to the suboccipital retrosigmoid approach for the removal of small acoustic neuromas that are confined primarily to the internal auditory canal and the region of the porus acusticus. In such patients, this approach offers the advantage of possible preservation of hearing.

The middle cranial fossa approach is also commonly used for decompression of the facial nerve in Bell's palsy, herpes zoster oticus, and longitudinal temporal bone fractures.

ANATOMICAL CONSIDERATIONS

Of principal importance in the middle fossa approach to the internal auditory canal is detailed knowledge of the complex course of the facial nerve and its anatomical relation to other vital structures. The facial nerve exits the brain stem at the pontomedullary junction just anterior to the vestibulocochlear nerve (CN VIII). The nervus intermedius emerges between cranial nerves VII and VIII and then becomes incorporated within the sheath of VII.

The facial nerve follows a rostrolateral course through the cerebellopontine cistern, emerging through the porus of the internal auditory canal of the temporal bone.

Other important structures in the cerebellopontine cistern include the anterior inferior cerebellar artery and the veins of the middle cerebellar peduncle. The anterior inferior cerebellar artery passes near or between cranial nerves VII and VIII, where it usually bifurcates into rostral and caudal trunks.

On entering the internal auditory canal the facial nerve occupies the anterosuperior quadrant of this channel for 8 to 10 mm. Then it enters the fallopian canal at the fundus of the internal auditory canal. The internal auditory canal is anterior to the plane of the superior semicircular canal.

The intratemporal bone course of the facial nerve has three distinct anatomical regions: the labyrinthine, tympanic, and mastoid segments. The labyrinthine segment is shortest (about 4 mm), extending from the meatal foramen to the geniculate ganglion. This segment travels anterior, superior, and lateral, forming an anterior medial angle of 120 degrees with the internal auditory canal portion.

The basal turn of the cochlea is closely related to the fallopian canal and lies anteroinferior to the labyrinthine segment of the facial nerve. Figure 1 shows the cochlea in relation to the internal auditory canal and other important structures within the petrous bone.

At the lateral end of the labyrinthine segment lies the geniculate ganglion, and it is at this point that the nerve makes an abrupt posterior change in direction, forming an acute angle of about 75 degrees. Extending anteriorly from the geniculate ganglion, the greater superficial petrosal nerve exits the temporal bone through the hiatus of the facial canal. The hiatus of the facial canal also contains the vascular supply to the geniculate ganglion.

The tympanic, or horizontal, segment of the nerve is about 11 mm long, running between the lateral semicircular canal superiorly and the stapes inferiorly, forming the superior margin of the fossa ovale. Between the tympanic and mastoid segments, the nerve gently curves inferiorly for about 2 to 3 mm.

The mastoid, or vertical, segment is the longest intratemporal portion of the nerve, measuring about 13 mm. As the facial nerve exits the stylomastoid foramen at the anterior margin of the digastric groove, an adherent fibrous sheath of dense vascularized connective tissue surrounds it. The stylomastoid artery and veins are within this dense sheath.

The cochlear nerve lies in the anteroinferior quadrant of the internal auditory canal, and the superior and inferior vestibular nerves lie in the posterior superior and inferior quadrants of the canal. The vertical crest (Bill's bar) separates the facial nerve from the vestibular nerve in the lateral extent of the internal auditory canal.

SPECIAL SURGICAL CONSIDERATIONS

Continuous facial nerve monitoring is carried out throughout the operation. It is essential to have the ipsilateral side of the face exposed for inspection by the nurse during the procedure. Taping the endotracheal tube to the other side of the mouth facilitates this observation.

POSITION

The patient is placed supine on the operating table with the head turned so that the involved temporal bone is upward. The hair is shaved 6 to 8 cm above and anterior to the ear and 2 cm posterior to it. The surgeon is seated at the head of the table with the instrument nurse at the anterior side of the patient's head (Figure 2A). After preparation, the side of the face is draped using an abdominal, clear, noniodinated plastic adhesive drape. Electromyographic needle electrodes can be placed in the orbicularis oculi and oris muscles and attached to electromyographic equipment for auditory feedback of neural activity throughout the surgical procedure.

INCISION

Three choices of scalp and temporalis muscle incisions are described. In Figure 2B, a trap-door incision is shown that is based posteriorly. The dotted line shows the extension of the inferior portion of the incision behind the ear if exposure of the mastoid is required. With this scalp incision, the underlying temporalis muscle incision is made as shown, with its base anteriorly.

Figure 3A shows an alternative trap-door incision. It is 6 × 8 cm and inferiorly based. If exposure of the mastoid is necessary, the inferior limb of the incision can be carried postauricularly (see Figure 3A, dashed line). The skin flap is elevated to expose the temporalis muscle and fascia. A 4 × 4-cm temporalis fascia graft is harvested for use during closure of the internal auditory canal dural defect. An anteriorly based trap-door incision is used to elevate the temporalis muscle and periosteum. Staggering the levels of the muscle and skin incisions provides for a double-layer watertight closure at the completion of the procedure.

Figure 3B shows a third alternative for the incision in performing the middle fossa approach. The exposure that can be obtained with this single curved incision is more limited, and access to the mastoid area is not possible.

OPERATIVE PROCEDURE

The temporal root of the zygoma is exposed during elevation of the temporalis muscle. This landmark represents the level of the floor of the middle fossa. Dural fish hooks are placed in the skin and temporalis muscle flaps for retraction. A 3 × 5-cm bone flap for facial nerve decompression or a 4 × 5-cm bone flap for tumor excisions, centered above the temporal root of the zygoma, is fashioned with a medium cutting burr. It is important to keep the anterior and posterior margins of the craniotomy parallel to facilitate placement of the self-retaining retractor.

Sometimes branches of the middle meningeal artery are embedded within the inner table of the skull; therefore, elevation of the bone flap must be performed in a controlled manner. Bipolar coagulation and bone wax are used to control bleeding. Elevation of the dura from the floor of the middle fossa can be one of the most difficult steps. Blunt dissection and magnification greatly facilitate dural elevation. The dura is elevated from the posterior to anterior direction to prevent injury to an exposed geniculate ganglion and greater superficial petrosal nerve. Bipolar coagulation is used to cauterize dural reflections within the petrosquamous suture before transection with a scissors.

The elevation proceeds until the petrous ridge is identified medially and the arcuate eminence, meatal plane, and greater superficial petrosal nerve are exposed anteriorly. The tip of a self-retaining (House-Urban or Fisch) retractor is placed at the petrous ridge anterior to the arcuate eminence and medial to the meatal plane (Figure 4A). A medium diamond burr and a suction-irrigation apparatus are used to identify the blue line of the superior semicircular canal (see Figure 4B). A preoperative Stenver's-projection radiograph helps to determine the level of the superior semicircular canal in relation to the floor of the middle fossa (Figure 5).

Drilling begins posterior to the arcuate eminence over the mastoid air cells until the dense yellow bone of the otic capsule is identified. Otic capsule bone is slowly removed until the blue outline of the superior semicircular canal is seen. The internal auditory canal is located by removing bone within a 60-degree angle anterior to the blue line of the superior semicircular canal and with the vertex based at the superior semicircular canal ampulla. This dissection is continued until about 180 degrees of the internal auditory canal is exposed for facial nerve decompressions (see Figure 4C) or 270 degrees of the internal auditory canal is exposed for schwannomas (see Figure 4D).

Because of the proximity of the superior semicircular canal and the basal turn of the cochlea, only about 120 degrees of the circumference of the internal auditory canal can be safely removed in its lateral 5 mm or so. The facial nerve occupies the anterosuperior portion of the internal auditory canal. Laterally, the vertical crest (Bill's bar) marks the division between the superior vestibular nerve and the meatal foramen containing the facial nerve.

At the entrance to the fallopian canal is the most narrow and delicate portion of the facial nerve and, consequently, the most challenging portion of the dissection. At the meatal foramen, the facial nerve turns anterior and slightly superior. The basal turn of the cochlea can be within 1 mm inferiorly and the ampulla of the superior semicircular canal can be directly posterior to the nerve.

The labyrinthine segment is followed to the geniculate ganglion. If the facial nerve needs to be exposed distal to the geniculate ganglion, the tegmen tympani is removed with care to avoid injury to the head of the malleus and incus. The tympanic segment is easily seen to turn abruptly posterior, and it is followed to where it courses inferior to the lateral semicircular canal. It is advisable to leave a thin shell of bone covering the nerve until its entire course is identified. The final layer of bone is removed by small blunt elevators.

The nerve is tightly confined within the labyrinthine segment of the fallopian canal. Larger curettes should be avoided to prevent compression injury. If the nerve is to be decompressed, a neurolysis is the final step. A disposable microscalpel (Beaver No. 5910) is used to slit the periosteum and epineural sheath.

CLOSURE

At the end of the procedure, a free temporalis muscle graft is placed within the internal auditory canal and a corner piece of the bone flap is fashioned to cover the defects in the tegmen tympani and the internal auditory canal (Figure 6). This prevents herniation of the temporal lobe into the middle ear or internal auditory canal. The temporalis fascia previously harvested is placed over the free bone graft to help seal the dural defect at the internal auditory canal and prevent the leakage of CSF. The squamosal craniotomy bone flap is replaced, and the temporalis muscle is closed with interrupted absorbable sutures.

The skin is closed in layers with particular care in closing the galea. No drain is placed. A mastoid-type pressure dressing is applied.

RECOMMENDED READING

Fisch, U.: Surgery for Bell's palsy. Arch. Otolaryngol. 107:1–11, 1981.

Fisch, U., Mattox, D.: Microsurgery of the Skull Base. New York, Thieme Medical Publishers, 1988.

Gantz, B.J.: Intraoperative facial nerve monitoring. Am. J. Otol. (Suppl.) 6:58–61, 1985.

Gantz, B.J., Gmur, A., Fisch, U.: Intraoperative evoked electromyography in Bell's palsy. Am. J. Otolaryngol. 3:273–278, 1982.

Ge, X.X. Spector, G.J.: Labyrinthine segment and geniculate ganglion of the facial nerve in fetal and adult temporal bones. Ann. Otol. Rhinol. Laryngol. 90(85):1–12, 1981.

House, W.: Surgical exposure of the internal auditory canal and its contents through the middle cranial fossa. Laryngoscope 71:1363–1385, 1961.

Jackson, C.G., Johnson, G.D., Hyams, V.J., Poe, D.S.: Pathologic findings in the labyrinthine segment of the facial nerve in a case of facial paralysis. Ann. Otol. Rhinol. Laryngol. 99:327–329, 1990.

Yamamoto, E., Fisch, U.: Experiments on facial nerve suturing. ORL 36:193–204, 1974.

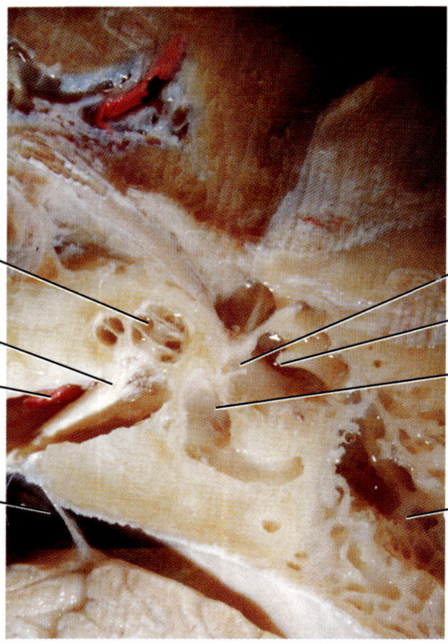

Figure 1. Cadaver dissection showing important anatomical structures in the petrous bone and the internal auditory canal.

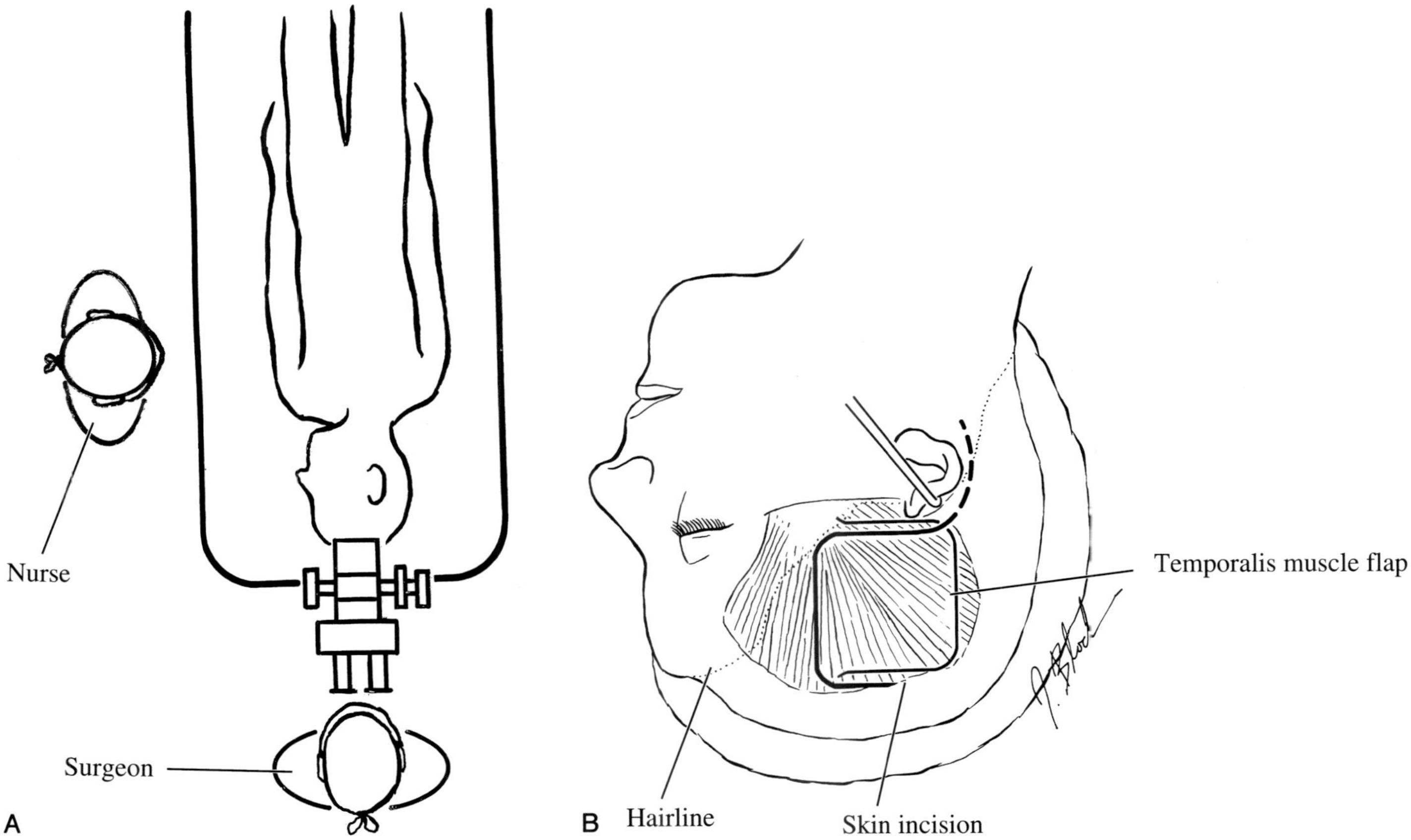

Figure 2. *A*, Patient position and placement of surgical team. *B*, Posteriorly based trap-door scalp incision. The dotted line shows the extension of the scalp incision that is required to reach the mastoid area. The temporalis muscle flap is shown based anteriorly.

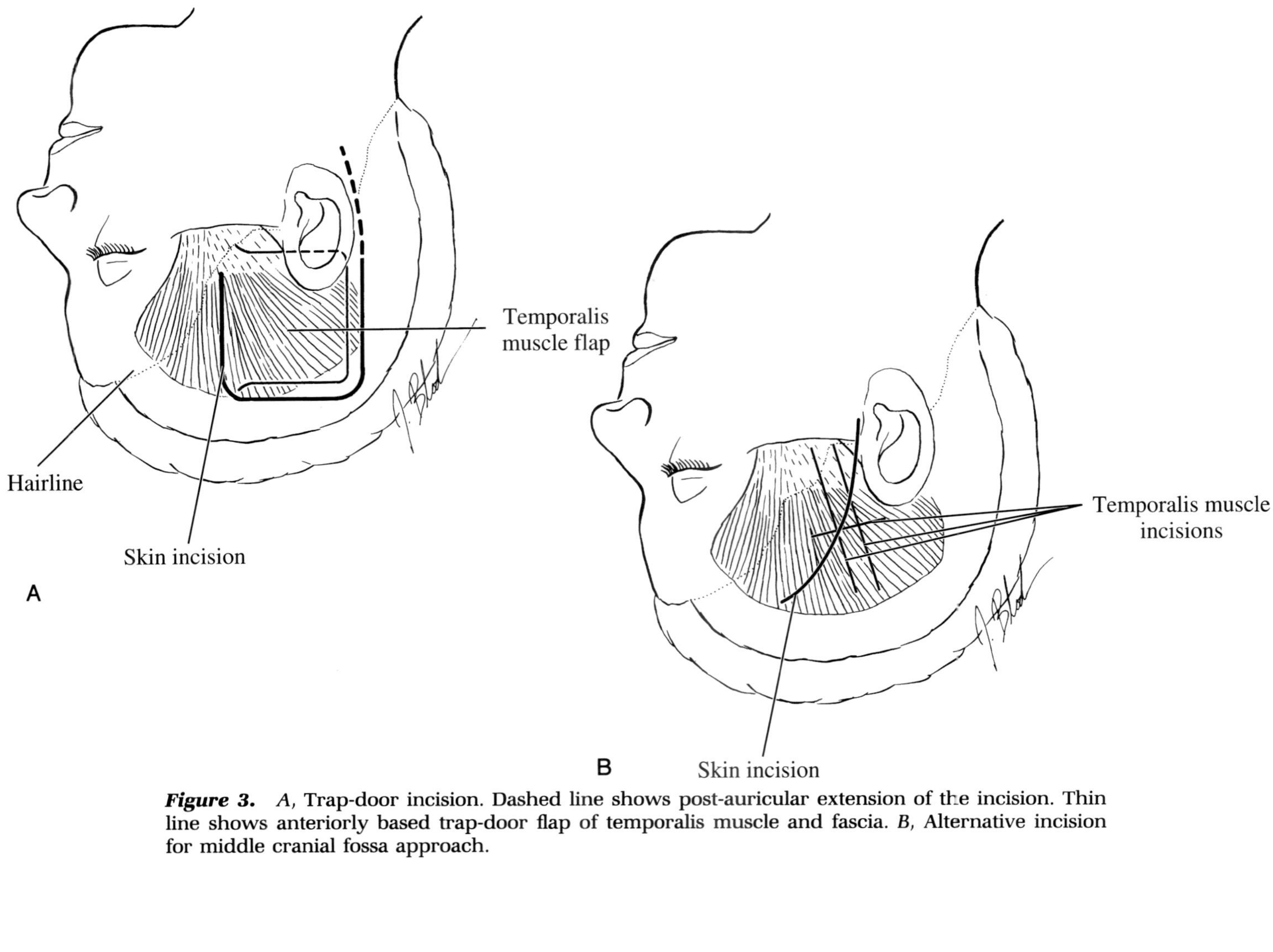

Figure 3. *A*, Trap-door incision. Dashed line shows post-auricular extension of the incision. Thin line shows anteriorly based trap-door flap of temporalis muscle and fascia. *B*, Alternative incision for middle cranial fossa approach.

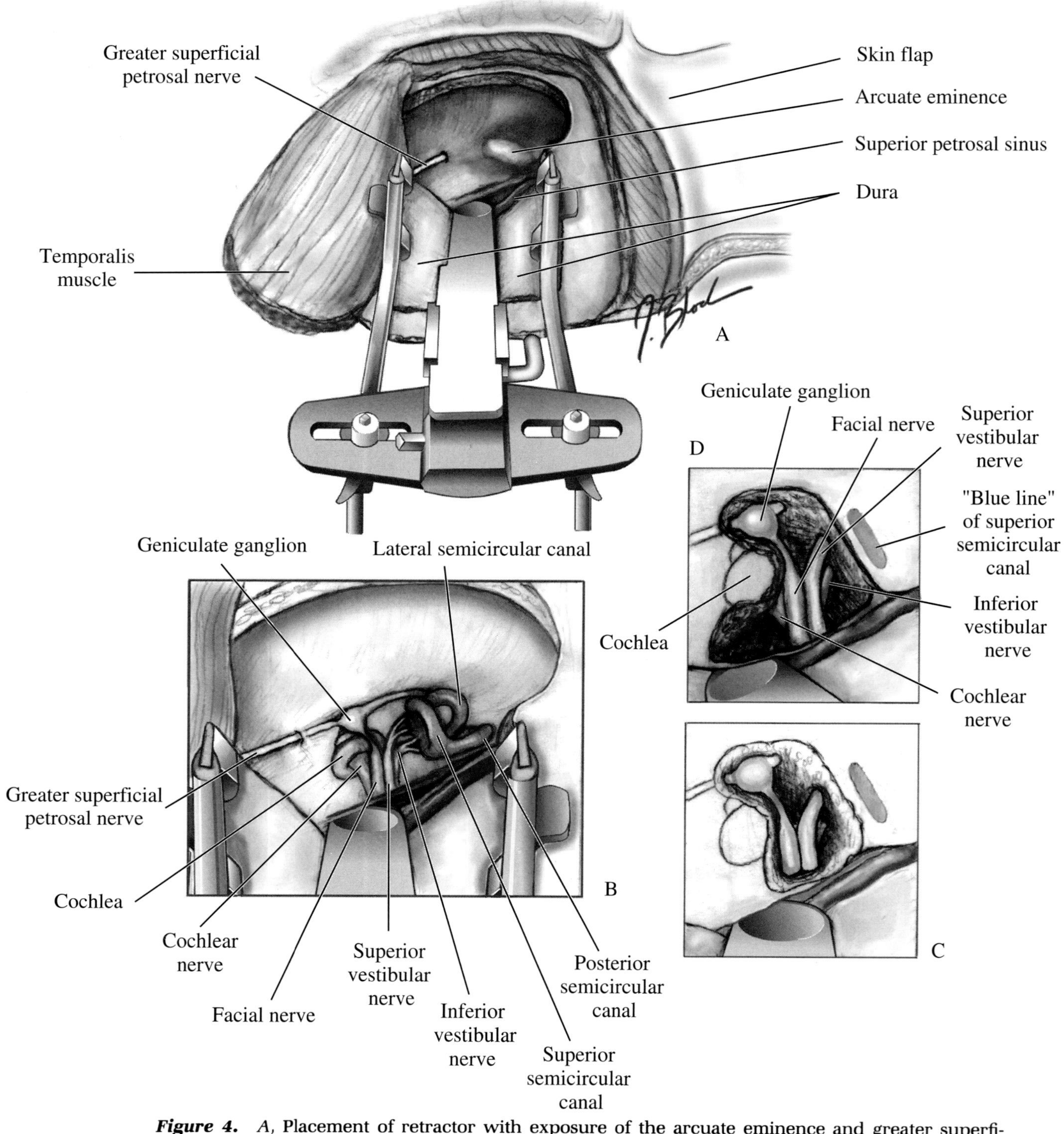

Figure 4. *A,* Placement of retractor with exposure of the arcuate eminence and greater superficial petrosal nerve. *B,* Identification of blue line of the superior semicircular canal. *C,* Drilling of the internal auditory canal to 180 degrees for facial nerve decompression. *D,* Drilling of the internal auditory canal to 270 degrees for excision of schwannomas.

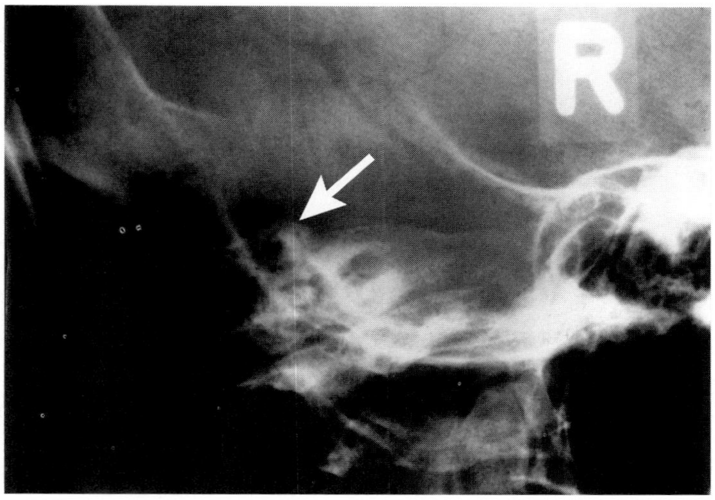

Figure 5. Stenver's-view radiograph to show the superior semicircular canal in relation to the floor of the middle fossa (*arrow,* pneumatized space above superior semicircular canal).

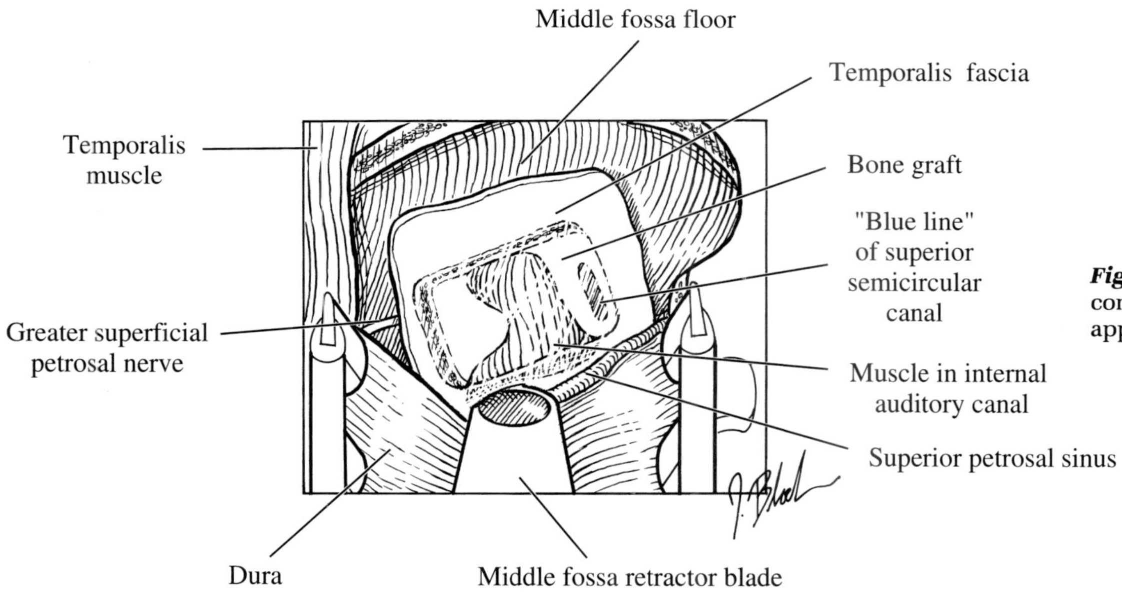

Figure 6. Postoperative reconstruction after middle fossa approach.

9 Transsphenoidal Approach

Wesley A. King

INDICATIONS

The transsphenoidal approach is the procedure of choice for the removal of tumors of the sella that are still largely confined to this space. It is also indicated for removal of some tumors of the parasellar area. Pituitary tumors with substantial intracranial extension can engulf important structures and should be treated using a transcranial approach.

For transsphenoidal surgery, there are several alternative approaches to the sphenoid sinus. These include the transnasal paraseptal, sublabial-transseptal, and paranasal transethmoidal approaches. For processes that are largely located in the sella, the sublabial or transnasal approach is used. With extreme involvement of the paranasal sinuses, the paranasal transethmoidal exposure is of benefit.

POSITION

Proper positioning is essential in transsphenoidal surgery to ensure adequate exposure of the sphenoid sinus structures, to minimize bleeding, and to maximize the surgeon's comfort. It is also crucial in helping to ensure that the operative dissection remains midline.

The patient is positioned supine with the head elevated to 30 degrees, turned 20 degrees toward the surgeon, and flexed toward the opposite shoulder (Figure 1).

The head is placed in a head immobilizer or, alternatively, supported with a padded ring. We prefer the latter because this allows subtle movement of the operative field intraoperatively without the need for microscope repositioning. The nurse stands next to the surgeon, and the asssistant is positioned at the head of the table (see Figure 1).

OPERATIVE PROCEDURE

We describe in this chapter the sublabial approach for transsphenoidal surgery.

A sublabial incision positioned on the gingival mucosa well above the teeth is made extending between the canine teeth (Figure 2).

Periosteal elevators are used to elevate the mucosa off the maxilla. After the pyriform apertures are identified and defined, the inferior mucosa within each aperture is elevated along the premaxilla, forming inferior tunnels (Figure 3).

The cartilaginous septum is exposed using sharp dissection, and a submucosal tunnel is elevated along its left side. Fibrous adhesions at the base of the cartilage must be divided sharply, allowing the septum to be disarticulated from the nasal spine and maxillary ridge. The cartilage can then be hinged to the patient's right side. Increased exposure may require enlargement of the pyriform apertures with rongeurs or removal of the nasal spine (Figure 4).

Posteriorly, the mucosa is elevated from both sides of the bony septum, which subsequently is fractured, removed, and saved. Under microscopic magnification, the characteristic keel appearance of the vomer is seen during this phase (Figure 5).

The anterior wall of the sphenoid sinus is confirmed by identifying the ostea, located superolaterally, or with a lateral radiograph. The sinus is opened widely, and all mucosa is removed from within it to prevent troublesome bleeding. Placement of the speculum within the sphenoid sinus should be avoided because fracture of the sphenoid bone can result in injury to the optic nerve, cranial nerves, and carotid artery. After the mucosa is removed, the bulge of the sella is readily apparent and, typically, is thinned by the tumor. If necessary, the bone of the sella can be fractured with a small osteotome or removed with a diamond drill, exposing the medial extent of each cavernous sinus (Figure 6). In rare cases, the sphenoid sinus is incompletely pneumatized, requiring removal of bone with a high-speed drill to expose the sella.

The dura is incised in a cruciate manner after coagulating it with the bipolar electrocautery (Figure 7). Intercavernous venous channels that extend across the sella frequently result in brisk bleeding when the dura is incised. The bleeding can be controlled by grasping both leaves of the dura with the bipolar forceps and coagulating.

Important anatomical relations in the transsphenoidal approach are seen in Figures 8 through 12. Pituitary adenomas usually are soft and can be readily removed with bayonetted ring curettes. Intermittent Valsalva maneuvers by the anesthesiologist expedite tumor removal by elevating the subarachnoid fluid pressure, which is transmitted to the tumor capsule, displacing tumor tissue downward.

After the bulk of the tumor is removed, the sella is inspected systematically and the pituitary gland itself is examined. If the tumor capsule prolapses into the sphenoid sinus or cerebrospinal fluid leakage occurs, fascia lata or adipose tissue and fibrin glue may be used to occlude the communication to the subarachnoid space and support the diaphragma sellae. The floor of the sella can be reconstructed with the bony septum previously removed. After complete hemostasis is achieved, the speculum is removed and the sublabial mucosa is closed with interrupted absorbable sutures.

Petroleum jelly–covered gauze is packed into each nasal passage and left in place for 48 to 72 hours.

In the case of extensive dural defect, lumbar cerebrospinal fluid drainage for 2 to 3 days is advisable.

CAVERNOUS SINUS EXTENSION OF TUMORS

Some tumors extend in the lateral direction, requiring surgical entry into the medial cavernous sinus. In these cases, the surgeon must be familiar with the important anatomical structures adjacent to the sella before proceeding with surgery (see Figures 11 and 12). The structures most at risk include the internal carotid artery and its intracavernous branches as well as cranial nerves to extraocular muscles.

Sometimes better exposure of the medial wall of the sphenoid sinus and cavernous sinus is necessary in these situations. This can be gained by enlarging the pyriform aperture or by removing the medial maxillary sinus wall contralateral to the involved cavernous sinus (Figures 13 and 14) and directing the speculum laterally.

Tumors that involve the medial cavernous sinus typically obliterate the venous channels and can be removed piecemeal using microdissectors. These instruments can be gently used to remove the tumor around the carotid artery with special care to avoid injury to the ocular muscle nerves, particularly the abducens nerve.

Significant venous bleeding is not a problem until the final stages of tumor removal as the patent part of the sinus is exposed. As with other approaches to the cavernous sinus, the tumor should be removed in an organized manner and bleeding controlled with carefully placed oxidized cellulose and pressure.

RECOMMENDED READING

Balagura, S., Tindall, G.: Technique of transsphenoidal microsurgery. Contemp. Neurosurg. 3(24): 1982.

Eisele, D., Flint, P., Janas, J., et al.: The sublabial transseptal transsphenoidal approach to sellar and parasellar lesions. Laryngoscope 98:1301–1308, 1988

Tindall, G., Herring, C., Clark, R., et al.: Cushing's disease: Results of transsphenoidal microsurgery with emphasis on surgical failures. J. Neurosurg. 72:363–369, 1990.

Tucker, H., Hahn, J.: Transnasal, transseptal sphenoidal approach to hypophysectomy. Laryngoscope 92:55–57, 1982.

Welbourn, R.: The evolution of transsphenoidal pituitary microsurgery. Surgery 100(6):1185–1189, 1986.

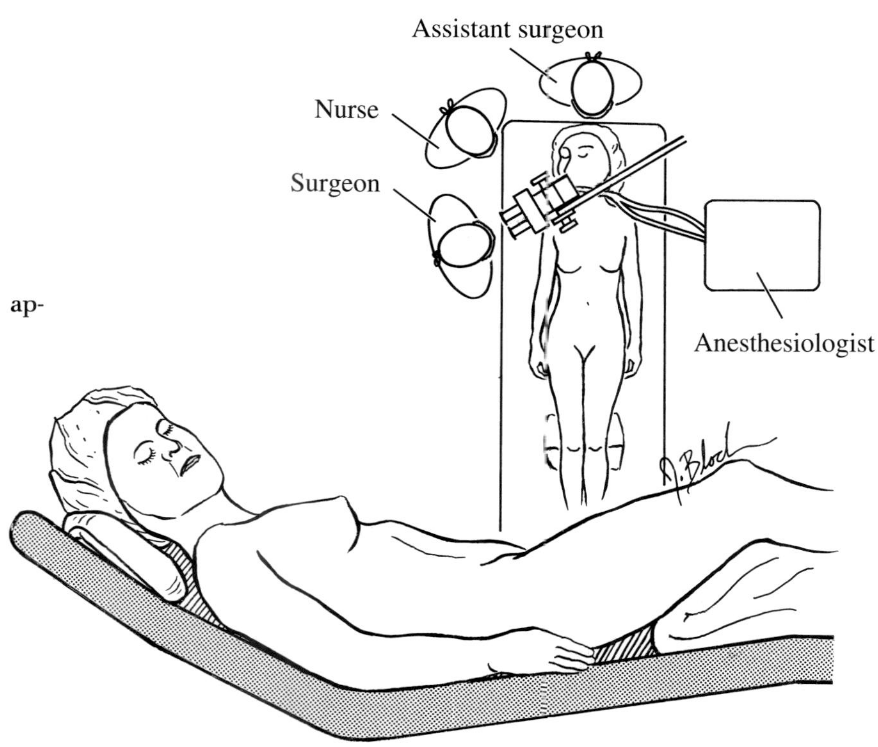

Figure 1. Patient position for transsphenoidal approach.

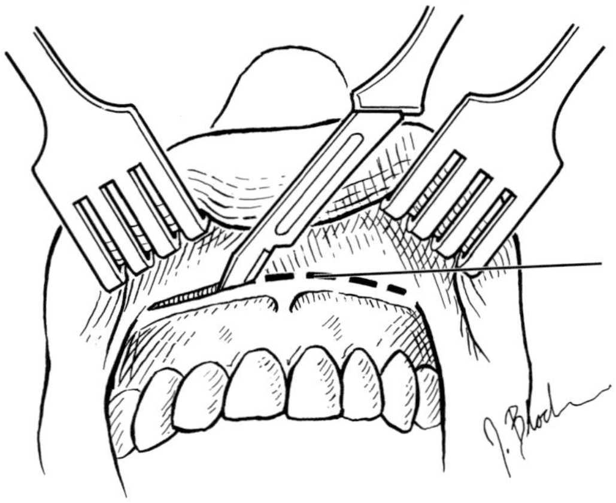

Figure 2. Sublabial incision.

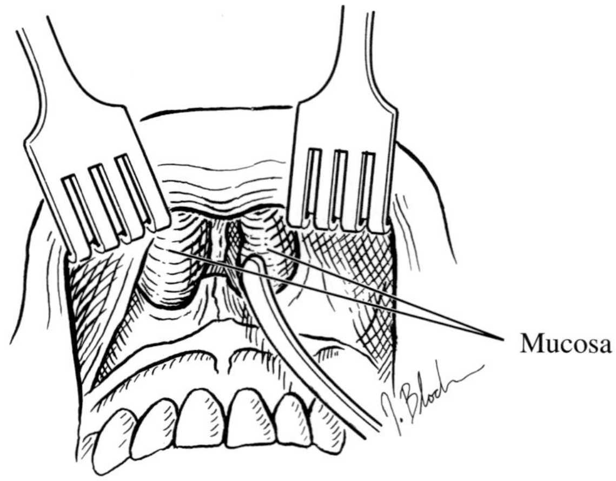

Figure 3. Elevation of the inferior mucosa within each aperture.

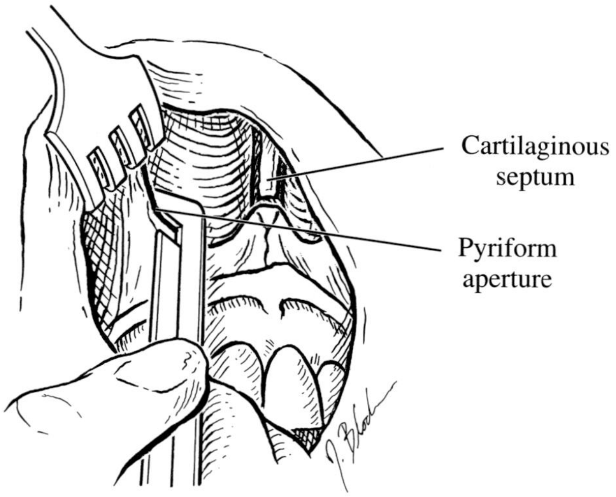

Figure 4. Enlargement of the pyriform apertures.

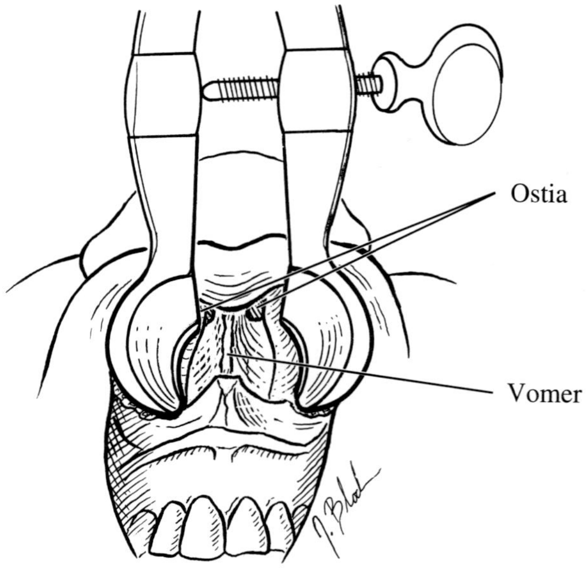

Figure 5. Visualization of the characteristic keel of the sphenoid sinus.

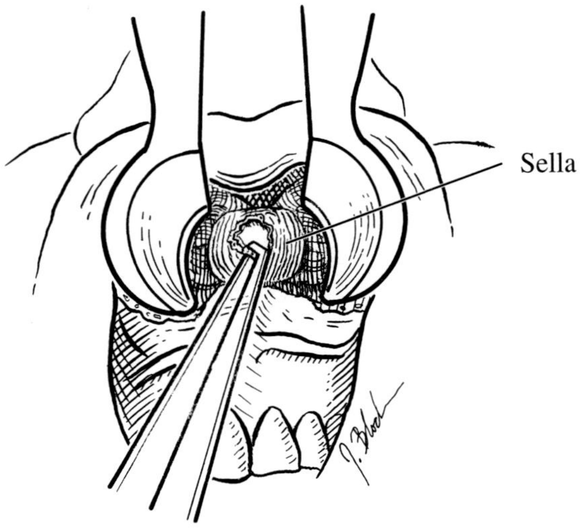

Figure 6. Removal of the floor of the sphenoid sinus.

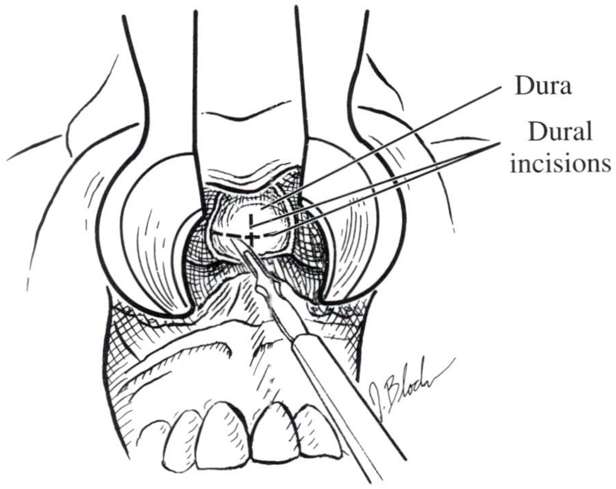

Figure 7. Incision of dura over the floor of the sella.

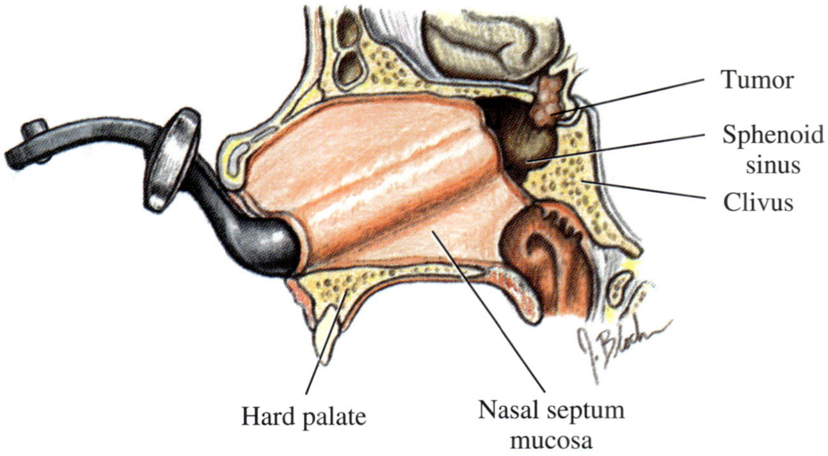

Figure 8. Overview of the transsphenoidal approach (lateral projection).

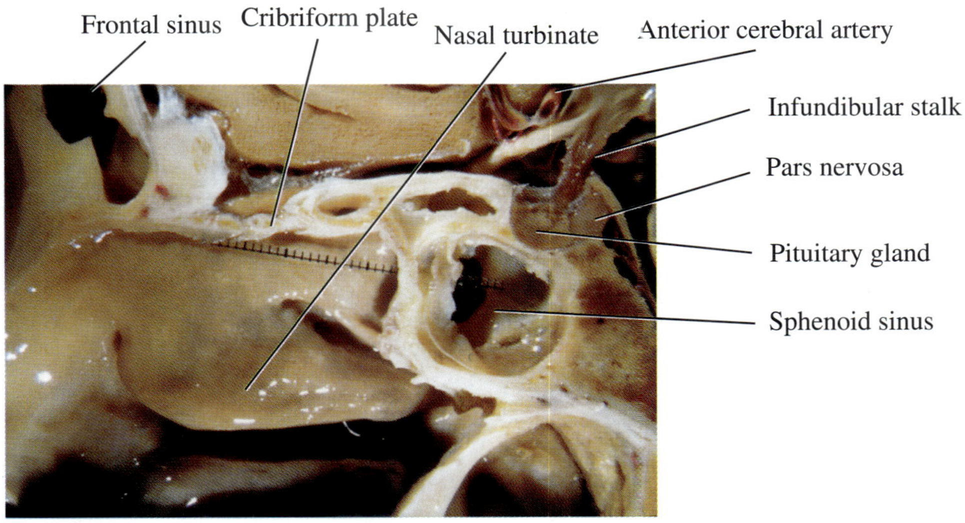

Figure 9. Cadaver dissection showing anatomical relations to sella (lateral projection).

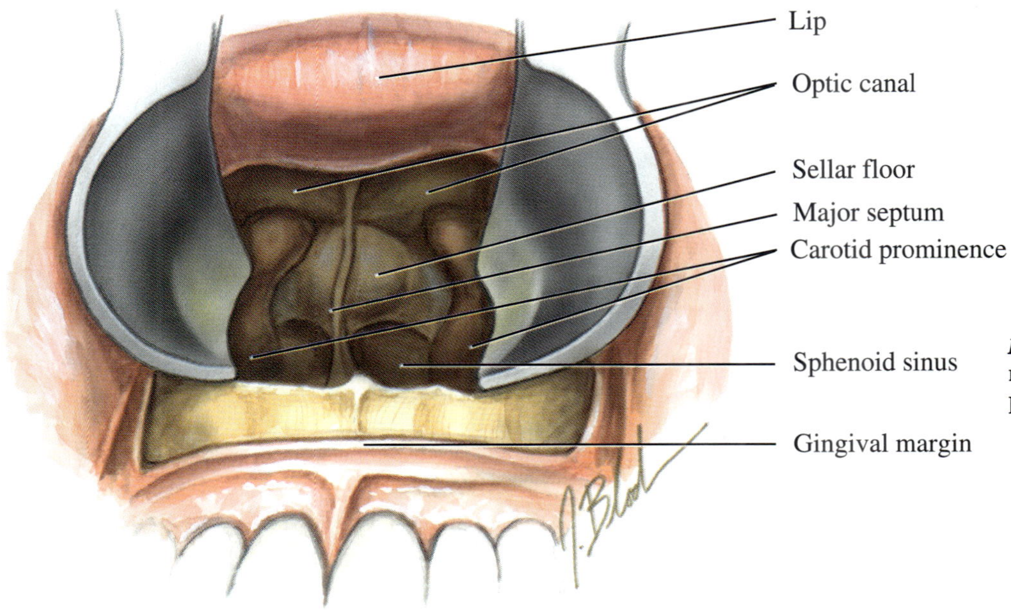

Figure 10. Overview of the transsphenoidal approach (anterior transnasal projection).

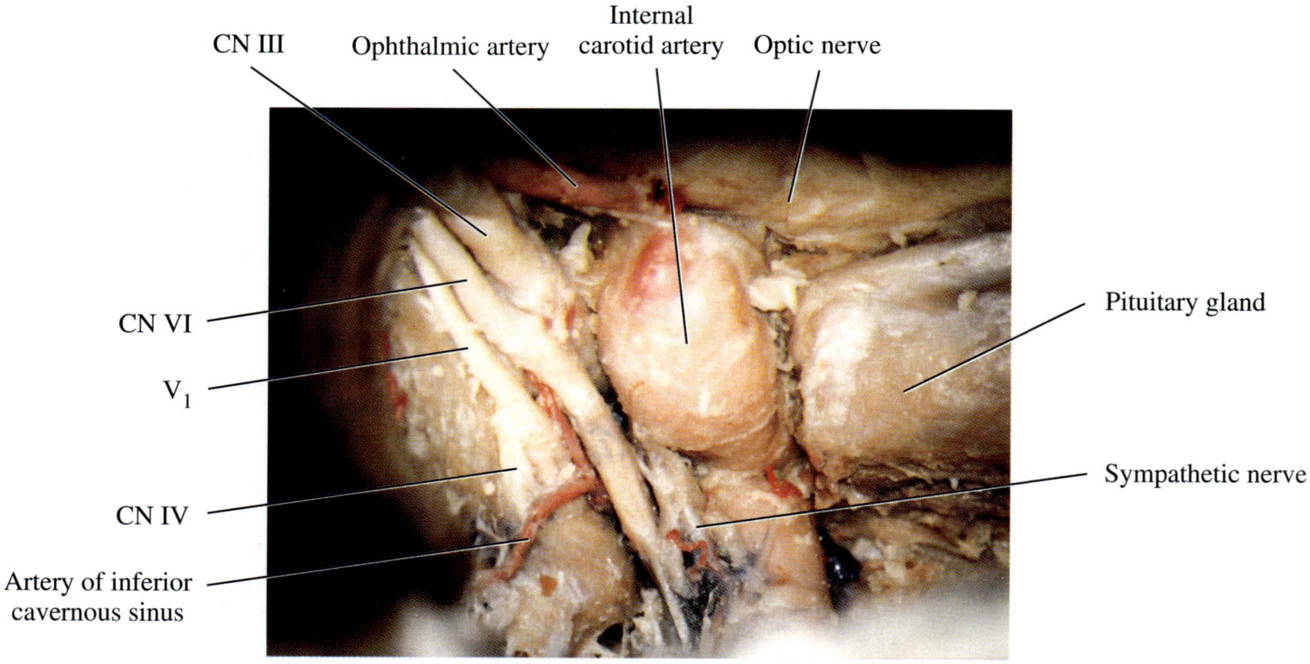

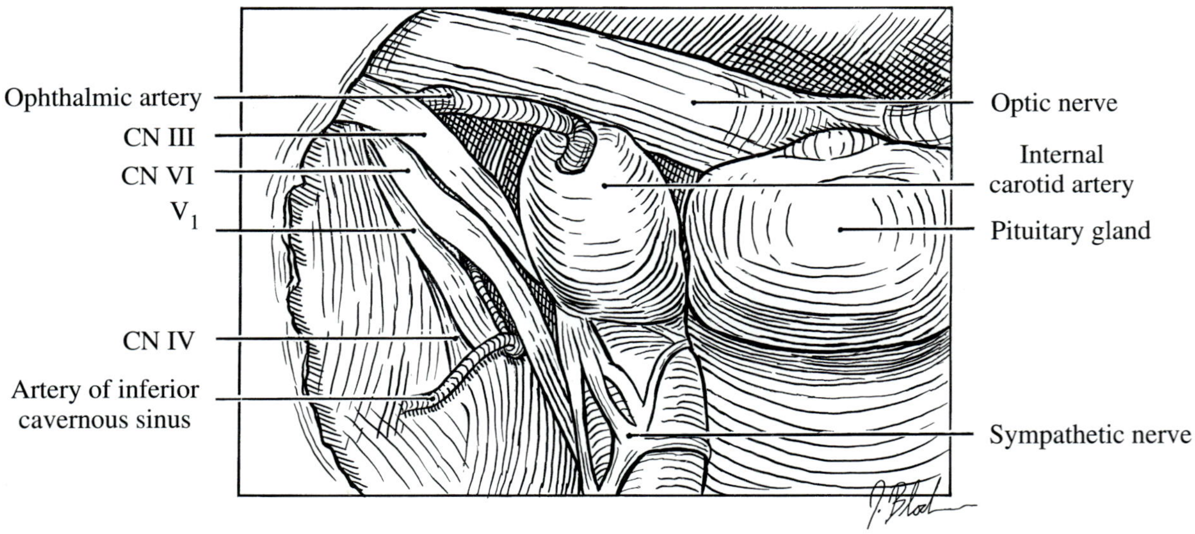

Figure 11. Important anatomical structures lateral to sella.

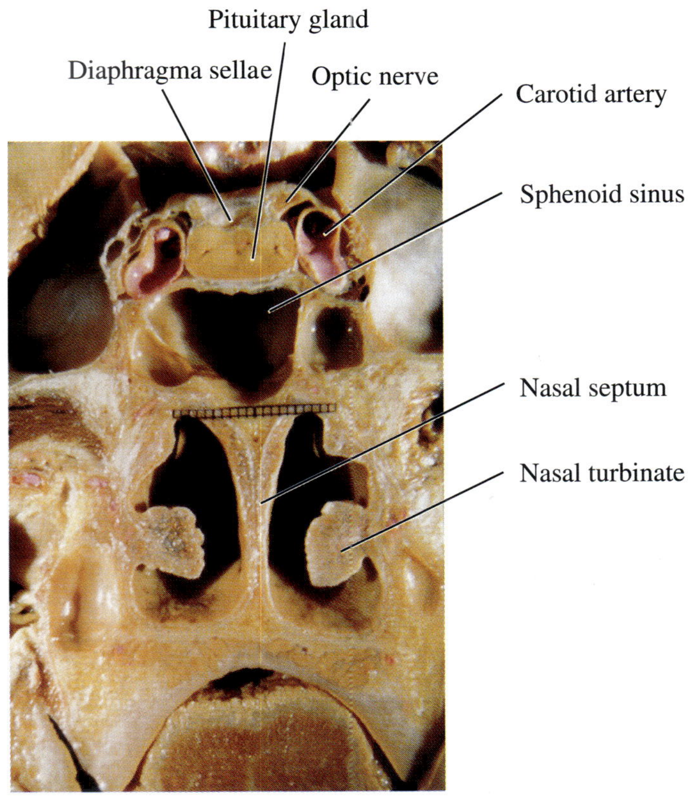

Figure 12. Cadaver dissection showing carotid artery and cavernous sinus relations to sella.

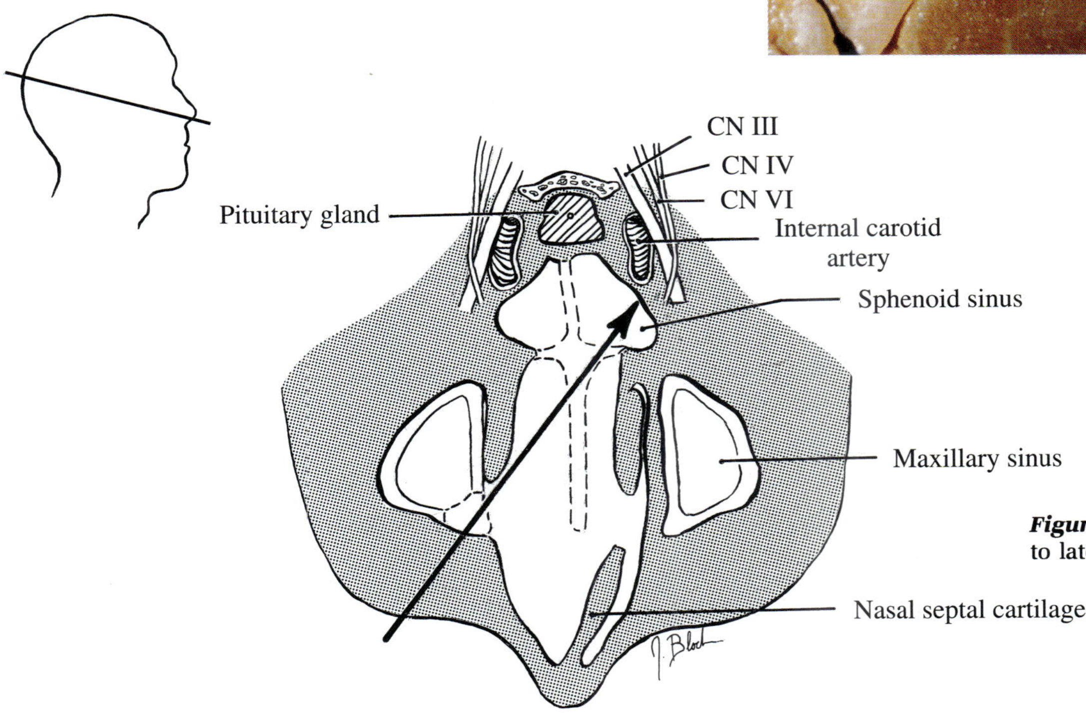

Figure 13. Axial view of approach to lateral parasellar area.

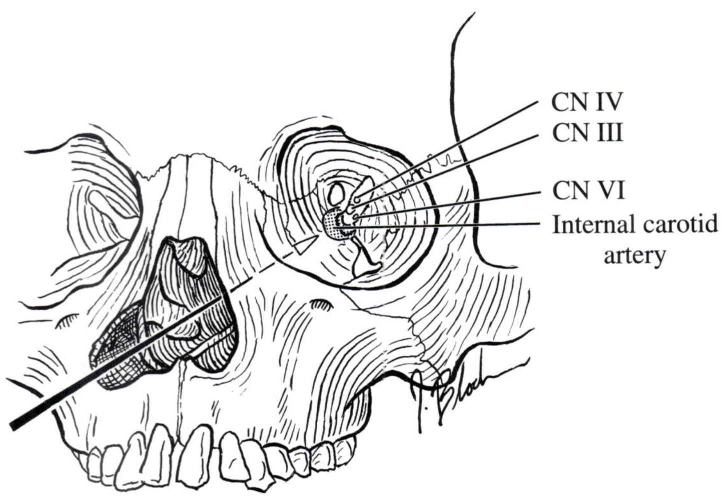

Figure 14. Removal of medial maxillary wall for approach to lateral parasellar area.

II

SPECIAL SURGICAL APPROACHES TO THE CRANIAL BASE

10 Subtemporal-Transzygomatic Approach

POSITION

The patient is positioned either on his or her side or supine with a sandbag elevating the shoulder to facilitate turning of the head. The head is placed in a headholder in three-point fixation and positioned parallel to the floor. The head is elevated 15 degrees above the level of the heart, and the vertex is tilted slightly downward to increase exposure of the subtemporal area of the middle fossa (Figure 1).

INCISION

A preauricular skin incision beginning at the level of the zygomatic arch 1 cm anterior to the tragus is carried upward curving first slightly posteriorly above the ear and then anteriorly toward the midpupillary line (Figure 2). The incision is carried 2 cm below the zygomatic root in front of the ear. Care is taken to avoid facial nerve branches. A scalp flap is developed in the subgaleal plane (Figure 3), and the main trunk of the superficial temporal artery is preserved. The temporalis fascia is incised several millimeters inferior to its bony attachment along the temporal line. The temporalis muscle is incised anteriorly and posteriorly, dissected from the temporal squama and then retracted inferiorly.

An incision in the periosteum of the zygomatic arch is made, and a subperiosteal dissection is carried from its anterior to its posterior extent. The masseter muscle attachment to the inferior border of the zygomatic arch and the fascial attachment of the temporal muscle to its superior border are released. The zygomatic arch is now cut at its anterior and posterior ends. The tendinous attachment of the temporalis muscle to the coronoid process is now exposed. After incision of the temporalis muscle along a line 1 cm below its insertion along the temporal line and subperiosteal dissection of the muscle from the temporal bone are completed, the muscle flap is retracted inferiorly (Figure 4).

CRANIOTOMY

Placement of one or more burr holes is followed by a connecting osteotome bone cut and elevation of a free temporal bone flap. The size of the cranial opening is dictated by the operative procedure to be done. The inferior retraction of temporalis muscle and dislodged segment of zygomatic bone offers increased exposure of the floor of the temporal fossa as well as its junction with the anterior cranial fossa. This low placement of the inferior extent of the craniotomy flap removes all bony obstruction to a flat viewing angle along the anterior and middle extent of the middle cranial fossa floor. By removing all bony obstruction to this angle of approach, the need for temporal lobe retraction is markedly reduced. Extradural visualization of the foramen rotundum, ovale, spinosum, and greater superficial petrosal nerve is possible with minimal elevation of the middle fossa dura and the temporal lobe. If necessary, the intrapetrous portion of the internal carotid artery can be unroofed.

The middle meningeal artery is the most important anatomical landmark in the beginning of epidural subtemporal exposure. This artery should be followed to the foramen spinosum. Medial to this, the foramen ovale can be identified, through which the third division of the trigeminal nerve runs. In case the carotid artery needs to be exposed, the surgeon can continue with bone drilling just posterior and medial to the foramen ovale. Ventral or anterior to this foramen, further bone resection leads the surgeon automatically to the foramen rotundum with the second division of the trigeminal nerve. By remaining between the second and third divisions of the fifth cranial nerve, the surgeon can cross the infratemporal fossa and reach the superior part of the clivus as well as the lateral wall of the sphenoid sinus without sacrificing nerves or vessels.

DURAL INCISION

Incision of the dura in a low transverse manner offers access to the intracranial internal carotid artery, cavernous sinus, Meckel's cave, and anterior and middle incisural space. Structures of the middle cranial fossa skull base and the tentorial notch are shown in the cadaver dissection in Figure 5.

CLOSURE

Dural closure is carried out in a watertight manner with 4-0 nylon in a running lock stitch. Tack-up sutures of 4-0 silk are placed at several points to support the dura to the pericranium or bone and prevent epidural hematoma formation. This is especially important if extradural dissection has been carried out.

The free bone flap is secured in place with three or four sutures of 0 black silk placed through small drill holes in the cranium and adjacent bone flap. Temporalis muscle and fascia are closed anatomically using 3-0 absorbable suture. The scalp closure is with monofilament nylon or skin staples.

RECOMMENDED READING

Al-Mefty, O.: The supraorbital-pterional approach to skull base lesions. Neurosurgery 21:474–477, 1987.

Ammirati, M., Ma, J., Becker, D., et al.: Transzygomatic approach to the tentorial incisura: Surgical anatomy. J. Skull Base Surg. 2(3):161–166, 1992.

Hakuba, A., Liu, S., Nishimura, S.: The orbitozygomatic infratemporal approach: A new surgical technique. Surg. Neurol. 26:271–276, 1986.

Sekhar, L.N., Schramm, V.L., Jones, N.F.: Subtemporal-preauricular infratemporal fossa approach to large lateral and posterior cranial base neoplasms. J. Neurosurg. 67:488–499, 1987.

Yasargil, M.G., Reichmann, M.V., Kubik, S.: Preservation of the fronto-temporal branch of the facial nerve using the interfacial temporalis flap for pterional craniotomy. J. Neurosurg. 67:463–466, 1987.

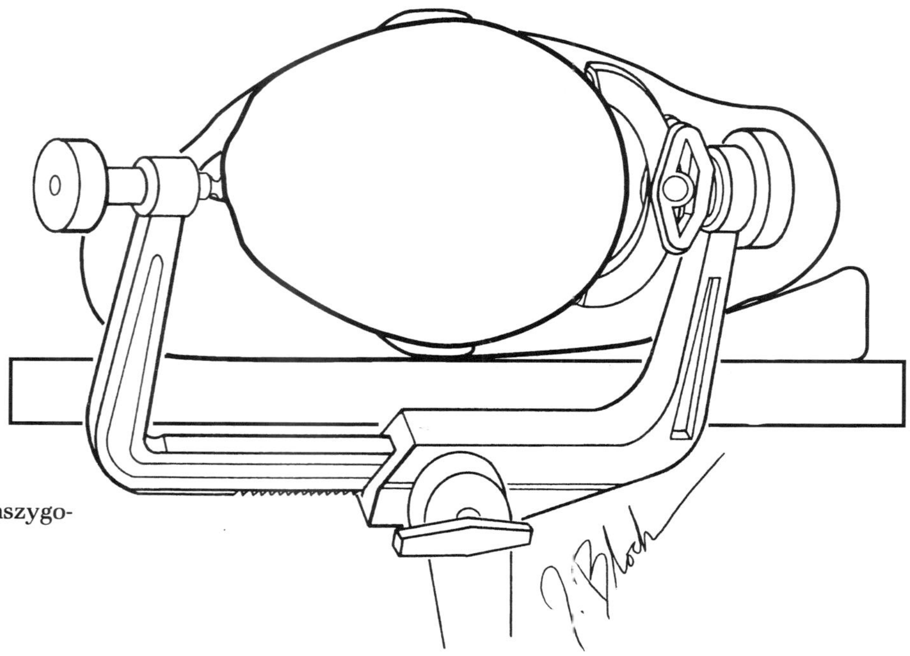

Figure 1. Patient position for subtemporal-transzygomatic approach.

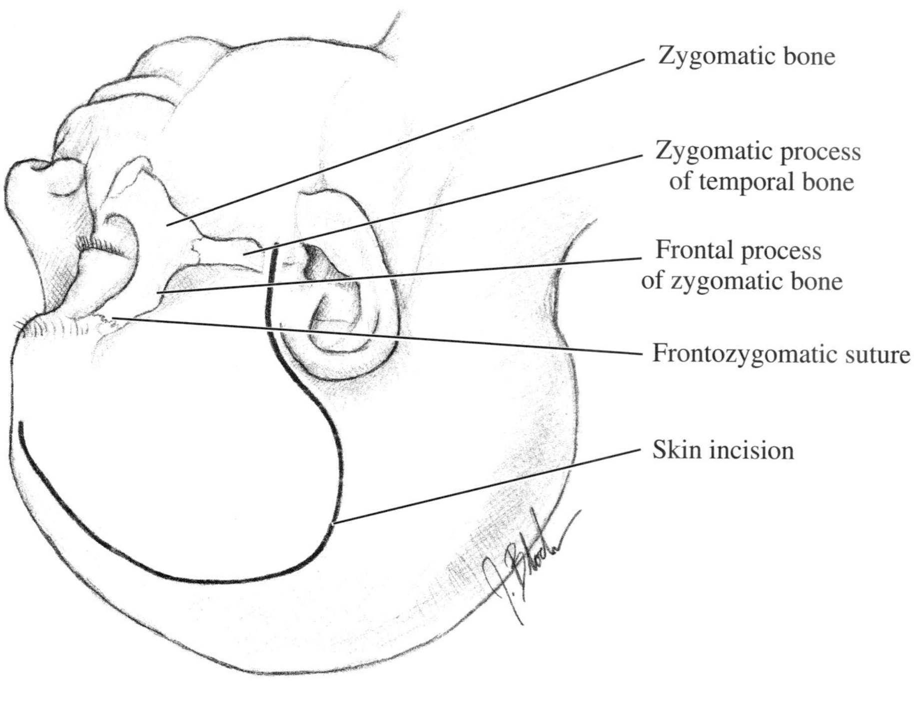

Figure 2. Scalp incision.

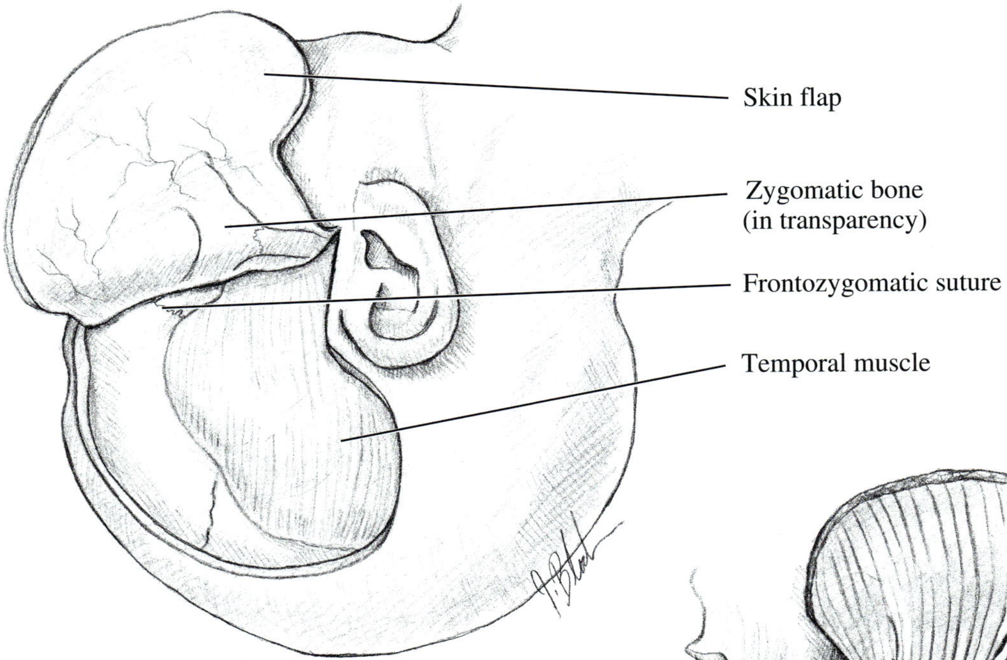

Figure 3. Retraction of the scalp flap.

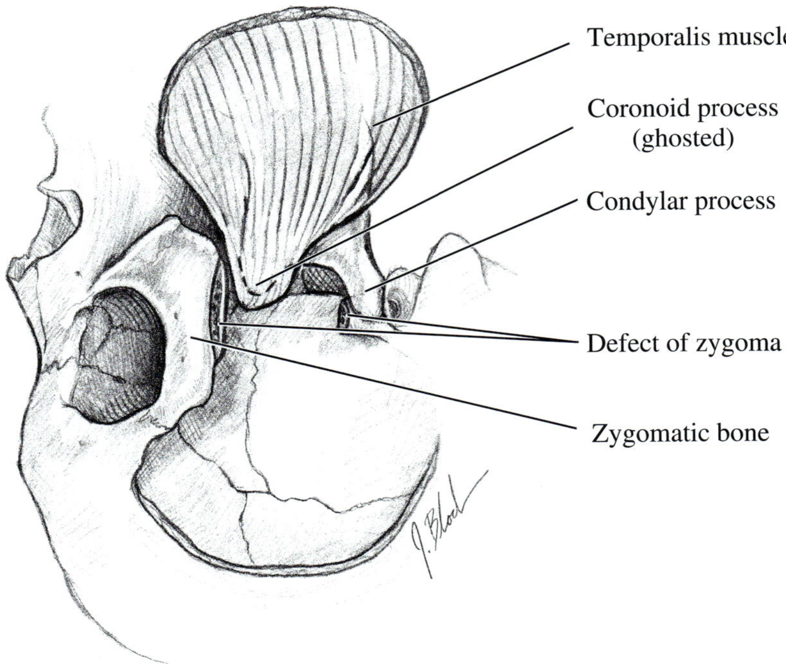

Figure 4. Inferior retraction of the temporalis muscle flap after anterior and posterior section of the zygomatic arch.

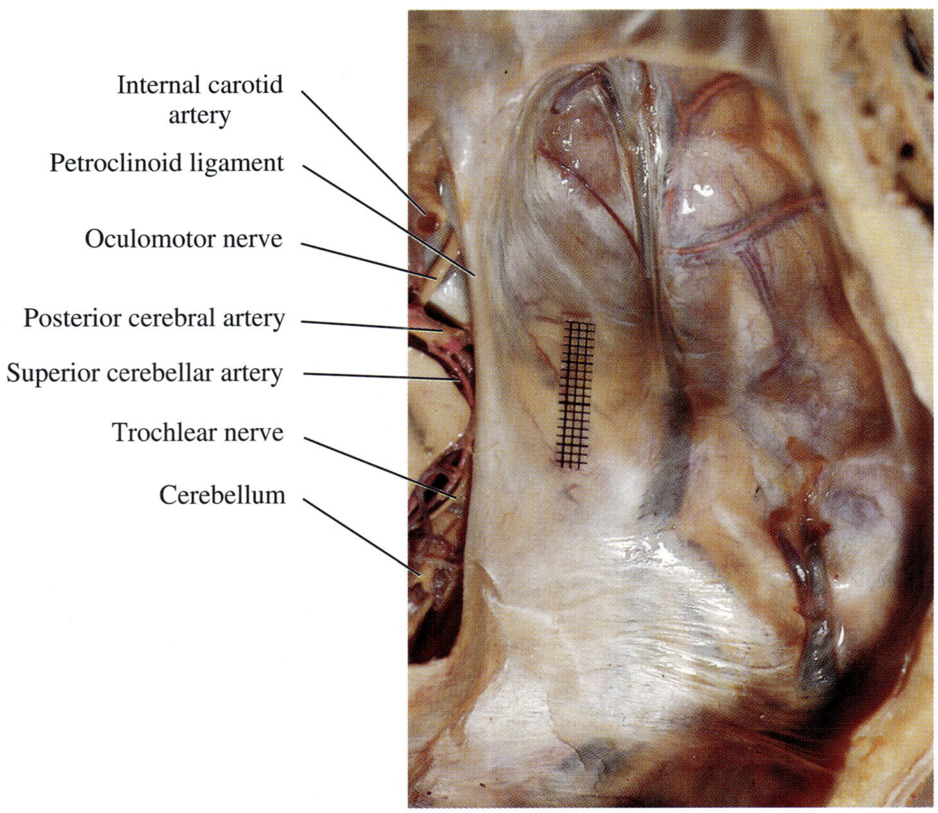

Figure 5. Cadaver dissection showing the middle fossa floor and tentorial notch.

Lateral Approach to the Middle Skull Base 11

(Temporal-Infratemporal Fossa, Carotid Artery, and Jugular Foramen)

ANATOMICAL CONSIDERATIONS

Three lateral approaches to the middle skull base have been described by Fisch and are designated as Types A, B, and C. These are approaches to the temporal-infratemporal fossa as well as to the region of the carotid artery in the petrous bone and the jugular foramen. For those pathological entities that may require surgery in these areas, we distinguish between (A) the lateral approach to the temporal-infratemporal fossa and (B) the lateral approach to the petrous bone and jugular foramen. In an extensive tumor extension, both regions are dissected together.

The anatomy of the petrous bone and the middle fossa skull base and specifically of the region of the jugular foramen is especially complex. Figure 1 shows the anatomical relations that are important in approaching tumors that involve the jugular foramen and the carotid canal. The tip of the mastoid process (see Figure 1) is used as the key point of orientation. Extending anteroinferiorly from this point is the sternocleidomastoid muscle. Deep to it, the posterior belly of the digastric muscle identified as the sternocleidomastoid muscle is retracted posteriorly. Emerging from under the posterior belly of the digastric muscle are the external carotid artery and the internal jugular vein. Between these two major vascular structures, cranial nerves IX, X, XI, and XII can be seen as they exit their skull base foramina (see Figure 1).

Figure 2 shows the deeper anatomical plane at the level of the jugular bulb with a partial mastoidectomy having been done and with the sigmoid sinus exposed. The facial nerve (CN VII) is shown transposed anteriorly. The parotid gland is also slightly retracted anteriorly.

In Figure 3, further mastoid drilling is in evidence with the internal carotid artery exposed as it enters the carotid canal. Relations of the lower cranial nerves and the posterior fossa dura to the jugular foramen are shown.

Figure 4 demonstrates the anatomical features of the middle skull base with the detachment of the zygoma and with reflection of the temporal muscle. The more complex deep anatomy of the region of the temporomandibular joint is shown in Figure 5 with exposure of the glenoid fossa. Medially, V3 can be identified as it exits the foramen ovale, with the middle meningeal artery just posterior as it passes into the foramen spinosum. The anatomical relations between the internal carotid artery and the jugular bulb–sigmoid sinus can be seen. The facial nerve is shown dissected free and transposed anteriorly.

In Figure 6, the pterygoid process is shown detached along with a section of V3 and the middle meningeal artery to expose the vomer and clivus. The dissection has now reached the lateral extent of the pharynx.

Even further anterior dissection of the middle skull base exposes V2 as it exits the foramen rotundum, the maxillary artery, and the sphenoid and maxillary sinuses (Figure 7). The orbit is also shown, having been opened. In Figure 8, the nasal cavity has been exposed and the lateral nasopharynx has been opened. The periorbita has been extensively exposed as well.

INDICATIONS

Approach to the Temporal-Infratemporal Fossa

The infratemporal fossa is unique in terms of skull base tumors because of the wide extent available for tumor growth and expansion. Tumors that arise primarily in the infratemporal fossa can easily spread anteriorly to the pterygoid fossa, the parasellar area, the inferior orbital fissure, and, eventually, the maxillary sinus and the pharynx. Posteriorly, these tumors may extend to the petrous apex as well as to the internal carotid artery, jugular bulb, and jugular vein. Medially, tumors may extend to the clivus.

These infratemporal fossa tumors may also extend intracranially to involve the temporal lobe, tentorial incisura, brain stem, and cranial nerves as they exit the brain stem. Tumors that are primarily clival, jugular foramen, or parasellar or located in the pterygopalatine fossa and pharynx are removed by appropriate other approaches to the cranial base as described in this atlas.

Approach to the Carotid Artery and Jugular Foramen

The indications for approach to the posterior middle skull base, particularly to the region of the jugular foramen and carotid canal, are rare. When they do occur, they require special knowledge of the anatomy and understanding of the clinical aspects of the petrous bone. Operative procedures for excision of tumors in this complex and difficult location usually are combined efforts by the neurosurgical and head and neck surgical teams.

In our experience, the most common tumors that are encountered in the region of the jugular foramen are meningiomas, neurinomas, and paragangliomas. Less commonly, clivus chordomas, epidermoids, and skull base carcinomas are seen in this area.

POSITION

The patient is placed in the supine position with the head sharply turned 70 degrees away from the side of the planned operation. The surgeon is seated at the head of the operating table, facing the patient's occiput, and the scrub nurse is directly opposite the surgeon.

The patient's abdomen and thigh are prepared sterilely and draped to allow harvest of abdominal fat pad grafts and fascia lata for use in cranial base reconstruction later. Hair is shaved from the side of the head, and the scalp, ear, posterior face, and neck are prepared sterilely and draped.

INCISION

For the approach to the temporal-infratemporal fossa (the anterior approach), a reverse question mark skin incision is made. The incision is started at the midpupillary line and extended posteriorly and then curved inferiorly to a point 1 cm anterior to the tragus. The incision is then curved along the inferior aspect of the earlobe to end along the midportion of the anterior margin of the sternocleidomastoid muscle (Figure 9, incision A).

The scalp flap is reflected in the subgaleal space in the usual manner and retracted anteriorly. The temporalis muscle is left attached unless it is involved by tumor and must be excised. The zygomatic arch is sectioned anteriorly and posteriorly and then its midportion is deflected downward with its masseter muscle attachment, which has been released from the ramus of the mandible.

A mandibulotomy is done by temporary displacement of the condyle. If more extensive exposure is needed, the vertical ramus of the mandible is partially removed.

The lateral approach to the middle fossa skull base depends on extradural access. The dura of the middle cranial fossa becomes a primary landmark in maintaining orientation during removal of tumors in this area. By following any exposed dura medially, the central skull base can be reached.

Subcutaneous dissection is continued inferiorly with care exercised to avoid injury to the facial nerve. The main trunk of the facial nerve and its superior branches are then exposed and traced peripherally through the parotid gland.

If more extensive posterior exposure of the infratemporal fossa is needed, a second incision (see Figure 9, incision B) is made. This retroauricular incision extends from a point behind the ear downward, curving anteriorly below the earlobe to join the previous incision along the mid-anterior border of the sternocleidomastoid muscle.

During subcutaneous dissection, efforts are made to spare the greater auricular nerve. The anterior margin of the sternocleidomastoid muscle is identified and followed to its insertion at the mastoid tip. The inferior aspect of the parotid gland and the posterior belly of the digastric muscle are exposed. The facial nerve is identified as it exits the stylomastoid foramen.

Before visualizing the tumor, it is important to expose the internal jugular vein, internal carotid artery, and cranial nerves IX, X, XI, and XII. Mastoidectomy is now completed, the digastric muscle is displaced anteriorly and inferiorly, and the sternocleidomastoid muscle is retracted posteriorly. The external auditory canal can be transected at the level of the bony cartilage junction and a blind sac closure done.

At this point, tumors that are located primarily within the infralabyrinthine space can be effectively exposed. For tumors that extend more medially with anterior extension to involve the clivus and the petrous portion of the carotid artery, it may be necessary to extend the infratemporal fossa approach posteromedially. This may be necessary in tumors such as chordoma and sarcoma of the clivus as well as in dermoid and epidermoid tumors that are in the petroclival area and extend to the temporal bone to involve the intrapetrous portion of the carotid artery and the region of the jugular bulb and foramen.

APPROACH TO THE CAROTID ARTERY AND THE JUGULAR BULB

To approach the petrous portion of the carotid artery and the jugular foramen, the retroauricular incision shown in Figure 9B is used. The greater auricular nerve is kept intact, if possible, for later use as a graft in case of injury to the spinal accessory nerve. After subcutaneous dissection, the sternocleidomastoid muscle is separated from its attachment to the mastoid process and the posterior belly of the digastric muscle is detached from the digastric groove. Cranial nerves IX, X, XI, and XII are identified (see Figure 3) between the internal jugular vein and the carotid artery. The dissection follows these structures to the jugular foramen and the carotid canal at the skull base. Figure 10 shows the relationship of these vessels as demonstrated in a cadaver dissection.

The facial nerve is carefully identified as it exits the stylomastoid foramen in the tympanomastoidal fissure above and anterior to the digastric muscle.

Further temporal bone drilling is carried to the fallopian canal inferior to the labyrinth and cochlea to allow preservation of hearing and vestibular function. The lateral semicircular canal and facial canal are opened if necessary. The facial nerve can be completely mobilized and transposed anteriorly. In cases of neurinomas and other processes that do not involve the fallopian canal, the facial nerve is left within the canal.

In those cases of extensive pathologies that require a subtotal or total petrosectomy, the bony external auditory canal, tympanic membrane, malleus, incus, and stapes arch are removed.

If the tumor extends intracranially into the posterior fossa, a lateral suboccipital craniectomy is performed and the transverse and sigmoid sinuses are exposed. The jugular bulb and sigmoid sinus are mobilized to their exit through the jugular foramen.

The shining agamous of the mandibula is distracted anteriorly, and the carotid artery is identified as it enters the petrous bone. A key landmark in the identification of the carotid artery within the temporal bone is the eustachian tube. By carefully drilling open the medial wall of the eustachian tube, the lateral wall of the carotid canal can be found. Once located, the internal carotid artery can be exposed throughout its infratemporal course and into the region of the cavernous sinus. The jugular vein as it exits the jugular bulb, along with the lower cranial nerves, is identified and protected.

At this stage of the dissection, the tumor usually is evident. If the tumor extends more medially, the jugular vein and the sigmoid sinus can be ligated using silk sutures after anterior and posterior incision of the dura, provided that preoperative angiography has demonstrated satisfactory venous drainage contralaterally. After ligation of the jugular vein, the jugular bulb can be excised to expose cranial nerves IX, X, and XI and to allow dissection of tumor away from them.

In cases of extensive giant tumors that reach the tentorial notch and supratentorial space, the dura is opened anterior to the sigmoid sinus and the tentorium cerebelli can be transected above the transverse sinus.

If the jugular bulb and sigmoid sinus are not infiltrated by the tumor, they can now be mobilized and gently retracted along with the transverse sinus and the cerebellar hemisphere posteriorly to expose the cerebellopontine angle and the region of the tentorial notch. The important anatomical relationships of the cranial nerves in this area are demonstrated in Figure 11A and B. After the cerebellopontine angle cistern is opened to allow drainage of cerebrospinal fluid, the tumor usually is well exposed and excision can begin.

While keeping the lower cranial nerves in constant view, the extracranial portion of the tumor is removed piecemeal under the operating microscope with high magnification. After removal of the extracranial tumor mass and intracapsular decompression, the remaining tumor is dissected from the jugular foramen while maintaining the integrity of cranial nerves IX, X, XI, and XII.

Chemodectomas arise from cells in the adventitia of the jugular bulb and extend into the lumen of the sigmoid sinus and downward into the internal jugular vein. In these cases, the sigmoid sinus must be ligated superiorly and the internal jugular vein inferiorly below the tumor and the mass excised en bloc.

Meningiomas, neurinomas, and other tumors at the jugular foramen are dissected free from the jugular bulb and sinus, and this vascular channel is left intact if possible.

An example of a tumor that can be removed through this lateral approach to the middle and posterior skull base, and specifically the region of the jugular foramen and cerebellopontine angle, is shown in Figures 12 through 16. This is the case of a neurinoma of the jugular foramen.

In Figure 12, a bone defect caused by this tumor is demonstrated by a computed tomographic bone window. The large jugular foramen neurinoma is further demonstrated in the computed tomographic image shown in Figure 13. Figure 14 shows photographs of magnetic resonance imaging scans that demonstrate the location of the large neurinoma in relation to the cerebellopontine angle and the internal carotid artery.

The exposure of the caudal cranial nerves, including the facial nerve, is shown in the operative photograph in Figure 15. This figure also shows the lateral suboccipital craniectomy as well as the partial mastoidectomy. Figure 16 shows the tumor bed after tumor removal.

CLOSURE

It is important to achieve meticulous hemostasis before closure in dealing with these often highly vascular tumors. In the case of jugular foramen exposure and displacement of the jugular bulb along with the sigmoid sinus, these structures are returned to their normal anatomical position and the dura is approximated at several strategic points with interrupted sutures of 4–0 nylon. Watertight closure of the dura with a running suture of 4–0 nylon is then completed. If necessary, a graft of lyophilized dura or fascia lata is used.

In reconstruction of the posterior exposure, the mastoid air cells and mastoid antrum as well as the eustachian tube when open are covered with a portion of the digastric muscle and sealed with fibrin glue. The sternocleidomastoid muscle is reattached to soft tissues in its normal anatomical position to complete the reconstruction.

A careful subcutaneous tissue and galeal closure is done using 0 Vicryl followed by skin closure using monofilament 3-0 nylon sutures or staples.

In the anterior temporal-infratemporal fossa approach, if the dura has been opened, it requires a watertight dural closure. If necessary, a dural defect is reconstructed with a graft of lyophilized dura or fascia lata (Figure 17). The method of choice for additional repair in this area is a vascularized, pedicled temporalis muscle or temporalis fascia graft.

The zygomatic arch is wired back in anatomical position to help maintain the original facial contour.

A careful subcutaneous and galeal closure is done using 0 Vicryl followed by skin closure using monofilament nylon or staples.

Postoperative lumbar drainage is maintained for 5 days, and intraoperative antibiotic coverage is continued for 10 days.

RECOMMENDED READING

Fisch, U.: Infratemporal fossa approach for glioma tumors of the temporal bone. Ann. Otol. Rhinol. Laryngol. 91:474–479, 1982.

Fisch, U.: The infratemporal fossa approach for nasopharyngeal tumors. Laryngoscope 93:36–44, 1983.

Fisch, U., Fagan, P., Valavanis, A.: The infratemporal fossa approach for the lateral skull base. Otolaryngol. Clin. North Am. 17:513–552, 1984.

Fisch, U, Mattox, D.: Microsurgery of the Skull Base. New York: Thieme Medical Publishers, 1988.

Fisch, U., Pillsbury, H.C.: Infratemporal fossa approach to lesions in the temporal bone and base of the skull. Arch. Otolaryngol. 105:98–107, 1979.

Gardner, G., Cocke, E., Robertson, J., et al.: Combined approach surgery for removal of glomus jugular tumors. Laryngoscope 87:665–688, 1977.

Kempe, L.: Glomus jugular tumors. *In:* Youmans, J. R. ed.: Textbook of Neurological Surgery, vol. 5. Philadelphia: W.B. Saunders Co., 1990, pp. 3285–3298.

Samii, M., Bini, W.: Surgical Strategy for Jugular Foramen Tumors. Surgery of Cranial Base Tumors. New York: Raven Press, 1993.

Samii, M., Draf, W.: Surgery of the Skull Base: An Interdisciplinary Approach. Berlin: Springer-Verlag, 1989.

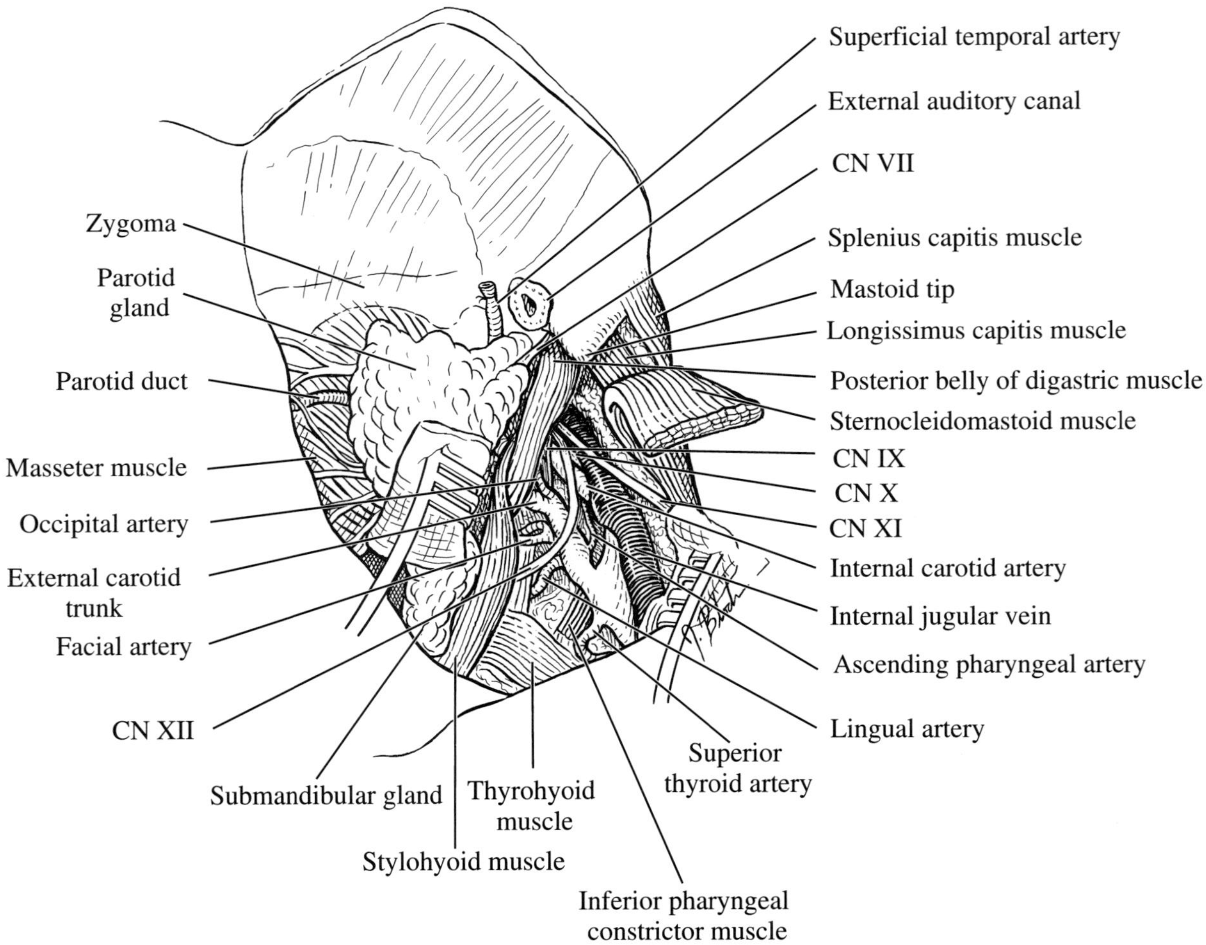

Figure 1. Carotid artery and jugular vein with cranial nerves IX, X, XI, and XII.

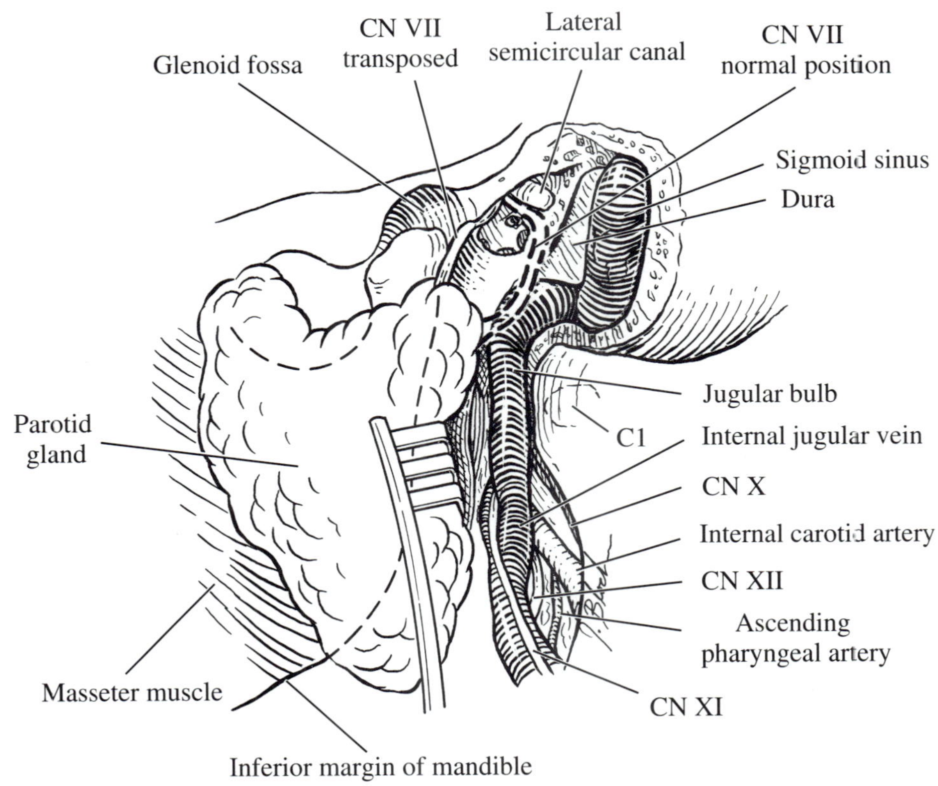

Figure 2. Deeper anatomical plane showing jugular bulb and partial petrosectomy.

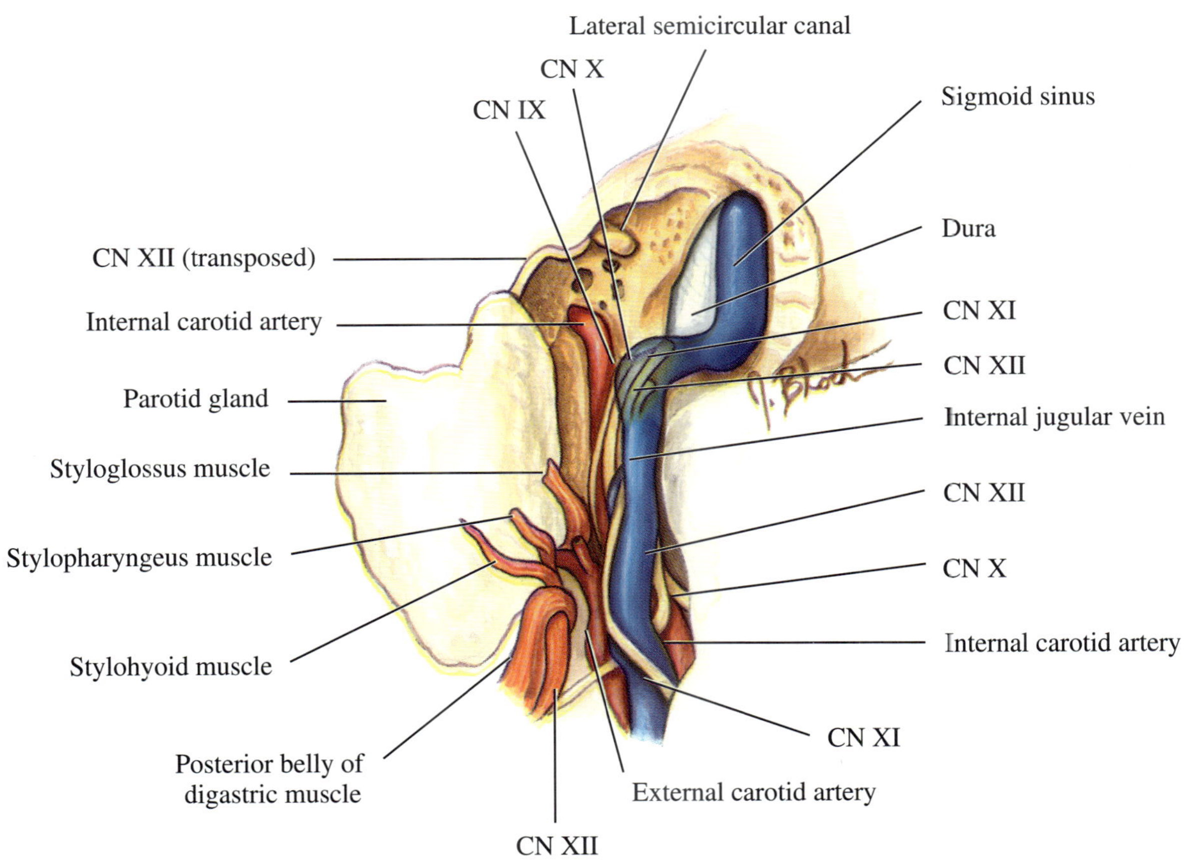

Figure 3. Carotid artery shown exposed in carotid canal after further mastoid drilling.

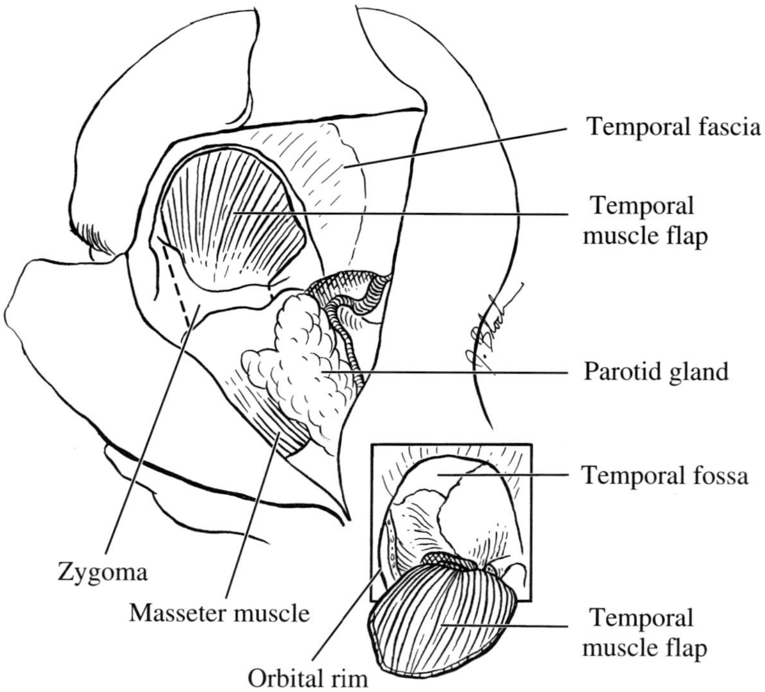

Figure 4. Detachment of the zygoma with reflection of the temporal muscle.

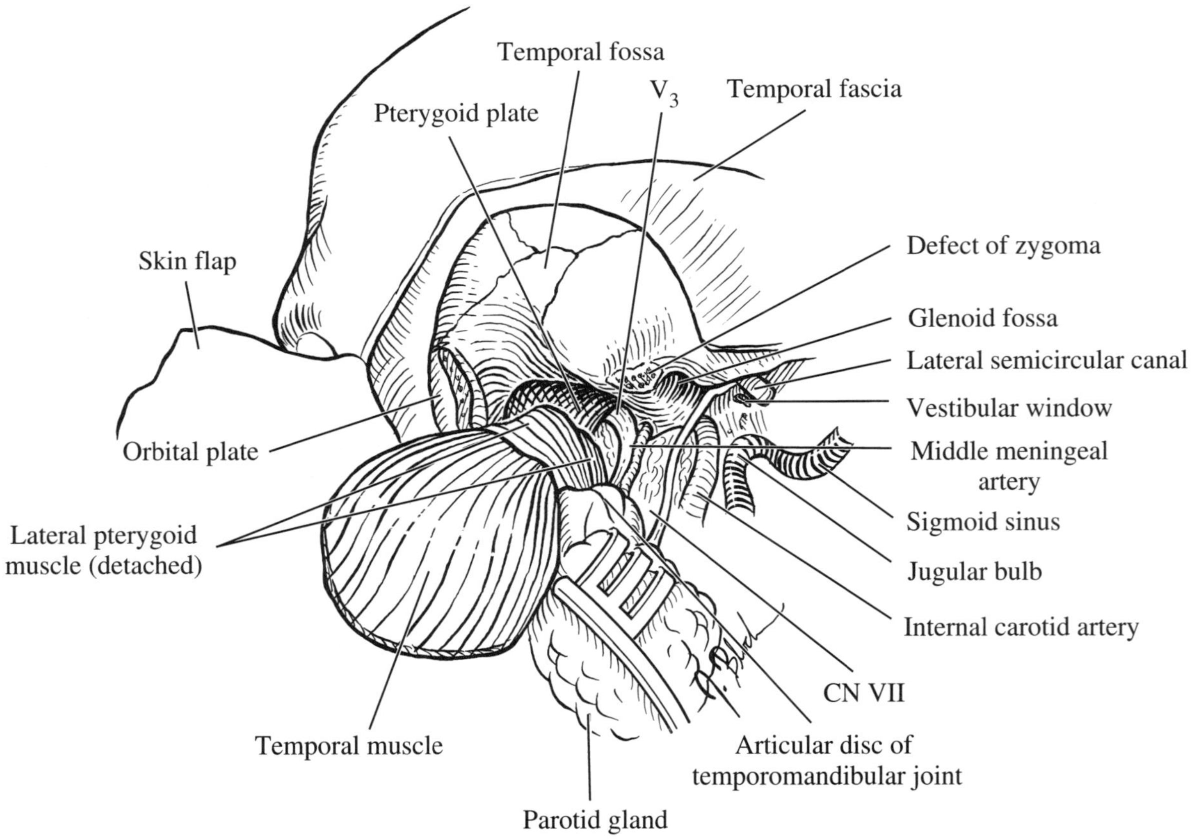

Figure 5. Deep anatomy of the region of the temporomandibular joint with exposure of the glenoid fossa.

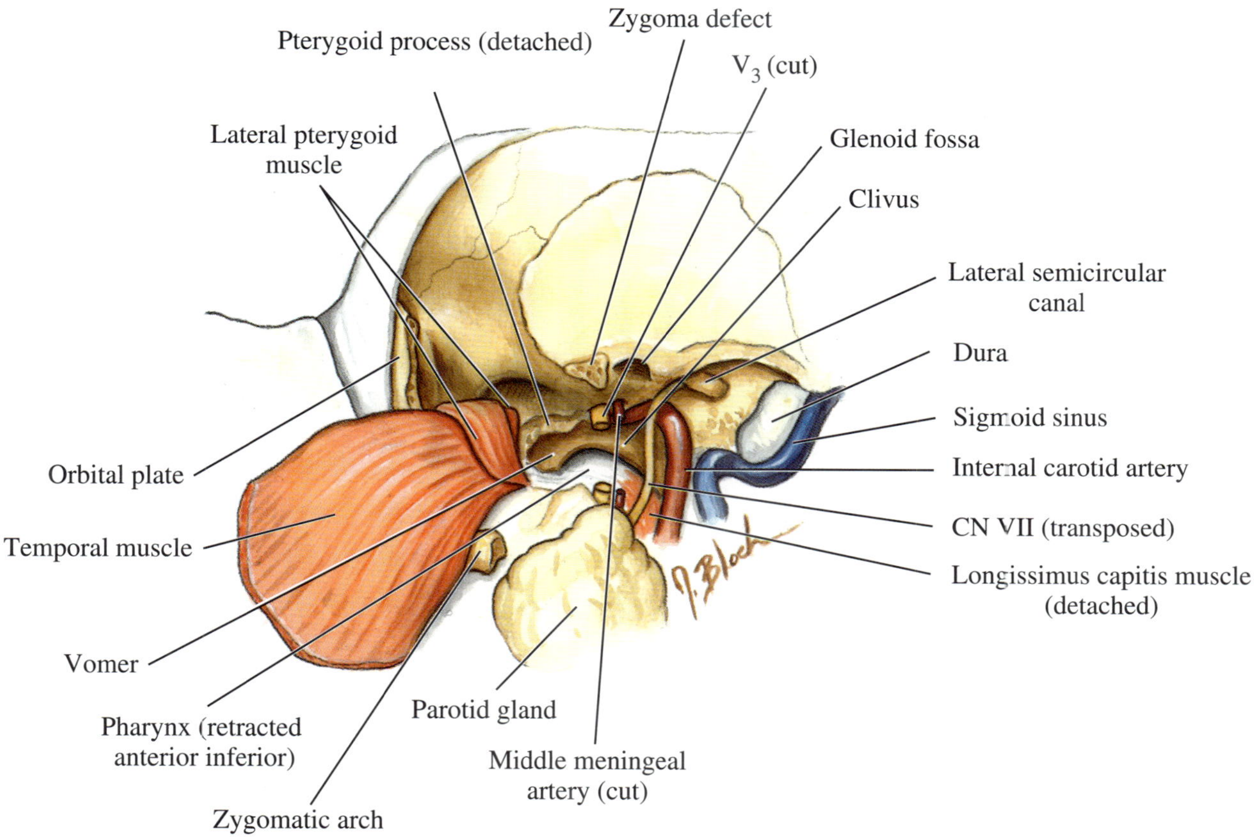

Figure 6. **Exposure of the pterygoid process shown detached along with section of V3 and the middle meningeal artery to expose the vomer and clivus.**

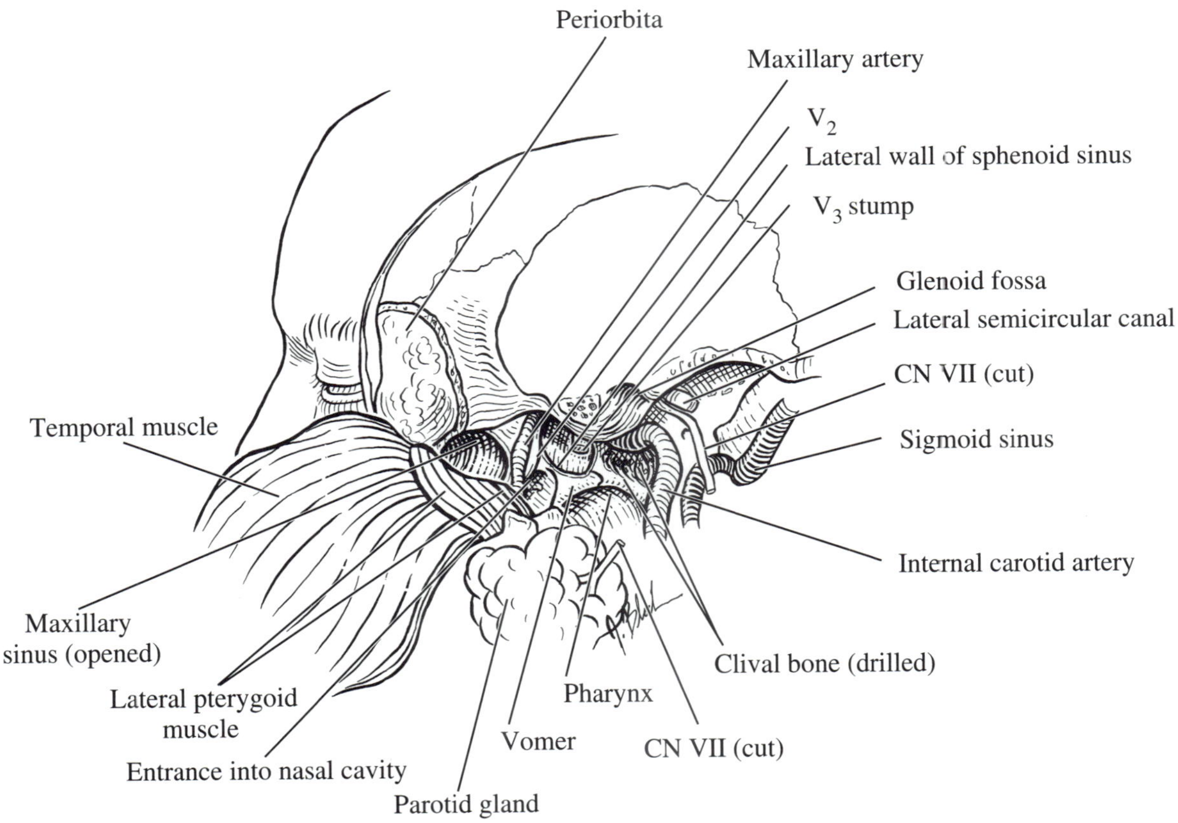

Figure 7. **Anterior dissection of the middle skull base to expose V2. Sphenoid and maxillary sinuses are shown open.**

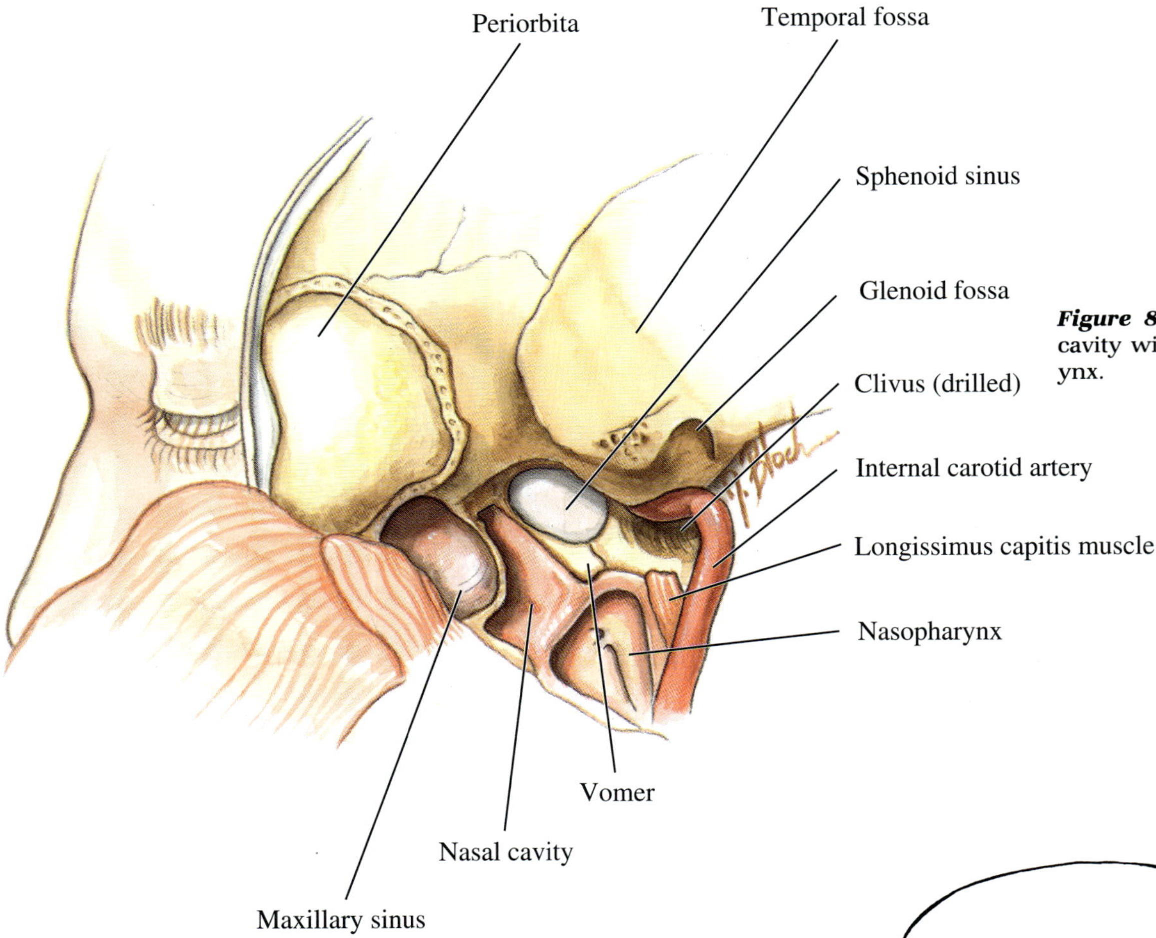

Figure 8. Exposure of the nasal cavity with open lateral nasopharynx.

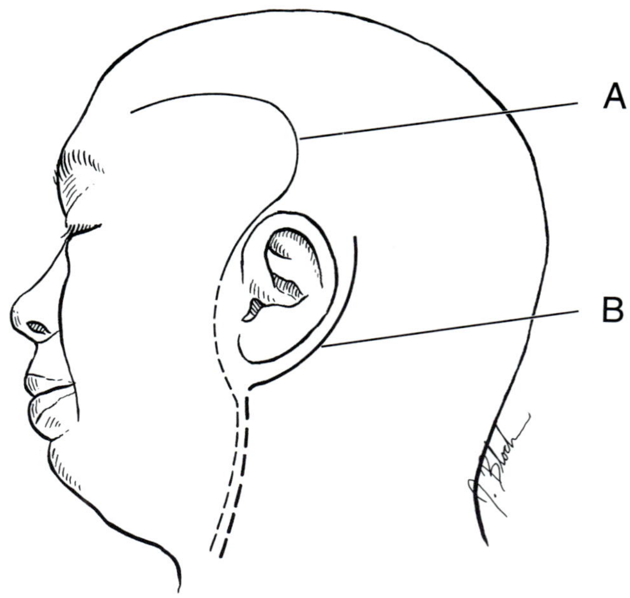

Figure 9. Incision A. Approach to temporal-infratemporal fossa. Incision B. More extensive approach to temporal-infratemporal fossa.

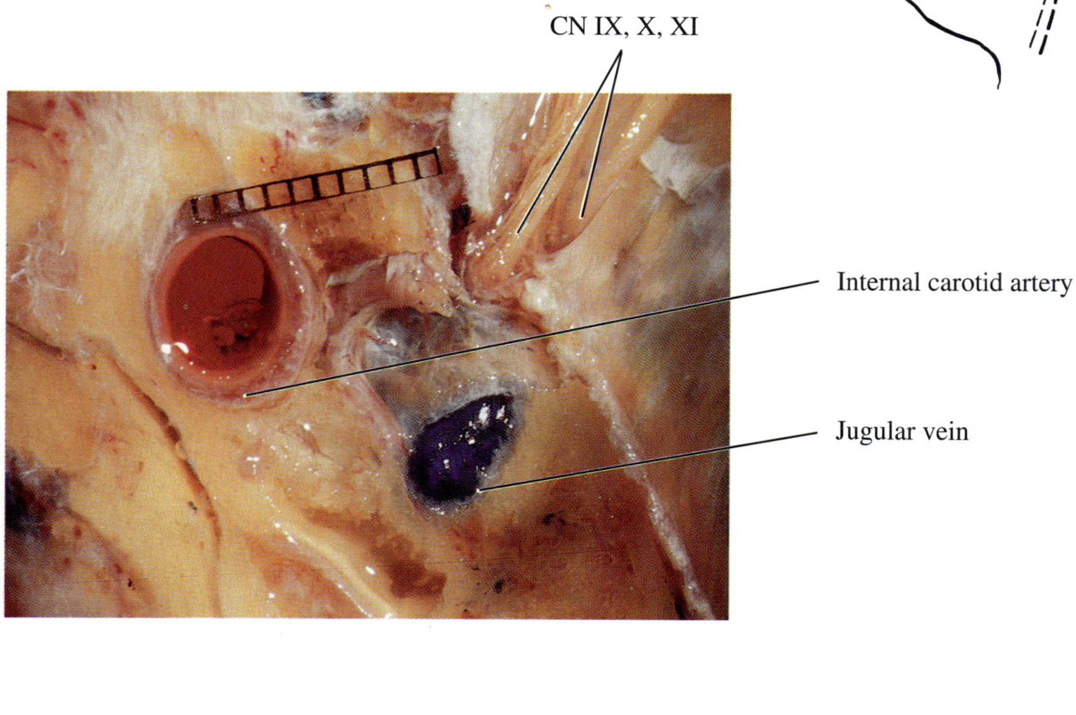

Figure 10. Cadaver dissection showing relation of the carotid artery to the jugular bulb at the skull base.

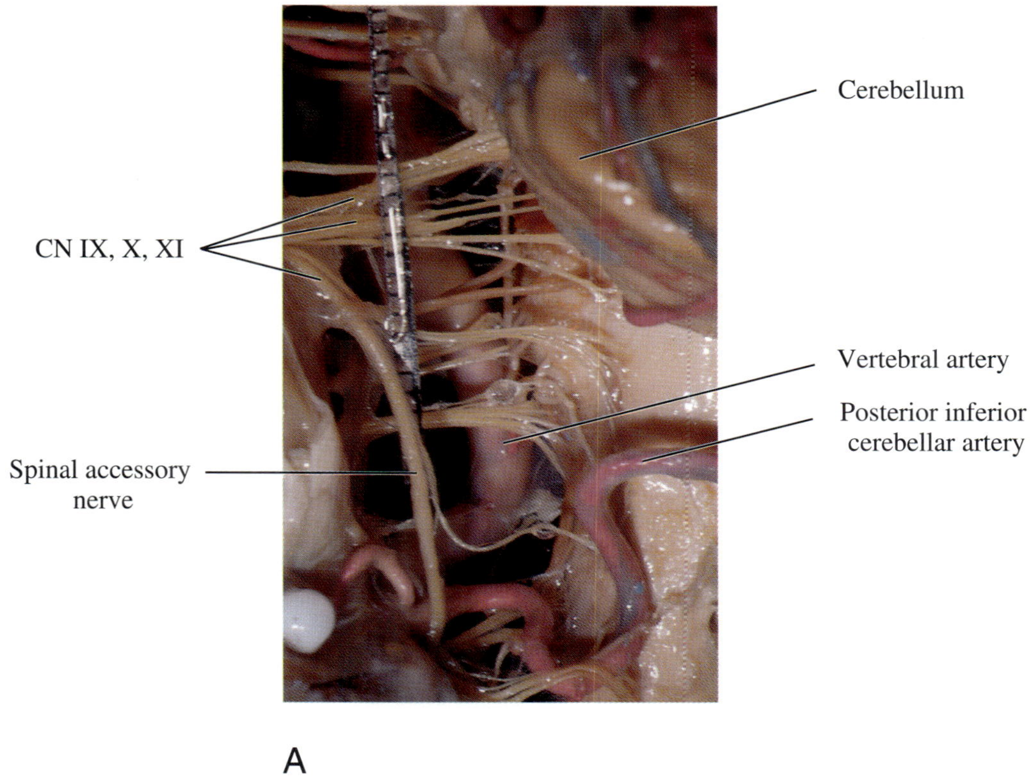

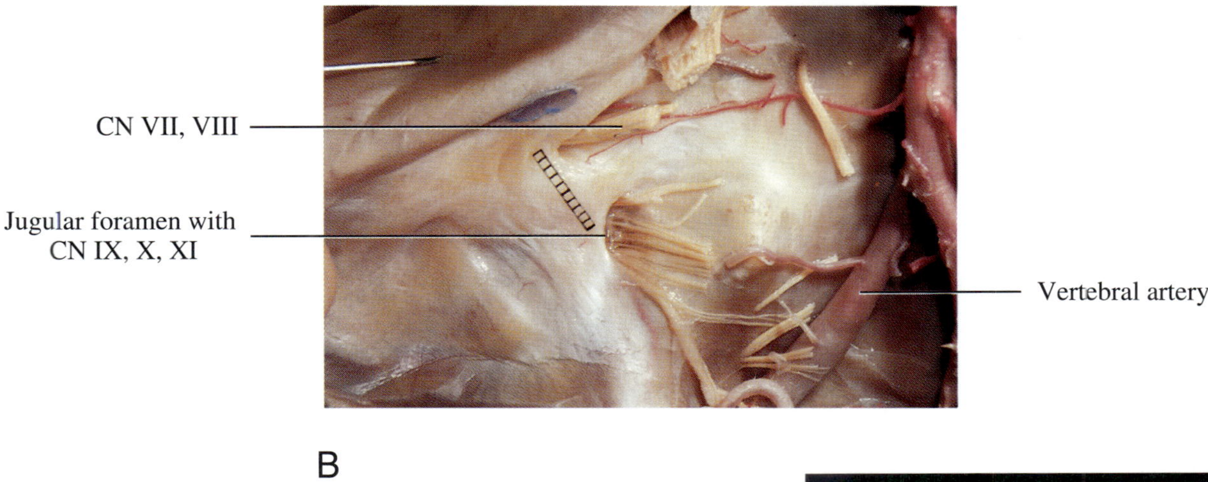

Figure 11. *A.* Anatomical relations in the cerebellopontine angle. *B.* Cranial nerves V, VI, VII, and VIII and the vertebral artery in relation to the jugular foramen and cranial nerves IX, X, and XI.

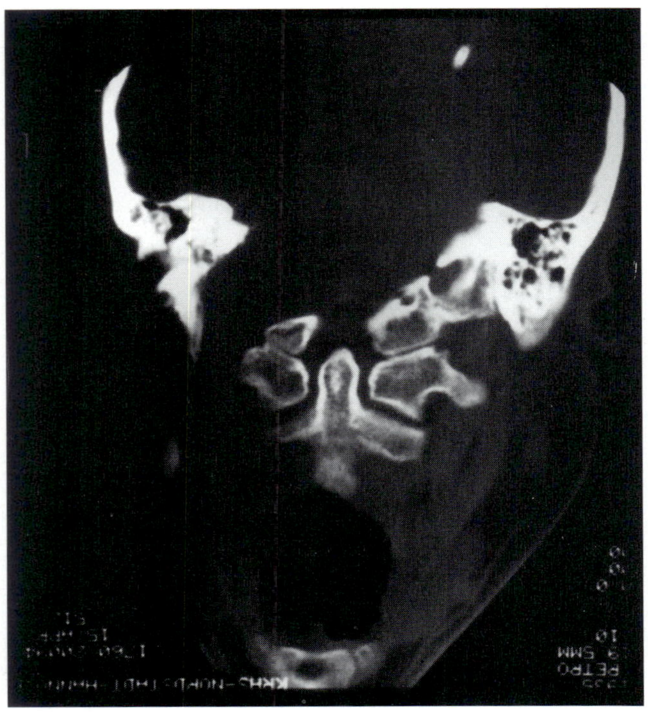

Figure 12. Computed tomographic bone window showing bone defect.

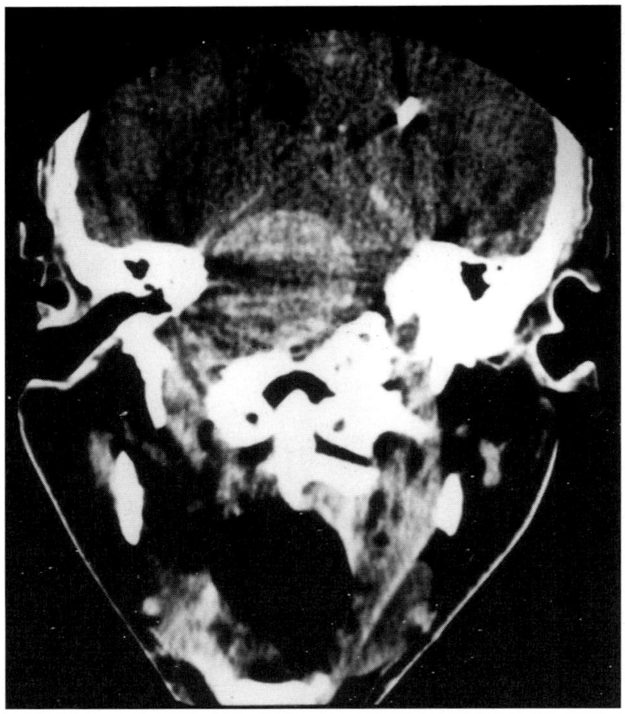

Figure 13. Computed tomographic image showing large jugular foramen neurinoma.

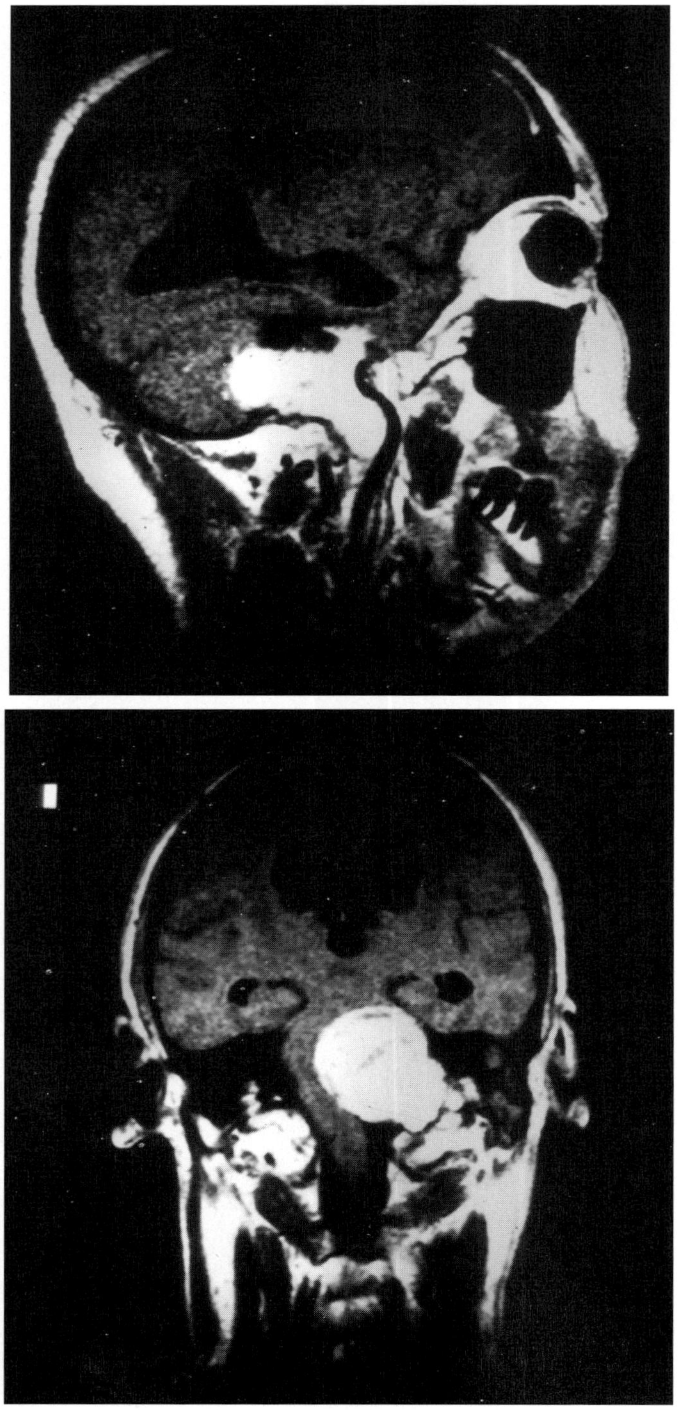

Figure 14. Magnetic resonance imaging scan images showing location of large neurinoma in relation to cerebellopontine angle and internal carotid artery.

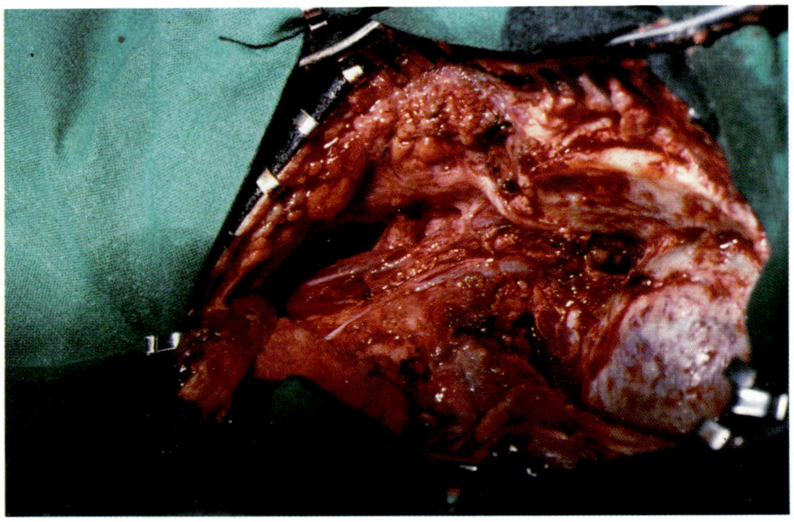

Figure 15. Operative photograph showing exposure of caudal cranial nerves.

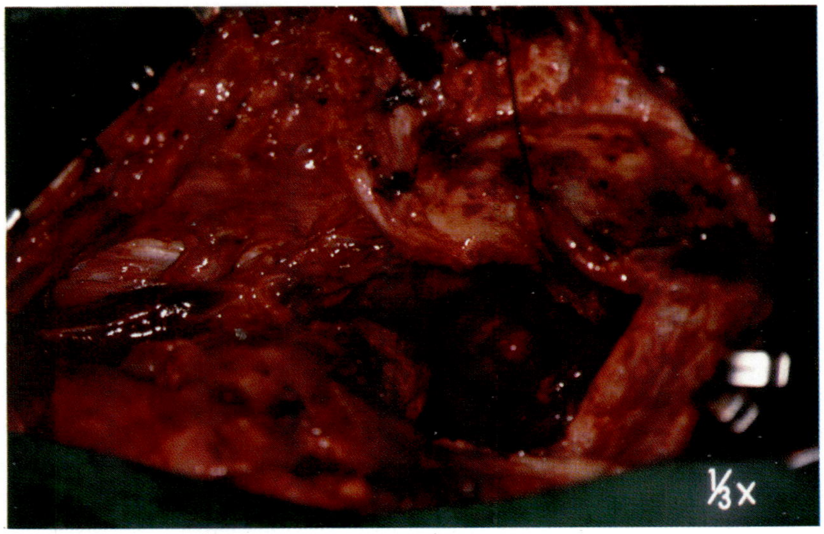

Figure 16. Operative photograph of tumor bed after tumor removal.

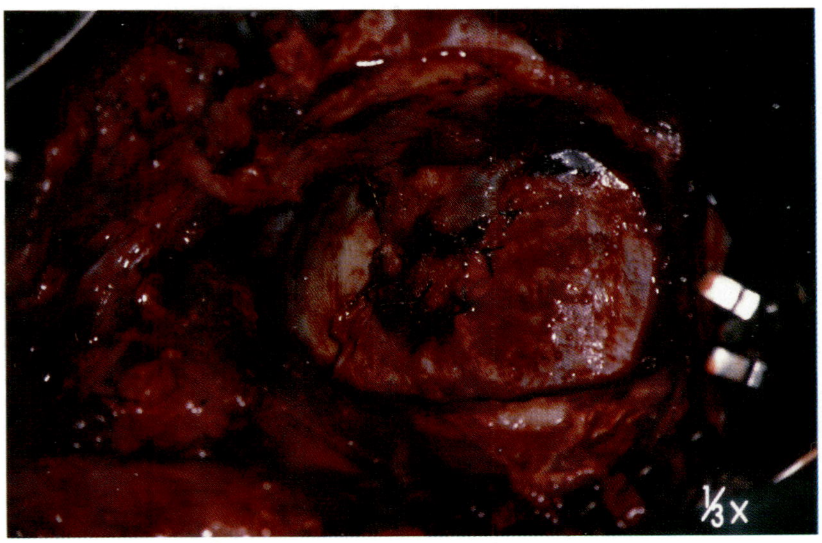

Figure 17. Closure of dural defect with lyophilized dura graft.

12 Lateral Approach to the Craniocervical Junction

INDICATIONS

The lateral approach to the craniocervical junction is used for tumors that involve the anterior or lateral aspect of the foramen magnum, the middle and lower clivus, the jugular foramen, and the hypoglossal foramen. This approach also provides access to the occipital condyle and the lateral rim of the foramen magnum for bone-invading tumors. It is the standard approach for intracranial aneurysms that arise from the vertebral artery or the vertebrobasilar junction. Microsurgical endarterectomy of the intradural segment of the vertebral artery is also performed through this exposure.

An alternative approach to the region of the jugular foramen is the standard retromastoid suboccipital craniectomy as described in Chapter 4. This standard approach does not provide the wide exposure of the vertebral artery, foramen magnum, and clivus available through the lateral approach to the craniocervical junction.

POSITION

The patient may be placed in the semisitting position (Figure 1) or modified park bench position (Figure 2), depending on the surgeon's preference. The usual precautions are taken to avoid nerve or skin injury at pressure points and to maintain the head at a level slightly higher than the heart to prevent venous congestion and to promote cerebrospinal fluid drainage. Head position is maintained in a headholder in three-point fixation.

With the patient in the semisitting position, the head is turned 30 degrees toward the side of the lesion and gently flexed relative to the neck. In the modified park bench position, the head is rotated 15 degrees downward (away) from the side of the lesion and also flexed 15 degrees.

ANATOMICAL CONSIDERATIONS

Because the lateral approach to the craniocervical junction constitutes a caudal extension of the standard lateral suboccipital craniectomy, certain anatomical features in this area are defined. Figure 3 shows the superficial muscle layer in relation to the placement of the skin incision. The sternocleidomastoid, splenius capitis, and trapezius muscles are demonstrated.

Figure 4 shows the relationship of the muscles to the greater and lesser occipital nerves, greater auricular nerve, and transverse cervical nerve as well as the external branch of the accessory nerve.

In Figure 5, the deep anatomical structures at the craniocervical junction are shown. The greater occipital nerve is identified in relationship to the obliquus capitis superior, obliquus capitis inferior, and the rectus capitis posterior major muscles, which form a triangle traversed by the arch of C1 and the vertebral artery. With these muscles removed (Figure 6), the arch of C1 and the hemilamina of C2 are exposed and the upward course of the vertebral artery as it passes through the foramen transversarium is demonstrated. The vertebral artery is seen to penetrate the posterior atlanto-occipital membrane. The atlanto-occipital joint and the atlantoaxial joint are demonstrated as well.

Figure 7 shows the lateral suboccipital craniectomy with exposure of the sigmoid sinus laterally and with removal of the rim of the foramen magnum and hemilaminectomy of C1. Figure 8 shows the dura opened with the cerebellum slightly elevated and the intracranial portion of the caudal cranial nerves exposed. The vertebral artery, anterior inferior cerebellar artery, medulla, and the upper cervical cord are visible.

INCISION

The skin incision for the approach is similar to that used for the lateral suboccipital craniectomy but is extended caudally to the level of C2, exposing the arch of C1 and C2 on one side. Alternatively, a lazy-S incision or an inverted L or J incision may be used.

The muscles discussed in Figures 3 through 5 are transected and detached from the occipital bone, arch of C1, and hemilamina of C2. A self-retaining retractor is introduced to expose the deep muscles. This muscle layer, made up of the semispinalis, splenius capitis, and splenius cervicis muscles, is also incised and separated from bony attachments.

Laterally, the tip of the mastoid process and the transverse processes of C1 and C2 are palpated and exposed. The deep muscle layers are incised with care exercised to avoid entry into the vertebral artery. The C1-C2 joint is identified, and the vertebral artery is then exposed along the superior margin of the arch of C1. The posterior arch of C1, hemilamina of C2, and medial portion of the C1-C2 joint are removed. If needed, the C2 spinal nerve is transected close to its dural entry point. The venous plexus surrounding the vertebral artery can cause troublesome bleeding and is therefore coagulated with bipolar cautery.

CRANIOTOMY

While protecting the exposed vertebral artery, a suboccipital craniectomy is completed that extends as far laterally as the sigmoid sinus and includes removal of the lateral rim of the foramen magnum and the medial C1-C2 joint, if needed. The craniectomy is done as described for the lateral suboccipital (retrosigmoid) approach. It is then extended caudally with removal of the lateral rim of the foramen magnum. It is important to expose the margin of the sigmoid sinus and to follow it caudally to the posterior aspect of the jugular foramen. In most intradural processes at the craniocervical junction, there is no need to remove any part of the condyle or the C1-C2 joint. In cases in which additional exposure is needed, the posterior one-third of the atlanto-occipital condyle is drilled away.

DURAL OPENING

The dura is opened over the midportion of the posterior fossa. This dural opening is carried superiorly and laterally to the level of the transverse sinus and inferiorly, crossing the craniospinal junction and continuing laterally to the vertebral artery entrance zone and inferiorly to the level of C2. The lateral dural margin is then retracted maximally to afford exposure of the entire craniovertebral junction (see Figure 8). This excellent exposure is further demonstrated in the intraoperative photograph shown in Figure 9, which was done for the purpose of a vertebral artery endarterectomy.

A further example of a lesion that can be approached through the lateral approach to the craniocervical junction is the hemangioblastoma demonstrated in vertebral angiography images in Figure 10. The intraoperative exposure of this tumor is seen in Figures 11 and 12. Figure 13 shows the tumor bed after complete removal.

In Figure 14, a hypoglossal schwannoma is shown at the craniocervical junction, as exposed by the lateral approach. Figure 15 is a magnetic resonance imaging scan of a foramen magnum meningioma, and Figure 16 shows the tumor intraoperatively as seen through the lateral approach to the craniocervical junction.

CLOSURE

Before closure, the anesthesiologist is asked to give several jugular compressions to demonstrate unidentified venous bleeding. It is important to look for such bleeding points over the cerebellum as well because torn bridging veins may not be in evidence in the semisitting position.

Dural closure is completed using 4-0 nylon in a running locking stitch. The muscles are closed in layers with 0 Vicryl, and a good subcutaneous closure is completed followed by monofilament nylon or staples in the skin.

RECOMMENDED READING

George, B., Dematons, C., Cophigno, J.: Lateral approach to the anterior portion of the foramen magnum. Surg. Neurol. 29:484–490, 1988.

Heros, R.: Lateral suboccipital approach for vertebral and vertebrobasilar artery lesions. J. Neurosurg. 64:559–562, 1986.

Meyer, F., Ebersold, M., Reese, D.: Benign tumors of the foramen magnum. J. Neurosurg. 61:136–142, 1984.

Shucart, W., Kleriga, E.: Lateral approach to the upper cervical spine. Neurosurgery 6:278–281, 1980.

Spetzler, R., Grahm, T.: The far-lateral approach to the inferior clivus and the upper cervical region: Technical note. Barrow Neurological Institute Quarterly, Vol. 6, No. 4, 1990.

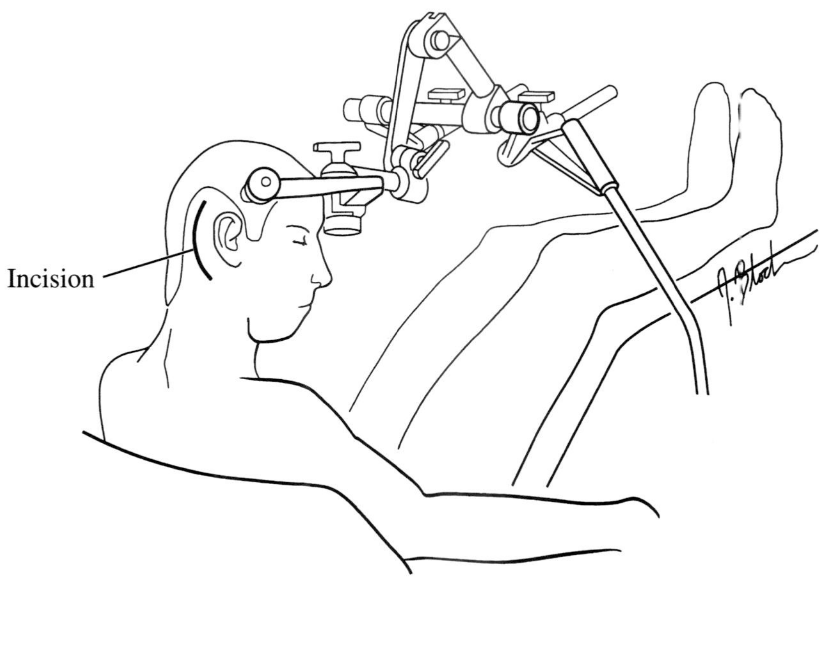

Figure 1. Semisitting position.

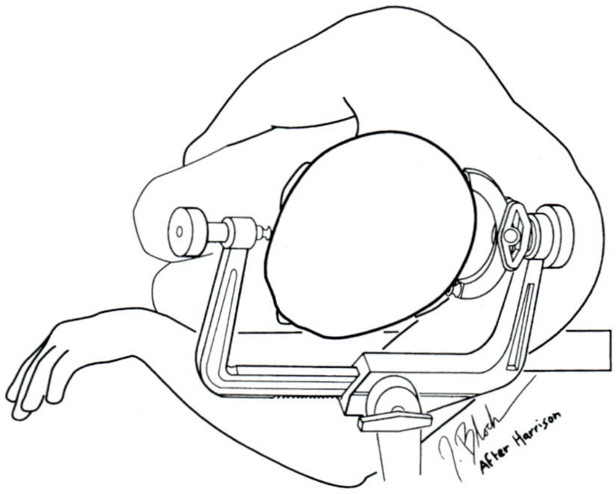

Figure 2. Modified park bench position.

Figure 3. Scalp incision for lateral approach, with demonstration of underlying muscle layers.

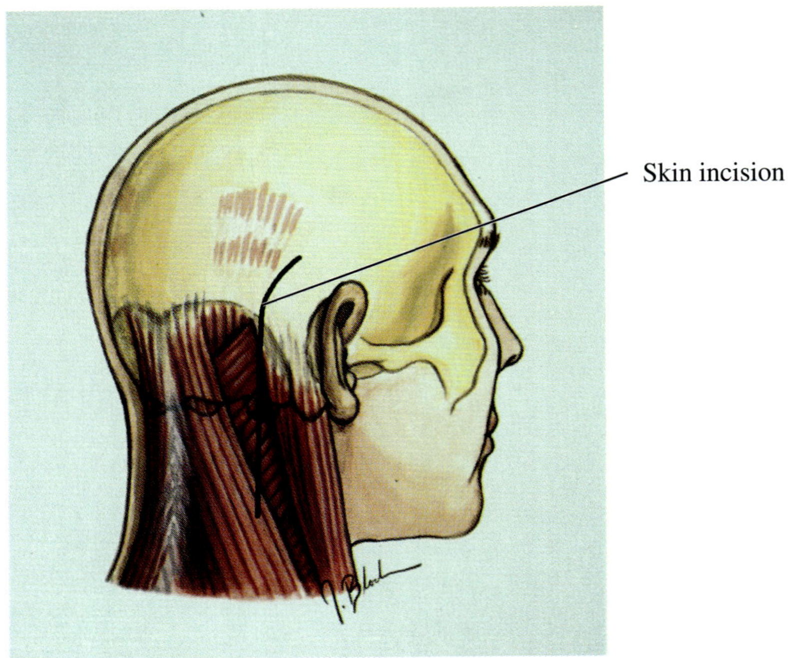

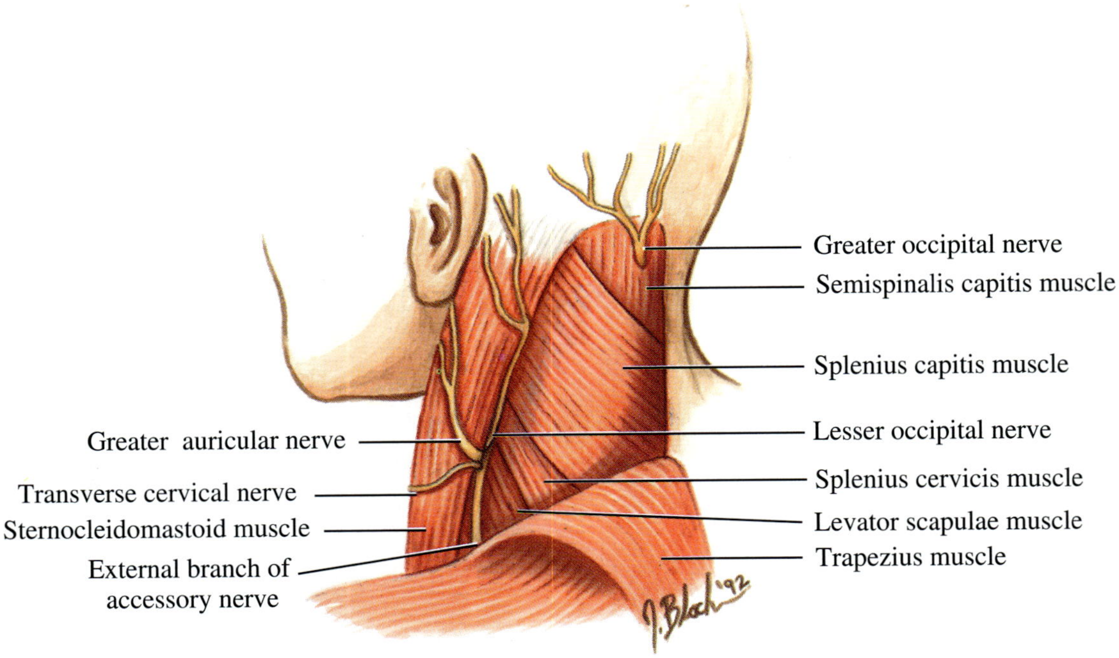

Figure 4. Deep cervical muscle layer with penetration of the semispinalis muscle by the greater occipital nerve.

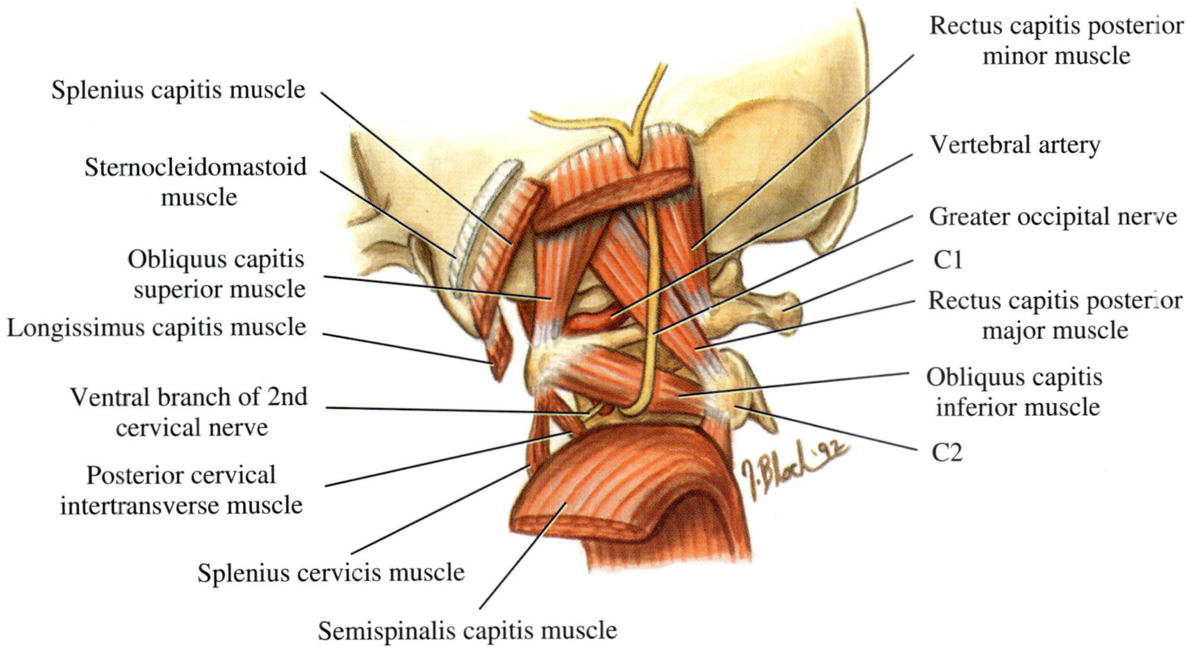

Figure 5. **Greater occipital nerve as it circles the inferior border of the obliquus capitis inferior muscle.**

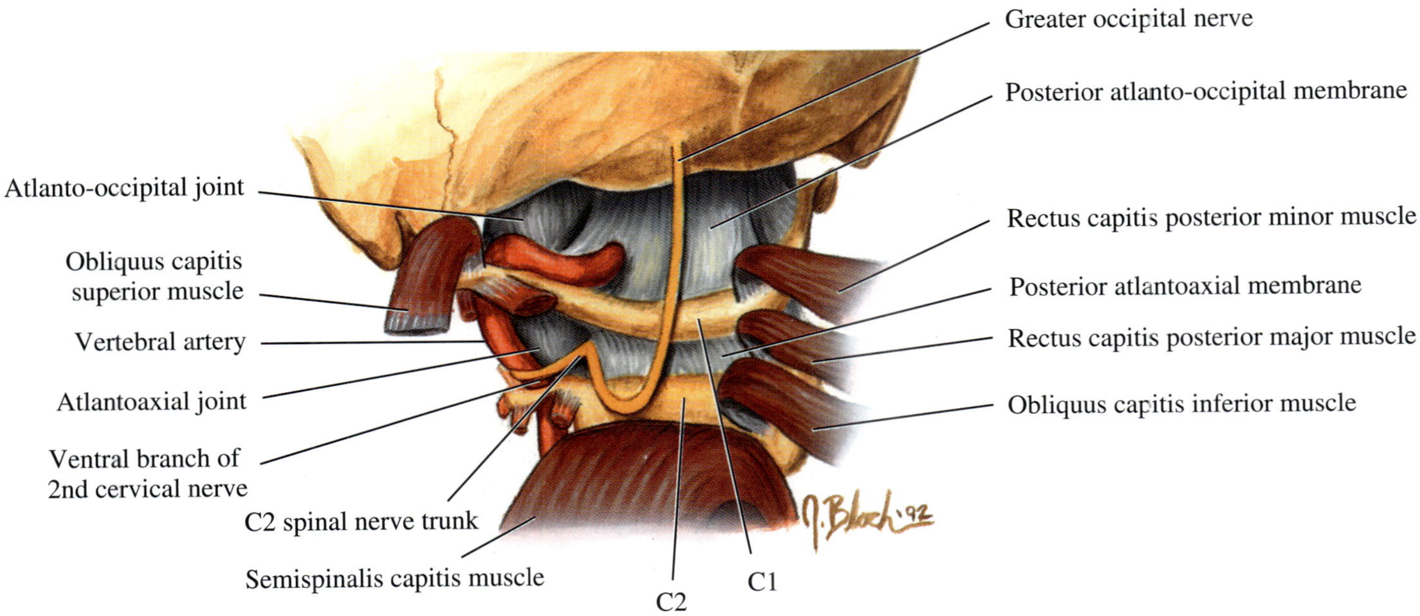

Figure 6. **Anterior branch of the C2 spinal nerve as it crosses the vertebral artery. Demonstration of the course of the vertebral artery at the craniocervical junction.**

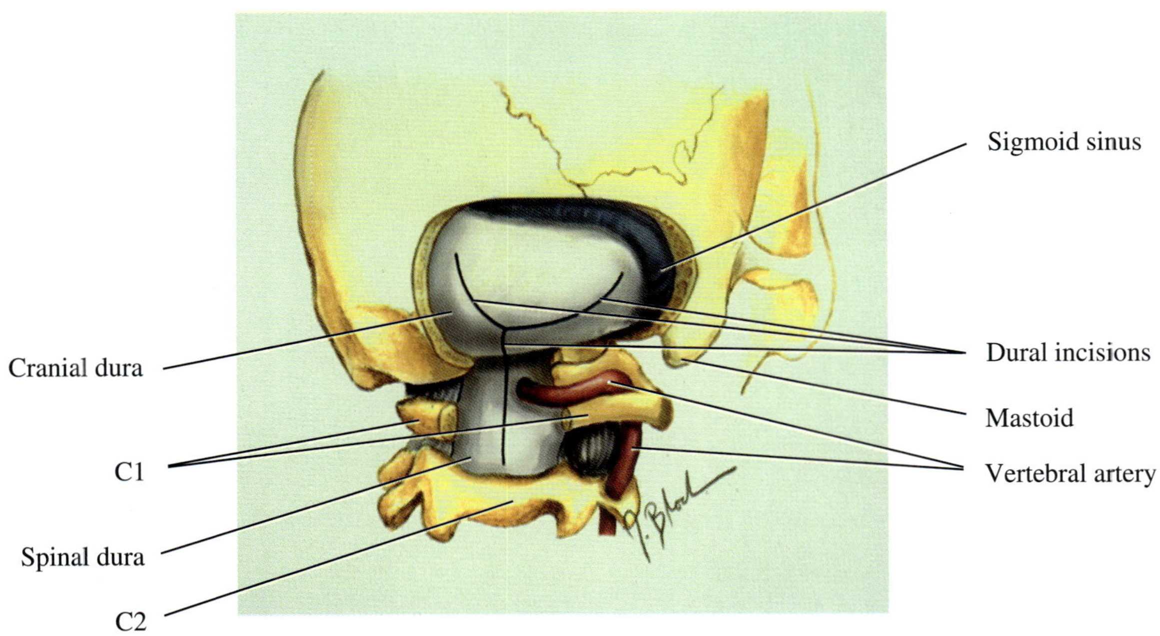

Figure 7. **Suboccipital craniectomy with removal of the lateral rim of the foramen magnum and medial C1-C2 joint.**

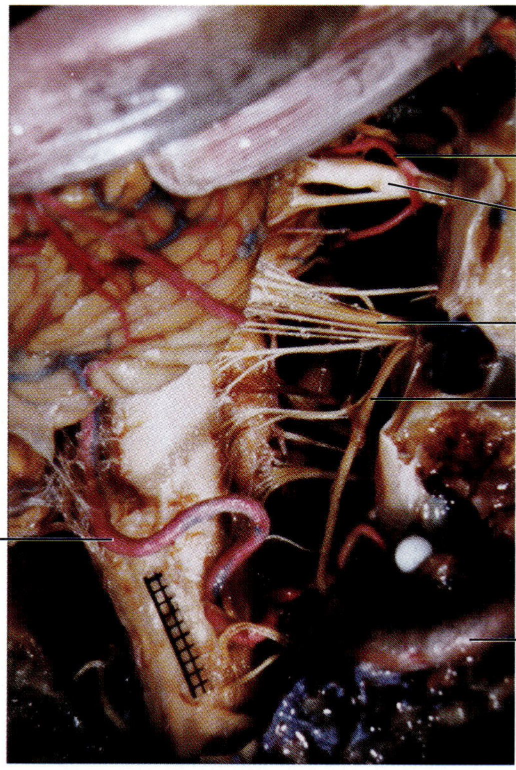

Figure 8. Cadaver dissection showing dura open with exposure of the entire craniocervical junction.

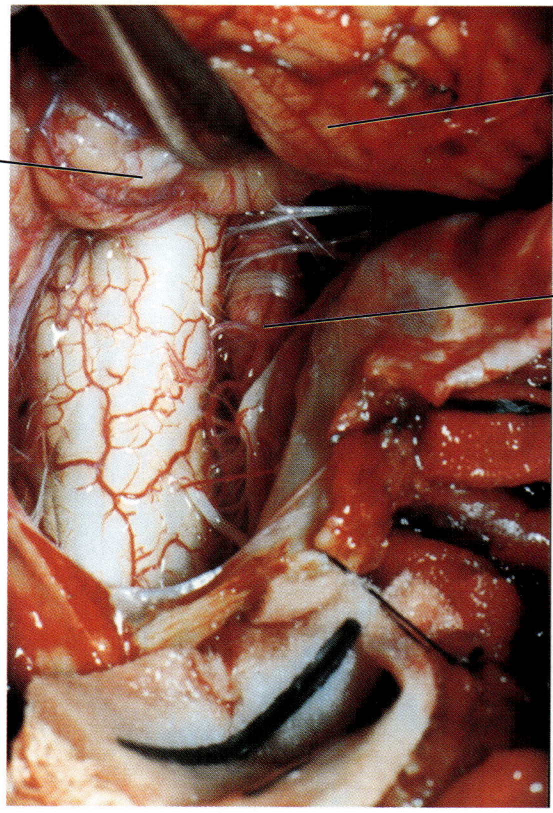

Figure 9. Intraoperative photograph showing lateral craniocervical junction exposed.

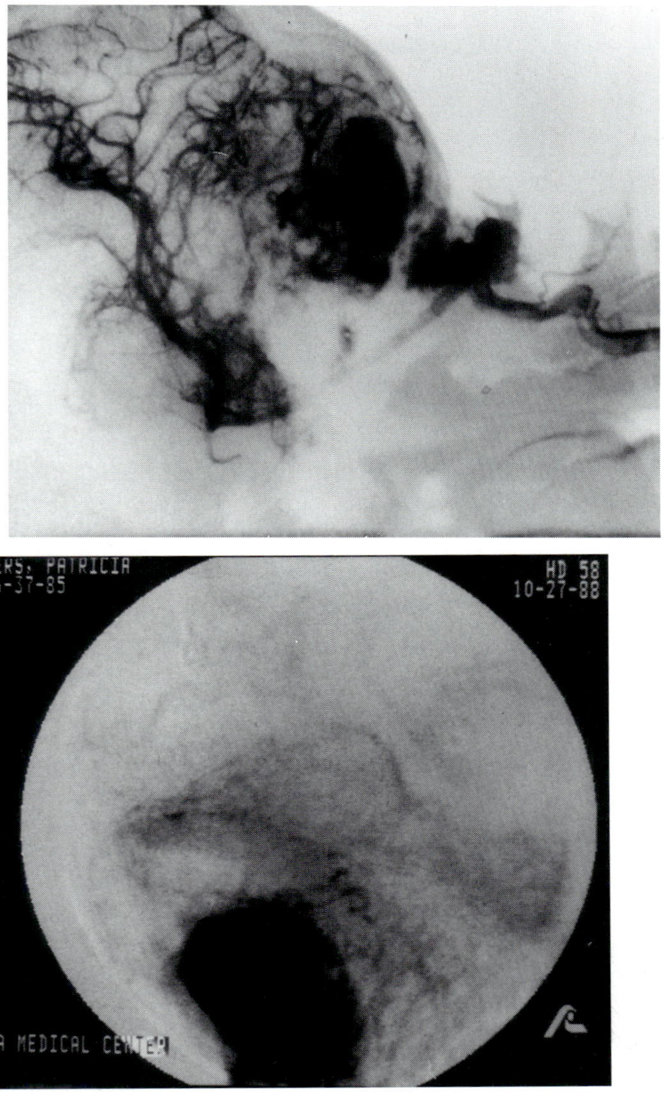

Figure 10. Vertebral angiography images showing tumor blush from a large hemangioblastoma at the craniocervical junction.

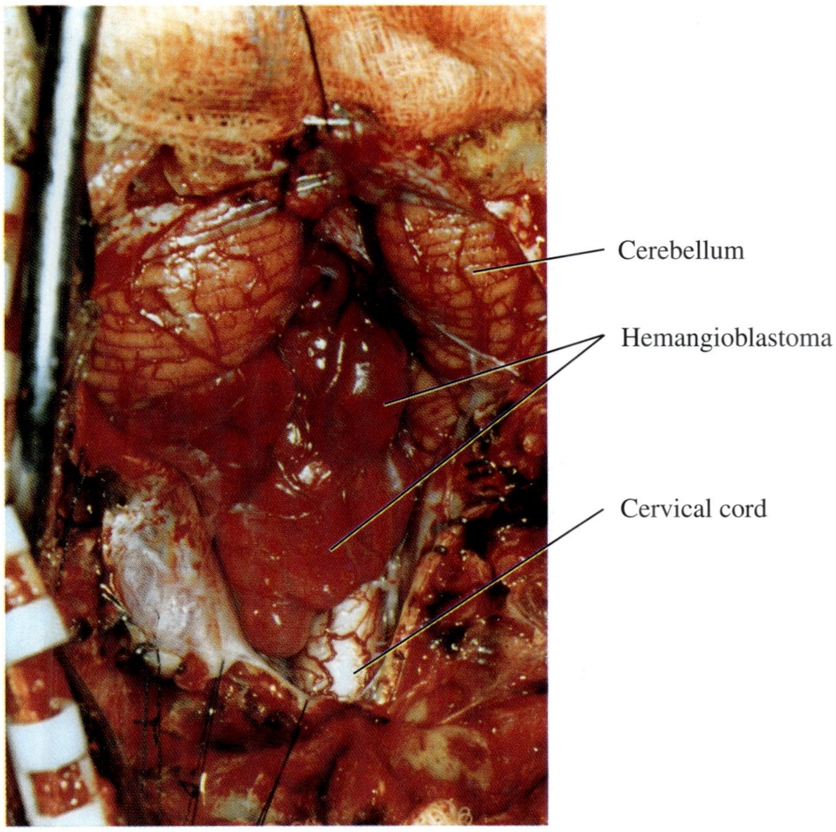

Figure 11. Intraoperative photograph of hemangioblastoma with displacement of cerebellum and upper cervical cord.

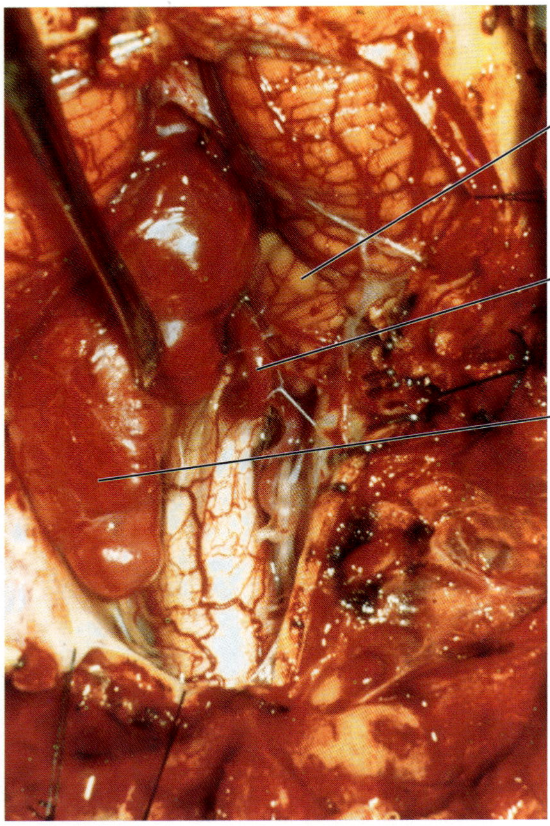

Figure 12. Posteromedial displacement of tumor mass with exposure of dilated feeding vessel.

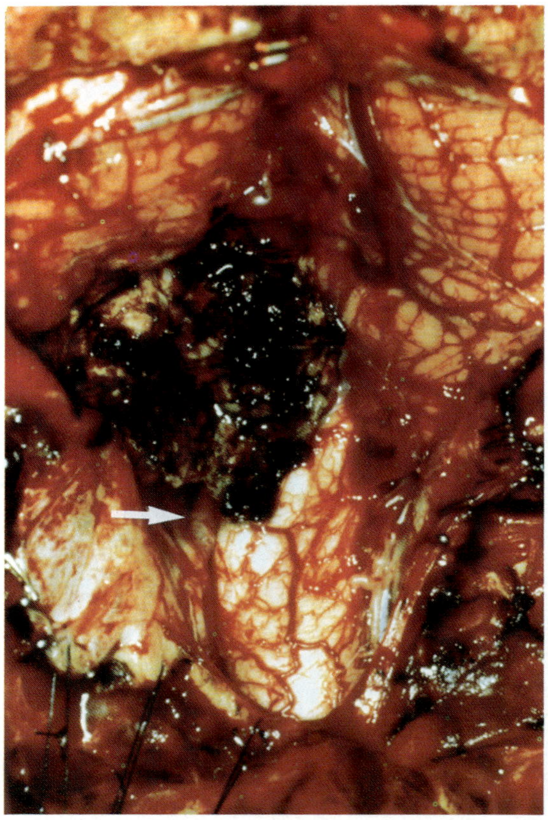

Figure 13. Tumor bed exposed after total removal of the hemangioblastoma (arrow points to vertebral artery).

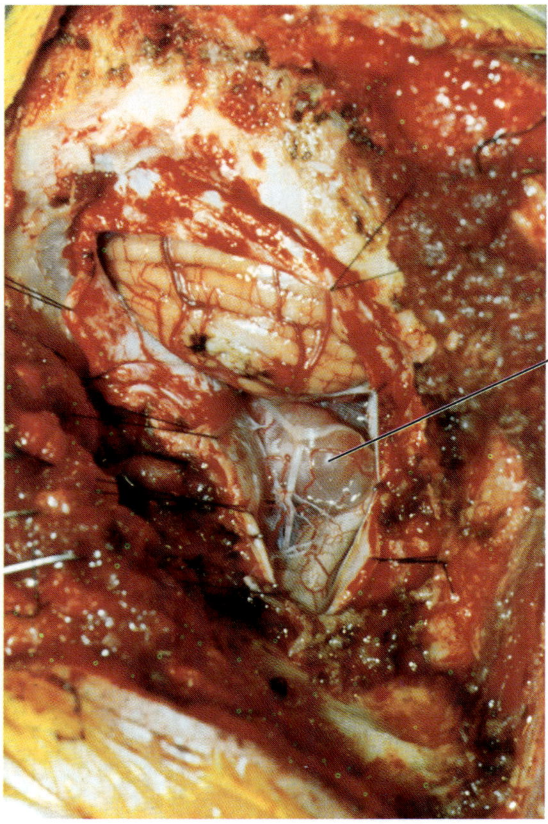

Figure 14. Hypoglossal schwannoma at the craniocervical junction, exposed by lateral approach.

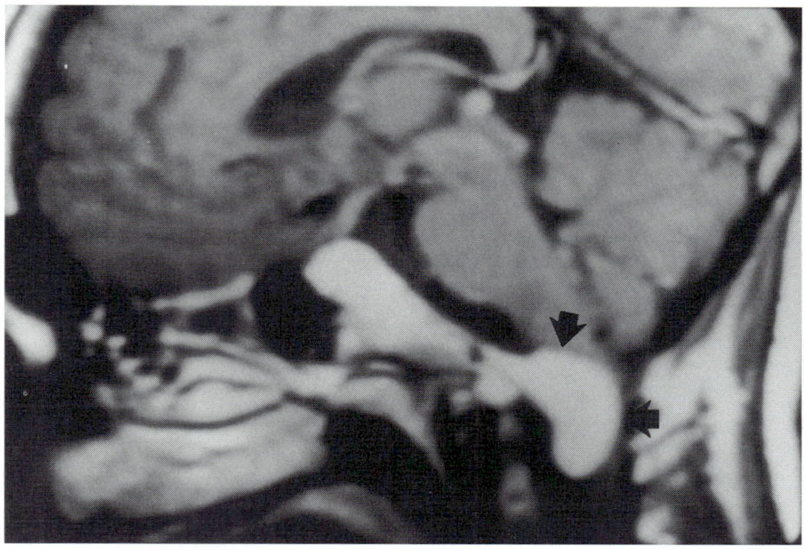

Figure 15. Magnetic resonance imaging scan showing a foramen magnum meningioma (see arrows).

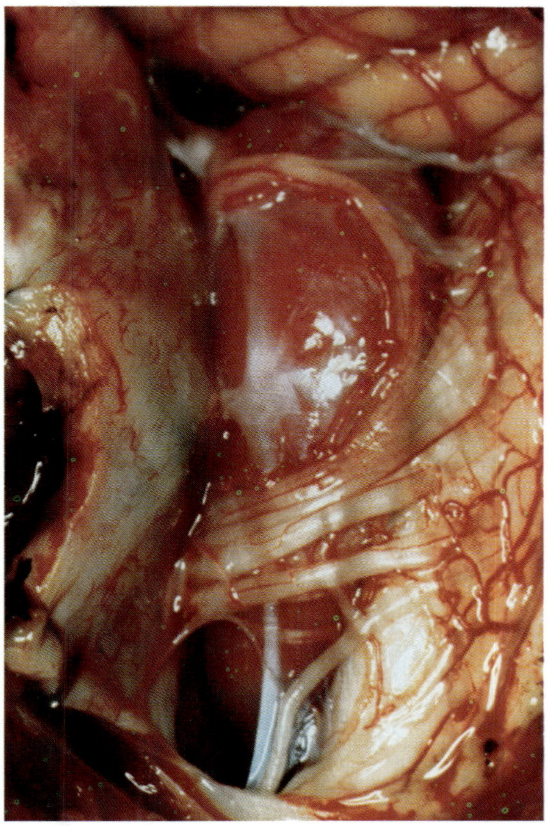

Figure 16. Intraoperative photograph of the tumor shown in Figure 15, as exposed by the lateral approach to the craniocervical junction.

13 Pre–Sigmoid Sinus Approach

Mario Ammirati

INDICATIONS

The pre–sigmoid sinus avenue to the petroclival region should be reserved for lesions that are centered in the lateral incisural space and extend infratentorially to the upper and mid-clivus. It is also useful in approaching the anterior aspect of the posterior pyramis and then extending supratentorially to the medial aspect of the middle fossa (parasellar area, medial aspect of the greater wing of the sphenoid, and the anterior aspect of the anterior pyramis). The advantages of such an approach are the decreased amount of brain retraction needed to reach the target areas and the multiangled approach to lesions that is afforded. Its potential hazards, apart from neurovascular injuries, lie in the possibility of iatrogenic hearing loss resulting from the extensive pyramidal drilling necessary to execute the approach.

In selected cases, a partial or total petrosectomy may be performed with increased exposure but at the expense of deliberate hearing sacrifice.

A combined supra-infratentorial-transsigmoid approach to the petroclival area, as popularized by Malis and Symon, gives the perception of a greatly increased exposure because the sigmoid sinus is out of the way and because the presigmoid and retrosigmoid compartments are joined. When the presigmoid approach is combined with a retrosigmoid approach, the exposure is similar.

The main advantage of the transsigmoid approach rests in the fact that the vein of Labbé is superiorly retracted along with the temporal lobe and the transverse sinus. This reduces the inevitable stretching of the vein of Labbé, which accompanies the presigmoid approach when the vein is tethered to the transverse sinus during retraction of the temporal lobe. The main disadvantage of the transsigmoid approach is the requirement for transection of the sigmoid sinus.

POSITION

The patient is positioned semisitting with the head turned 30 degrees toward the side of the lesion. Flexion of the head is carried to a point where two fingers may be introduced between the patient's chin and the sternum.

Flexion-extension x-ray films of the cervical spine are advisable to rule out abnormal craniovertebral or vertebral motion. The usual additional precautions taken with the semisitting position are used (e.g., right atrium catheter, appropriate padding of pressure points).

INCISION

A curvilinear skin incision starting 2 cm above the upper part of the ear is carried posteriorly along the temporal line and then curved downward in a linear manner to the suboccipital area, about 2 cm posterior to the mastoid process (Figure 1).

A subgaleal scalp flap is raised over the temporal muscle, which is released from its bony attachments and retracted anteriorly. A standard paramedian muscle dissection is performed in the suboccipital area.

CRANIOTOMY

A temporal and suboccipital craniotomy is performed extending to but not over the transverse sinus, which is skeletonized using rongeurs. The transverse sinus–sigmoid sinus junction is exposed together with the medial border of the sigmoid sinus all the way to the point where the sigmoid sinus slopes anteriorly to become the jugular bulb.

Using a high-speed air drill with a carbide bit, an extensive mastoidectomy is done with exposure of the full length of the sigmoid sinus as low as the jugular bulb. Care must be taken to preserve the operculum of the endolymphatic sac and the endolymphatic duct inside the vestibular aqueduct.

The posterior wall of the petrous pyramid is drilled away using a high-speed air drill with a diamond bit. The drilling is continued in a lateral-medial direction up to the porus acusticus and as far as possible in a postero-anterior direction without entering the posterior semicircular canal or the fallopian canal.

The distance between the anterior border of the sigmoid sinus and the posterior semicircular canal varies from a few millimeters to 1 cm or more. At this stage, the transverse and sigmoid sinuses and the posterior portion of the superior petrosal sinuses are well exposed (Figure 2). The dura is then cut in a T-shaped manner with the short arm located supratentorially above the transverse sinus and the long arm, infratentorially in front of the sigmoid sinus.

The entrance of the vein of Labbé into the transverse sinus is then located, and the vein is dissected from its arachnoidal sleeve as much as possible. The temporal lobe is then gently retracted superiorly. The superior petrosal sinus is located at the junction of the long and short arms of the T. The sinus is transected close to its entrance into the transverse sinus–sigmoid sinus junction after clips or ligatures have been applied. The tentorium is then cut a few millimeters medial to the superior petrosal sinus toward the petrous apex. The tentorium is also cut in a lateral-medial direction anterior to and parallel with the transverse sinus (Figure 3).

Care must be taken not to injure the trochlear nerve during this maneuver. Gentle superior retraction of the temporal lobe is maintained while the sigmoid sinus and the cerebellum are retracted medially. The position of the tumor is now exposed, and its relation to the local neurovascular structures can be assessed and tumor removal can begin. The cranial nerves and the major vessels within the cerebellopontine angle, as visualized through a presigmoid approach, are shown in Figure 4. The same structures are visualized with a cadaver dissection exposing the cerebellopontine angle, as seen in Figure 5.

Removal of the tumor is carried out with the use of the ultrasonic aspirator and standard microsurgical techniques. When operating on benign extra-arachnoidal tumors, such as meningiomas, it is critical to continuously assess the relations between the neoplasm and the arachnoid. Whenever the tumor-arachnoid interface is absent, tumor removal becomes extremely problematic and neurovascular injury can easily occur.

An operative case using the presigmoid approach for removal of a pontine cavernous angioma is shown in Figures 6 through 9. Figure 6 shows the bony exposure with the sigmoid sinus in view. In Figure 7, the dura has been opened anterior to the sigmoid sinus with dissection along the petrous ridge developed. Aspiration of the cavernous angioma from the pons is seen in Figure 8, and in Figure 9, the pons has been decompressed and the angioma cavity is visible. Note is made of the excellent exposure of the cerebellopontine angle and pons through this approach.

CLOSURE

At the end of the procedure, the dura is approximated with interrupted sutures of 4–0 nylon and then closed in a watertight manner using a running lock stitch of 4–0 nylon. If there is a dural defect that cannot be closed primarily, a graft of fascia lata or lyophilized dura is sutured in place to achieve watertight closure.

The muscle and overlying soft tissues are then closed in layers as usual. In case of a dural defect in which a duraplasty has been necessary, lumbar spinal drainage is used for 3 to 5 days.

RECOMMENDED READING

Al Mefty, O., Fox, J.L., Smith, R.R.: Petrosal approach for petroclival meningiomas. Neurosurgery 22:510–517, 1988.

Ammirati, M., Samii, M.: Pre-sigmoid sinus approach to petroclival meningiomas. Skull Base Surgery, 124–128, 1992.

Hakuba, A., Nishimura, S., Jo Jang, B.: A combined retroauricular and preauricular transpetrosal-transtentorial approach to clivus meningiomas. Surg. Neurol. 30:108–116, 1988.

Malis, L.I.: Surgical resection of tumors of the skull base. *In* Wilkins, R.H., Rengachary, S.S., eds.: Neurosurgery. Vol. 1, New York: McGraw-Hill, 1985, 1011–1021.

Samii, M., Ammirati, M.: The combined supra-infratentorial presigmoid sinus avenue to the petroclival region. Surgical technique and clinical applications. Acta Neurochir. (Wien) 95:6–12, 1988.

Samii, M., Ammirati, M., Mahran, A., et al.: Surgery of petroclival meningiomas. Report of 24 cases. Neurosurgery 24:12–17, 1989.

Spetzler, R., Daspit, P., Pappas, C.T.E.: The combined supra- and infratentorial approach for lesions of the petrous and clival regions: Experience with 46 cases. J. Neurosurg. 76:588–599, 1992.

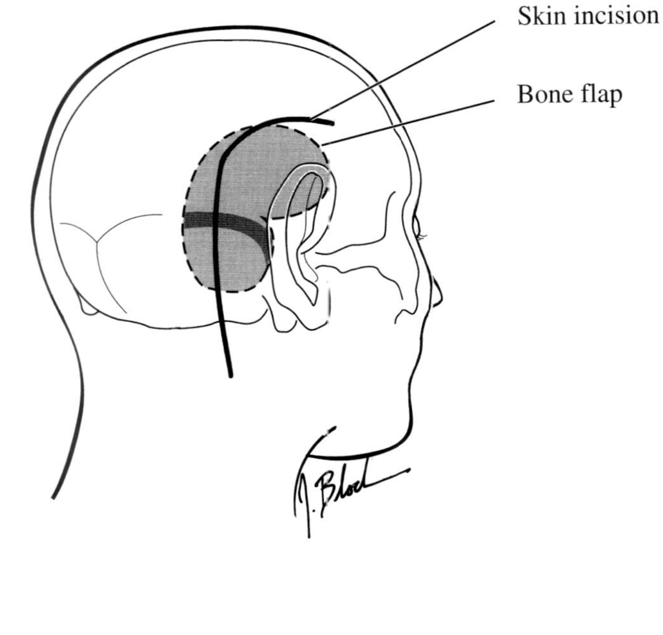

Figure 1. Scalp incision.

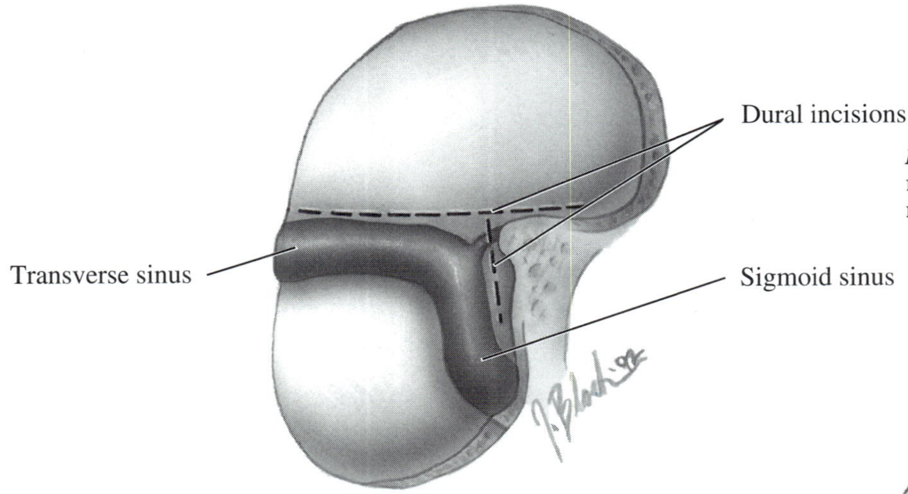

Figure 2. Exposure of the transverse and sigmoid sinuses and the posterior portion of superior petrosal sinus.

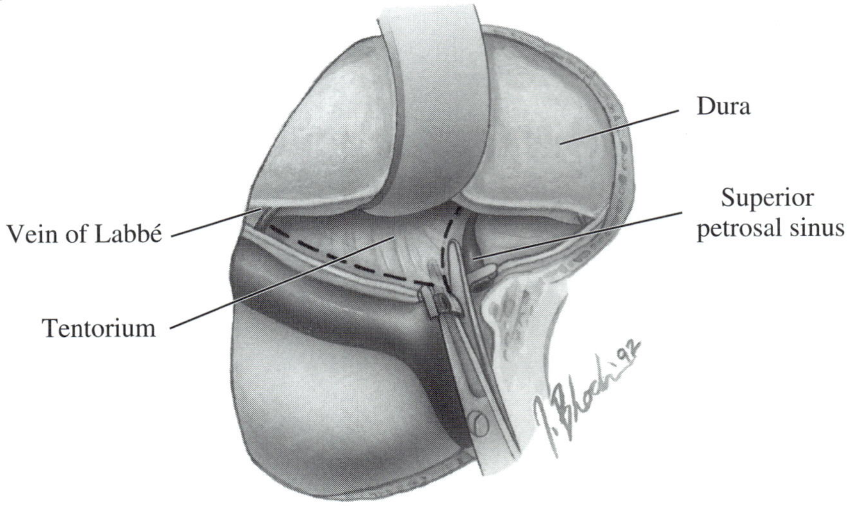

Figure 3. Transection of the tentorium in a lateral-medial direction.

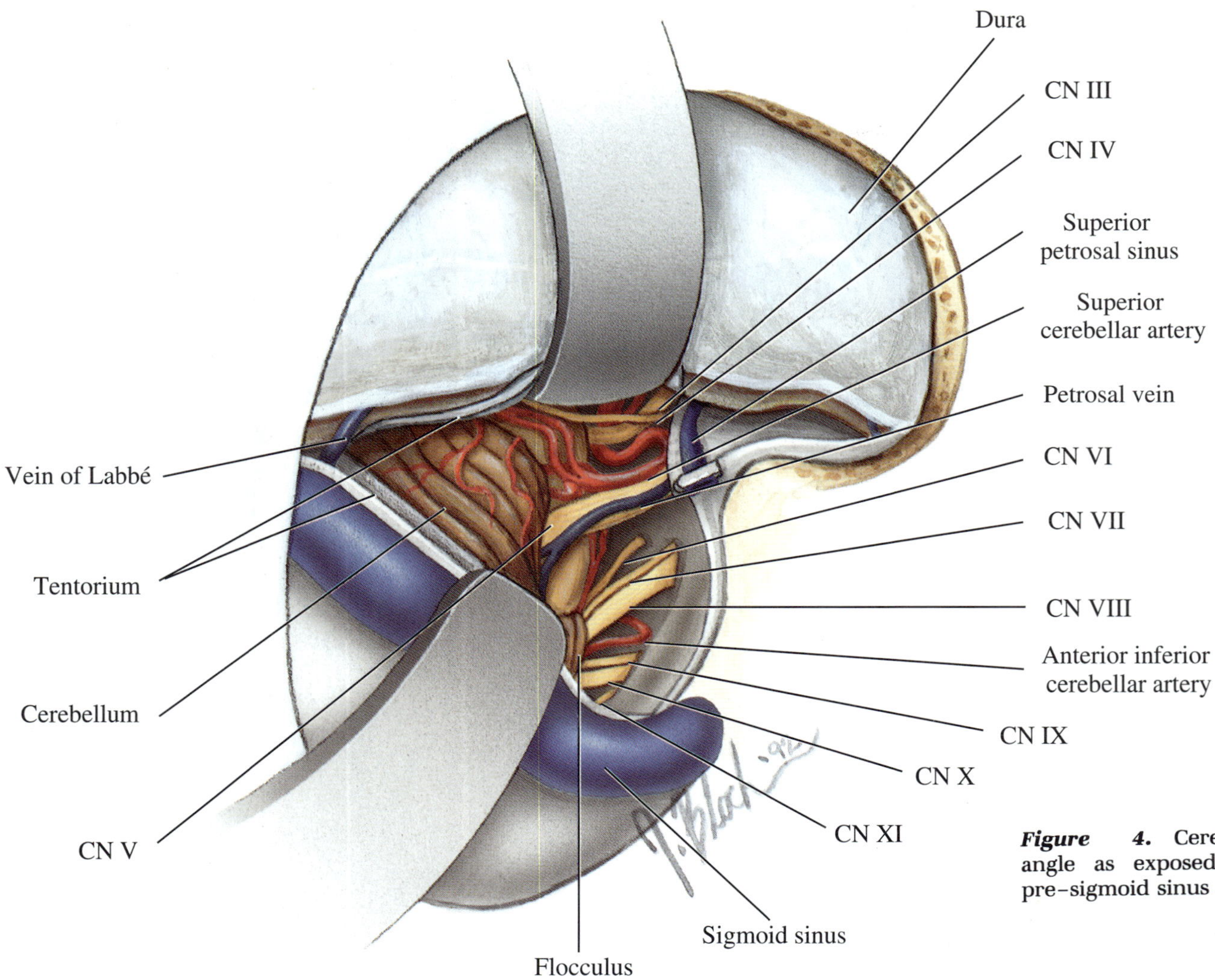

Figure 4. Cerebellopontine angle as exposed through a pre-sigmoid sinus approach.

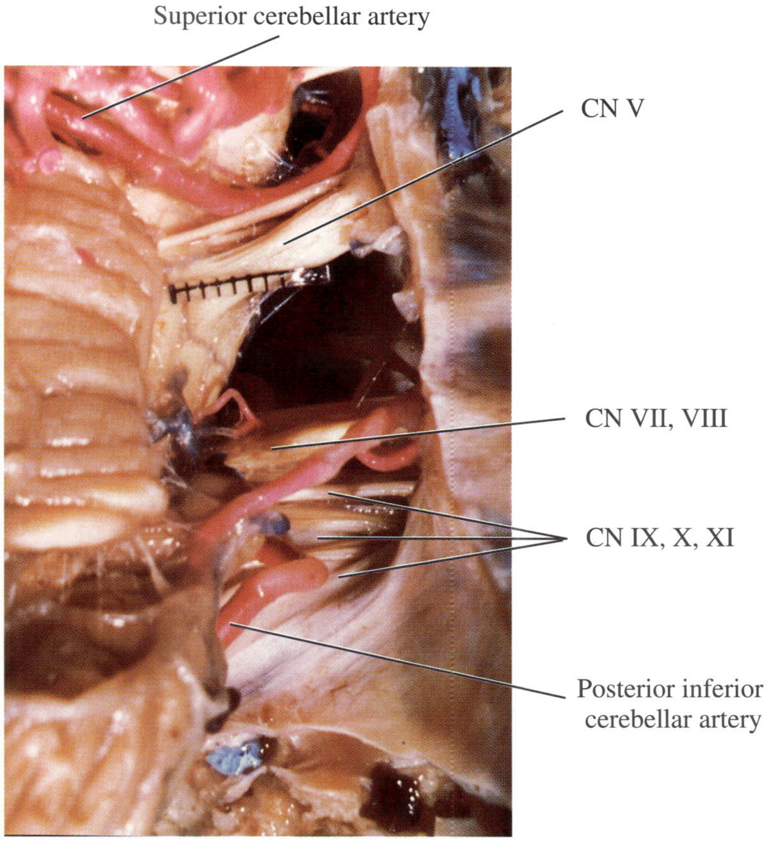

Figure 5. Cadaver dissection specimen showing the important anatomical details of the cerebello-pontine angle.

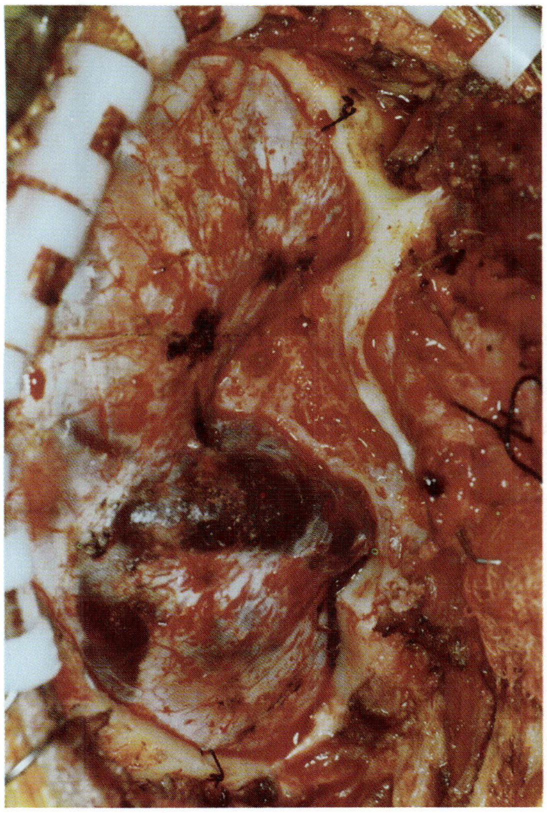

Figure 6. Supratentorial and infratentorial dura and transverse and sigmoid sinuses exposed after completion of the craniotomy.

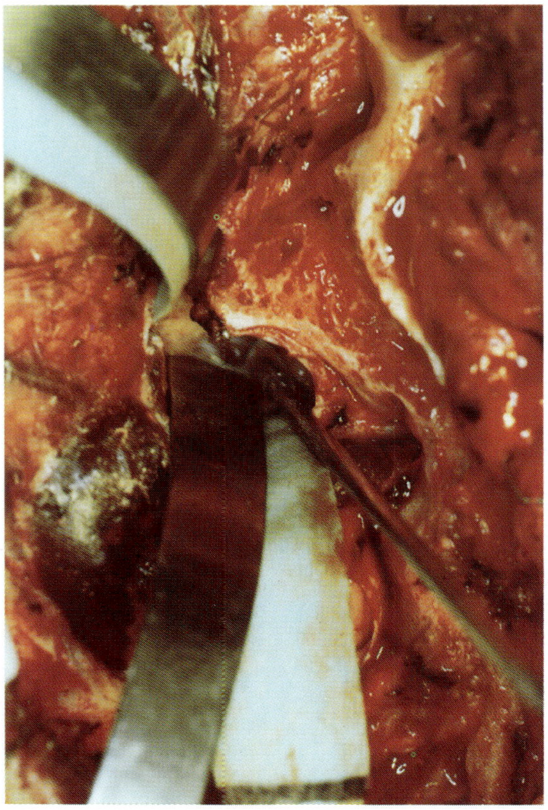

Figure 7. Initial exposure of the cerebellopontine angle after opening of the dura.

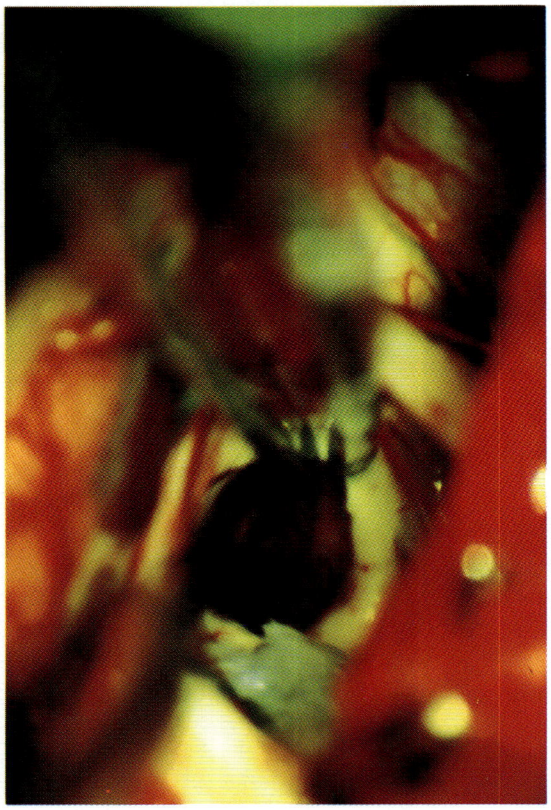

Figure 8. Under high magnification, drainage of the pontine cavernous angioma contents is seen.

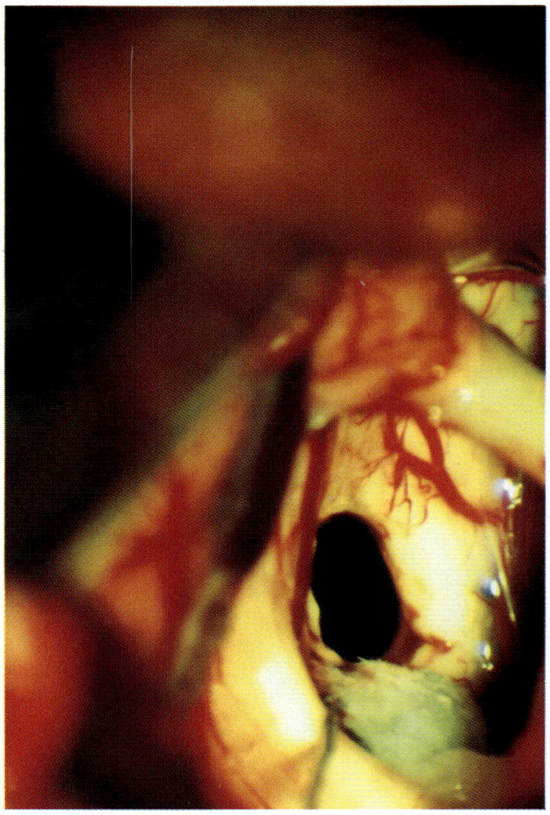

Figure 9. Excellent exposure of the pons and the empty cavernous angioma cavity.

Subtemporal Transtentorial Approach 14

Neil Martin

INDICATIONS

The subtemporal transtentorial approach is a deeper extension of the standard subtemporal approach and is appropriate for the removal of tumors of the petroclival area. It is also useful for approaching aneurysms of the basilar tip. The primary advantage of this extended subtemporal exposure is that it allows the use of a more anterior angle of approach and widened visualization of the interpeduncular area, the basilar apex and upper trunk, the ventral lateral brain stem, and the upper petroclival area. The disadvantages of this approach to the skull base are the limited exposure that is afforded, and the potential for injury to the cochlea, facial nerve, trochlear nerve, and important bridging veins, which could lead to damage of the temporal lobe because of venous congestion. The angle of approach is not optimal to visualize the clivus or the posterior surface of the petrous bone.

Other approaches have been used to reach this area. The transsylvian approach requires no skull base or tentorial dissection but provides a narrow, deep exposure that is suitable only for lesions in the region of the basilar apex. The posterolateral transpetrous approaches (presigmoid, retrolabyrinthine, translabyrinthine, transcochlear) provide improved exposure of the posterior surface of the petrous bone, internal auditory canal, jugular foramen, and mid- and lower clivus. These approaches do not provide optimal exposure of the ventrally located structures at the incisura, particularly the upper basilar artery.

The variations of the extended subtemporal approach are used for pathologies that require an anterolateral approach at various levels. The zygomatic arch is divided and reflected for all these variations. The transtentorial variation is suited for lesions that involve the interpeduncular fossa and the basilar artery apex. The posterior transcavernous extension is used when the transtentorial exposure must be increased anteriorly. The transpetrous extension is added when the pathology involves the ventral or ventrolateral surface of the upper pons or the basilar artery trunk at the level of the anterior inferior cerebellar arteries.

The extradural exposure of the petrous apex that is obtained with this approach is particularly well suited for lesions that infiltrate or involve the apex of the petrous bone. The bony anatomical relations of this area can be seen in Figure 1.

OPERATIVE PROCEDURE

Patient positioning, scalp incision, and basic subtemporal craniotomy are the same as described and shown for the subtemporal approach (Chapter 3). An exception is that the head is rotated so that the midline forms an angle of about 15 to 20 degrees with the horizontal plane (with the nose elevated). Figure 2 shows the position of the head and the craniotomy exposure. The scalp incision is carried 2 cm below the zygomatic root in front of the ear. Care is taken to avoid facial nerve branches. The lateral surface of the zygomatic arch is exposed subperiostially and divided at the lateral aspect of the orbit and at its posterior root. The temporal fascia is divided along the frontozygomatic junction and the superior temporal line. The temporalis muscle is elevated from the temporal fossa, and the muscle and attached zygomatic arch are reflected inferiorly. A free craniotomy flap is cut that extends to the floor of the middle cranial fossa. This removes all bony obstruction to a flat viewing angle along the anterior and middle extent of the middle cranial fossa floor. By removing all bony obstruction to this angle of approach, the need for temporal lobe retraction is markedly reduced.

Depending on the location, extension, and type of the pathology, the surgeon has to decide between purely intradural, transtentorial exposure and stepwise exposure of the intraosseous structures of the middle skull base epidurally before the dura is incised. In my experience, most pathological entities in the middle fossa can be excised completely without exposure of the carotid artery, facial nerve, trigeminal nerve, semicircular canals, or cochlea in the middle fossa. However, only by transecting the tentorium and the superior petrosal sinus and performing a limited bony resection of the petrous apex is the surgeon able to achieve a radical removal of some large tumors in this area.

In Figure 3, the anatomical relations for these exposures are shown by the drawing of an exaggerated retraction of the temporal lobe.

In the rare situation of a tumor that infiltrates or destroys primarily the petrous bone, I prefer extradural exposure of the lesion and dissection of the carotid artery and the surrounding structures in the petrous bone. For example, cholesterol granuloma, infiltrative meningioma, fibrous dysplasia, chordoma, and chondrosarcoma may require such extradural exposure.

For the rare extradural exposure, the middle fossa dura is separated from the middle cranial fossa floor, and the dura and temporal lobe are gently elevated. The landmarks of the middle cranial fossa floor are identified. The first landmark is the middle meningeal artery as it exits the foramen spinosum (Figure 4A). The artery should be cauterized and sectioned (Figure 4B). Medial to the foramen spinosum, the foramen ovale with the exiting third division of the trigeminal nerve is identified. The greater superficial petrosal nerve runs in the dura from the geniculate ganglion within the petrous bone anteromedially to cross over the third division of cranial nerve V. Traction injury to the greater superficial petrosal nerve must be avoided because this can result in facial nerve palsy. If necessary, the carotid artery can be exposed just posteromedial to the foramen ovale by careful drilling with a diamond burr (Figure 4C). It is important to recognize that the bony roof of the carotid canal is absent in some patients, and the canal is enclosed only with a membranous layer. The eustachian tube, which runs just lateral to the horizontal segment of the petrous carotid artery, should be protected. A length of about 10 to 12 mm of the internal carotid artery can be exposed. Exposure of the internal carotid artery is an important initial step because this forms the inferior extent of the petrous apex bone removal (shown partially completed in Figure 4C). The important anatomical relations in the middle and posterior fossa skull base are further demonstrated in the cadaver dissection shown in Figure 5.

The dura is elevated medially and posteriorly to expose the petrous ridge. The area between the foramen ovale anteriorly and the cochlea posterolaterally can be drilled away to offer further access to the posterior fossa and to tumors in this petroclival area. Care must be exercised to avoid entering the cochlea and the internal auditory canal as well as injuring the carotid artery within the petrous bone.

For the much more common intradural transtentorial exposure of the petroclival area and interpeduncular fossa, the drilling of the middle fossa is not necessary in all cases. After the conventional temporal craniotomy, the dura is opened in a low transverse manner and reflected superiorly. A moist cottonoid is placed against the temporal lobe, which is then gently elevated to visualize the tentorial edge (after ventricular or lumbar cerebrospinal fluid drainage). The tentorial notch is identified, as shown in the intraoperative photograph in Figure 6, and the tentorium is elevated so that the course of the trochlear nerve can be identified. The entry point of cranial nerve IV into its dural tunnel at the edge of the tentorium is located. The tentorium is coagulated and divided 1 to 2 cm posterior to the fourth nerve entry point. The tentorial incision is extended laterally to the superior petrosal sinus. The triangular tentorial flap is retracted anterolaterally to expose the orifice of the dural tunnel of the trochlear nerve. Using sharp dissection with a curved scissors or an arachnoid knife, this dural tunnel is opened anteriorly to the area where cranial nerve III enters the lateral wall of the cavernous sinus (Figure 7).

Once the dural tunnel is open, the trochlear nerve can be freed from the tentorium. By freeing the trochlear nerve, the tentorial flap can be reflected another 1 to 2 cm farther anteriorly. Additional anterior reflection of this flap is possible if the lateral extent of the tentorial incision is carried through the superior petrosal sinus (which can be doubly clipped, or packed with Surgicel, and divided) and into the roof of Meckel's cave. Traction sutures through the tentorial flap can be sewn to the dura of the anterolateral middle cranial fossa floor. The exposure opened by the retraction of the tentorial flap provides excellent visualization of the interpeduncular and prepontine cisterns between the trochlear nerve and the trigeminal nerve root. Slight temporal lobe retraction adds exposure of the basilar artery apex above and below cranial nerve III. The exposure between the trochlear and trigeminal nerves allows the surgeon to visualize the basilar artery as far caudally as 1 cm below the superior cerebellar artery, the trigeminal nerve root entry zone, the ventrolat-

surface of the upper pons. This approach is much broader than the standard subtemporal approach. Access to the lower basilar artery for temporary clipping during aneurysm clipping is much improved.

The key step in this approach is dissection of cranial nerve IV from the edge of the tentorium. Without this dissection, the tentorium can be reflected forward only far enough to expose the lateral surface of the midbrain and pons without providing optimal exposure of the basilar artery. Even delicate dissection of the trochlear nerve from the tentorial edge causes a superior oblique palsy. If the nerve is not traumatized and is left anatomically intact, this condition is almost always transient.

Taking the trigeminal nerve as the landmark between the brain stem and the tentorium, the surgeon is able to distinguish two compartments for further exposure. The first can be opened anteromedially to the trigeminal root. The tentorium between the fourth and fifth cranial nerves is excised (Figure 8A).

For the posterolateral compartment, the superior petrosal sinus must be coagulated and cut to resect the tentorium and the dura around the petrous bone (Figure 8B). Figure 9 shows this area with a portion of the tentorium excised and a portion of the petrous apex drilled away. In doing the partial petrosectomy, care is exercised to avoid injury to the carotid artery and cochlea. Figure 10 shows a cadaver specimen that demonstrates the important anatomical features in the region of the petrous ridge and tentorium.

Subtemporal transtentorial exposure offers

the possibility for removal of pathological entities in the middle fossa with extension into the infratentorial space. This approach is limited in exposure. Anterior partial petrosectomy is being replaced by the posterior presigmoid transtentorial approach.

CLOSURE

After achieving careful hemostasis, the dura is closed with approximation with interrupted 4-0 nylon sutures followed by a running suture closure of 4-0 nylon. The dura is tacked up to the pericranium and temporalis muscle and fascia with 4-0 black silk sutures at strategic points. The free craniotomy bone flap is secured in place at three or four points with 0 nylon sutures passed through drill holes in the bone. The temporalis muscle and fascia and the galea are closed with interrupted sutures of 3-0 Vicryl, and the skin is closed with 3-0 monofilament nylon sutures or skin clips.

RECOMMENDED READING

Andrews, J., Martin, N., Black, K., et al.: Middle cranial fossa transtemporal approach to the intrapetrous internal carotid artery. Skull Base Surgery 1:142–146, 1991.

Hakuba, A., Nishimura, S.: A combined retroauricular and preauricular transpetrosal-transtentorial approach to clivus meningiomas. Surg. Neurol. 30:108–116, 1988.

Harsh, G., Sekhar, L.: The subtemporal, transcavernous, anterior transpetrosal approach to the upper brainstem and clivus. J. Neurosurg. 77:709–717, 1993.

Kawase, T., Shiobara, R., Toya, S.: Anterior transpetrosal-transtentorial approach for sphenopetroclival meningiomas; surgical method and results in 10 patients. Neurosurgery 28(6):869–876, 1991.

Kawase, T., Toya, S., Shiobara, R., Mine, T.: Transpetrosal approach for aneurysms of the lower basilar artery. J. Neurosurg. 63:857–861, 1985.

Samii, M., Ammirati, M., Mahran, A., et al.: Surgery of petroclival meningiomas: Report of 24 cases. Neurosurgery 24(1):12–17, 1989.

Sen, C., Sekhar, L.: The subtemporal and preauricular infratemporal approach to intradural structures ventral to the brain stem. J. Neurosurg. 73:345–354, 1990.

Shiokaw, Y., Saito, I., Aoki, N., Mizutani, H.: Zygomatic temporopolar approach for basilar artery aneurysms. Neurosurgery 25:793–797, 1989.

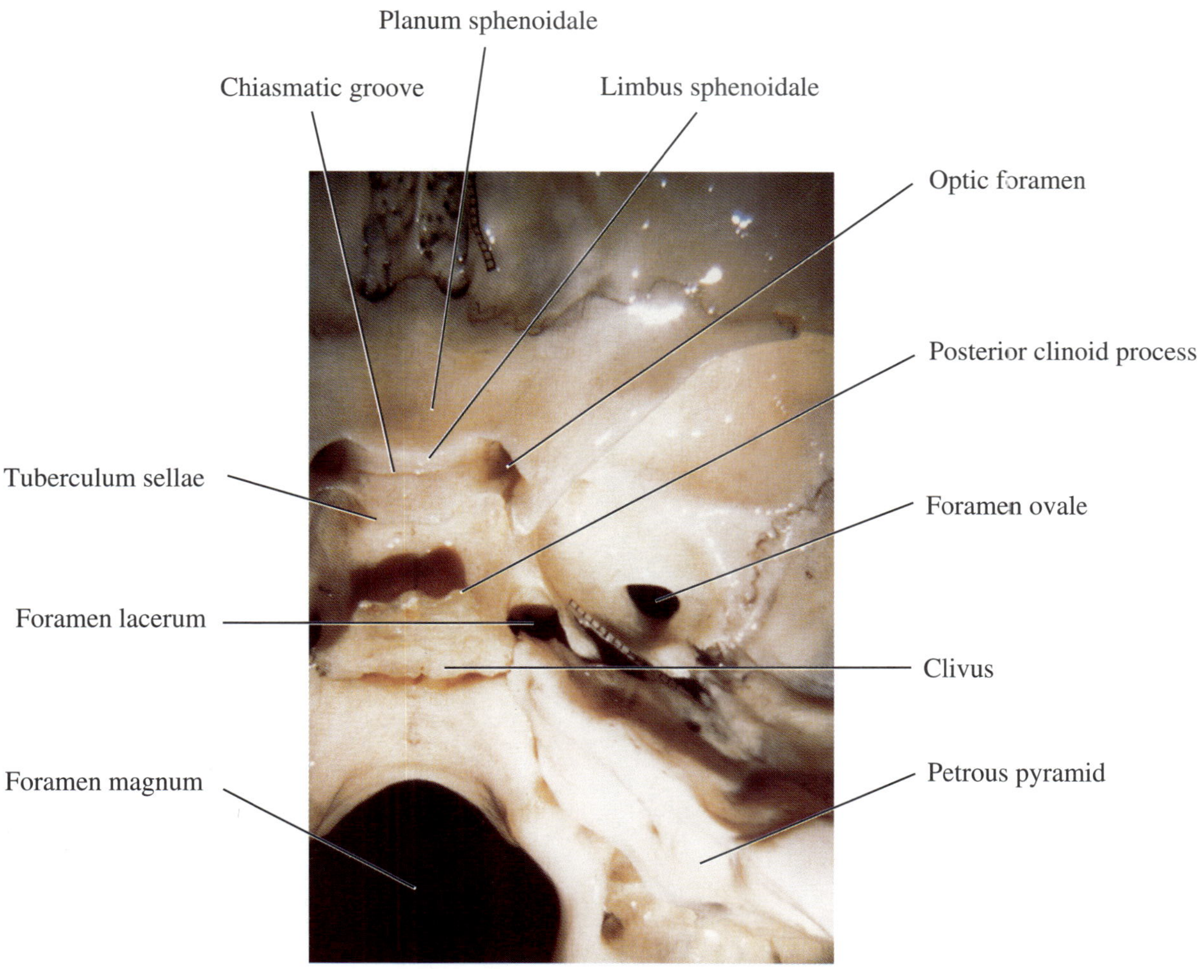

Figure 1. Skull specimen showing the important bony structures and relations of the middle fossa floor and petrous bone.

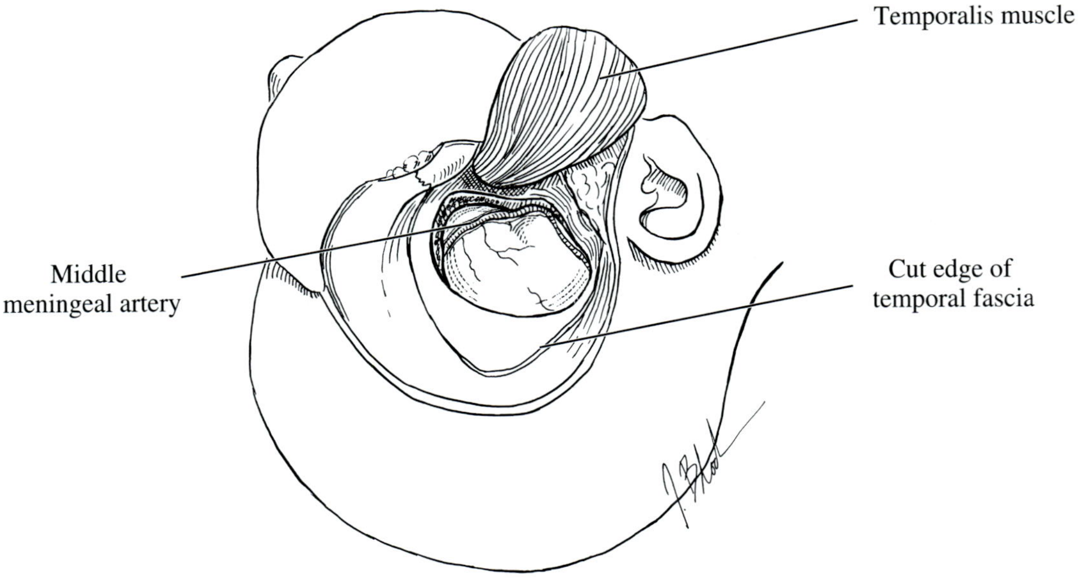

Figure 2. Position of patient's head with operative incision. The temporalis muscle is reflected after sectioning of the zygomatic arch. The craniotomy is carried to the floor of the middle fossa.

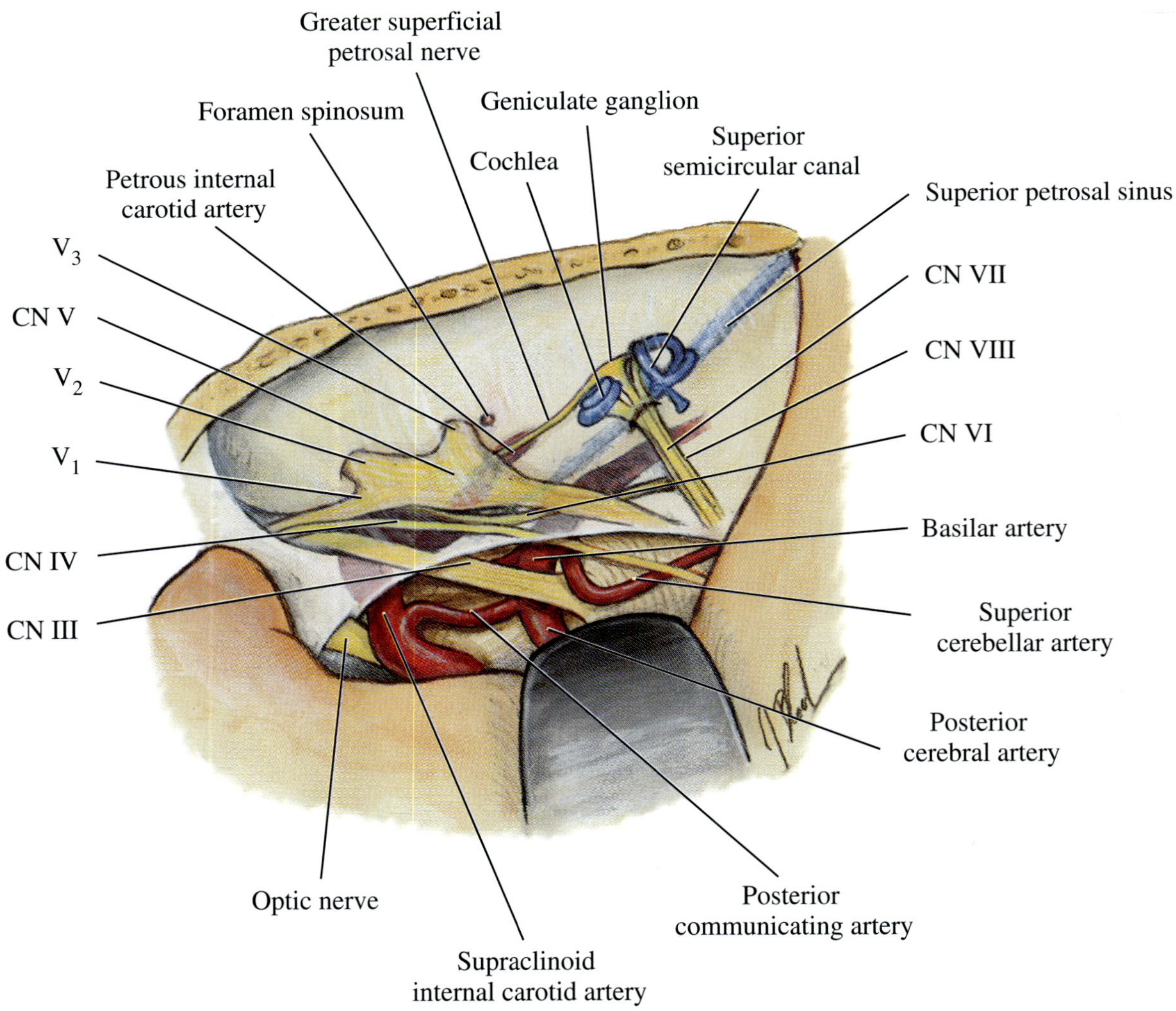

Figure 3. Anatomical relations at the tentorial notch and in the middle fossa skull base and petrous bone.

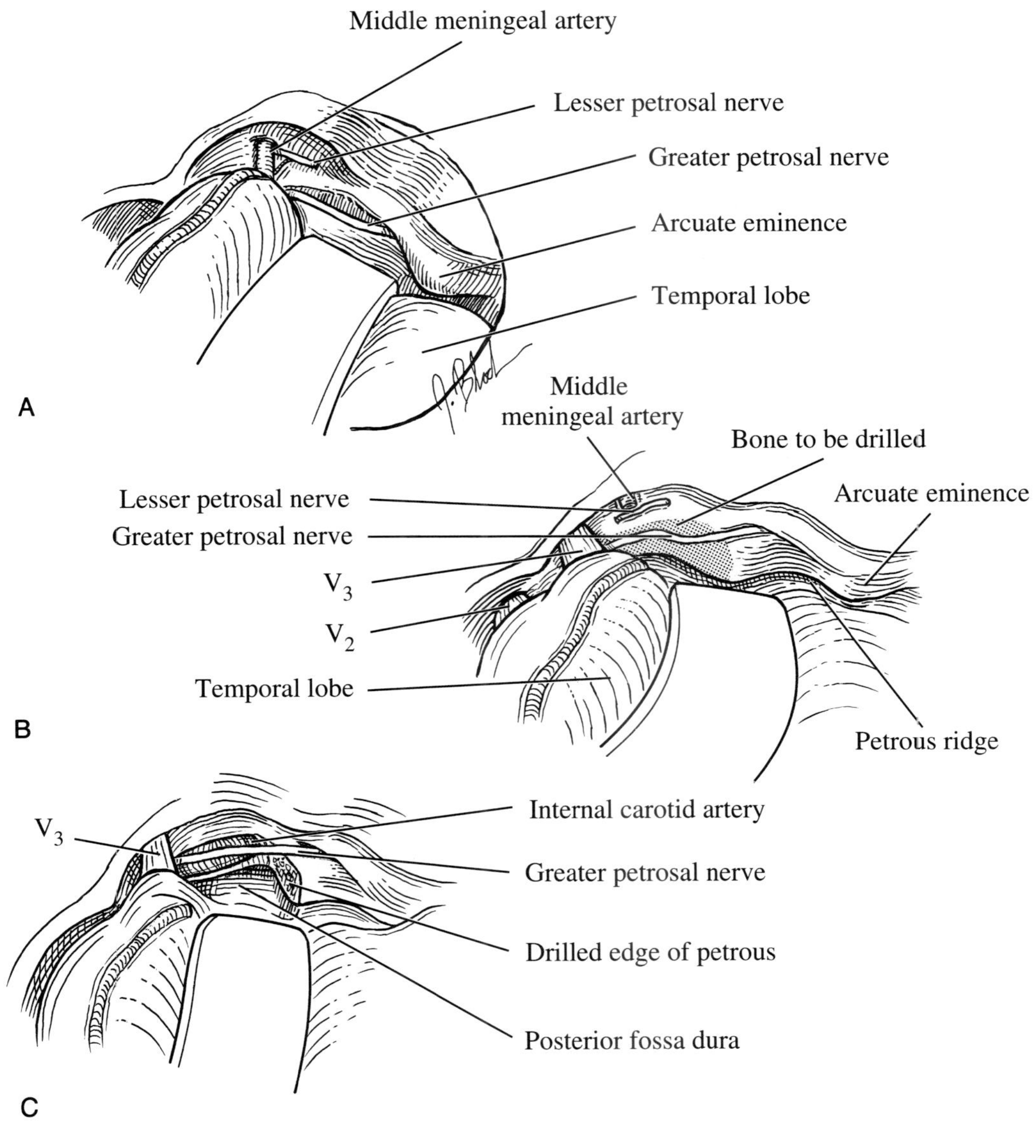

Figure 4. Anatomical relations of the posterior middle fossa floor and region of tentorial notch. A. Middle meningeal artery arcuate eminence. B. Middle meningeal artery sectioned and greater superficial nerve exposed. C. Part of posterior petrous ridge drilled away and carotid artery exposed.

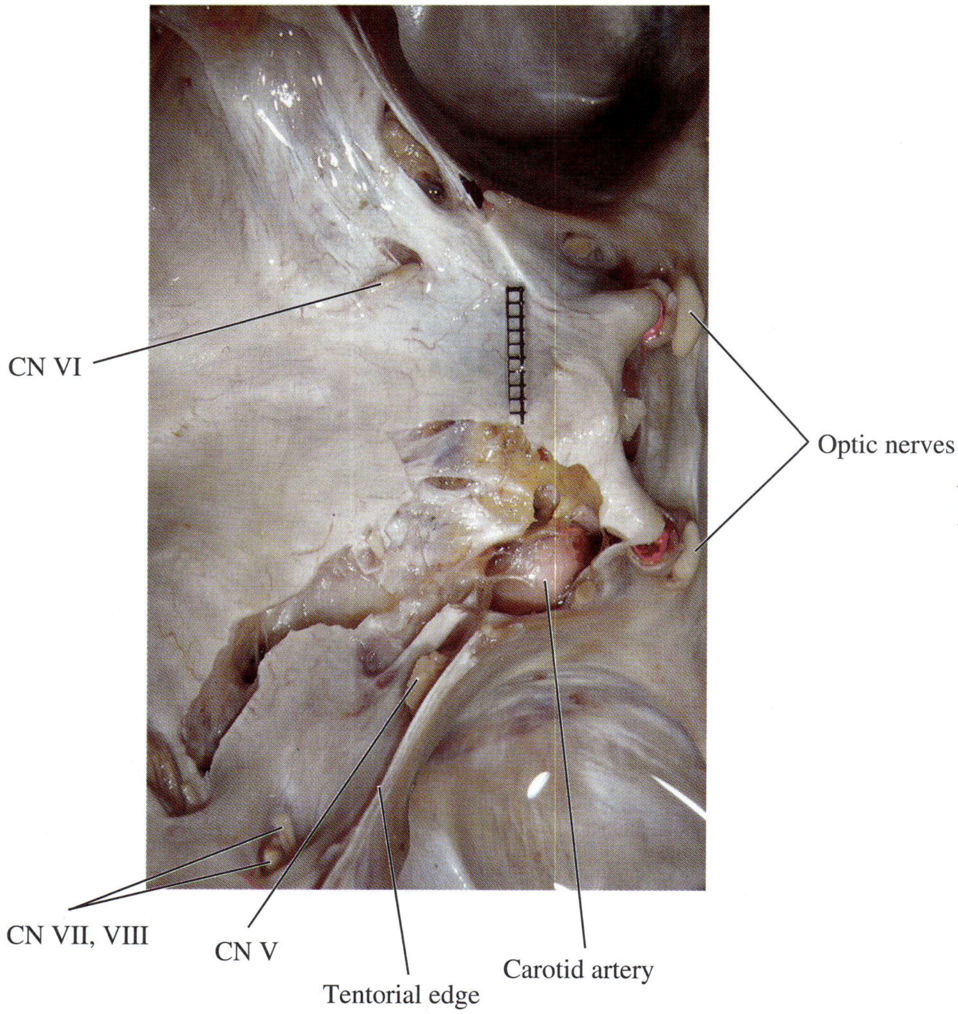

Figure 5. Cadaver dissection showing the tentorial notch area and important cranial base structures.

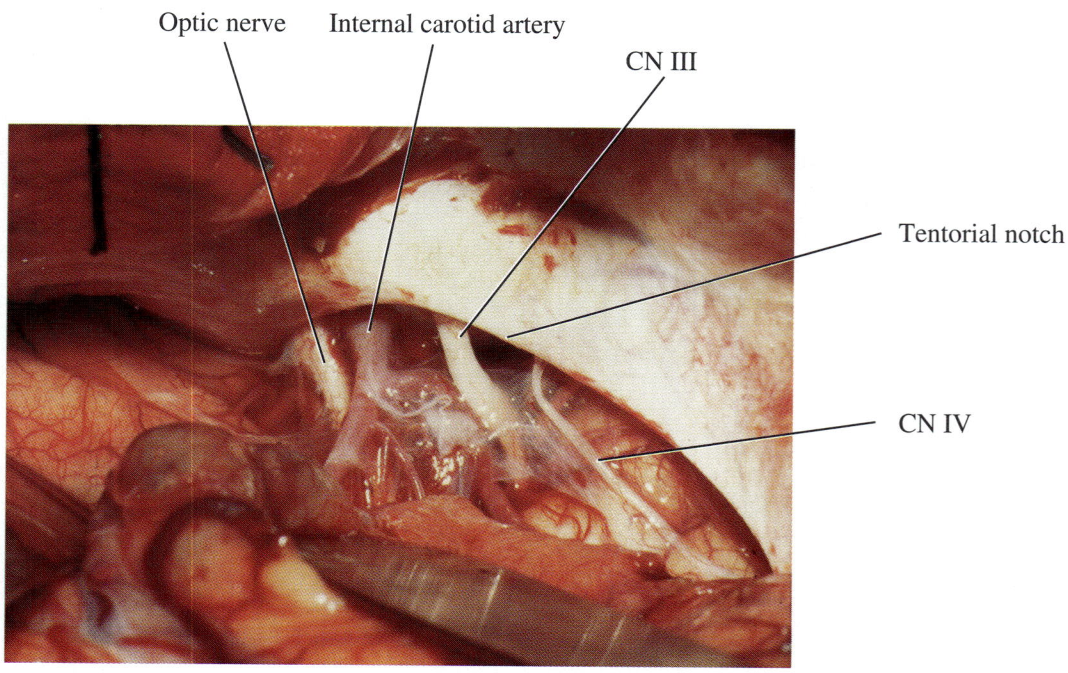

Figure 6. Anatomical relations through an intradural approach to the tentorial notch (retraction of the temporal lobe is exaggerated in this case of hemispherectomy).

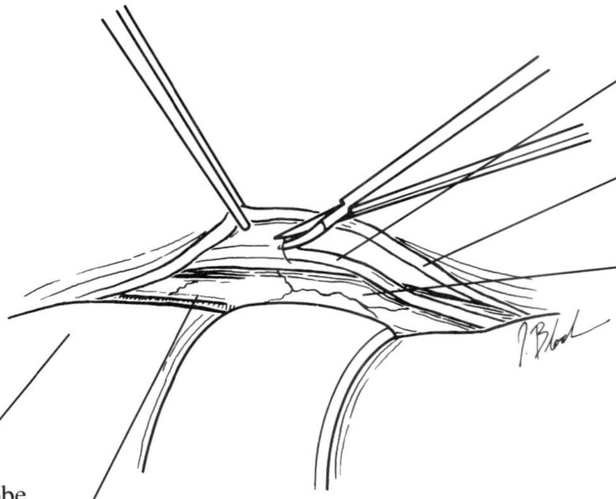

Figure 7. Opening of dura at the point of entry of cranial nerve IV.

Transtentorium-Posterior Transcavernous

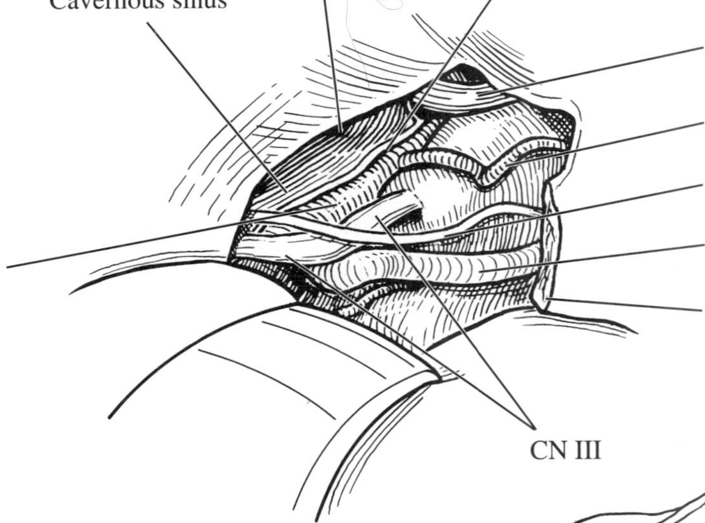

A

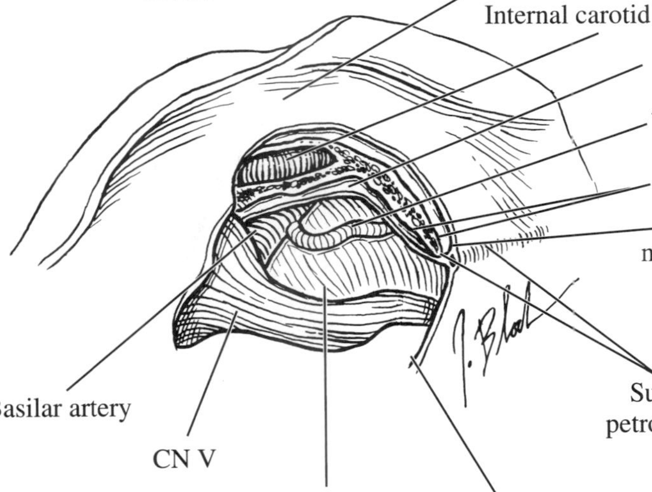

B

Transtentorium-Transpetrous

Figure 8. Anterior compartment structures (A) and posterior compartment structures (B).

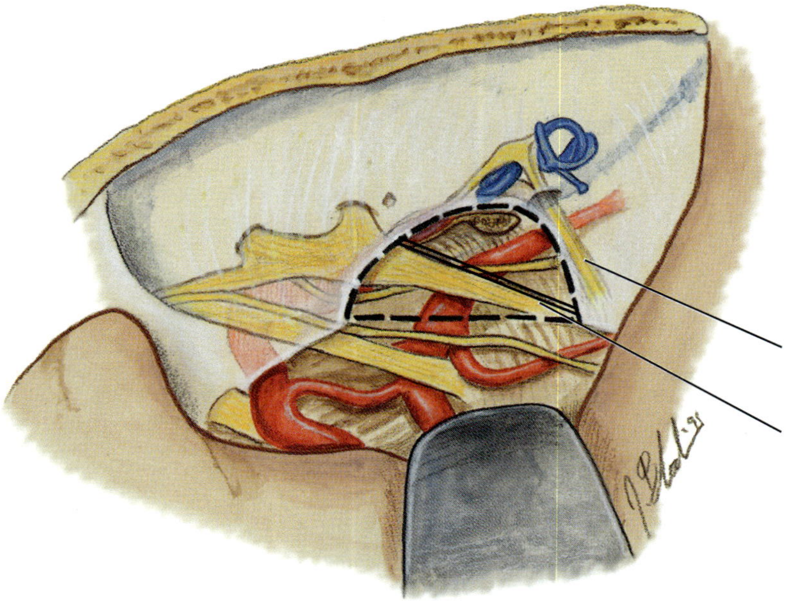

Figure 9. Anatomical relations with a portion of the tentorium excised and part of the petrous apex drilled away.

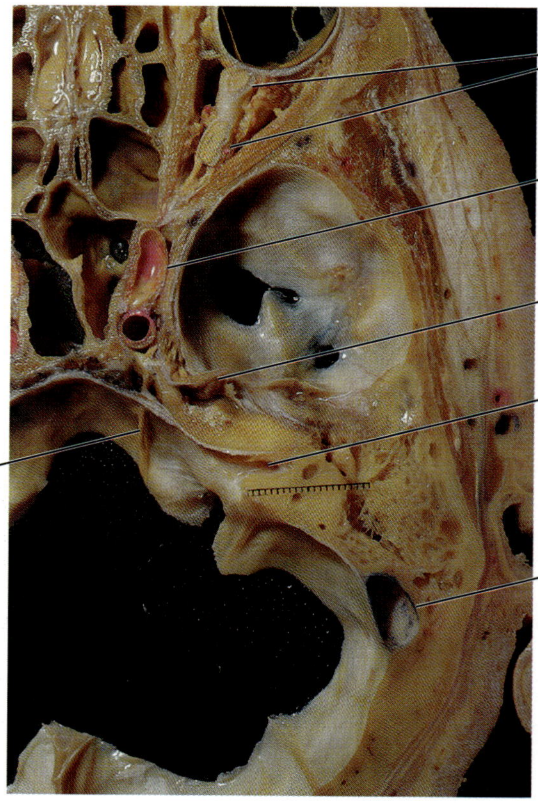

Figure 10. Cadaver dissection specimen showing the anatomical structures in the area of the petrous ridge and tentorial notch.

Transfrontal Basal Approach 15

INDICATIONS

The transfrontal basal approach is indicated for skull base tumors or other lesions that predominantly involve the anterior skull base as well as paranasal sinuses. It offers a more extensive exposure to the midline processes.

POSITION

The patient is positioned supine with the head fixed in the headholder in three-point fixation and placed in slight extension. The head is elevated 15 degrees above the level of the heart to promote venous drainage.

INCISION

A bicoronal scalp incision is made extending from the zygoma at a point 1 cm anterior to the tragus of the ear on each side. The incision is made behind the patient's hairline, if possible, for cosmetic reasons. Periosteum is separated from the frontal bone and dissected with the galea, and the scalp flap is reflected anteriorly over the face. Dissection is continued low enough to expose the orbital rim. The supraorbital nerves are preserved with removal of a small segment of surrounding orbital rim, if necessary.

CRANIOTOMY

The procedure for the bilateral subfrontal approach is described in Chapter 1.

The transfrontal basal approach can be used for extradural or intradural exposure of the anterior midline skull base. For such processes as fibrous dysplasia, osteofibroma, and traumatic lesions, exposure is adequate with an extradural approach. The dura is separated from the anterior skull base, posterior wall of the frontal sinus, crista galli, cribriform plates, roof of the ethmoidal cells, planum sphenoidale, and both orbital roofs. The posterior limit of this exposure is the sphenoid wing (Figure 1). Bony anatomical features of the anterior cranial fossa floor are shown in Figure 2.

The next step is the approach to the paranasal sinuses. Depending on the location and extent of the pathological process, it is necessary to enter the frontal, ethmoidal, and sphenoid sinuses. In some cases, it is necessary to decompress the optic nerve, or nerves, within the optic canal.

With this exposure, the surgeon has access to the entirety of the paranasal sinuses as well as the sella turcica, clivus, and medial extent of the petrous bone (Figure 3).

If necessary, both orbits can be exposed with removal of the orbital roof or medial orbital walls (Figure 4).

In case of dural involvement and intradural extension, such as anterior skull base meningiomas with intracranial and extracranial extensions, the intradural exposure is indicated.

DURAL OPENING

Bifrontal basal incision of the dura with double ligation and transection of the superior sagittal sinus is carried out. Protection of the brain with moist cottonoids is followed by the introduction of brain spatulas and gradual elevation of the frontal lobes to expose the tumor.

In the case of large intracranial tumor extension, two general principles are considered to avoid unnecessary brain compression. First, gradual resection of the tumor from anterior to posterior direction, starting at the deepest level of the tumor in the anterior fossa, is accomplished. Second, the lateral exposure of the tumor is developed to a point where the cistern can be identified and opened along the lateral portion of the sphenoid wing to achieve additional decompression.

After complete intradural tumor removal, the procedure of extradural tumor excision can be followed as described earlier.

CLOSURE

After removal of tumor, any defect in the dura is closed in a watertight manner using a pedicle of pericranium from the frontal scalp or a pedicle of temporal muscle with the use of 4-0 nylon sutures. If the pericranial flap or temporal muscle is not available, fascia lata or lyophilized dura may be used. If there is a small dural defect in the midline, the surgeon can use the dura of the orbital roof with rotation toward the midline and with covering of the open paranasal sinuses. The defect of the orbital roof can then be replaced with lyophilized dura or fascia lata.

The reconstruction of bony defects of the floor of the anterior fossa is completed with autogenous bone grafts or with methyl methacrylate, depending on the size of the area to be repaired (Figure 5).

In small and middle-sized openings, reconstruction is not necessary. In addition to the pericranial flap, we use fascia lata or lyophilized dura as a second layer to produce a more substantial repair that protects against the possibility of late brain herniation.

For protection against any complication, the following steps have to be considered. (1) All mucosa of the paranasal sinuses that could create mucoceles should be removed. (2) In extensive involvement of the paranasal sinuses by tumor, thus requiring excision of ethmoidal cells, and with a large opening to the nasal cavity, temporary packing to support the dural repair is indicated. Gauze impregnated with antibiotic ointment is used for packing. In patients with minor imvolvement of the paranasal sinuses, the complete packing against the repair is not necessary, but adequate sinus drainage to the nasal cavity must be maintained. Postoperative lumbar cerebrospinal fluid drainage for up to 7 days is also essential.

The free bone plate is replaced. The bone is held in place with 0 silk sutures tied through drill holes in the bone. The galea is closed with 2-0 Vicryl. The scalp is closed with 4-0 nylon with a running lock stitch.

RECOMMENDED READING

Blacklock, J., Weber, R., Lee, Y.: Transcranial resection of tumors of the paranasal sinuses and nasal cavity. J. Neurosurg. 71:10–15, 1989.

Derome, P., Akerman, M., Anquez, L., et al.: Spheno-ethmoidal tumors. Excision possibilities and surgical repair. Neurochirurgie (Suppl.) 18:1–164, 1972.

Jackson, I., Marsh, W., Hide, T.: Treatment of tumors involving the anterior cranial fossa. Head Neck Surg. 6(5):901–913, 1984.

Persing, J., Jane, J., Levine, P., Cantrell, R.: The versatile frontal sinus approach to the floor of the anterior cranial fossa. J. Neurosurg. 72:513–516, 1990.

Schramm, W., Myers, E., Maroon, J.: Anterior skull base surgery for benign and malignant disease. Laryngoscope 89:1077–1091, 1979.

Sekhar, L., Nanda, A., Sen, C., et al.: The extended frontal approach to tumors of the anterior, middle, and posterior skull base. J. Neurosurg. 76:198–206, 1992.

Uttley, D., Moore, A., Archer, D.: Surgical management of midline skull-base tumors: A new approach. J. Neurosurg. 71:705–710, 1989.

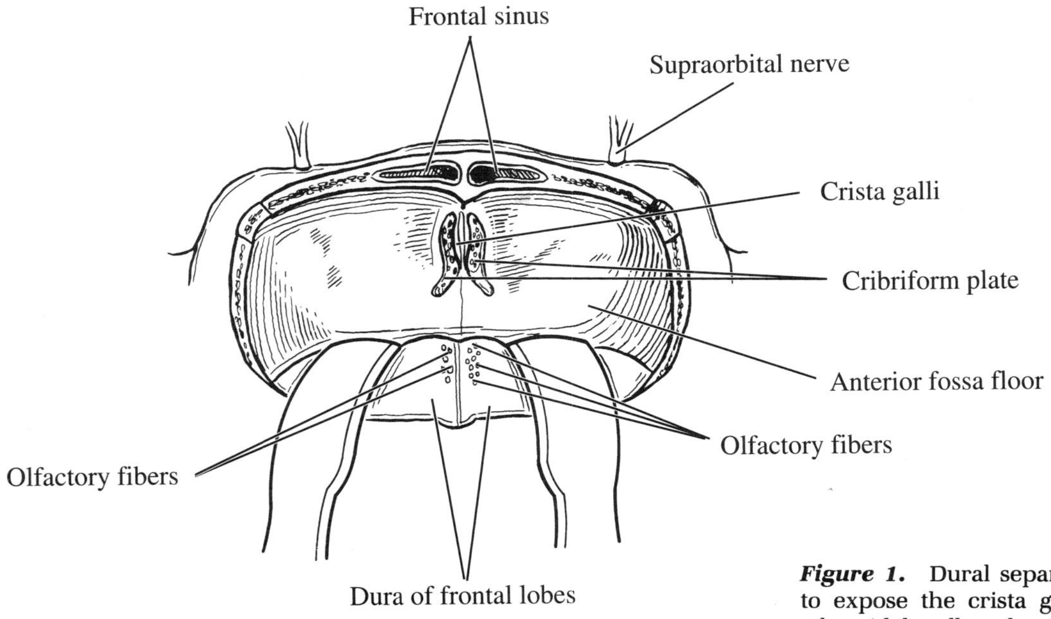

Figure 1. Dural separation from the anterior skull base to expose the crista galli, cribriform plates, roof of the ethmoidal cells, planum sphenoidale, and both orbital roofs.

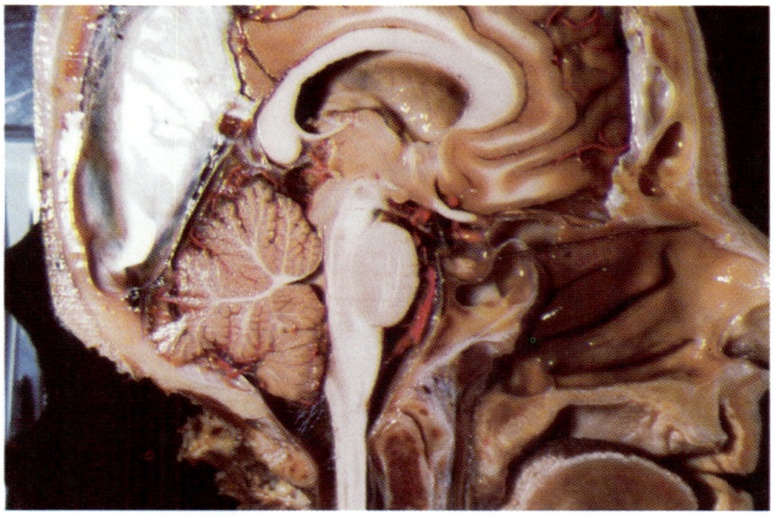

Figure 2. Skull specimen showing anterior cranial fossa features.

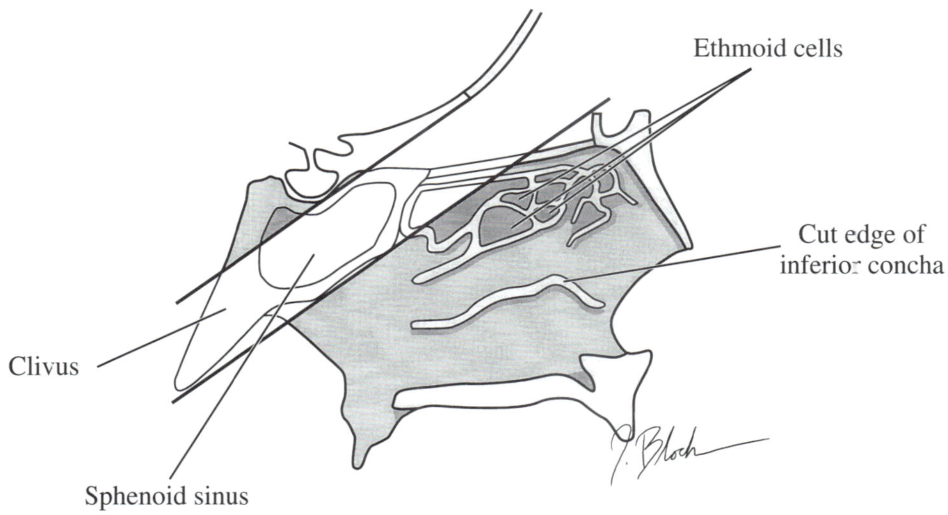

Figure 3. Exposure of the paranasal sinuses, sella turcica, and clivus.

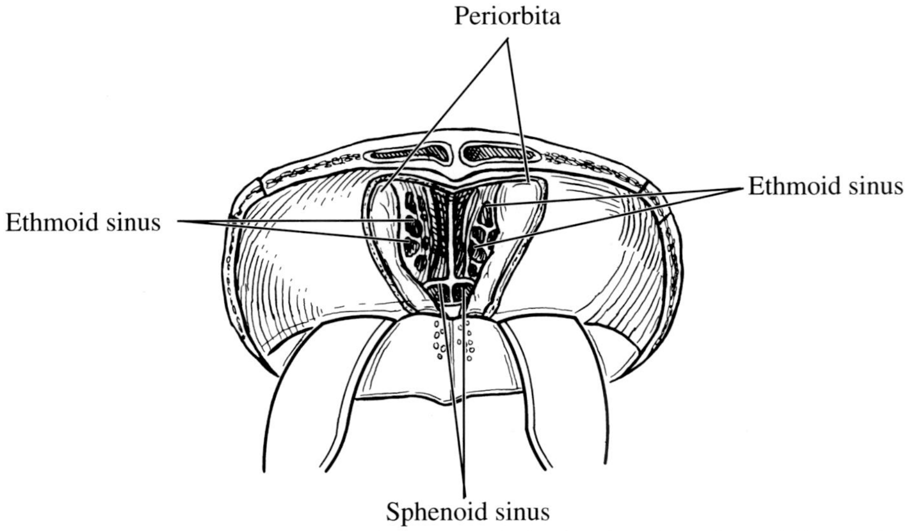

Figure 4. Exposure of both orbits by removal of orbital roofs and medial orbital walls.

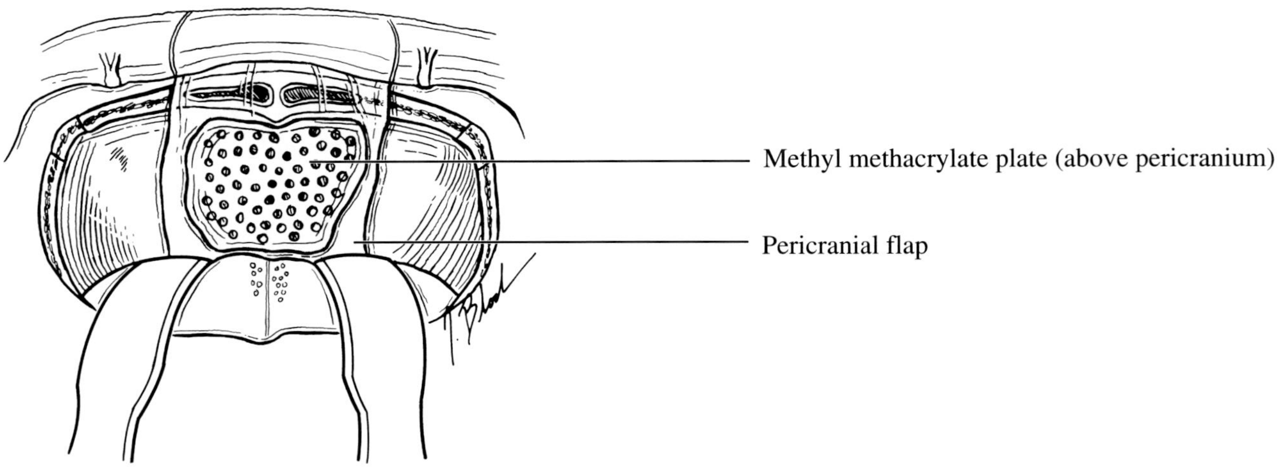

Figure 5. Reconstruction of anterior fossa floor with methyl methacrylate.

Bifrontal Orbital Approach 16

INDICATIONS

The bifrontal orbital approach is indicated for anterior skull base processes with involvement of both orbits, such as in some skull base meningiomas and bilateral optic nerve gliomas with intracranial and intraorbital extension.

POSITION

The patient is positioned supine with the head immobilized face up in three-point fixation in the headholder. The head is elevated 15 degrees above the level of the heart and the head and neck extended 15 degrees to optimize exposure of the anterior skull base and the orbits.

INCISION

A bicoronal scalp incision is made that extends from a point 1 cm anterior to the tragus of the left ear, over the root of the zygoma, and to the vertex at the bregma and ends in the same position anterior to the right ear. Subgaleal dissection is completed and carried low down to expose the orbital rims and the nasion anteriorly and the keyhole position anterolaterally. The scalp flap is retracted with multiple fish hooks attached to a fixed retractor to maintain this low anterior exposure. The pericranium is dissected from the superior orbital rim with the supraorbital nerve preserved by the drilling of a small bony plate containing the supraorbital foramen. The periorbita is carefully separated from the roof and the upper lateral wall of the orbit.

CRANIOTOMY

Burr holes are placed bilaterally in the keyhole position. This is followed by the placement of a low midline burr hole overlying the frontal sinus above the glabella. On entering the frontal sinus, its membrane is stripped downward and displaced against the sinus ostea. The keyhole burr hole is properly positioned to allow entry into the floor of the anterior fossa bilaterally. A high-speed drill is used to open the lateral orbital roof. Two burr holes are placed adjacent to the superior sagittal sinus at a point 2.5 to 5 cm above the glabella.

After stripping away the dura, the burr holes are connected superiorly with the craniotome. Next, the crucial placement of the orbital bone cuts is accomplished. From the keyhole on each side, a Gigli saw guide is passed to the low frontal burr hole, and a Gigli saw is used to cut across the orbital roof, inferior to the orbital rim, bilaterally. If correctly done, this results in a single-piece bifrontal orbital free bone flap (Figure 1A). The bone flap is lifted away to expose the frontal dura bilaterally as well as the periorbita of both orbits (Figure 2A). Figure 1B shows the free bone flap removed in this approach. Figure 2B shows the extradural exposure achieved. Additional orbital roof can be

posure posteriorly to the orbital apex and to expose the optic nerves. This epidural frontal orbital approach can be combined with an intradural exposure in cases of intradural tumor expansion.

CLOSURE

The frontal sinus is closed with a vascularized pedicled pericranium flap that is laid over the frontal sinus and then sutured to the dura. The free craniotomy flap is replaced and held firmly with 0 silk sutures passed through small drill holes at four points (Figure 3).

The burr holes are covered using methyl methacrylate for cosmetic purposes. The galea is closed with 3-0 Vicryl, and the scalp is closed with 4-0 nylon or skin clips.

RECOMMENDED READING

Blacklock, J., Weber, R., Lee, Y., et al.: Transcranial resection of tumors of the paranasal sinuses and nasal cavity. J. Neurosurg. 71:10–15, 1989.

Jackson, I.: Craniofacial osteotomies to facilitate resection of tumors of the skull base. *In* Wilkins, R. and Rengachary, S. eds.: Neurosurgery Update I. New York: McGraw-Hill, 1990, 277–291.

Jane, J., Park, T., Pobereskin, L., et al.: The supraorbital approach: Technical note. Neurosurgery 11(4): 537–541, 1982.

Persing, J., Jane, J., Levine, P., et al.: The versatile frontal sinus approach to the floor to the anterior cranial fossa: Technical note. J. Neurosurg. 72:513–516, 1990.

Uttley, D., Moore, A., Archer, D.: Surgical management of midline skull-base tumors: A new approach. J. Neurosurg. 71:705–710, 1989.

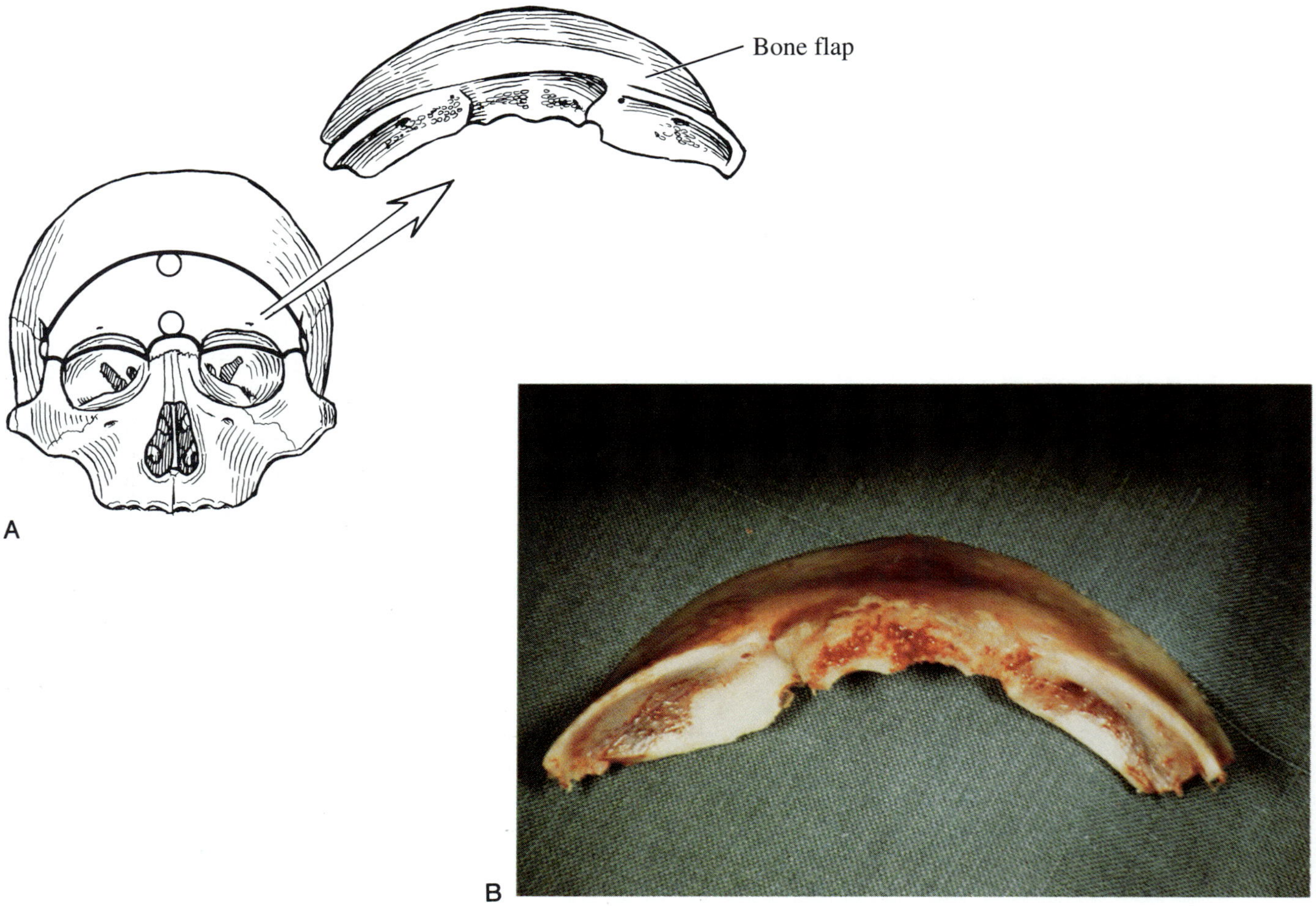

Figure 1. A. Extent of bifrontal orbital bone flap. B. Free bone flap.

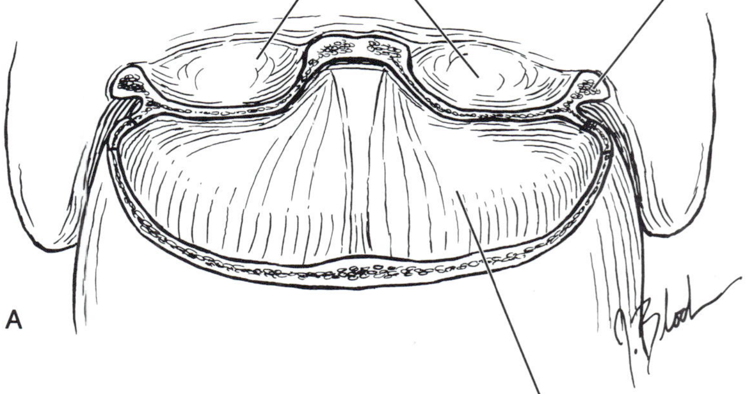

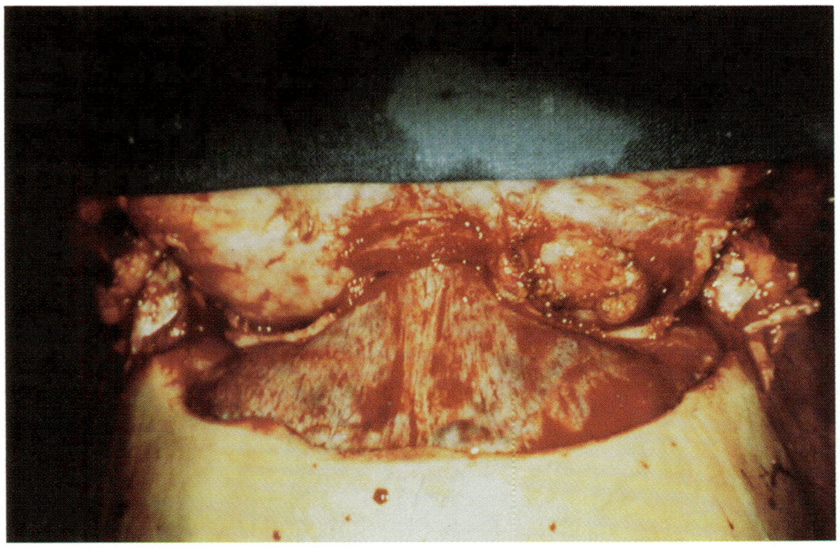

Figure 2. *A*, Exposure of frontal dura and periorbita of both orbits. *B*, Extradural exposure.

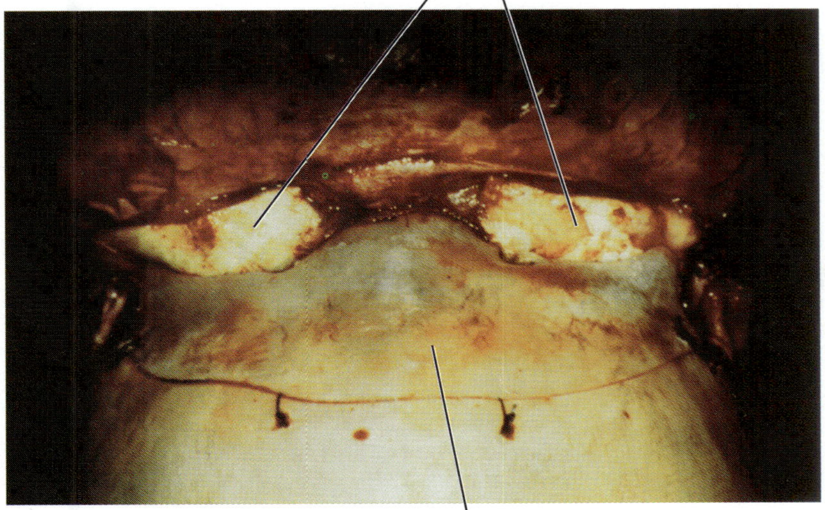

Figure 3. Replacement of bifrontal orbital bone flap.

17 Frontal-Temporal-Orbital Approach (With Approaches to the Cavernous Sinus)

POSITION

The patient is positioned supine with the head slightly extended and turned 30 degrees away from the side to be operated. The head is secured in position in a headholder with three-point fixation (Figure 1).

INCISION

To provide necessary low access to the frontal, orbital, and suprasellar regions, a bicoronal scalp incision is preferred. The superficial temporal artery is preserved in the scalp flap.

The incision (see Figure 1) extends from the zygomatic arch anterior to the tragus on the ipsilateral side to the opposite superior temporal line. The scalp flap is dissected from the skull and retracted forward to expose the orbital rim (Figure 2). The periosteum is preserved with the scalp on its vascular pedicle for dural and sinus closure. Exposure of the superior and lateral orbital rim above the zygomatic arch is achieved.

A cuff of temporal muscle is incised below on the superior temporal line, leaving a cuff of fascia for closure, and then the muscle is elevated from the skull and the frontal-zygomatic process (see Figure 2).

CRANIOTOMY

Burr holes are placed in the keyhole position, low in the temporal fossa and immediately above the nasion lateral to the midline. The supraorbital nerve is dissected from its foramen, and the periorbita is elevated from the bony orbit. The dura is separated intracranially and a Gigli saw is passed beneath the frontal lobe, as shown in Figure 2, and the burr holes are connected while protecting the orbital contents with a malleable retractor blade. A high-speed craniotome is used to complete the craniotomy.

The frontal and temporal lobes together with the dura are elevated. Drilling of the sphenoid ridge is continued with a high-speed drill and a diamond burr. As the medial portion of the sphenoid ridge is reached, drilling is continued cautiously to avoid injury to the optic nerve and the carotid artery.

Additional bone is removed from the orbit, lateral wall of the optic foramen, and lateral portion of the anterior clinoid process (Figure 3). The central part of the anterior clinoid process is then drilled from inside, after the dura has been opened, while preserving a thin outer shell of cortical bone. This remaining thin sheet of bone is then carefully lifted away from the optic nerve.

The supraclinoid portion of the internal carotid artery is identified as it courses lateral to the optic nerve. It completes its posterior course after emerging from the dural ring, and the carotid artery bifurcates into the anterior and middle cerebral arteries (Figure 4). The anterior choroidal artery and posterior communicating branches are seen extending posteriorly from the internal carotid artery. Figure 5 shows the position of the structures within the cavernous sinus relative to the open sylvian fissure and major arterial branches in this area.

The anterolateral surface of the cavernous sinus dural wall is now exposed. The method of entry into the cavernous sinus depends on the size and nature of the lesion to be removed. It is necessary to completely understand the anatomical relations of the cavernous sinus and the structures contained within before operating in this area (Figure 6).

The dura that forms the lateral wall of the cavernous sinus is composed of two layers. Posteriorly, the trochlear nerve (CN IV) enters the cavernous sinus below and medial to the free edge of the tentorium. The oculomotor nerve (CN III) enters through the dural folds between the posterior clinoid process and the tentorial edge formed by the petroclinoid ligament. The ophthalmic (V_1) and maxillary (V_2) divisions of the trigeminal nerve are positioned within the cavernous sinus, lateral to the trochlear and abducens (CN VI) nerves. V_1 and V_2 lie between the two layers of dura that make up the lateral wall of the sinus. On incising the outer layer of this dural wall, these two cranial nerve branches can be identified.

In removing intracavernous lesions from a lateral approach, the point of entry may best be determined by the way in which the cranial nerves within the sinus are displaced by the tumor mass. After identification of these nerves, orientation should be possible and tumor excision can proceed. Electrical stimulation can be helpful in identifying the nerves.

Care must be exercised to avoid injury to the intracavernous carotid artery. Because it has its own dural sheath, it usually can be separated from the tumor capsule.

Entry into the cavernous sinus through its superior surface has the advantage of avoiding the cranial nerve branches that are positioned between the dural layers laterally. The carotid artery is vulnerable from this avenue of approach and must be protected during dissection. With this in mind, the safest way to enter the sinus superiorly is to begin the dural incision at the point of the dural ring and then follow the carotid artery into the cavernous sinus in a retrograde manner.

In past years, fear of uncontrollable venous bleeding kept many neurosurgeons from attempting removal of cavernous sinus lesions. Experience has shown that venous bleeding is usually not of major concern, and can be easily controlled by gently packing with Surgicel gauze.

Of more serious concern is possible entry into the intracavernous carotid artery. For this reason, proximal and distal control is advisable before attempting surgery within the cavernous sinus. This control can be achieved by exposing the carotid artery within the neck before the craniotomy and by being prepared for temporary clipping of the carotid artery in its supraclinoid portion.

In the occasional case in which violation of the intracavernous carotid artery is such that suturing is not enough to control bleeding, the artery may need to be clipped. Placement of a vein graft from the intrapetrous carotid artery to its supraclinoid portion has been recommended by some surgeons. Alternatively, a superficial temporal to middle cerebral artery bypass may be done. The reconstruction of the carotid artery in a case of insufficient collateral circulation carries a high risk of hemiplegia or even death, and for this reason, this procedure must be definitely indicated.

More posteriorly placed cavernous sinus lesions may be approached inferiorly. This can be done by first exposing the intrapetrous carotid artery and then following the artery into the cavernous sinus from below. Sacrifice of the mandibular branch of the trigeminal nerve is necessary to gain the exposure needed for this approach, and this usually is not done unless it has already been destroyed by tumor. Access to the entire cavernous sinus is not possible by this inferior approach.

CLOSURE

The frontal sinus mucosa is dissected free and displaced downward into the ostea. Macerated muscle is packed to fill the sinus cavity. The pericranium is placed over the sinus and then sutured to the dura along the sphenoid ridge. The dura is approximated with interrupted sutures and then closed with a running suture of 4-0 nylon.

The bone flap, including the orbital rim, is replaced with miniplates to reestablish anatomical position. The temporal muscle and fascia are sutured to the temporalis cuff on the bone flap. The galea is closed with 3-0 Vicryl, and the skin is closed with monofilament nylon or skin staples.

RECOMMENDED READING

Al-Mefty, O., Smith, R.: Surgery of tumors invading the cavernous sinus. Surg. Neurol. 30:370–381, 1988.

Hakuba, A.: Orbitozygomatic infratemporal approach for parasellar meningiomas. *In* Schmidek, H. H. (ed): Meningiomas and Their Surgical Management. Philadephia: W. B. Saunders Co., 1991, pp. 451–458.

Hakuba, A., Liu, S., Nishimura, S.: The orbitozygomatic infratemporal approach: A new surgical technique. Surg. Neurol. 26:271, 1986.

McDermott, M., Durity, F., Rootman, J., Woodhurst, W.: Combined frontotemporal-orbitozygomatic approach for tumors of the sphenoid wing and orbit. Neurosurgery 26(1):107–116, 1990.

Sindou, M., Alaywan, M.: Orbital and/or zygomatic removal in an approach to lesions near the cranial base. Surgical technic, anatomic study and analysis of a series of 24 cases. Neurochirurgie 36(4):225–233, 1990.

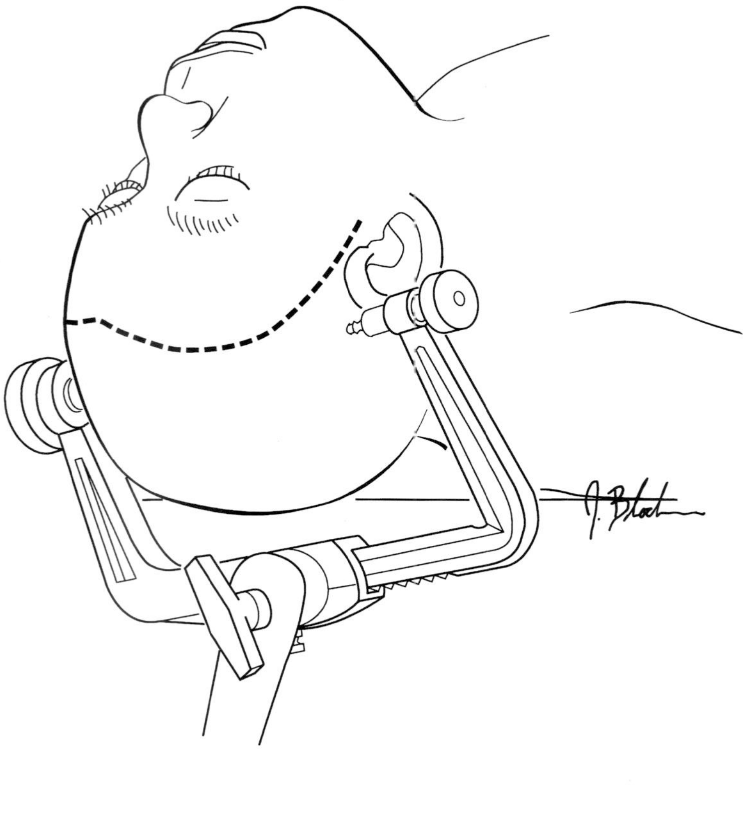

Figure 1. Patient position.

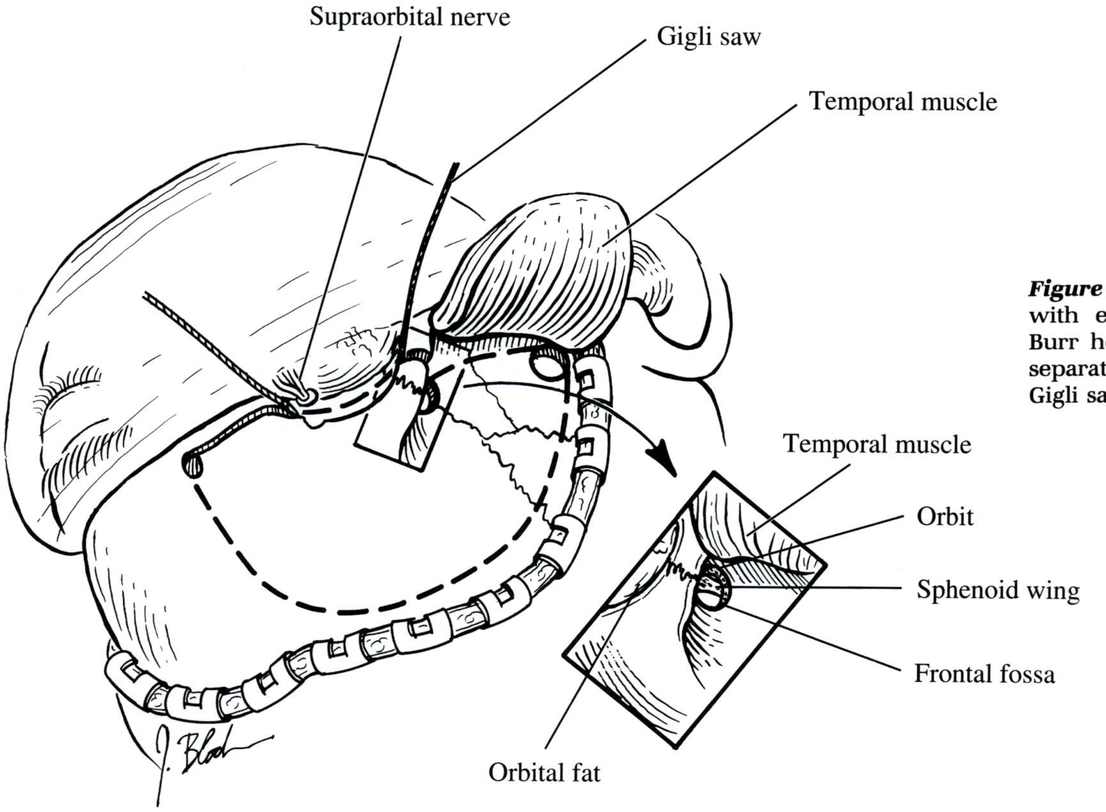

Figure 2. Reflection of scalp flap with exposure of supraorbital rim. Burr hole placement is shown, with separation of dura and passage of Gigli saw.

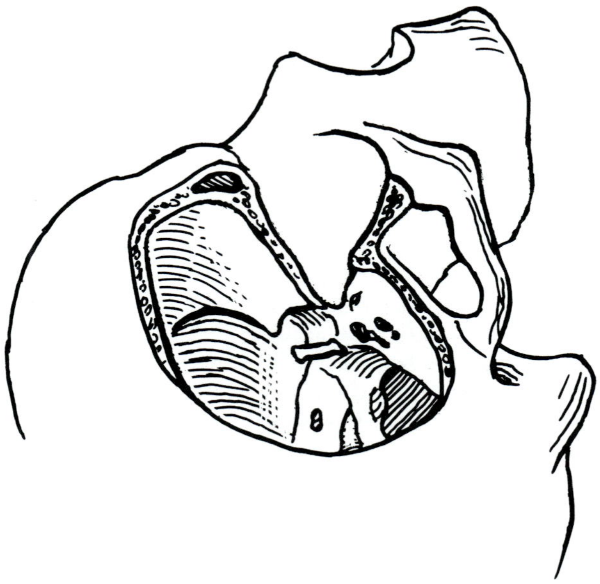

Figure 3. Exposure after extensive drilling of anterior cranial fossa and orbital bone to expose orbits; cranial nerves I, II, III, IV, and V; and internal carotid arteries.

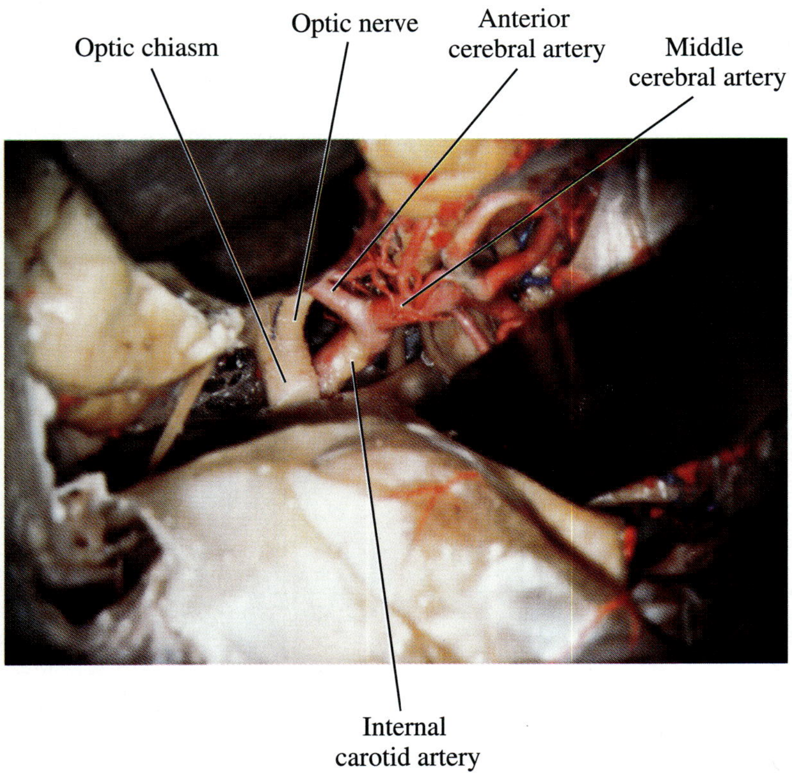

Figure 4. Cadaver dissection specimen to demonstrate the carotid artery bifurcation, middle and anterior cerebral arteries, and relation to optic nerve and chiasm.

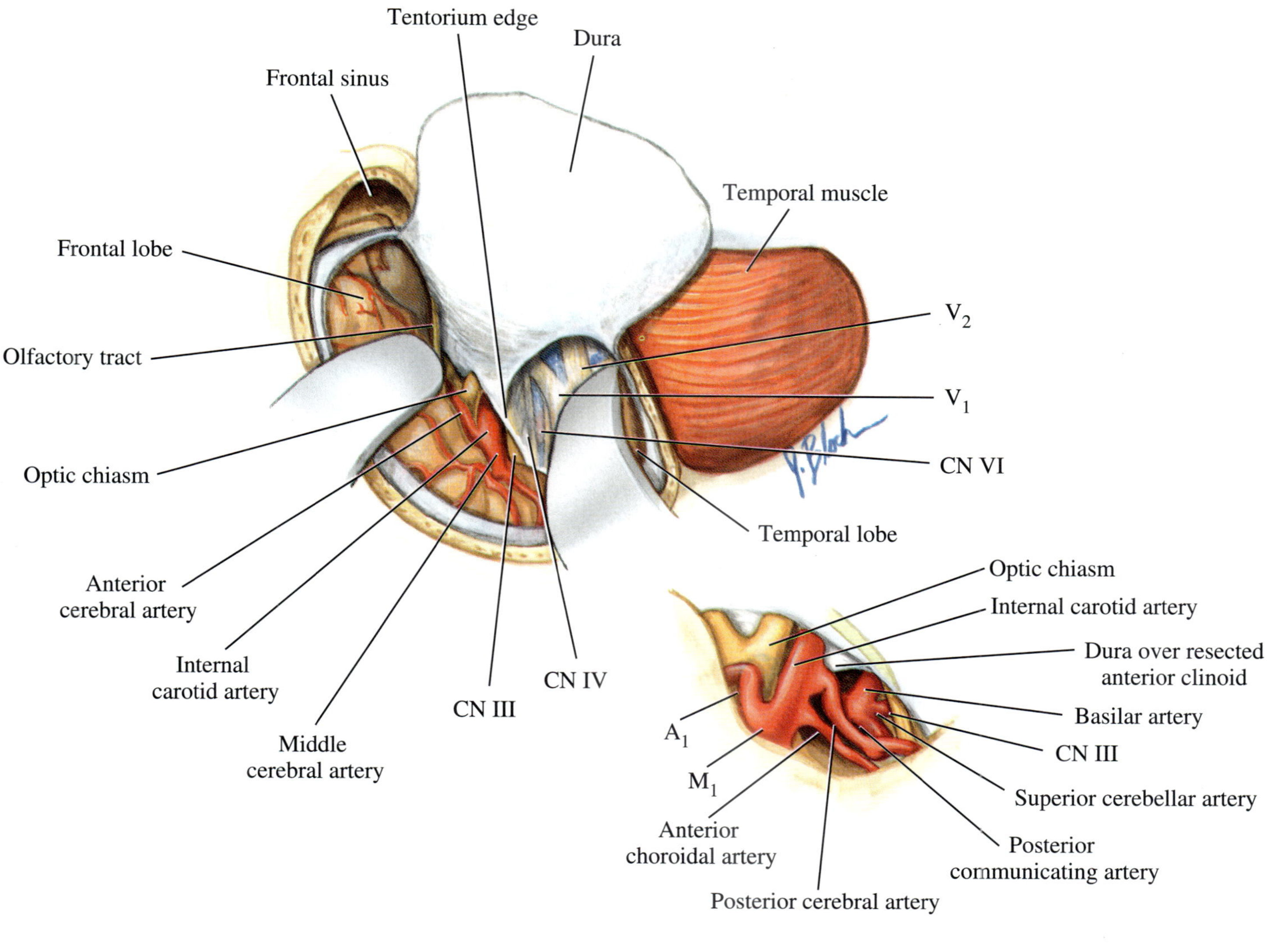

Figure 5. Anterior choroidal and posterior communicating arteries extend from the carotid arteries to the posterior cerebral arteries and basilar artery complex. The relation of the cavernous sinus to surrounding structures is shown.

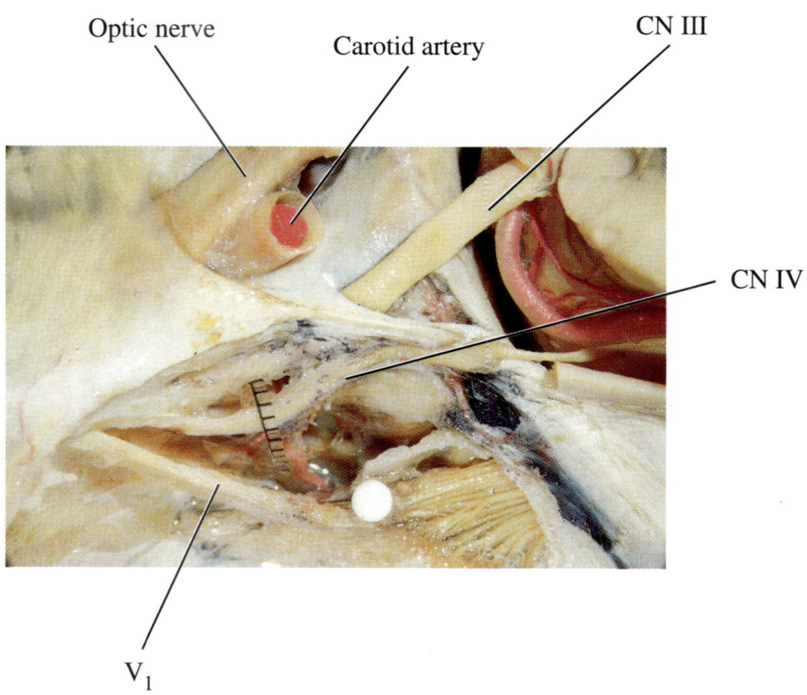

Figure 6. Cadaver dissection showing cavernous sinus opened with carotid artery and cranial nerve branches exposed.

18 Sublabial Transnasal Transmaxillary Sphenoidal Approach to the Sella and Clivus (Modified Midface Degloving)

INDICATIONS

The transnasal-transmaxillary midface degloving exposure is used for those benign or low-grade malignant tumors at the skull base that predominantly involve the clivus. This exposure may also be used in the removal of lesions of the sphenoid, sellar, and parasellar regions. Figure 1 shows computed tomographic and magnetic resonance imaging of a clival tumor that might be removed with this approach.

POSITION

The patient is placed supine in a semirecumbent position with the head slightly elevated and supported on a circular foam cushion in a neutral position. The head is slightly extended. Nonrigid fixation allows intraoperative adjustment of the position of the head. The surgeon stands at either the right or the left side of the patient, depending on the position and extension of the tumor. The best visualization can be obtained by standing on the side opposite the maximum extent of the tumor. The operating microscope usually is positioned on the side opposite the surgeon.

INCISION

The gingival mucosa is infiltrated along the hard palate with lidocaine with epinephrine. The upper lip is retracted, and a sublabial incision is made along the gingival sulcus extending to the lateral maxillary buttress (Figure 2). The periosteum and soft tissues are elevated to expose the maxillary arch, anterior walls of the maxillae, and infraorbital foramina (Figure 3). The infraorbital nerves are preserved, and the anterior nasal spine is partially removed. At this point, the exposure is similar to an extended transsphenoidal approach (see Chapter 9). The next step is to perform unilateral or bilateral Caldwell-Luc sinusotomies (Figure 4). Most of the anterior wall of the maxillary antrum is removed, taking care not to go beyond the lateral buttress. Then the medial maxillary wall is removed on one or both sides (Figure 5A, unilateral opening; Figure 5B, bilateral opening). The anterior ethmoidal cells are entered through the Caldwell-Luc opening and removed. The floor of the orbit is identified and protected. The inferior and superior attachments of the medial maxillary buttress are cut with a 4-mm chisel (Figure 6).

Using heavy, curved scissors, the mucosa of the lower meatus is transected to the posterior pole of the lower turbinate. Using the same scissors, by placing the lower blade into the dissected ethmoid, the upper cut is completed at the root of the middle turbinate. In this cut, the lacrimal duct is dissected free and transected. On completion of this maneuver, the inferior two-thirds of the medial wall of the maxilla is removed, permitting clear visualization of the entire septum. The cartilagenous septum is then dislocated from the maxillary crest after an incision is made separating it from its attachment to the bony septum. The cartilagenous septum must retain its mucoperichondrium on both sides and remains suspended from the dorsum of the nose. The mucosa overlying the bony septum is now easily separated from the vomer and perpendicular plate of the ethmoid and deflected superiorly on both sides. The bony septum is then removed as in the standard transsphenoidal approach. At this point, a contralateral medial maxillectomy is performed. It is best to preserve as much medial wall mucosa and turbinates as possible, provided they do not interfere with the necessary exposure. Mucosal conservation reduces postoperative crusting.

Peripheral ethmoidal cells are removed as needed. The cartilagenous septum is then swung to the side opposite the major extent of the lesion and secured into the soft tissues with a silk suture. At this point, a large Gelpi-type self-retaining retractor (two Gelpi retractors for bilateral exposure) is used to maintain the soft tissues of the midface in a retracted position (Figure 7). The lower jaws of the self-retaining retractors are best anchored in the lower teeth.

On completion of these steps, the anterior wall of the sphenoid, pterygomaxillary fossae, and clivus are brought into view. The exposure beyond this point is determined by the location and extent of the tumor. When necessary, the anterior walls of the sphenoid sinus are opened widely and its mucosa removed (see Figure 7). If tumor extension requires removal of the floor of the sella turcica, this can be done at this time (Figure 8).

The clival bone is exposed after excision of the clival mucosa (Figure 9). A high-speed drill is used to remove the clival bone as needed for exposure. The clivus has numerous venous channels that connect with the cavernous sinuses. Bleeding from these may be controlled with bone wax and gentle packing with Surgicel.

Final removal of the posterior cortical wall of the clivus is done with small Kerrison rongeur forceps to expose the dura overlying the brain stem. Extradural lesions along the clivus are well exposed through this approach, and intradural lesions can be exposed through a midline dural incision.

EXTENDED MAXILLOTOMY

For clival lesions above the hard palate, the sublabial transnasal-transmaxillary approach as described usually is sufficient. If the lesion extends both above and below the hard palate, an extended maxillotomy technique may be necessary. For this procedure, a sublabial incision as described previously is used.

The incision is made along the gingival sulcus overlying the maxilla and extended from the central incisor to a point behind the second molar. The lip and the skin of the face overlying the maxilla are then elevated to expose the anterior and lateral walls of the maxilla, pyriform aperture, infraorbital foramen and nerve, and malar bone and masseter muscle.

The masseter muscle is detached at its malar attachment, and a wedge of malar bone is removed for further exposure of the lateral pterygoid plate and internal maxillary artery. The mucosa of the hard palate is incised behind the teeth from the central incisor and extended to join the retromolar incision.

The mucosa of the hard palate is then elevated toward the midline (Figure 10). The greater palatine artery is coagulated and divided. The mucosa of the hard palate as well as the soft palate, anterior tonsillar pillar, tonsil, and pharynx may then be retracted medially and elevated from the prevertebral fascia. The pterygoid muscles can be divided to expose the lateral pterygoid plate where the internal maxillary artery can then be mobilized (Figure 11). The bony walls of the maxilla and the hard palate are cut with an oscillating saw, and the maxilla can be rotated laterally while maintaining a vascular pedicle to the maxilla.

Additional exposure can be gained by removal of more of the malar bone to include the inferior orbital rim, middle and superior turbinates, ethmoid sinus, anterior sphenoidal sinus, posterior nasal septum, and pterygoid plates at their attachment to the body of the sphenoid.

A vertical midline incision is made through the soft tissue of the posterior wall of the nasopharynx extending from the sphenoid sinus to the foramen magnum. Additionally, a transverse incision can be made from the sphenoid sinus lateral to the nasopharyngeal wall and posterior to the eustachian tube.

Further exposure is achieved with an incision extending from the lateral pharyngeal wall through the anterior tonsillar pillar to the retromolar incision with retraction of the anterior tonsillar pillar, tonsil, and soft palate toward the midline (Figure 12). The pharyngeal wall incision is extended inferiorly to the level of the hyoid bone. The superior constrictor muscle, prevertebral fascia, longus capitis muscle, and anterior longitudinal ligaments can be divided and separated from the bony skull base. The roof of the maxilla, infratemporal fossa, nasal septum, clivus, region of the foramen magnum, foramen lacerum, and lateral pharyngeal muscle to the level of C1-C3 can be exposed through this approach. In Figure 13, the clivus, foramen magnum, and C1 can be seen.

CLOSURE

In the transnasal-transmaxillary procedure, closure is accomplished with a free fascia lata graft overlying the surgical defect. Alternate adipose tissue and fascia layers may be used in larger defects. When possible, fascia is anchored to the retained mucosa with interrupted 3-0 absorbable sutures. Careful packing with 1-inch antibiotic-impregnated petrolatum gauze is critical to support the closure. The gauze is used to pack both maxillary defects and the nose after the septum is set free and reanchored to the maxillary crest. The latter step is accomplished by placing one or more 2-0 absorbable sutures through the inferior edge of the septum into the midline maxillary mucosa, followed by packing of the nasal passages (Figure 14). The gingival buccal incision is closed with two 3-0 continuous Vicryl sutures. The packing should stay in place for 5 to 7 days after surgery.

A moustache dressing is applied to the nose. The patient is maintained in a 45-degree semisitting position during the initial 72 hours after surgery.

For the extended maxillotomy approach, the maxilla is replaced and secured in position with miniplates. The pharyngeal mucosa is closed with 4-0 absorbable suture. Closure of the nasal mucosa is similar to that described in Chapter 9. A vascularized temporalis muscle flap can be used for reconstruction if needed.

RECOMMENDED READING

Casson, P., Bonnano, P., Converse, J.: The midface degloving procedure. Plast. Reconstr. Surg. 53:102–106, 1974.

Cocke, E.W., Jr., Robertson, J.H., Robertson, J.T., et al.: The extended maxillotomy and subtotal maxillectomy for excision of skull base tumors. Arch. Otolaryngol. Head Neck Surg. 116:92, 1990.

Decker, R., Malis, L.: Surgical approaches to midline lesions at the base of the skull. Mt. Sinai J. Med. 37:84–102, 1970.

Miller, R., Woodson, G., Neely, J., Murphy, E.: A surgical approach to chordomas at the base of the skull. Otolaryngol. Head Neck Surg. 90:251–255, 1982.

Price, J.: The midfacial degloving approach to the central skull base. Ear Nose Throat J. 65:174–180, 1986.

Rabadan, A., Benedetti, D., Conesa, H., et al.: Transmaxillary transnasal approach. An anatomomicrosurgical model. *In* Samii, M. (ed.): Surgery of the Sellar Region and Paranasal Sinuses. Heidelberg: Springer-Verlag, 1991, pp. 453–467.

Rabadan, A., Conesa, H.: Transmaxillary-transnasal approach to the anterior clivus: A microsurgical anatomical model. Neurosurgery 30(4):473–481, 1992.

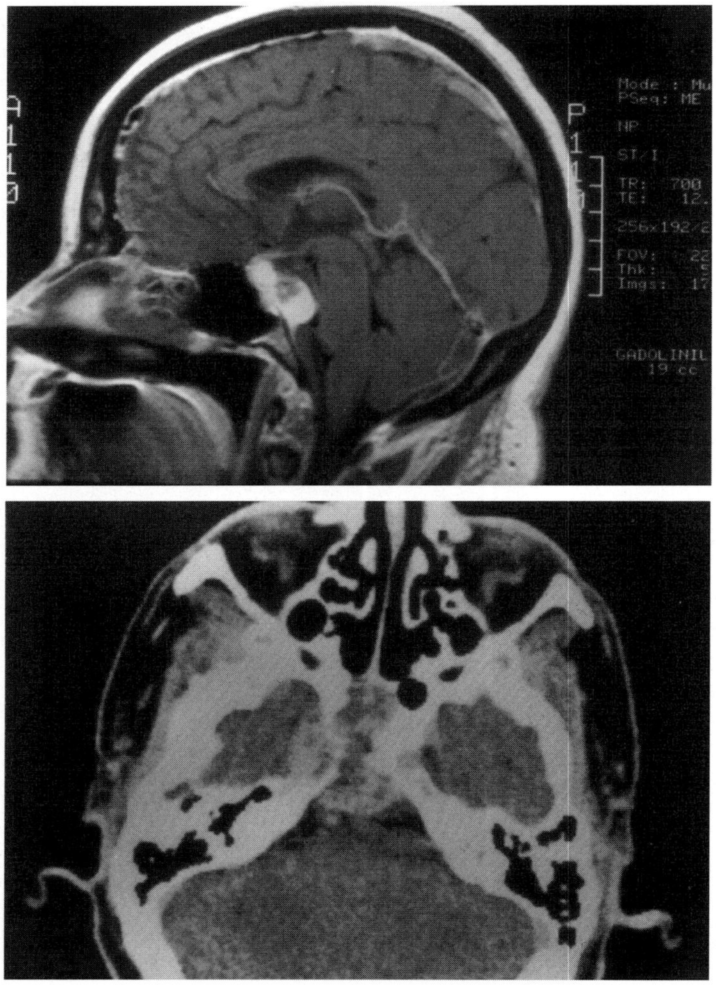

A

B

Figure 1. *A.* Post-gadolinium T_1-weighted sagittal MR image showing a chordoma of the upper clivus with extension into the sellar region. *B.* Axial computed tomographic scan of same patient shown in A, demonstrating extensive bone destruction of the upper clivus.

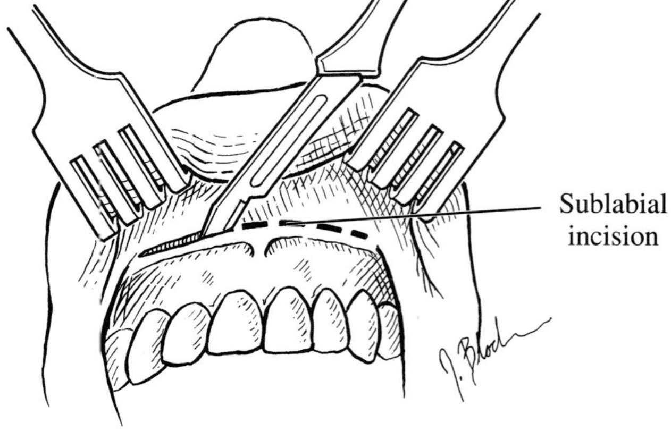

Figure 2. Sublabial incision.

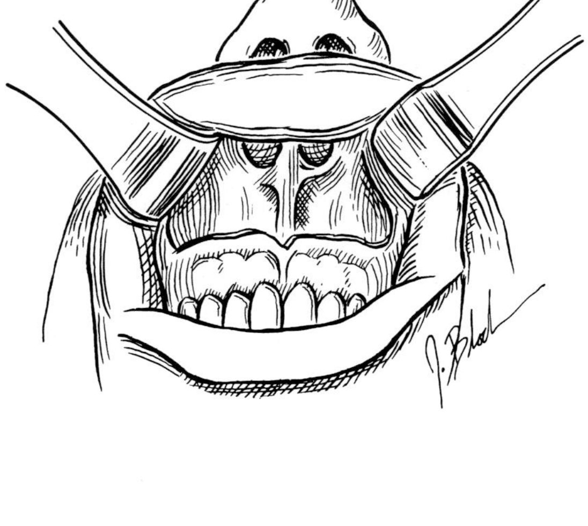

Figure 3. Exposure of the maxillary arch, anterior walls of the maxillae, and infraorbital foramen.

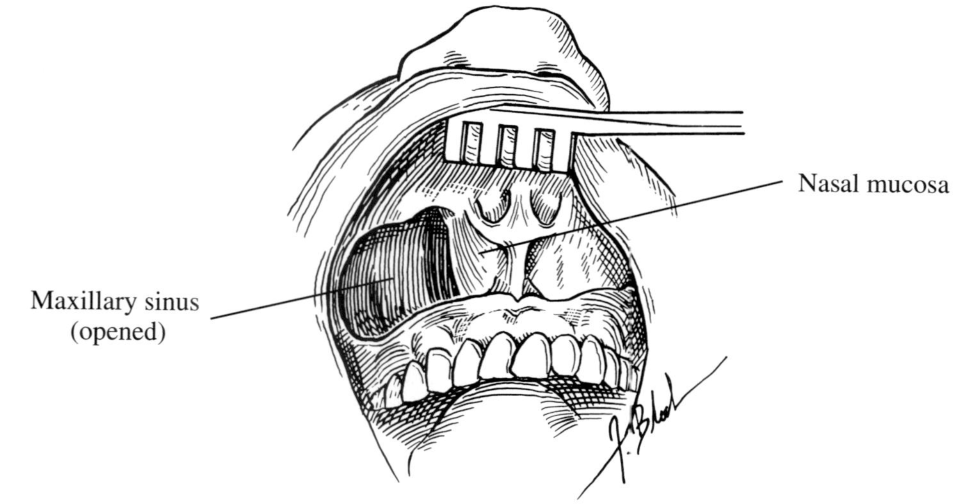

Figure 4. Unilateral Caldwell-Luc procedure.

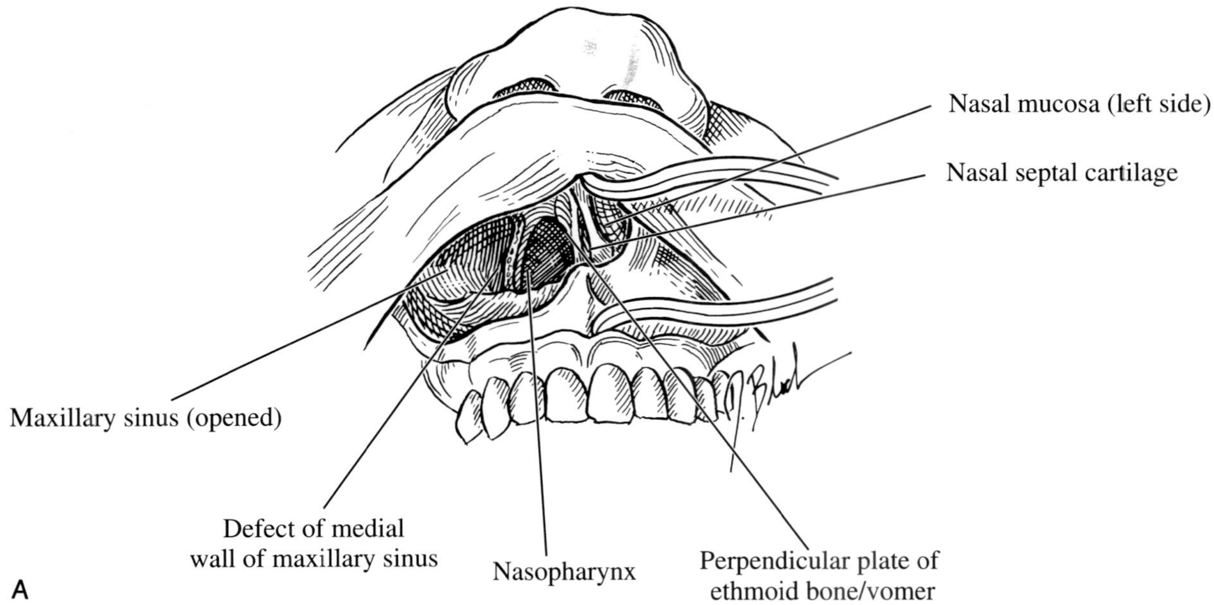

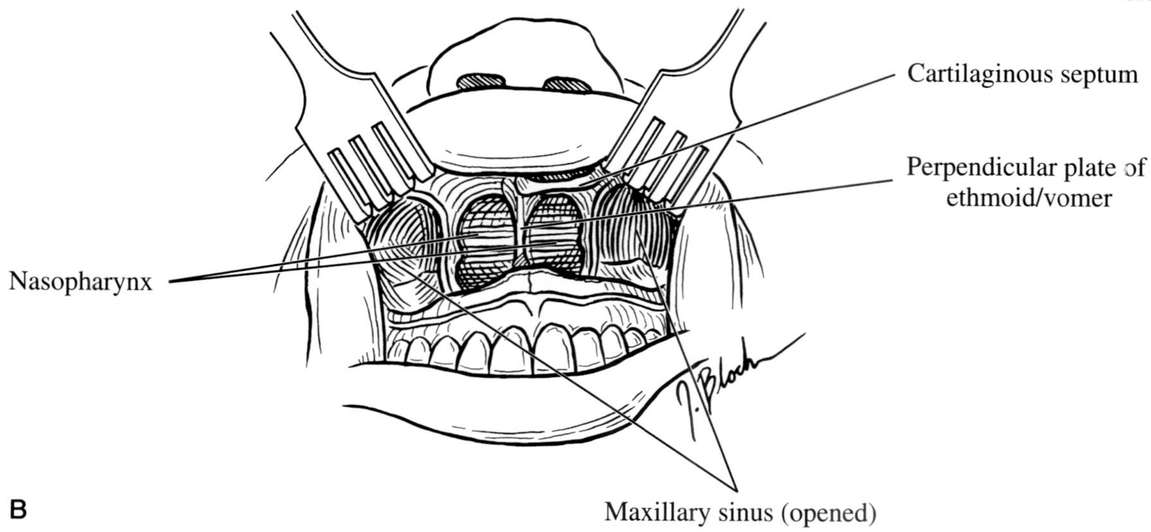

Figure 5. *A.* Removal of medial maxillary wall (unilateral). *B.* Removal of medial maxillary wall (bilateral).

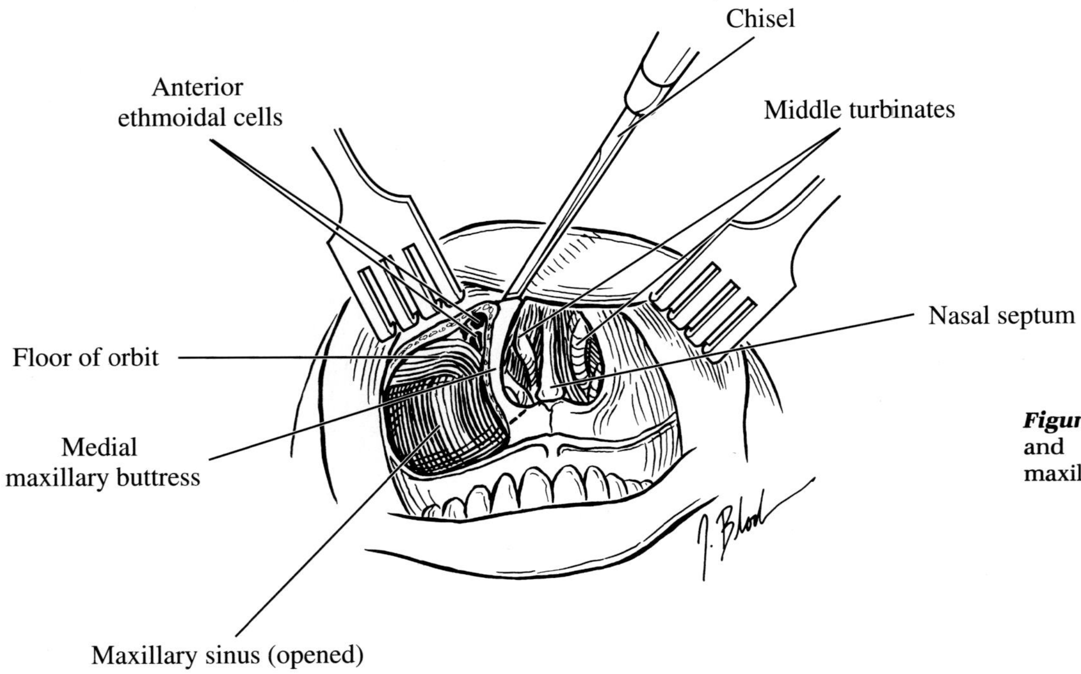

Figure 6. Cutting of the inferior and superior attachments of the maxillary buttress.

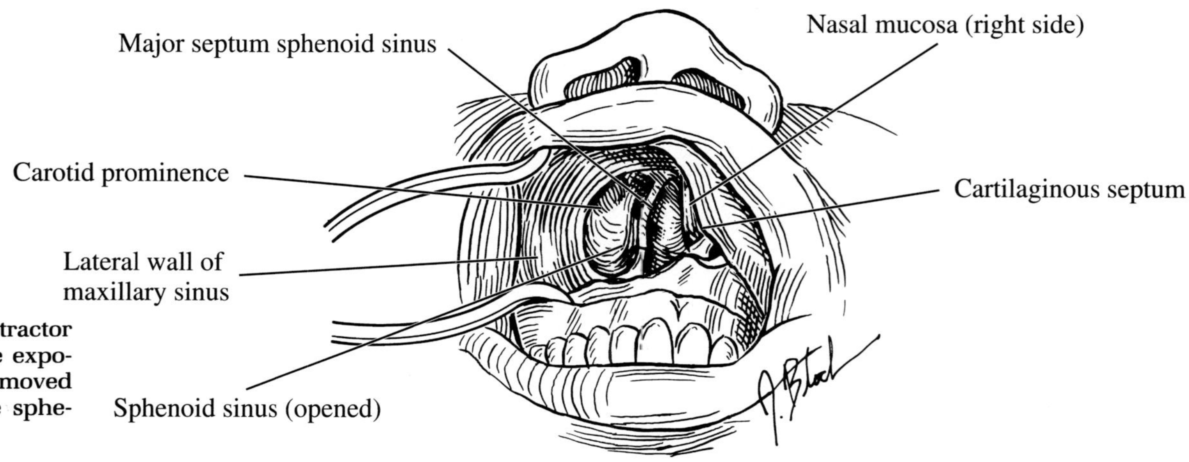

Figure 7. Gelpi retractor maintaining soft tissue exposure. Mucosa is removed from the walls of the sphenoid sinus.

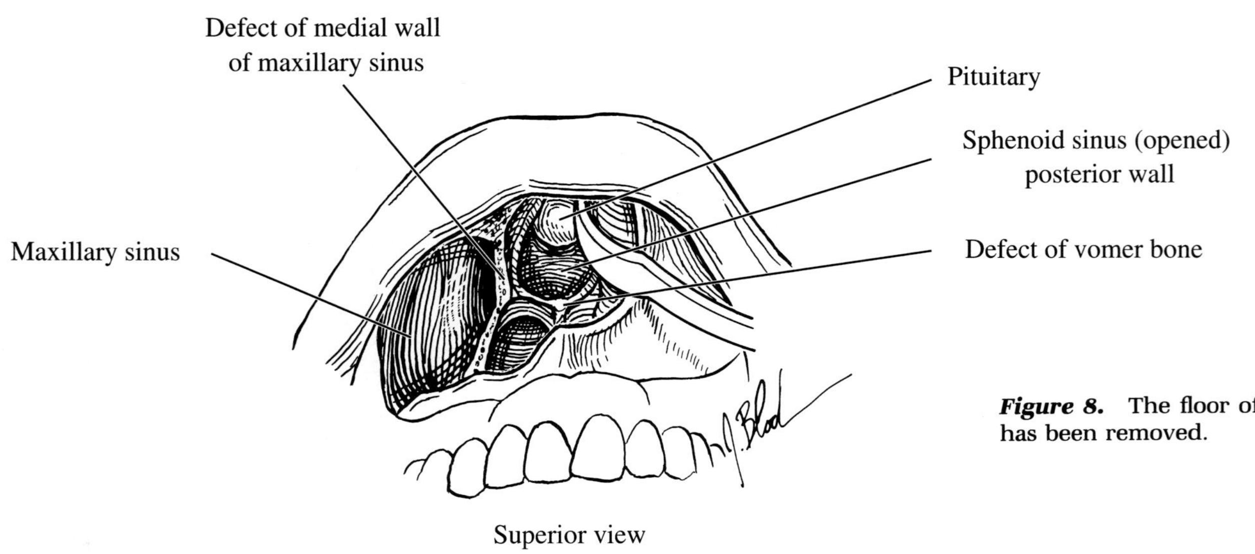

Figure 8. The floor of the sella turcica has been removed.

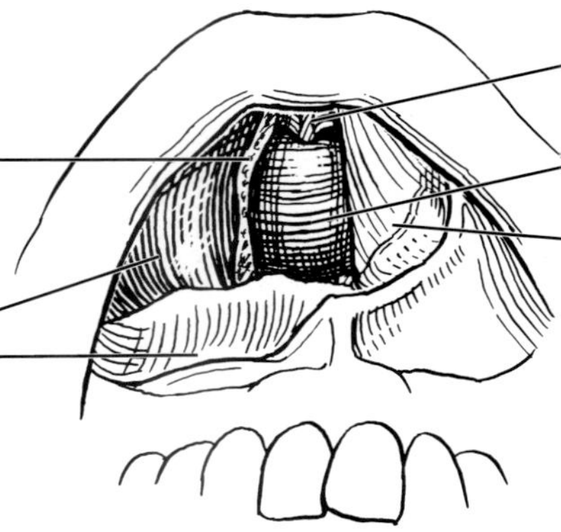

Figure 9. Exposure of the clivus after excision of the clival mucosa.

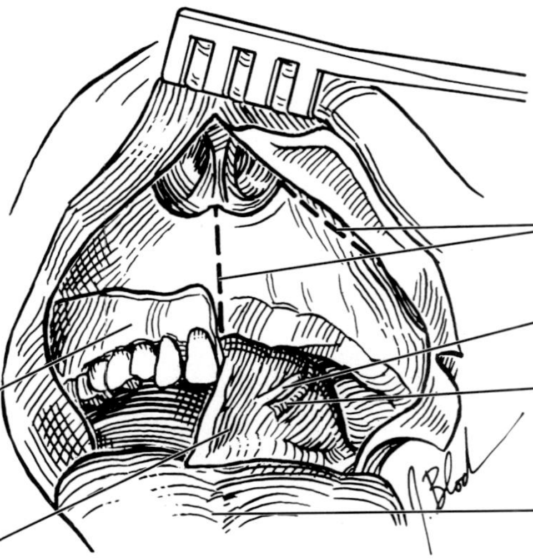

Figure 10. Elevation of the mucosa of the hard palate toward the midline.

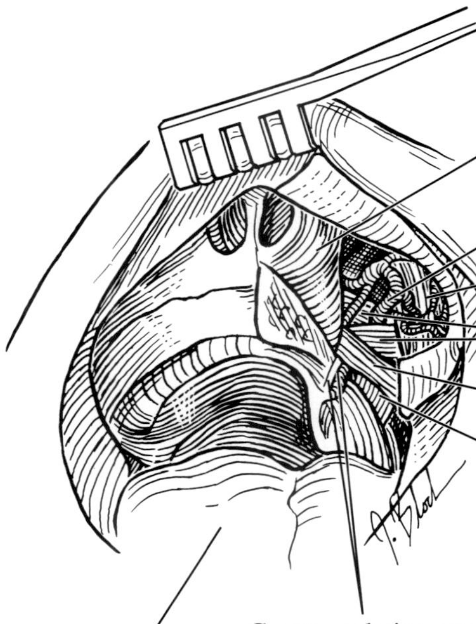

Figure 11. Pterygoid muscles are shown. The internal maxillary artery and its branches are exposed.

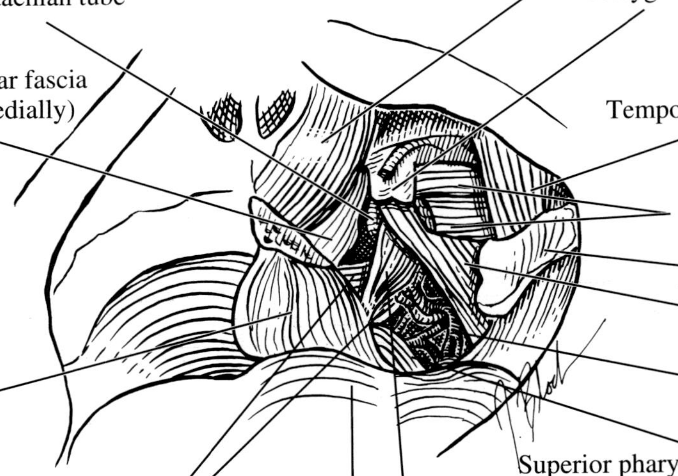

Figure 12. Mucosa is retracted toward the midline to expose the pterygoid plate.

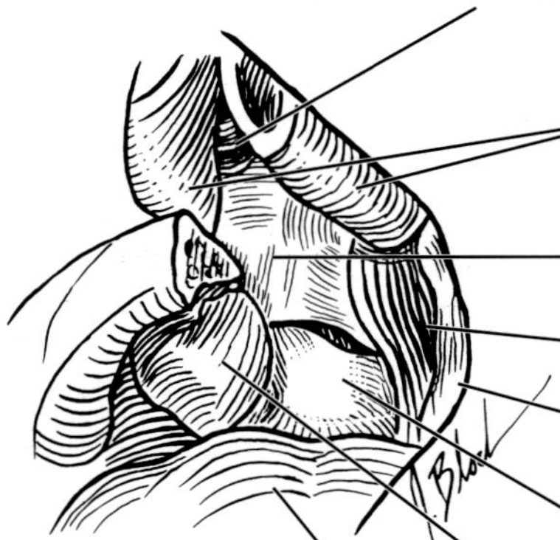

Figure 13. Exposure of the clivus, foramen magnum, and C1. The longus capitis muscle has been retracted laterally.

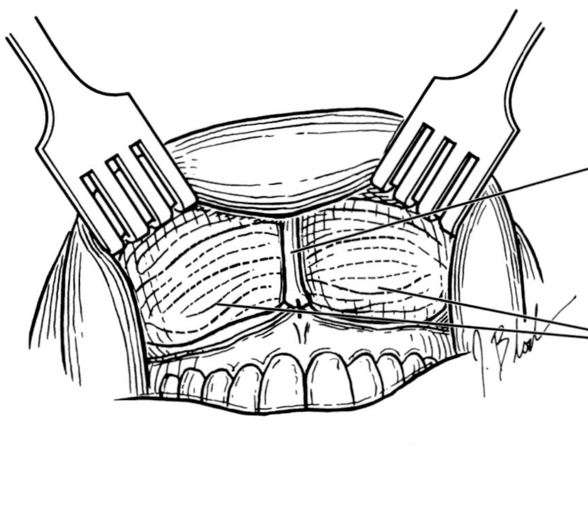

Figure 14. Reapproximation of the inferior edge of the septum to the midline maxillary mucosa.

Ethmoidal Sphenoidal Approach to the Sella and Clivus 19

INDICATIONS

The ethmoidal sphenoidal approach to the sella and clivus may be useful for the excision of skull base tumors that arise in the ethmoid or sphenoid sinus or along the clivus. It primarily offers extracranial access to these areas.

POSITION

The patient is placed in the supine position with the head slightly elevated and supported on a circular foam cushion and turned 15 degrees toward the side of the operation. The head is elevated 30 degrees above the level of the heart. Bilateral protective tarsorrhaphies are done, and the face is prepared.

INCISION

An incision is made from the inferior margin of the eyebrow and curved gently downward, following the curvature of the lateral nose, and ending at the crease of the nostril. It is positioned midway between the bridge of the nose and the inner canthus of the eye (Figure 1). The incision is deepened to the periosteum, which is separated from the bone to expose the medial and inferior orbit.

EXPOSURE

The periorbita and the orbital contents are retracted laterally. The lacrimal sac and lacrimal duct are identified and preserved medially, and the inferior wall of the frontal sinus is opened. Next, the ethmoid sinus is opened and the bone of the ethmoid air cells is progressively removed until the sphenoid sinus is entered. The anatomical relationship of the ethmoid and sphenoid sinuses to the clivus is shown in Figure 2.

An extensive exposure of the interior of the entire sphenoid sinus is achieved by removal of sphenoid septae along with the anterior wall and floor (Figure 3). For removal of clival tumors, additional removal of the clivus is done as needed. The septum has to be transected and displaced laterally. The optic nerve and carotid artery as well as other structures within the cavernous sinus must be protected. The posterior ethmoid artery must be identified at its foramen and left intact. Dissection beyond this important landmark can result in injury to the optic nerve. The anterior knee of the carotid artery can be exposed on the ipsilateral side. Care is exercised to avoid entry into the contralateral carotid artery as the midline is crossed.

Additional exposure can be obtained with a medial maxillectomy if needed for removal of larger tumors. This consists of removing the medial wall of the maxillary sinus as far laterally as the infraorbital foramen. Medially, the turbinates are removed as well.

Wide exposure of the tumor bed is now offered, extending from the nasal passages to the entire clivus.

CLOSURE

After achieving careful hemostasis, the wound is inspected for evidence of dural defect and cerebrospinal fluid leak. Openings in the dura are closed with fascia lata, lyophilized dura, muscle, or a piece of galea aponeurotica and then sealed with fibrin glue. The dural graft is supported by nasal packing, which is left for 5 to 7 days. The subcutaneous tissue layer is closed with 4-0 Vicryl, and the skin is closed with 4-0 nylon or Steri-Strips.

Postoperative lumbar spinal drainage is continued for 5 to 7 days to assist in avoidance of a cerebrospinal fluid leak.

RECOMMENDED READING

Cocke, E., Robertson, J.H., Robertson, J.T., Crook, J.: The extended maxillotomy and subtotal maxillectomy for excision of skull base tumors. Arch. Otolaryngol. Head Neck Surg. 116:92–104, 1990.

Lalwlani, A., Kaplan, M., Gutin, P.: The transsphenoethmoid approach to the sphenoid sinus and clivus. Neurosurgery 31 (6): 1008–1014, 1992.

Samii, M., Draf, W.: Surgery of the Skull Base: An Interdisciplinary Approach. New York: Springer-Verlag, 1989.

Samii, M., Knosp, E.: Approaches to the Clivus. New York: Springer-Verlag, 1992.

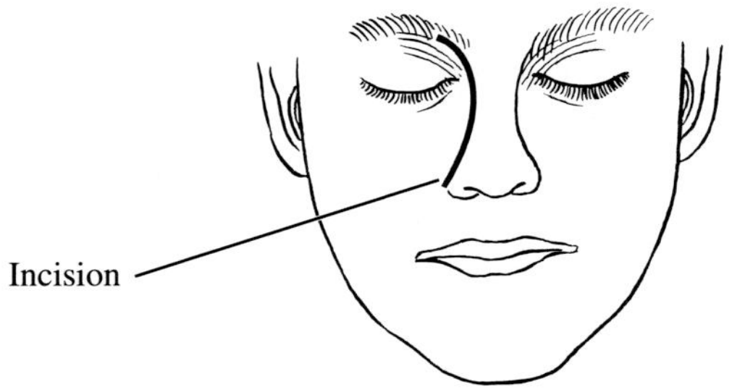

Figure 1. Facial skin incision (bilateral tarsorrhaphies have been done).

Figure 2. Extensive exposure of the sphenoid and ethmoid sinuses (lateral view).

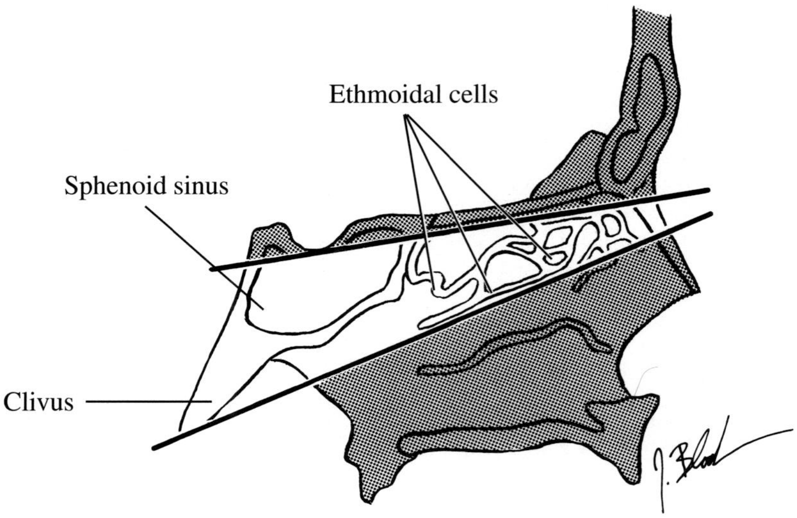

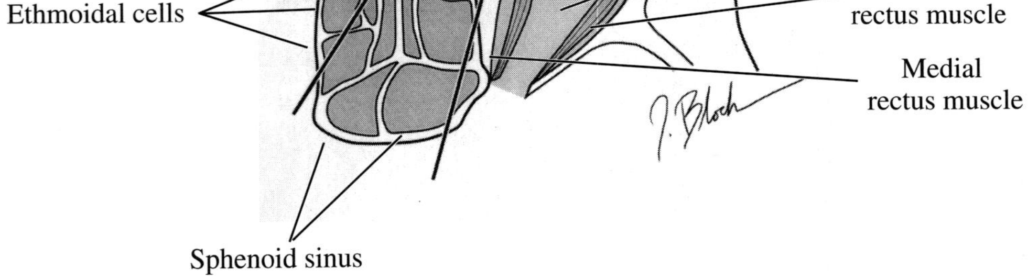

Figure 3. Extensive exposure of sphenoid and ethmoid sinuses (dorsal view).

20 Transoral Approach to the Clivus and C1–C2

J. Patrick Johnson

INDICATIONS

Transoral procedures are useful in approaching primarily midline lesions of the clivus, anterior craniocervical junction, and upper anterior cervical spinal canal. The transoral approach can be used for lesions that extend from the midclivus to the upper cervical spine at C2. It is limited in offering access to lesions that are not near the midline. The approach is useful for removing both intradural and extradural tumors and is now being used in the clipping of aneurysms of the basilar artery. Chordomas of the lower clivus and craniocervical junction are the most common neoplastic mass lesions removed through a transoral approach. It is also the procedure used for anterior cervical cord decompression in patients with advanced rheumatoid arthritis affecting the odontoid and its supporting ligamentous structures. Drainage of neurenteric cysts can also be done orally.

The operating microscope has provided the magnification necessary to operate through a relatively deep and limited exposure as well as the illumination necessary for such procedures.

PATIENT POSITION

The patient is placed in the supine position with the head in extension. The supine position is used for delayed two-stage procedures, and the patient is placed flat with appropriate padding. For transoral surgery that is followed by immediate second-stage posterior occipital-cervical fixation, the patient is placed in a lateral position. In this way, the oral procedure can be followed by posterior fixation without having to move the patient intraoperatively.

When the lateral position is used, the patient is placed facing the surgeon with the head secured in a Mayfield-Kees headholder and held in a neutral position. The table can then be rotated and redraped for immediate posterior occipital to cervical fusion.

Fiberoptic nasal tracheal intubation is necessary when the patient has evidence of craniocervical junction instability or a stenotic cervical spinal canal.

OPERATIVE PROCEDURE

The face, oral cavity, and nasopharyngeal region are prepared with topical iodine, and sterile drapes are applied. The oropharynx is protected with vaginal packing to prevent blood and irrigation fluid from entering the stomach. The transoral retractor is then placed in the oral cavity as shown in Figure 1.

The tongue is depressed inferiorly with the retractor, and the endotracheal tube is moved into the lateral oropharynx. The midline of the posterior pharyngeal wall and uvula are infiltrated with 1% lidocaine with epinephrine for hemostasis.

The anterior tubercle of C1 can be palpated and verified with a lateral radiograph. The operating microscope is brought into position, and the entire operative procedure is performed with microscopic magnification.

A paramedian or median incision can be made in the uvula and extended in the midline of the soft palate to the hard palate. Temporary sutures are placed to retract the bisected uvula laterally and out of the surgeon's field (Figure 2). The posterior pharyngeal wall is incised vertically in the midline, and the soft tissues can then be elevated over the anterior arch of C1 with a periosteal dissector. The self-retaining pharyngeal retractor is placed to expose the arch of C1 (Figure 3).

Exposure of the clivus in a cephalic direction and of the upper cervical region in a caudal direction may require extension of the midline incision.

Chordomas of the clivus are often exposed with the initial retraction of the pharyngeal soft tissues, but other pathologies that involve the odontoid or masses in the upper cervical region require removal of the anterior arch of C1. The arch of C1 and the odontoid can be drilled with a cutting burr, after which a diamond burr is used for final drilling of the posterior cortex of the bone (Figure 4). Drilling of the odontoid is done by removing bone in its center, converting it into a boat shape. The remaining cortical bone is then chipped out with small curettes or Kerrison rongeurs.

Intradural pathology requires a more extensive bone removal, and the dural opening is performed vertically in the midline. Figure 5 shows the basilar and vertebral arteries and the anterior surface of the pons and medulla exposure in a cadaver specimen. The anatomical relations along the posterior surface of the clivus and the cerebellopontine angle are shown in the cadaver dissection in Figure 6.

CLOSURE

Primary closure of the dura is often difficult, and fascia lata is the preferred grafting material. In addition to the specialized long instrumentation of the transoral set, we have found that the fine, extra-long gynecological needleholders with curved tip are useful for the closure.

The posterior pharyngeal wall is closed in two layers with the constrictor muscles and the pharyngeal mucosa. The uvula is closed in both anterior and posterior mucosal layers. Patients with preoperative instability or those undergoing resection of the odontoid and its supporting ligamentous structures may have increased instability and must be maintained in craniocervical fixation until definitive posterior occipital-to-cervical fusion is performed. Most patients can be extubated immediately, but some should remain nasotracheally intubated for 1 to 3 days, depending on the amount of pharyngeal swelling seen on lateral craniocervical radiographs.

RECOMMENDED READING

Crockard, H.A., Sen, C.N.: The transoral approach for the management of intradural lesions at the craniocervical junction: Review of 7 cases. Neurosurgery 28(1):88–97, 1991.

Di Lorenzo, N.: Transoral approach to extradural lesions of the lower clivus and upper cervical spine: An experience of 19 cases. Neurosurgery 24(1):37–42, 1989.

Hadley, M.N., Spetzler, R.F., Sonntag, V.K.: The transoral approach to the superior cervical spine. A review of 53 cases of extradural cervicomedullary compression. J. Neurosurg. 71(1):16–23, 1989.

Hayakawa, T., Yamada, K., Yoshimine, T.: Transoral transclival approach: Anatomical and technical notes. No Shinkei Geka. Neurol. Surg. 17(7):609–614, 1989.

Merwin, G.E., Post, J.C., Sypert, G.W.: Transoral approach to the upper cervical spine. Laryngoscope 101(7, Pt 1):780–784, 1991.

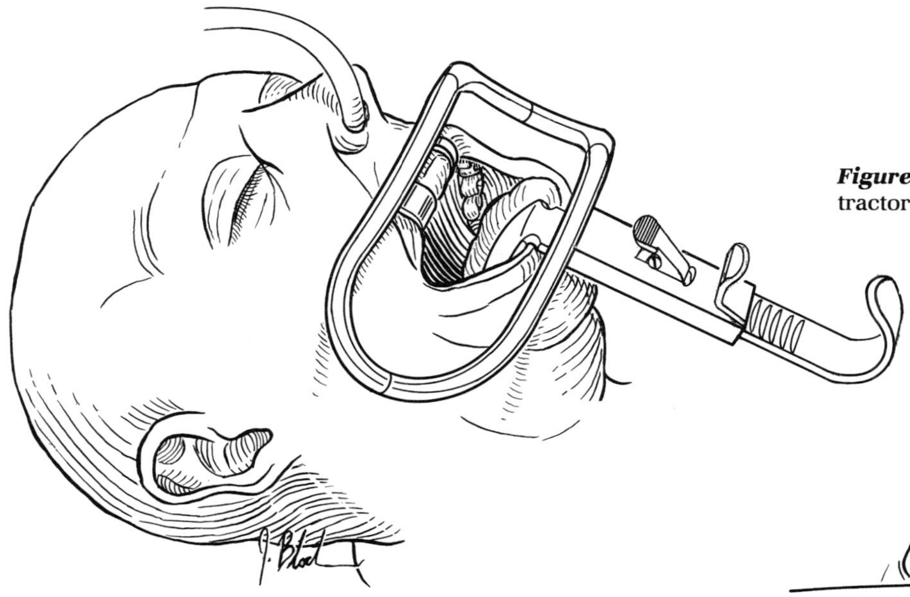

Figure 1. Placement of the Crockard transoral retractor and position of nasotracheal tube.

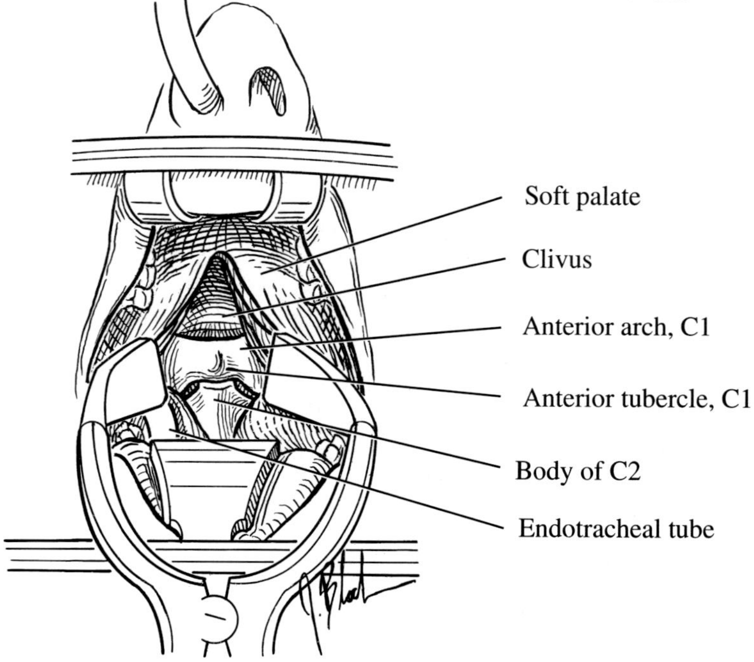

Figure 2. Paramedian incision of the uvula extended to the midline of the soft and hard palates and pharyngeal wall.

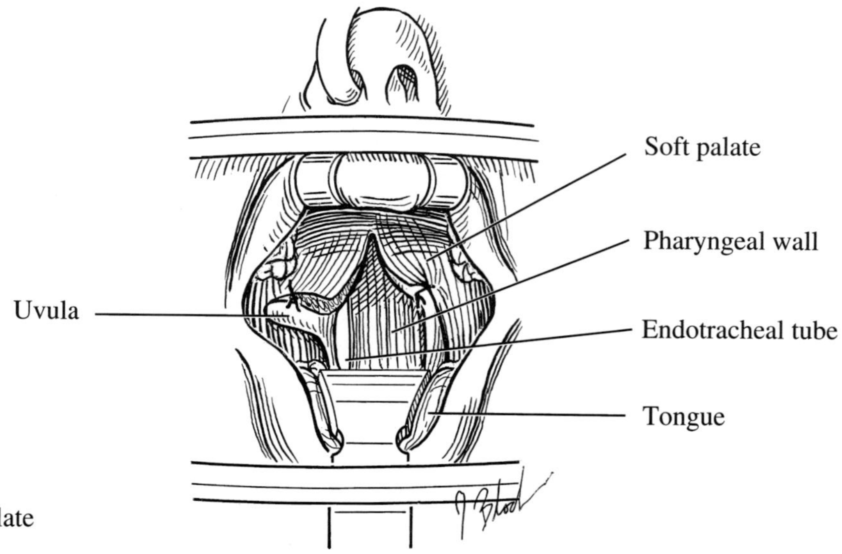

Figure 3. Placement of self-retaining pharyngeal retractor to expose the arch of C1.

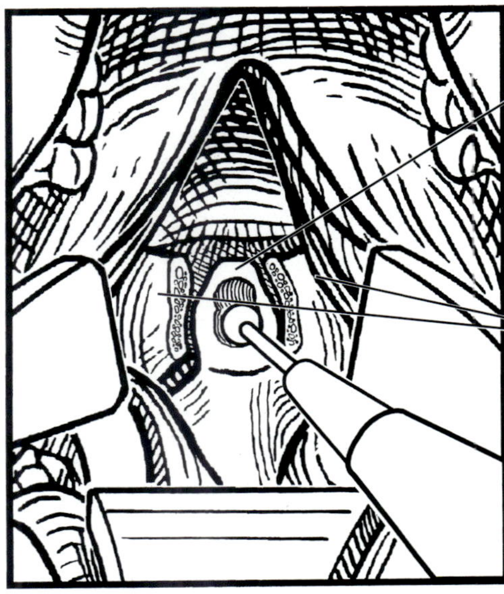

Figure 4. Drilling of the arch of C1 and the odontoid with a high-speed drill with a diamond burr.

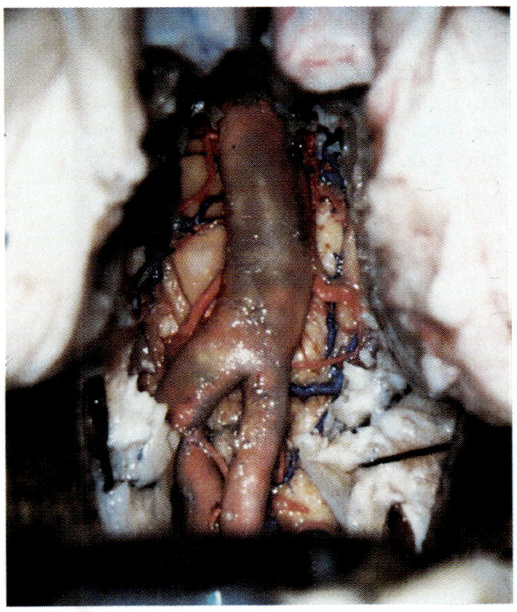

Figure 5. Brain stem and vertebrobasilar artery system after midline transoral exposure and dural opening.

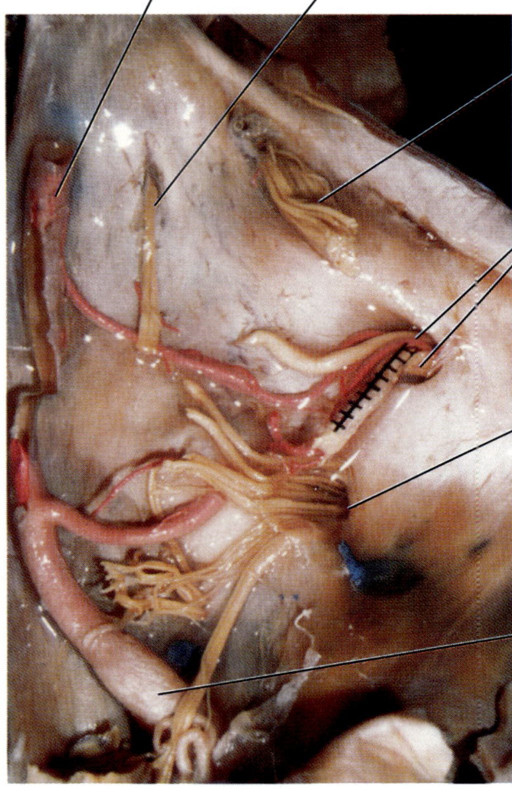

Figure 6. Anatomical relations along the posterior clivus and cerebellopontine angle as seen in a cadaver specimen.

21 Orbitotomy: Medial Approach
(Paranasal-Ethmoidal)

Howard R. Krauss *and* Robert Alan Goldberg

The medial orbital space may be entered by various means. A transconjunctival approach is appropriate for access to the medial intraconal space or for anterior optic nerve sheath decompression. A transcutaneous approach to the anterior medial and superior extraconal orbital space may be made by way of a number of incisions, including lid crease, subbrow, and modified Lynch. A transethmoidal approach is appropriate for pathology including the sinus or for exposure of the posterior medial and superior orbit for biopsy, excision of tumor, or decompression of the orbital apex.

In most cases, general anesthesia is preferred; selected cases may be performed with peribulbar or retrobulbar block with sedation. Standard ophthalmic preparation and draping are performed with the patient in the supine position.

TRANSCONJUNCTIVAL MEDIAL ORBITOTOMY

A lid speculum is used to maintain an open palpebral aperture. The assistant surgeon assures adequate moisturization of the cornea, positioning and protection of the globe, maintenance of hemostasis, and adequate retraction of tissues. The conjunctiva is opened at the limbus for 360 degrees or medially over at least 180 degrees with relaxing incisions, as needed. Tenon's capsule and the intermuscular septum are gently divided in the medial oblique quadrants, allowing procurement of the medial rectus muscle tendon with a muscle hook. A double-armed 5-0 or 6-0 Vicryl or Dexon suture with spatula needle is then woven through the full width of the tendon 1 mm posterior to its natural insertion, and a suture-locking loop is made superiorly and inferiorly. A blunt Westcott scissors is used to detach the tendon. A 4-0 silk suture is baseball-stitched through the scleral insertion site for use as a traction suture in maintaining abduction of the globe (Figure 1.) Sometimes a self-retaining Kennerdell medial orbital retractor is used. The operating microscope is now used. Medial retraction of the medial rectus muscle tendon and abduction of the globe reveal the posterior Tenon's capsule, which is opened for access to the medial intraconal space. Orbital fat is gently displaced with the use of cotton-tipped applicators. Bleeding most often resolves spontaneously and cauterization is avoided; when cauterization is used, it is bipolar with irrigation. Topical thrombin may be used. In performance of optic nerve sheath fenestration for pseudotumor cerebri, dural vessels must not be disturbed. Entry may be made into the subarachnoid space with a myringotomy blade (Figure 2) and the incision extended with a scissors. Subarachnoid adhesions are then lysed to allow adequate egress of cerebrospinal fluid, and several fenestrations may be made or a window of dura may be removed. Retractors are removed. The microscope is moved out of position. The silk traction suture is removed.

Closure

Closure is accomplished with reattachment of the medial rectus muscle tendon and reapproximation of the conjunctiva with interrupted 7-0 or 8-0 absorbable sutures.

TRANSCUTANEOUS MEDIAL OR ANTERIOR ORBITOTOMY

The approach is varied in accordance with the needs of the individual case. The skin incision may be a lid crease, subbrow (superior orbital rim), or modified Lynch (Figure 3). A lid crease incision offers the best cosmetic result but requires the greatest care to avoid damage to the levator aponeurosis and muscle; it offers an approach to the superior extraconal space, including the lacrimal gland. The subbrow approach may be preferred for access to the superior subperiosteal space. The modified Lynch approach gives more direct access to the medial wall, ethmoidal arteries, and medial extraconal space. In most cases, a solution with 1:200,000 epinephrine is injected subcutaneously to aid in the maintenance of a hemostatic field.

In the lid crease incision, a No. 15 Bard-Parker blade is used for the skin incision. Then, while the assistant distracts the lid inferiorly, 0.3- or 0.5-mm Castroviejo forceps and blunt Westcott scissors or Stevens tenotomy scissors are used to penetrate and open the orbicularis muscle in line with the skin incision.

A Desmarres retractor may then be used to retract the skin and orbicularis superiorly, exposing the superior orbital septum (Figure 4). The orbital septum is opened widely just inferior to the superior orbital rim, thus avoiding damage to the levator aponeurosis. Superior orbital fat then presents and is displaced during surgical exploration. If need be, fat may be excised, but traction must be minimized and bipolar cauterization may be used to reduce the risk of retrobulbar hemorrhage. Closure is accomplished with running 6-0 nylon or Prolene. Sutures are removed 4 days postoperatively.

In the subbrow incision, the surgeon seeks to avoid severance of the supratrochlear and supraorbital branches of cranial nerve V_1 when possible. Parallel supratrochlear and supraorbital arteries may also be present. At the supraorbital rim, the periosteum is incised, and a Freer elevator is used to enter the superior subperiosteal space. The trochlea is a cartilaginous pulley applied to the superonasal periosteum; reflecting it with the periosteum avoids damage to the action of the superior oblique muscle and tendon.

In the modified Lynch incision, one seeks to avoid severance of the angular artery or vein (Figure 5). The incision of periosteum is made anterior to the anterior lacrimal crest, thus allowing reflection of the medial canthal ligament and lacrimal drainage apparatus within the protective covering of periorbita. As the periorbita is elevated off the lamina papyracea, the anterior and posterior ethmoidal arteries are identified (Figure 6). If necessary, these arteries may be coagulated and severed to allow greater exposure. The arteries provide an important landmark, being at the level of the roof of the ethmoid sinus. This approach also allows access to the medial portions of the superior and inferior orbit. If periosteum is elevated off the orbital floor, the surgeon does this posterior to the nasolacrimal duct, thus avoiding damage to the lacrimal drainage apparatus.

At the conclusion of surgery, reapproximation of the periosteum with absorbable suture aids in the maintenance of superior oblique muscle and tendon function and normal medial canthal appearance.

TRANSETHMOIDAL ORBITOTOMY

The transethmoidal approach to the posterior medial and superior orbit may be used for biopsy, excision of tumor, or decompression of the orbital apex. The modified Lynch incision is used. Anterior and posterior ethmoidal arteries are identified, coagulated, and severed. The lamina papyracea is removed with rongeurs posterior to the lacrimal crest and inferior to the ethmoidal artery foramina. This is done posteriorly to the beginning of the optic foramen, and an external ethmoidectomy is carried out. The periorbita is then opened, allowing orbital exploration or decompression.

RECOMMENDED READING

Hurwitz, J., Freeman, J., Eplett, C., et al.: Ethmoidectomy decompression for the treatment of Graves' optic neuropathy. Can. J. Ophthalmol. 27:283–287, 1992.

McCord, C., Jr.: A combined lateral and medial orbitotomy for exposure of the optic nerve and orbital apex. Ophthalmic Surg. 9:58–66, 1978.

Rootman, J.: Diseases of the Orbit. A Multidisciplinary Approach. Philadelphia: J.B. Lippincott, 1988.

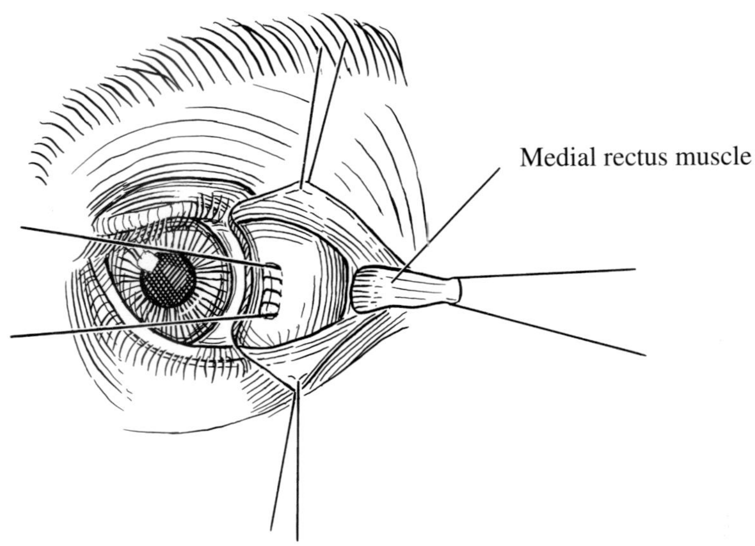

Figure 1. A 4-0 silk suture placed in the stump of the detached medial rectus muscle is used as a traction suture to rotate and displace the globe laterally.

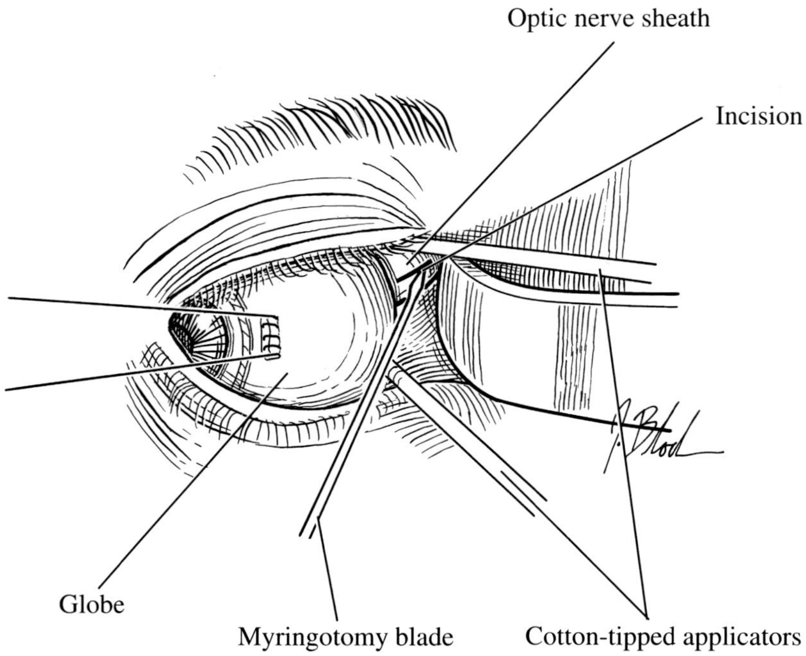

Figure 2. The optic nerve is exposed behind the globe, using blunt dissection. Entry through the optic nerve dura into the perineural subarachnoid space is made with a microscalpel.

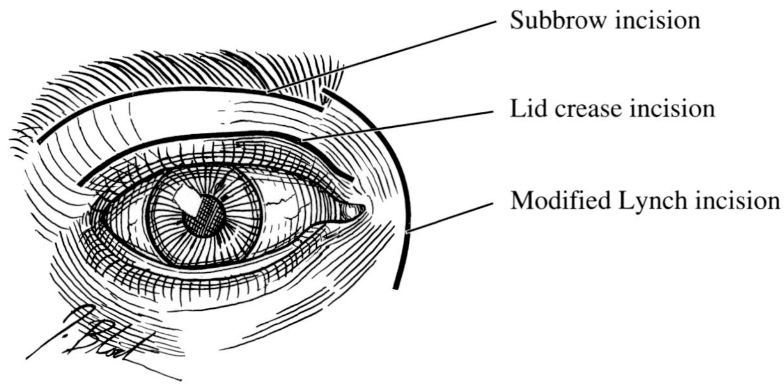

Figure 3. Cutaneous incisions for anterior orbitotomy.

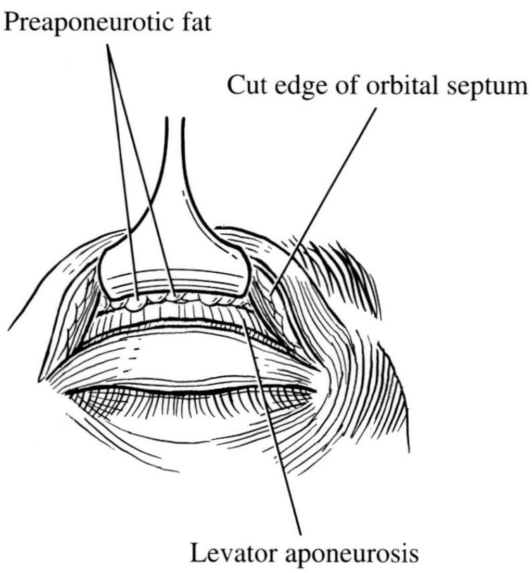

Figure 4. Retraction of skin and orbicularis superiorly with Desmarres retractor, exposing the superior orbital septum.

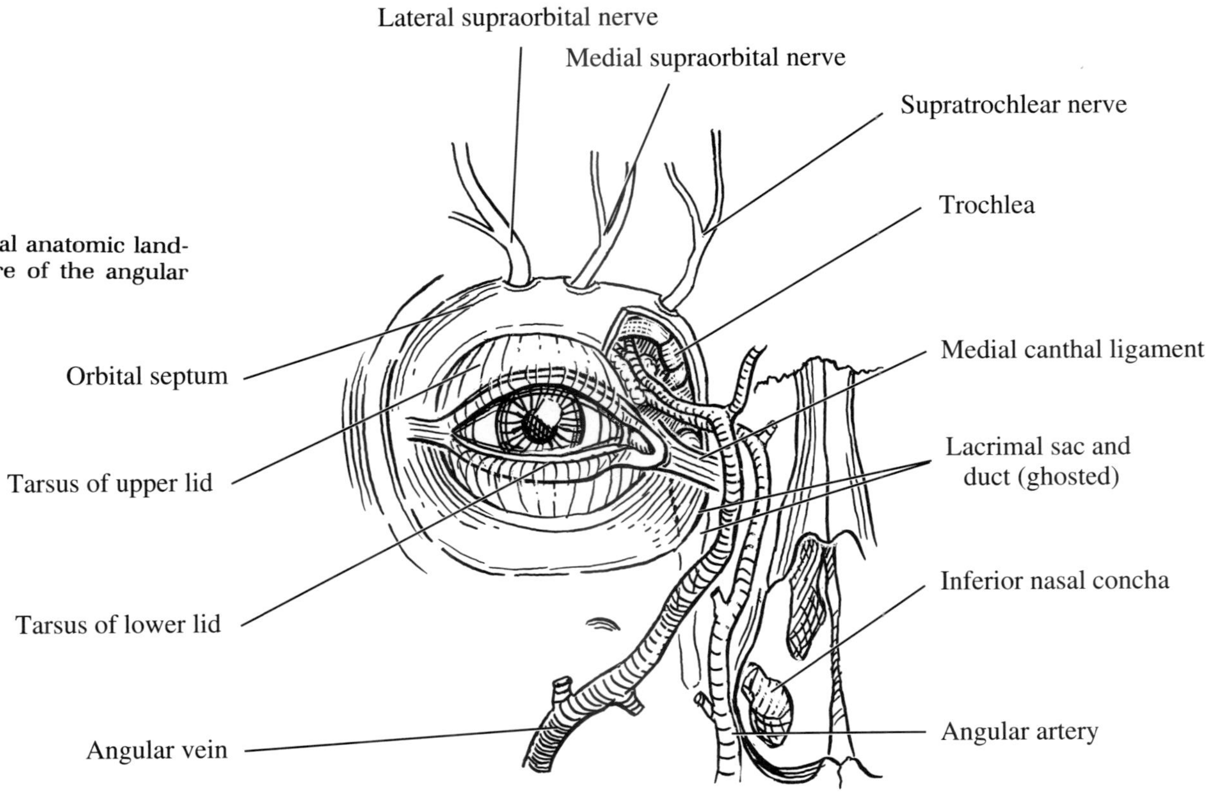

Figure 5. Periorbital anatomic landmarks with exposure of the angular artery and vein.

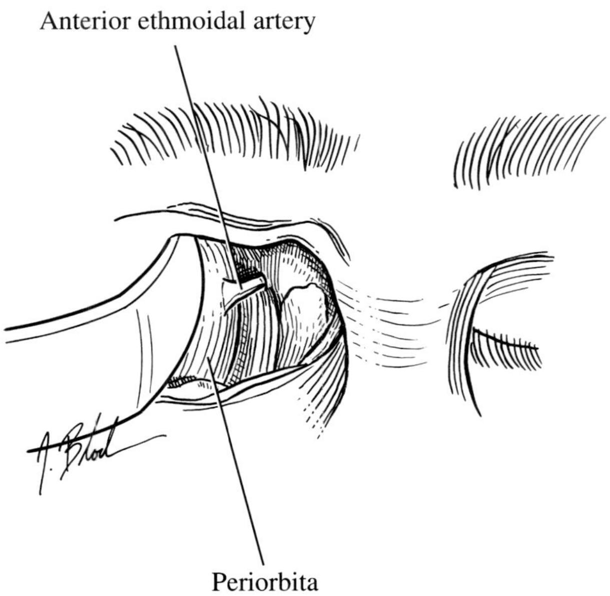

Figure 6. Identification of the anterior and posterior ethmoidal arteries after elevation of the periorbita from the lamina papyracea.

22 Orbitotomy: Lateral Approach

Howard R. Krauss *and* Robert Alan Goldberg

A lateral transconjunctival approach may be taken to the orbital floor. A lateral orbitotomy with bone flap may be performed for extended orbital exposure, and in some cases, a combined lateral and medial approach may be helpful.

TRANSCONJUNCTIVAL APPROACH

A lateral canthotomy is performed. The lateral aspect of the inferior lid is elevated, and the attachment of the inferior tarsal plate to the periosteum is severed. The lower lid is then reflected inferiorly, and the conjunctiva is opened from lateral to medial (Figure 1). The opening is *not* carried further medially than the punctum to avoid damage to the lacrimal drainage apparatus.

The opening is then taken deeper through the lower lid retractors and inferior orbital septum to the inferior orbital rim, where the periosteum is incised and elevated from the orbital floor. The infraorbital nerve usually is left protected in its canal to avoid postoperative malar anesthesia.

This approach allows complete access to the orbital floor and the anteroinferior medial orbit (Figure 2). It is most often used for repair of an orbital blowout fracture or for orbital decompression, but it is a useful approach to anterior extraconal inferolateral tumors as well.

Closure

At closure, the periosteum is reapproximated. Closure of the conjunctiva is optional. Reapproximation of the tarsal plate to the periosteum of the lateral orbital rim is critical to the restoration of normal postoperative appearance. This may be accomplished with 4-0 Vicryl. The skin of the lateral canthotomy is then closed with 6-0 nylon or Prolene.

LATERAL ORBITOTOMY WITH BONE FLAP

A Kronlein or modified Wright incision is performed (Figure 3). The lateral orbital rim is exposed. The periosteum is incised along the rim and then carried posteriorly in a T incision. The periosteum is elevated from the lateral orbital rim, temporalis fossa, and internal aspect of the lateral orbital wall (Figure 4). While protecting the orbit and temporalis with metal malleable retractors, osteotomies are made with an oscillating saw at the zygomaticofrontal suture and just above the zygomatic arch.

A drill may be used to complete the bone flap or the lateral wall may be carefully outfractured. The bone flap may be soaked in a dilute bacitracin solution while surgery is carried out. Bone wax is used as necessary for hemostasis.

Rongeurs and drills may be used to take the lateral wall posterior as far as required for posterior orbital exposure. Some cases benefit from exposure of the dura of the middle cranial fossa with bone removal to the lateral aspect of the superior orbital fissure.

A self-retaining lateral Kennerdell retractor often is used. The periorbita is opened longitudinally above or below the lateral rectus muscle, which is then identified, protected, and retracted superiorly or inferiorly, as needed. The superior, lateral, and inferior extraconal spaces and the entire intraconal space are thus visible.

Cautery within the intraconal space is avoided to minimize the risk of damage to vision or ocular motility. Fat is displaced with minimal traction. Moist cottonoid sponges under malleable retractors are useful in keeping fat out of the operative field. Cotton-tipped applicators serve as useful blunt dissectors. When desired, an operating microscope is used. Figure 5 shows the anatomical structures that are encountered in the lateral orbitotomy approach.

Closure

The deep lateral periorbita is closed with absorbable suture. The bone flap is cleared of adherent tissue and repositioned. A careful periosteal closure often obviates the need for fixation, but sutures may be passed through drill holes, or miniplates may be used to aid stabilization of the lateral orbital rim. Most cases do not require drains.

Combining approaches may be useful in cases that require enhanced medial orbital exposure in which the globe and orbital contents may be displaced laterally.

RECOMMENDED READING

Rootman, J.: Diseases of the Orbit. A Multidisciplinary Approach. Philadelphia: J.B. Lippincott, 1988.

Simonton, J., Garber, F., Ahl, N.: Margins of safety in lateral orbitotomy. Arch. Ophthalmol. 95:1229–1231, 1977.

Steward, W., Levin, P., Toth, B.: Orbital surgery. The technique of coronal scalp flap approach to the lateral orbitotomy [see comments]. Arch. Ophthalmol. 106:1724–1726, 1988.

Viale, G., Pau, A.: A plea for postero-lateral orbitotomy for microsurgical removal of tumors of the orbital apex. Acta Neurochir. (Wien) 90:124–126, 1988.

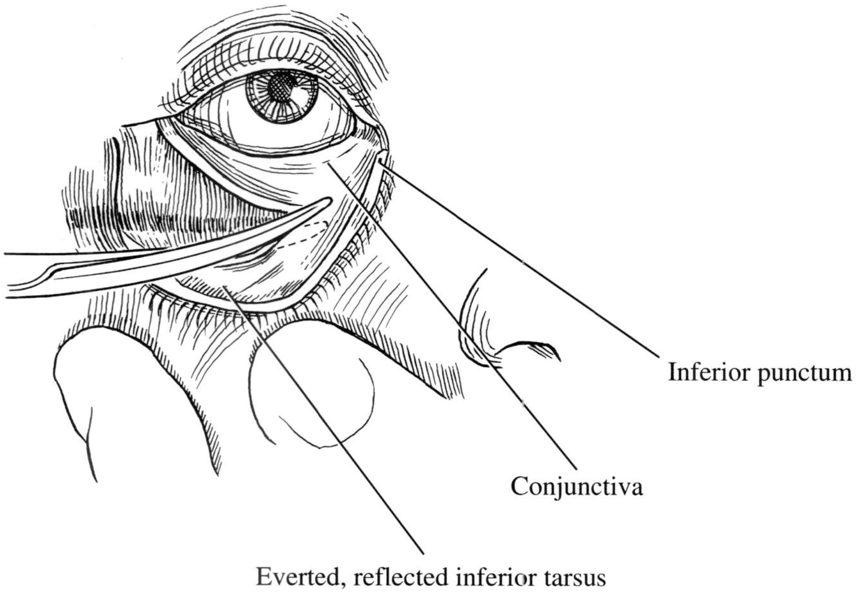

Figure 1. After a lateral canthotomy, the lateral aspect of the inferior lid is elevated and the attachment of the inferior tarsal plate to the periosteum is severed.

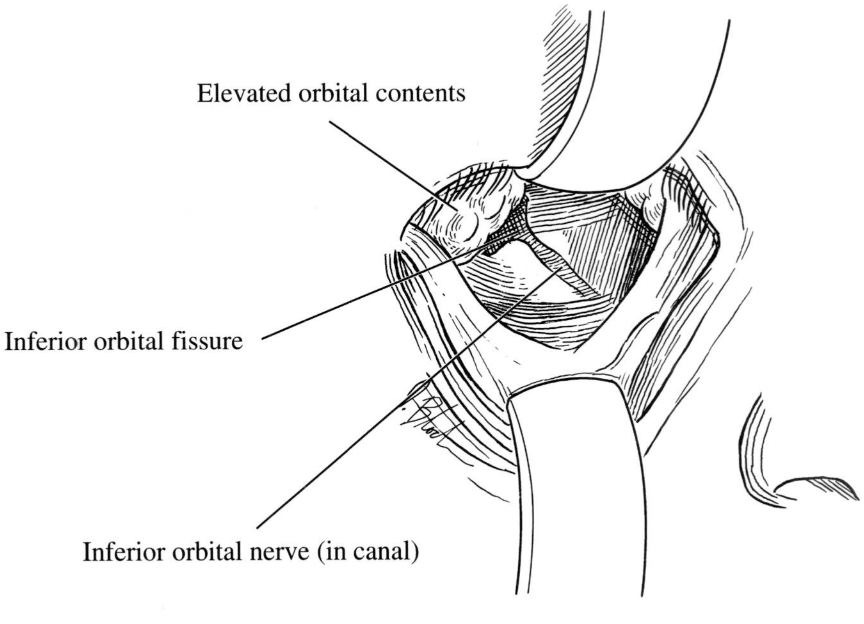

Figure 2. Exposure of the orbital floor and the anteroinferior medial orbit.

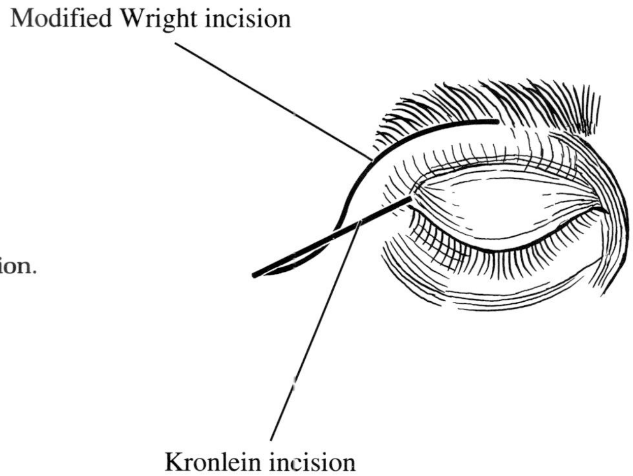

Figure 3. Kronlein or modified Wright incision.

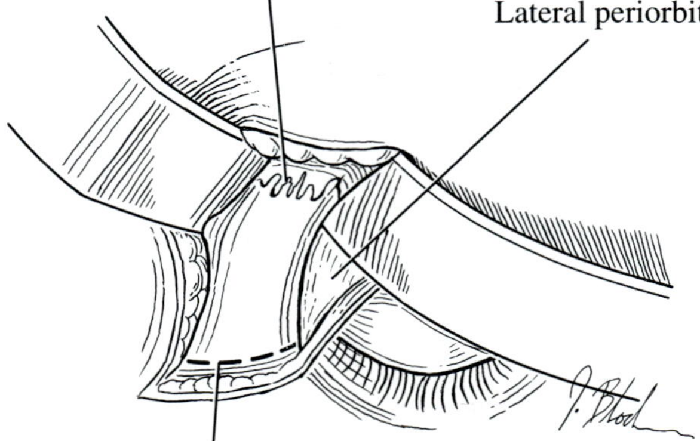

Figure 4. Elevation of periosteum from the lateral orbital rim, temporalis fossa, and internal aspect of the lateral orbital wall.

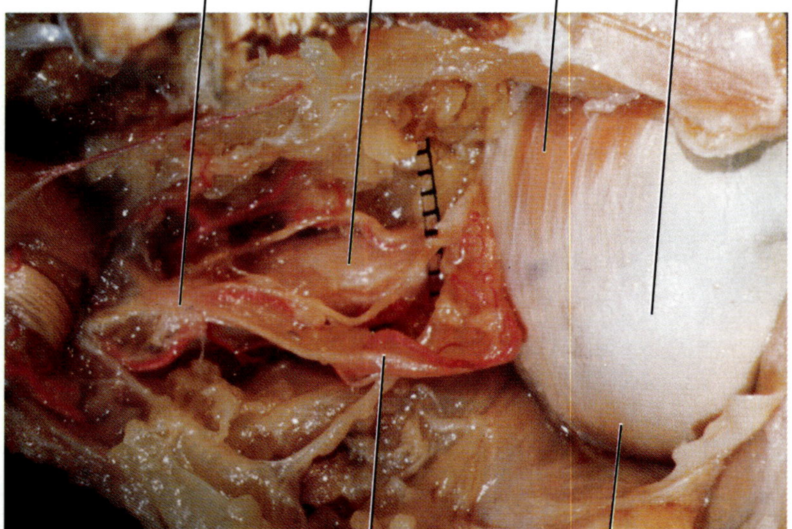

Figure 5. Cadaver dissection showing anatomical structures as encountered in the lateral orbital approach.

Orbitotomy: Cranial Approach (Frontal-Orbital) 23

Howard R. Krauss *and* Robert Alan Goldberg

The cranial approach is appropriate for lesions at the orbital apex or for lesions that involve both intracranial and orbital compartments. The craniotomy may be frontotemporal, pterional, or orbitocranial, with a one- or two-piece bone flap (see Chapter 16).

The orbitocranial bone flap provides several advantages, including improved access to the orbit as a consequence of removal of the orbital rim and preservation of the orbital roof as part of the flap, thus reducing the risk of postoperative ocular pulsation or dystopia.

The transcranial exposure allows access to all orbital compartments (Figure 1). The optic canal and superior orbital fissure are easily deskeletonized with drilling, if needed. The periorbita is opened longitudinally. Branches of cranial nerve V_1 in the superior extraconal space may be retracted. The fourth cranial nerve crosses the orbital apex superiorly on its way to the superior oblique muscle and is the most easily damaged nerve if not looked for and protected (Figure 2).

When needed, entry into the intraconal space is easiest by lateral distraction of the levator superior rectus complex, avoiding disturbance of the innervating third cranial nerve branches from below. At the orbital apex, there is a confluence of periorbita, extraocular muscles, and optic nerve sheath at the annulus of Zinn. When necessary, the annulus may be opened.

CLOSURE

Reapproximation of the periorbita reduces the risk of ocular pulsation. If the orbital roof has not been preserved as part of the bone flap, it may be replaced with split-thickness calvarial graft or molded acrylic or other alloplastic material may be used. If the frontal sinus has been entered, mucosa is extirpated, and the posterior wall of the frontal sinus may be removed and the orbitosinus region covered with pericranial flap.

RECOMMENDED READING

Blacklock, J.B., Weber, R.S., Lee, Y.Y., Goepfert, H.: Transcranial resection of tumors of the paranasal sinuses and nasal cavity. J. Neurosurg. 71:10–15, 1989.

Blinkov, S.M., Gabibov, G.A., Tcherekayev, V.A.: Transcranial surgical approaches to the orbital part of the optic nerve: An anatomical study. J. Neurosurg. 65:44–47, 1986.

Housepian, E.M.: Microsurgical anatomy of the orbital apex and principles of transcranial orbital exploration. Clin. Neurosurg. 25:556–573, 1978.

Leone, C.R., Jr., Wissinger, J.P.: Surgical approaches to diseases of the orbital apex. Ophthalmology 95:391–397, 1988.

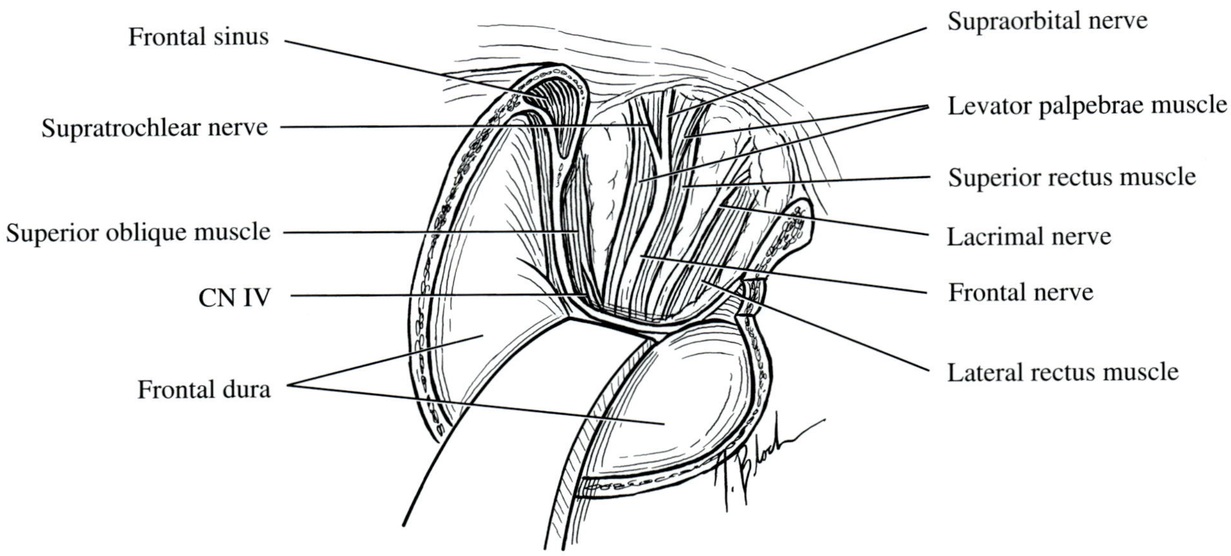

Figure 1. View of the superior orbital structures after removal of the bony orbital roof and superior periorbita. The frontal nerve (V_1) is the superior-most structure and overlies the levator superior rectus muscle complex. The superior oblique muscle lies medially (overlying the medial rectus muscle), and the lacrimal nerve and artery lie laterally (overlying the lateral rectus muscle.)

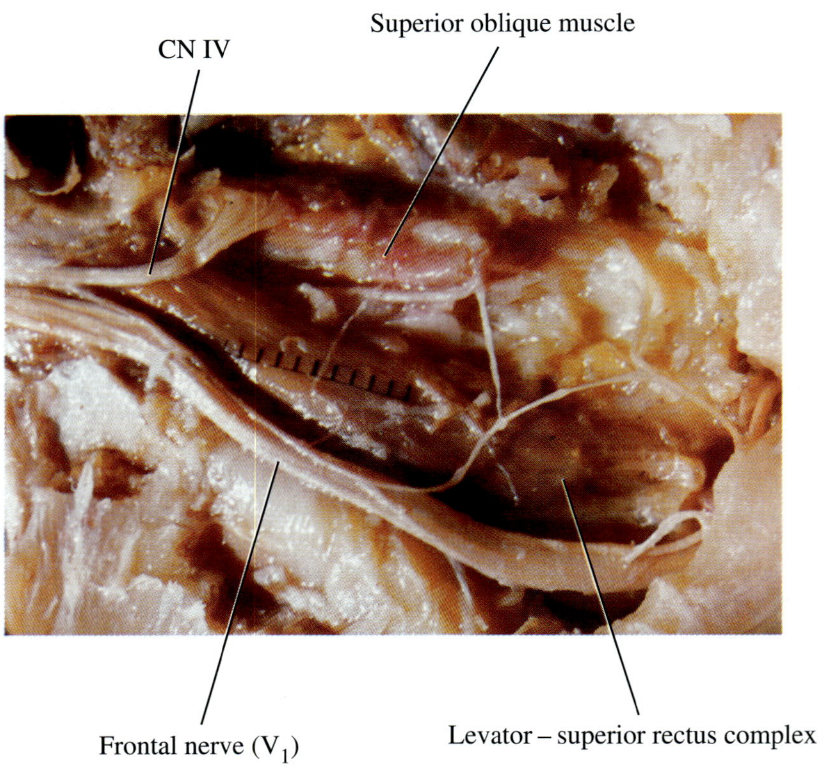

Figure 2. Cadaver dissection showing the anatomical structures as seen in the cranial (frontal-orbital) approach.

Orbitotomy: Caudal Approach 24

Robert Alan Goldberg *and* Rinaldo Canalis

INDICATIONS

Caudal orbitotomy is a useful approach for lesions of the posterior inferomedial orbit, particularly those that extend into the pterygopalatine fossa. Examples include orbital decompression for Graves' orbitopathy, inferomedial orbital tumors that involve the sinuses, and lesions of the inferior orbital nerve.

POSITION

The patient is placed in a semisitting position, which allows intraoperative fluids to drain out of the surgical field and enhances the surgeon's comfort. The patient's head can be additionally angled 30 degrees toward the surgeon, and venous compression leg dressings can be used to decrease venous pooling.

INCISION

A sublabial incision is made in the gingival recess to avoid the frenulum in the midline and Stensen's duct laterally (see Chapter 18, Figures 2 through 4). If the initial incision plane onto the face of the maxillary sinus leaves some connective tissue attached to the periosteum for a distance of 5 mm, this provides additional tissues to make a watertight closure, but the plane should then rapidly obey the periosteum as dissection proceeds superiorly to avoid entering the buccal fat pad.

OPERATIVE PROCEDURE

Gentle dissection reveals the infraorbital neurovascular bundle exiting in the subperiosteal plane from the inferior orbital foramen. Elevation of the flap with Army-Navy retractors allows wide visualization of the face of the maxillary sinus, which is then removed using osteotomes and rongeurs. Bone removal should be as generous as needed to provide adequate exposure; the bone surrounding the infraorbital canal can be carefully removed, if necessary. If the orbital floor and medial wall are to be removed, for example, in orbital decompression, care should be taken to avoid early rupture of the periorbita because the resulting spillage of orbital fat in the tight operative space of the sinuses will restrict subsequent visualization of the posterior structures.

Depending on the required exposure, additional bone can be removed, including the orbital floor, ethmoid sinus, and lamina papyracea; the posterior sinus wall for exposure of the pterygopalatine fascia; or the posterior ethmoid, superior palatine bone, and anterior wall of the sphenoid sinus for exposure of the orbital apex and optic canal ring (Figure 1). When working in the ethmoid and sphenoid sinuses from below, it is important to be aware of anatomical variations (preoperative coronal computed tomographic scans provide this information) to avoid inadvertent penetration of the fovea ethmoidalis or cribriform plate with subsequent cerebrospinal fluid leak (Figure 2). If dural penetration is recognized intraoperatively, control can be obtained using tissue glue, cyanoacrylate, fascia grafts, and local flaps, such as turbinate mucosal flaps.

The sublabial incision is closed carefully in a single layer to avoid postoperative formation of an oral antral fistula. Particularly in the case of orbital decompression, when downward prolapse of the orbital contents might occlude the sinus osteum, it is advisable to create a nasal antral window through which a 16F Foley catheter can be inserted and the balloon filled with 2 to 3 mL of sterile saline solution inside the maxillary sinus to act as a drain for the first 2 to 3 postoperative days.

POSTOPERATIVE MANAGEMENT

Intraoperative and postoperative prophylactic antibiotics are routinely used. Steroids are also used postoperatively in selected cases—for example, in inflammatory conditions such as Graves' orbitopathy or in cases of potential optic nerve compression.

Lemon glycerine swabs and mouthwash are useful for postoperative oral comfort. Sinus drains are left in for 3 to 5 days. Postoperative sinus lavage and drainage are occasionally needed if tissue edema and perhaps some preexisting sinusitis lead to late sinus opacification.

RECOMMENDED READING

Baylis, H., Call, N., Shibata, C.: The transantral orbital decompression (Ogura technique) as performed by the ophthalmologist: A series of 24 patients. Ophthalmology 97:1005–1010, 1980.

Calcaterra, T.: Paranasal sinus decompression of the orbit in Graves'. Ophthalmic Surg. 8:80–84, 1977.

De Santo, L., Gorman, C.: Orbital decompression in Graves' ophthalmopathy. Laryngoscope 84:637, 1974.

Ogura, J., Walsh, T.: The trans-antral orbital decompression operation for progressive exophthalmos. Laryngoscope 72:1078–1097, 1962.

Warren, J., Spector, J., Burde, R.: Long-term follow-up and recent observations on 305 cases of orbital decompression for dysthyroid orbitopathy. Laryngoscope 99:35–40, 1989.

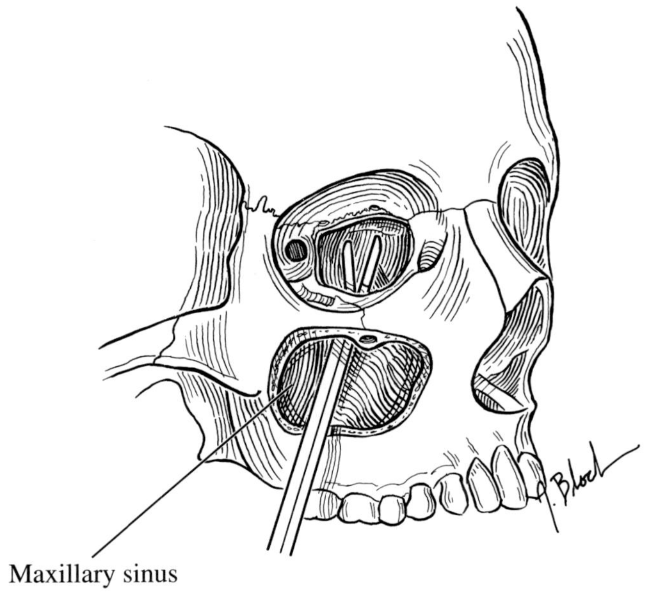

Figure 1. Schematic frontal view showing bony removal of medial wall and orbital floor for decompression or access for tumor removal in the inferomedial orbit.

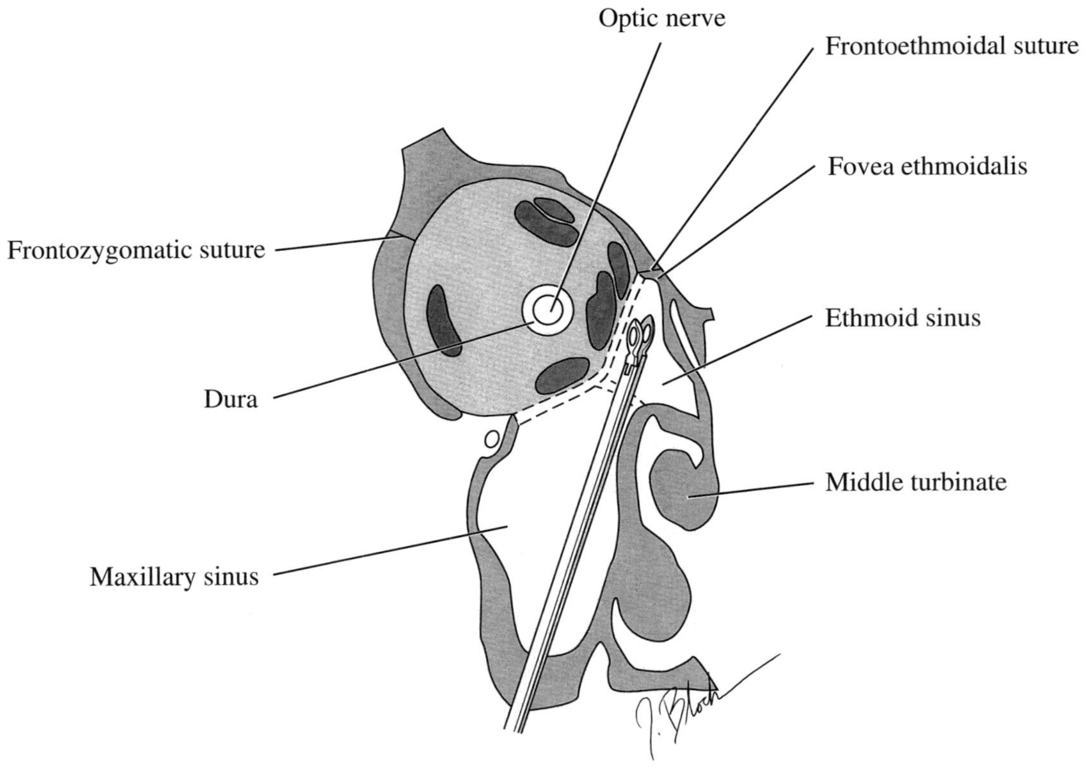

Figure 2. Caudal approach, coronal view. Bony removal in caudal approach to orbital decompression is shown. Care is taken to visualize and avoid damaging the fovea ethmoidalis at the roof of the ethmoid sinus, violation of which could lead to dural laceration.

Panoramic Orbitotomy 25

Robert Alan Goldberg *and* Howard R. Krauss

INDICATIONS

Panoramic orbitotomy is indicated whenever wide exposure of the orbital apex and adjoining structures is needed—for example, in the removal of a large meningioma of the sphenoid, orbit, and adjacent skull base. The approach differs from a standard transcranial orbitotomy primarily in the increased exposure, through the orbit, of the greater wing of the sphenoid and the lateral orbital apex and particularly the combined exposure of the cranial, pterygopalatine, infratemporal, and orbital fossae. Figure 1 shows structures as seen in a cadaver dissection, with special reference to the anatomical relations at the orbital apex.

POSITION AND INCISION

Patient positioning and initial incision and bony exposure are performed as in the frontal-temporal-orbital approach (see Chapter 17).

OPERATIVE PROCEDURE

The dissection laterally is carried along the temporalis fascia in a deep plane to avoid injury to the facial nerve. The zygomatic arch can be removed at this point if exposure of the inferior orbit in the region of the inferior orbital fissure is needed (Figure 2).

The periorbita is then dissected from the lateral orbital wall, exposing the greater wing of the sphenoid from the inferior orbital fissure to the superior orbital fissure, working within the orbit underneath the extended coronal flap. While the orbital contents are protected with a malleable retractor, the lateral wall and roof are removed with part of the zygomatic arch as a large bony unit. The superior orbital fissure can be further exposed above and below with rongeurs or drills (Figure 3). Figure 4 shows the exposure in a panoramic approach.

Wide exposure of the anterior and middle skull base, including the orbit and the infratemporal and pterygopalatine fossae, is obtained for further tumor resection or soft tissue work. At the end of the procedure, the orbital rim is replaced. The roof can be reconstructed of split inner table bone, if this is desired. Large roof defects (greater than one-half) may result in pulsatile proptosis and should probably be repaired.

SUMMARY

The panoramic orbitotomy extends the frontotemporal approach to access the lateral orbit from a different direction with a good overview of the infratemporal and pterygopalatine fossae. It is ideally suited for tumors that involve the orbital, pterygopalatine, and middle cranial fossae with or without extension along the orbital roof.

RECOMMENDED READING

Alaywan, M., Sindou, M.: Fronto-temporal approach with orbitozygomatic removal. Acta Neurochir. (Wien) 104:79–83, 1990.

Maroon, J., Kennerdell, J.: Surgical approaches to the orbit: Indications and techniques. J. Neurosurg. 60:1226–1235, 1984.

McDermott, M., Durity, F., Rootman, J., Woodhurst, W.: Combined frontotemporal-orbitozygomatic approach for tumors of the sphenoid wing and orbit. Neurosurgery 26:107–116, 1990.

Seifert, V., Dietz, H.: Combined orbito-frontal, subtemporal and infratemporal fossa approach to skull base neoplasms. Surgical technique and clinical application. Acta Neurochir. (Wien) 114:139–144, 1992.

Viale, G., Pau, A.: A plea for postero-lateral orbitotomy for microsurgical removal of tumours of the orbital apex. Acta Neurochir. (Wien) 90:124–126, 1988.

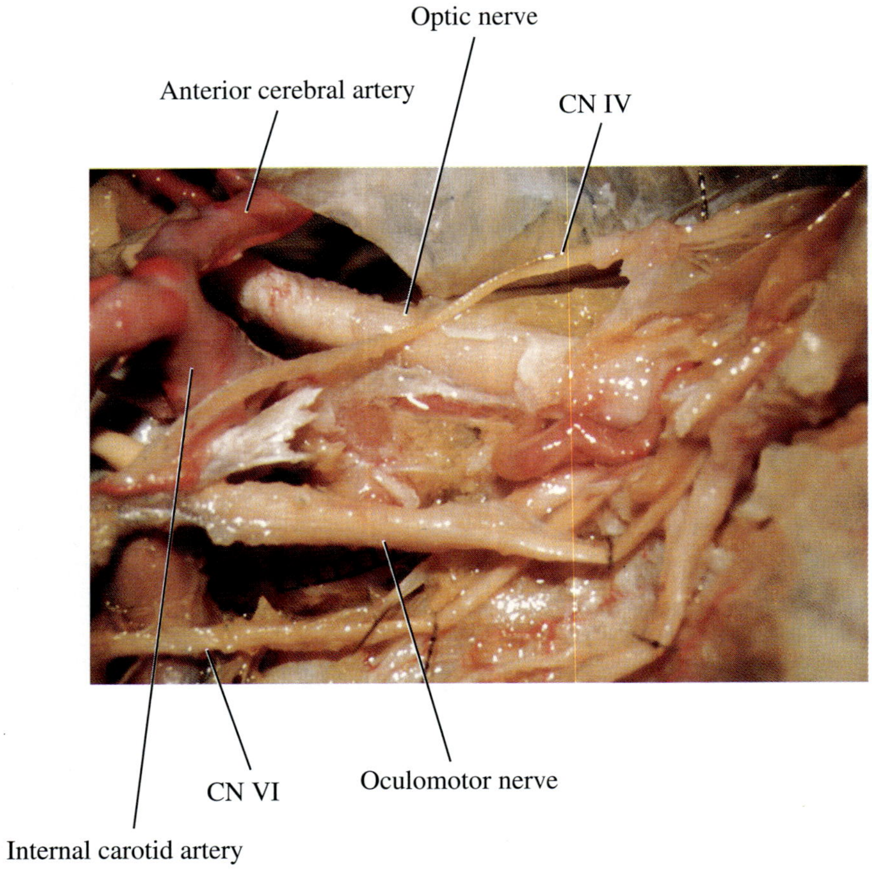

Figure 1. Cadaver dissection showing orbital anatomy with special reference to structural relations at the orbital apex.

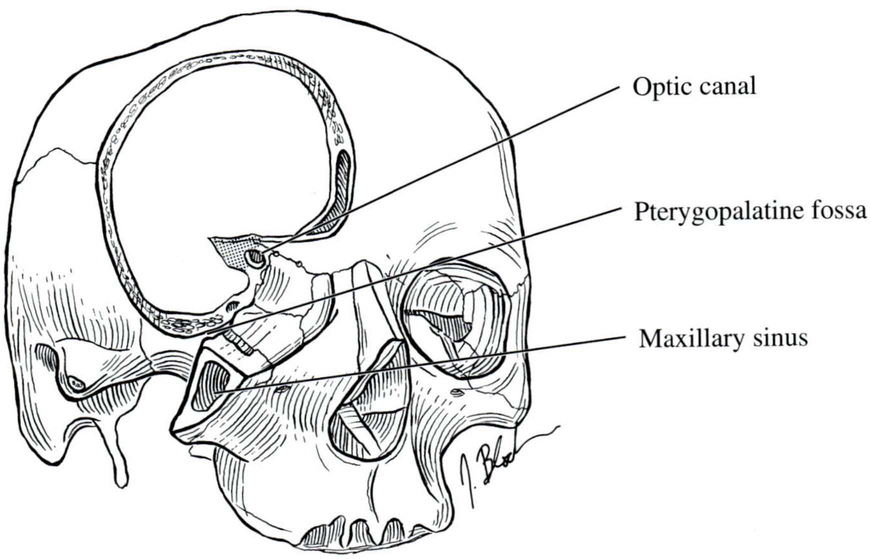

Figure 2. Schematic diagram of bony removal in panoramic orbitotomy, giving wide exposure of the orbit, pterygopalatine fossa, and skull base.

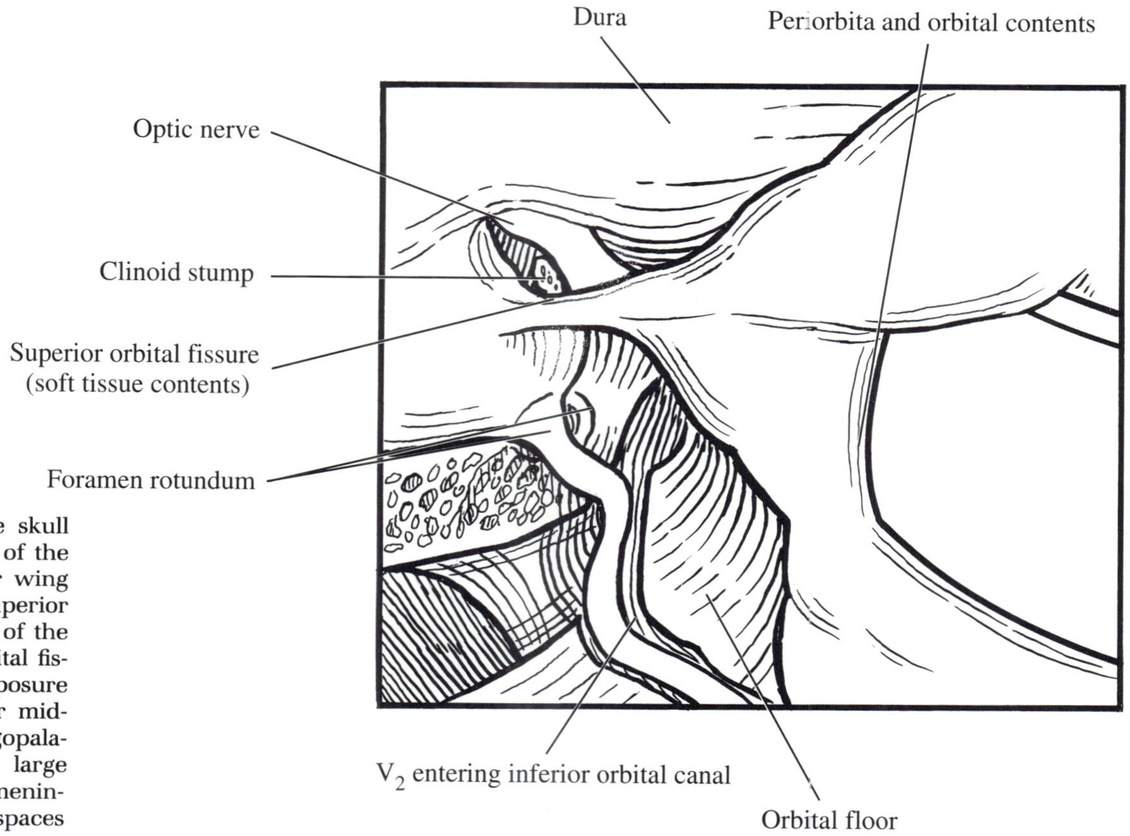

Figure 3. Exposure of the skull base. After further removal of the deep portion of the greater wing of the sphenoid to the superior orbital fissure (and removal of the lesser wing to the superorbital fissure, if necessary), wide exposure of the orbital apex, anterior middle cranial fossa, and pterygopalatine fossa is achieved. A large tumor—for example, a meningioma—involving these spaces can be removed.

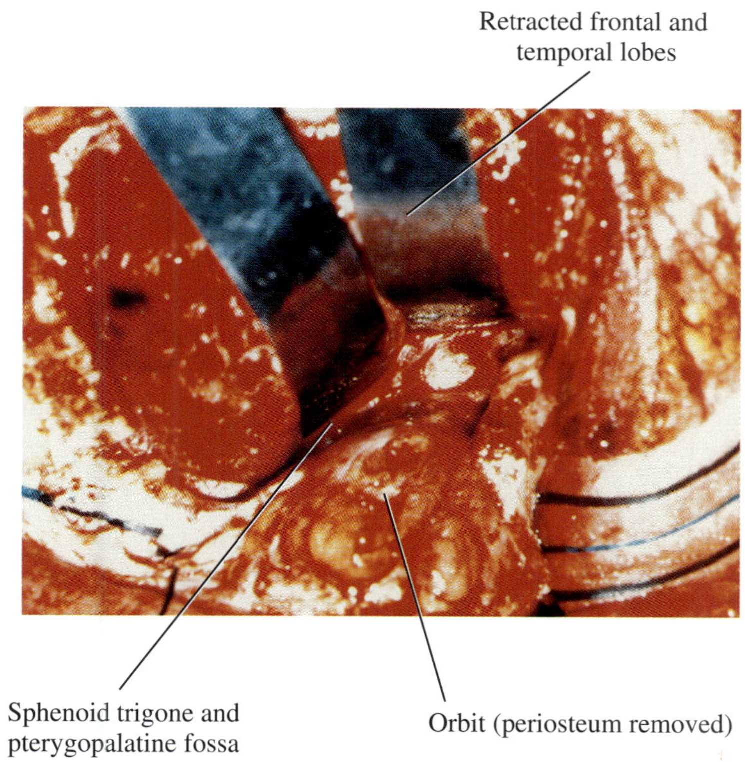

Figure 4. Exposure in a panoramic approach.

26 Transsphenoidal Optic Canal Decompression

Robert Alan Goldberg *and* Howard R. Krauss

INDICATIONS

Optic canal decompression by the transsphenoidal approach is indicated for traumatic optic neuropathy. It is also indicated for compressive intracanalicular optic neuropathy caused by tumor, callus formation, or osteopetrosis.

POSITION

The patient is placed in the semisitting or supine position with the head turned 30 degrees toward the surgeon on the side of the lesion to be decompressed.

PREPARATION

The nose is packed with cotton gauze that has been soaked in 4% cocaine and wrung out. Local anesthesia is instituted with the injection of 1:100,000 epinephrine into the medial canthal tissues to provide hemostasis during the initial wound entry. Intravenous broad-spectrum antibiotics are given at the beginning of the case, and if the patient is not already on intravenous steroids, these are also given at the beginning of surgery.

INCISION

A Lynch incision is made, and a subperiosteal medial orbitotomy is performed in standard manner, as described in Chapter 36. The anterior and posterior ethmoid arteries are clipped or cauterized, and great care is taken to avoid spilling orbital fat because this might compromise visualization at the orbital apex. The lamina papyracea is removed (Figure 1), and sufficient ethmoidal air cells are taken out to achieve good visualization directly into the sphenoid sinus. The sinus is entered through the thin wall of bone that separates the posteriormost ethmoid air cell from the sphenoid sinus. Careful preoperative study of the orbital and sinus imaging studies will obviate any surprises resulting from atypical sinus anatomy.

BONY CANAL DECOMPRESSION

Once the ethmoidectomy and the sphenoidotomy are completed, attention is turned toward identifying the bony landmarks of the optic canal. The anterior and posterior ethmoid arteries form an imaginary line that typically points directly to the beginning of the optic canal ring. Within the lateral wall of the sphenoid sinus, the optic canal often is visible as a bony prominence in the superior recess of the lateral wall, although the bony optic canal ring initially may block the view of this structure.

Using a high-speed 2- or 3-mm diamond burr in combination with microcurettes and rongeurs, the bony optic canal ring is removed. This exposes the periosteum overlying the annulus of Zinn, which has a characteristic vertical orientation to its striations (Figure 2).

Under direct visualization, the diamond burr is used to thin the bone overlying the optic canal (Figure 3). Care is taken to minimize thermal damage to the nerve by drilling under constant irrigation and minimizing the drilling to as little as required for exposure.

It is critical to work superiorly within the sphenoid sinus to avoid damage to the carotid artery, which often can be identified by a characteristic bulge more inferiorly located within the sinus. The medial portion of the canal roof can then be removed and the entire length of the canal back to the posterior wall of the sphenoid sinus opened. The dural sheath of the optic nerve can be incised with a sickle blade, if desired.

CLOSURE

Cerebrospinal leaks are addressed in the usual manner, using vascular periorbital or nasal septal flaps, if required. The cutaneous wound is closed in layers, taking care to approximate the deep tissues of the medial canthal tendon.

RECOMMENDED READING

Joseph, M., Lessell, S., Rizzo, J., Momose, K.: Extracranial optic nerve decompression for traumatic optic neuropathy. Arch. Ophthalmol. 108:1091–1093, 1990.

Kline, L., Morawetz, R., Swaid, S.: Indirect injury of the optic nerve. Neurosurgery 14:756–764, 1984.

Miller, N.: The management of traumatic optic neuropathy [editorial comment]. Arch. Ophthalmol. 108:1086–1087, 1990.

Newton, N., Jr., Baratham, G., Sinniah, R., Lim, A.: Bilateral compressive optic neuropathy secondary to bilateral sphenoethmoidal mucoceles. Ophthalmologica 198:13–19, 1989.

Niho, S., Niho, M., Niho, K.: Decompression of the optic canal by the transethmoidal route and decompression of the superior orbital fissure. Can. J. Ophthalmol. 5:22–40, 1970.

Nyak, S., Kirtane, M., Ingle, M.: Transethmoid decompression of the optic nerve in head injuries: An update. J. Laryngol. Otol. 105:205–206, 1991.

Osguthorpe, J.: Transethmoid decompression of the optic nerve. Otolaryngol. Clin. North Am. 18:125–137, 1985.

Sofferman, R.: Sphenoethmoid approach to the optic nerve. Laryngoscope 91:184–196, 1981.

Takahashi, M., Itoh, M., Kaneko, M., et al.: Microscopic intranasal decompression of the optic nerve. Arch. Otorhinolaryngol. 246:113–116, 1989.

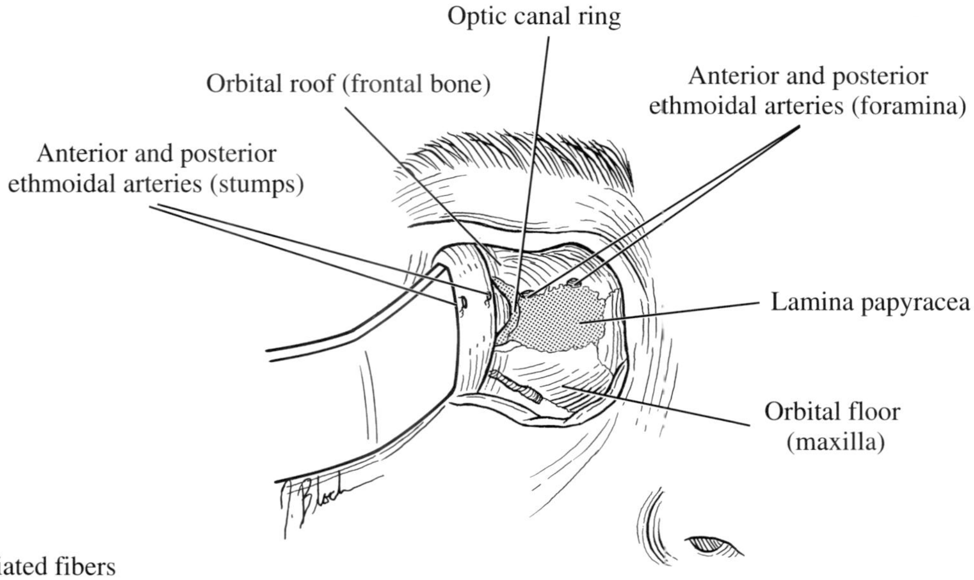

Figure 1. Extraperiorbital exposure of the bony medial orbital wall is performed through a Lynch incision (see Chapter 21, Figure 5). The anterior and posterior ethmoidal arteries have been identified and severed. The shaded bone indicates the portion of the lamina papyracea that is to be removed. The optic canal ring is visualized as a thickening of the medial orbital wall about 6 mm posterior to the posterior ethmoid artery.

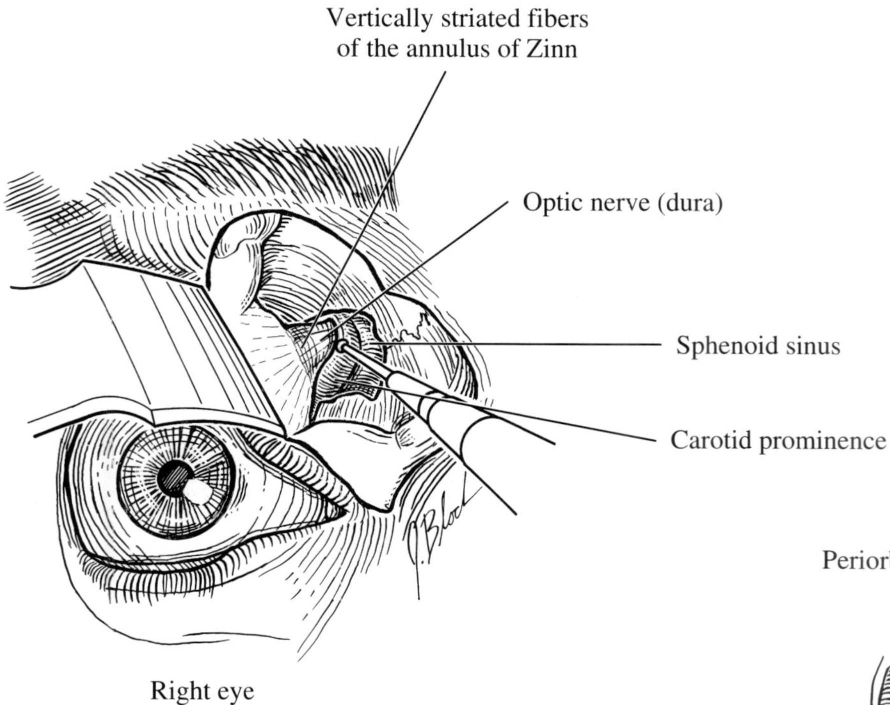

Figure 2. Bony exposure of the middle and posterior ethmoid sinus and opening of the anterior wall of the sphenoid sinus have been accomplished, exposing the bony optic canal running in the superior lateral wall of the sphenoid sinus. A diamond burr is used to remove the bony optic canal ring and then to remove bone posteriorly and superiorly along the bony optic canal, with care taken to avoid the carotid artery located inferiorly and posteriorly.

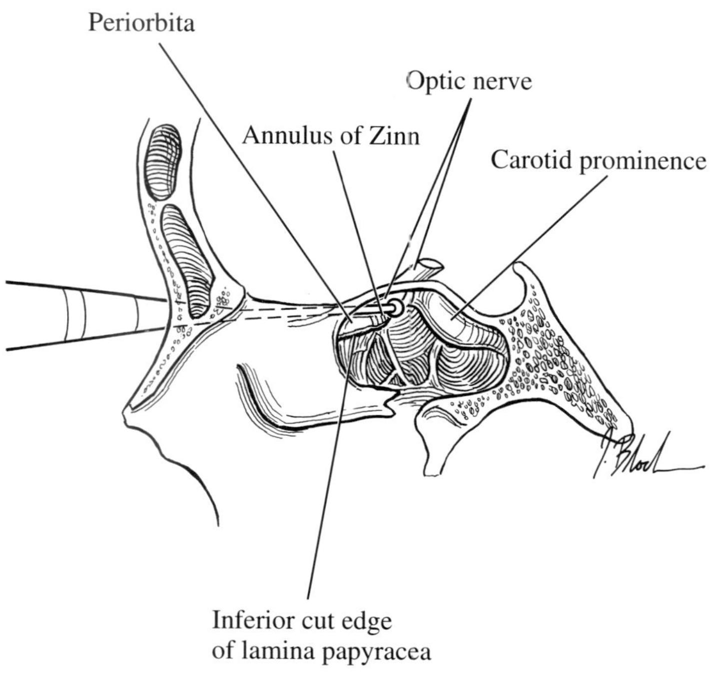

Figure 3. Schematic view of the lateral wall of the sphenoid sinus during transsphenoidal optic canal decompression. The optic canal runs in the superiormost aspect of the sphenoid sinus lateral wall. The carotid artery bulge can be seen in the lateral sphenoid sinus wall inferior and posterior to the optic nerve.

III

SPECIFIC CRANIAL BASE PATHOLOGY: PRINCIPLES OF SURGICAL APPROACHES

Meningiomas 27

Meningiomas arise from the cells that form the outer lining of the arachnoid membrane (arachnoidal cap cells), meningeal blood vessels, and fibroblasts of the meningeal stroma. The changing composition of these elements is responsible for the different histological types of meningiomas. More than 50 per cent of meningiomas are located at the cranial base (Figures 1 and 2). Intraventricular meningiomas (Figure 3) are explained by the presence of nests of arachnoidal cap cells associated with the choroid plexus, whereas ectopic meningiomas are thought to be related to the presence of ectopic arachnoidal cell inclusions.

By gross appearance, intracranial meningiomas are globular or lobulated, firm, and, occasionally, calcified or ossified ("brain stone"). Sometimes they invade adjacent dura and bone. Especially in cases of meningiomas growing en plaque, hyperostosis of the adjacent bone frequently occurs, even without true invasion by the tumor. The brain tends to be compressed by these tumor masses, but it is not invaded, with the exception of relatively rare malignant meningiomas.

HISTOLOGICAL TYPES

Meningiomas have been categorized in various manners by different authors. Generally included are the basic meningioma types defined by Zülch. Four major types of meningiomas are named, based on the predominant cell types seen microscopically: (1) meningotheliomatous, (2) transitional, (3) fibroblastic, and (4) angiomatous. Various subtypes will be listed in the revised International Histological Classification of Tumours by the World Health Organization (1979), including anaplastic (malignant) meningiomas and the newly introduced atypical meningiomas that have a moderately increased mitotic rate, cellular polymorphism (atypia), and a tendency to recurrence. Atypical meningiomas do not behave in a malignant manner, but a close follow-up of patients is recommended. The absence of progesterone receptors is more frequently seen in malignant and large meningiomas.

INCIDENCE

Meningiomas account for about 15 per cent of all primary intracranial neoplasms seen clinically. Although histologically benign in most cases, these tumors can be difficult to remove completely, especially when they are located at the cranial base.

More common in women than in men, with a ratio of 2:1, meningiomas present with a peak incidence at about age 45 years. No sexual prevalence can be found in malignant variants. Meningiomas rarely occur in children, constituting only 1.5 per cent of all primary intracranial tumors of childhood. Fifteen per cent of all meningiomas in children are intraventricular, a higher percentage than in adults.

CLINICAL PRESENTATION

The clinical presentation of skull base meningiomas is related to their topographical localization. Because these tumors typically grow slowly, they may reach a large size before they present clinically. Retrospectively, a history of headache of several years' duration can often be elicited. Some patients with meningiomas present with seizures.

CLINICAL DIAGNOSIS

Computed tomography (CT) is an effective instrument for diagnosing meningiomas and identifying the extent of their bone involvement or dural attachment. Its sensitivity has been reported to be as high as 96 per cent and its specificity about 90 per cent.

The "typical" CT scan appearance of a meningioma is that of a well-defined lesion that is moderately hyperdense in nonenhanced CT with respect to the brain parenchyma. The lesion enhances densely and homogenously after contrast infusion. Sometimes isodense and hypodense meningiomas are seen.

Nonenhanced magnetic resonance imaging (MRI) shows meningiomas poorly; enhanced MRI shows meningiomas more accurately than does CT. Because MRI poorly images bone, much detail concerning the relation between the tumor and adjacent bone (i.e., erosion, hyperostosis, invasion), readily available on CT, is not obtainable. MRI may be helpful in assessing the relation between meningiomas and major blood vessels, cranial nerves, brain tissue, and other cranial base structures. The meningeal sign ("dural tail sign") in MRI after administration of gadolinium consists of a distinct, flat enhancement of the dura adjacent to the tumor. The sign can be attributed to reactive fibrosis or vascularization or to extension of tumor along the dura or, eventually, to small tumor nodules extending flatly along the inner surface of the dura, rendering the total removal of the tumor more difficult (Figure 4).

Cerebral angiography retains its place as a major surgical adjuvant, showing main tumor feeders and the patency of the major cerebral arteries and dural sinuses. Another role of angiography is to identify those cases in which preoperative embolization may be desirable.

SURGICAL REMOVAL

If meningiomas can be totally removed (i.e., with a safety margin of the surrounding dura), the recurrence rate is low and the patient commonly is cured. Meningiomas occur in a number of predictable locations at the skull base (Figure 5). The surgical approach is dictated by the location, size, and dural attachment of the tumor and by the nature of involvement of adjacent structures.

Skull base meningiomas can be classified by location as follows:

1. Planum sphenoidale
2. Olfactory groove
3. Tuberculum
4. Anterior clinoidal
5. Sphenoid ridge (medial, middle, and lateral third)
6. Cavernous sinus
7. Meckel's cave
8. Tentorial
9. Clival
10. Petroclival
11. Cerebellopontine angle
12. Cerebellar convexity
13. Foramen magnum

Meningiomas located in these locations may be grouped as follows, with the preferred approach for removal as listed:

Subfrontal: Olfactory groove, planum sphenoidale, and tuberculum meningiomas

Pterional: Sphenoid ridge, anterior clinoidal, and cavernous sinus meningiomas

Orbito-frontal-zygomatic: Sphenoid ridge, orbital, and parasellar meningiomas

Subtemporal: Cavernous sinus, Meckel's cave, petroclival, and tentorial meningiomas

Pre–sigmoid sinus: Clival, petroclival, and cavernous sinus meningiomas

Retrosigmoid (lateral suboccipital): Tentorial, cerebellopontine angle, occipital, and petroclival meningiomas

Lateral craniocervical: Clival, foramen magnum, and jugular foramen meningiomas

General Principles

The surgeon has to distinguish the relation of tumor tissues to surrounding structures such as cranial nerves, vessels, brain, and adjacent bone. It is possible to differentiate, from a surgical point of view, between two types of meningiomas. One type of meningiomas are those that respect, during their growth, the arachnoidal sheath and only compress and displace soft tissues (Figure 6). These meningiomas can also engulf the arteries and nerves without infiltrating them. They are well encapsulated.

The second type includes those meningiomas that do not respect the arachnoidal sheath and infiltrate through the arachnoidal layer into neural tissues. The arterial walls are not spared by these tumors, which can grow through the adventitia muscularis and endothelium and even obliterate the vessel lumen.

If these facts are taken into consideration, the surgeon can easily understand that in the infiltrative type, the option of radical surgical removal without harming the patient is often nonexistent. The goal of surgery in such cases is careful and safe debulkment of the tumor mass to reduce intracranial pressure and the direct compression of neural structures. One of the potentials for disaster present during the debulking of these tumors exists when the surgeon does not have correct orientation of the location and course of important structures within the tumor mass.

In these types of meningiomas, it is essential in the beginning to expose the nerves and vessels adjacent to the tumor, if possible, and to follow them through the tumor tissue. The nerves or arteries cannot be dissected free from tumor completely, and some tumor tissue will remain attached to these structures. With careful dissection, the remaining tumor mass gradually can be removed. This is the only option in achieving debulking of meningiomas of this type without losing important function. We often are surprised to find that despite infiltration of cranial nerves, there is almost no functional deficit clinically.

In rare conditions, it may be necessary to sacrifice a cranial nerve, or nerves, to achieve radical surgical removal. Such an example might be an infiltrative cerebellopontine angle meningioma with growth into the internal auditory canal. In such a case, the facial nerve can be sacrificed. Immediate reconstruction with a nerve graft can follow with satisfying functional result. This decision can be made in case of complete functional loss of the eighth cranial nerve and if the vertebral artery, internal carotid artery, and posterior inferior cerebellar artery are not infiltrated.

Most meningiomas fall into the first group, in which the arachnoid plane has not been violated. Therefore, it is essential to know that in these types of meningiomas, the arachnoidal sheath is compressed and displaced but still definable. This phenomenon can be easily judged when the tumor is exposed. Primary debulkment of large meningiomas is fundamental for dissecting the tumor capsule from adjacent important structures.

One of the surgeon's hands holds the tumor capsule with an instrument while the other hand is used for the dissection of the arachnoid membrane. As long as we respect this *sacred* surgical tissue, we can avoid damage to surrounding structures adjacent to the tumor mass. We should avoid direct manipulation of the nerves and vessels, which might lead to interruption or functional deficit of the nerves or perforation of the arterial wall.

An understanding of the blood supply and

the extent of tumor attachment is essential before approaching meningiomas. The objective must be to remove tumor by debulking and lifting away from neural tissue rather than by retraction of neural tissue to facilitate removal of the meningioma as an intact tumor mass.

It is helpful to interrupt arterial blood flow to the tumor as early in the dissection as possible. Retraction of the brain should be avoided to reduce tissue damage as well as postoperative brain swelling.

With increasing knowledge from MRI and CT scanning procedures, we can clearly estimate the bony and dural involvement by meningiomas preoperatively. Therefore, we need to plan not only the removal of the tumor mass but also the complete resection of pathologically changed dura around the tumor matrix and involved bone. After removal of the tumor matrix, the interosseous part of the tumor is removed with a diamond drill. The drilling is carried far enough in all directions to expose normal bone. The important anatomical structures within the bone must be respected.

After tumor removal, a watertight dural closure is essential to avoid a postoperative cerebrospinal fluid fistula.

REMOVAL OF MENINGIOMAS OF THE OLFACTORY GROOVE, PLANUM SPHENOIDALE, AND TUBERCULUM SELLA

In Chapter 1, the patient positioning and basic outline for the subfrontal approach are presented. Whether to use a unilateral or bilateral scalp incision and the size of the bone flap to be turned are determined by the size of the tumor to be removed and the limits of its dural attachment.

For a bilateral approach, the dura is opened in a low transverse manner with ligation and section of the superior sagittal sinus as needed to extend the dural incision far enough to offer adequate surgical access. Meningiomas of the olfactory groove usually are in evidence either immediately on opening the dura or after gentle elevation of the frontal poles of the cerebral hemispheres.

Self-retaining retractors are introduced to elevate the brain and to allow access to the tumor. After tissue biopsy for frozen-section confirmation, the tumor is progressively removed by working at its base to control bleeding with bipolar cautery and bone wax as it is debulked with the ultrasonic aspirator or by suction and bipolar cautery. Care is taken to remove the tumor without placing unnecessary traction on the brain.

Piecemeal tumor debulking is continued until the mass has been reduced to its final point of attachment along the floor of the anterior fossa and the optic nerves and chiasm have been visualized and are completely decompressed. Then the final portion of the tumor is excised. Removal of the tumor from the area of the optic nerves and chiasm and the carotid arteries should be done using higher magnification with the operating microscope to avoid injury to these structures.

Figure 7 shows MRI scan images of a large meningioma of the olfactory groove with extension to the planum sphenoidale, tuberculum sella, and ethmoid and sphenoid sinuses. The CT scan image in Figure 8 shows extension of this tumor into the sphenoid sinus. Figure 9 shows a bifrontal craniotomy for removal of this tumor. The dura has been opened and the superior sagittal sinus has been ligated and transected. The frontal lobes are shown gently retracted, and the anterior aspect of the tumor is exposed. Figure 10 shows partial removal of the tumor with both optic nerves visible. In Figure 11, total removal of the intracranial portion of the tumor is seen and the sphenoid sinus has been opened. The tumor within the sphenoid sinus is elevated with forceps. Both optic nerves and the infundibular stalk are seen.

In Figure 12, the tumor has been completely removed from the paranasal sinuses. Figure 13 shows the dural defects covered by lyophilized dura after the paranasal sinuses have been packed with Xeroform gauze. The entire anterior skull base has been covered by pedicled pericranium and the suture line sealed with fibrin glue in Figure 14. Figure 15 shows postoperative CT scans demonstrating complete removal of this large olfactory groove meningioma.

Figure 16 shows MRI scan images of a tuberculum sella meningioma. In Figure 17, the meningioma is seen by a unilateral subfrontal approach and is noted to be compressing both optic nerves. Total removal of the tumor with preservation of the optic nerves and chiasm as well as the anterior cerebral arteries is seen in Figure 18. The tumor capsule was found to be intimately attached to these arteries.

REMOVAL OF MENINGIOMAS OF THE SPHENOID RIDGE AND ANTERIOR CLINOID

Sphenoid ridge and anterior clinoidal meningiomas can be easily exposed by the frontotemporal (pterional) approach, as described in Chapter 2. Most meningiomas of the lateral or middle third of the sphenoid ridge do not involve the important cranial nerves and vessels and can be easily removed by this approach. The pterional approach is especially useful in the surgical removal of meningiomas of the medial third of the sphenoid wing, anterior clinoid process, and cavernous sinus. These tumors usually involve the carotid artery and its branches as well as the optic nerve and chiasm and may even extend medially to the brain stem.

After completion of the initial pterional approach, the sylvian fissure is opened, facilitating the retraction of the frontal and temporal lobes and offering a more extensive view of the tumor superiorly. After the tumor is entered laterally, it is progressively debulked by piecemeal intracapsular removal. The tumor capsule can then be carefully dissected away from the middle cerebral artery under magnification to facilitate identification and preservation of its small branches.

With mobilization of the tumor capsule, dissection from the internal carotid artery as well as from the posterior communicating and anterior choroidal arteries and the optic nerve and chiasm can be carried out. Many of these tumors surround the carotid artery, and careful microdissection of tumor from the artery is necessary. Under higher magnification, the small amount of remaining tumor can be dissected away from the lateral wall of the cavernous sinus, oculomotor nerve, and optic nerve. Finally, its point of attachment along the anterior clinoid process and medial sphenoid ridge can be removed, and the lesser sphenoid wing can be partially drilled away with a diamond burr to remove tumor within the bone and lessen the likelihood of tumor recurrence.

Figure 19 shows the anatomical relations involved in a meningioma of the medial third of the sphenoid ridge and anterior clinoid process. CT scan images of such a meningioma of the right anterior clinoid process are shown in Figure 20, and in Figure 21 the placement of the frontotemporal craniotomy flap is demonstrated. In Figure 22, the dura has been opened and the sylvian fissure dissected. Figure 23 shows the sylvian fissure open and the anterior clinoid meningioma exposed. The tumor mass has been partially removed in Figure 24, and the olfactory nerve and anterior cerebral artery are exposed. Figure 25 shows the tumor matrix, including the anterior clinoid process, having been removed with a diamond drill. The optic nerve canal is open, and to achieve radical bony removal the sphenoid sinus is opened. In Figure 26, the dural defect around the optic canal and at the anterior clinoid process has been covered by a pericranial flap and sealed by fibrin glue.

REMOVAL OF MENINGIOMAS OF THE ORBITAL SPHENOIDAL, PARASELLAR AREA, CAVERNOUS SINUS, AND MECKEL'S CAVE

For removal of meningiomas of the orbital sphenoidal area, parasellar area, cavernous sinus, and Meckel's cave, the pterional approach is also the procedure of choice. In case of orbital tumor extension, the lateral wall of the orbit and/or orbital roof may be additionally removed. Figure 27 shows a CT scan image of a meningioma with involvement of the sphenoid ridge, orbit, and cavernous sinus. This tumor was removed by a pterional approach, and the entire sphenoid ridge and part of the temporal bone, along with the lateral wall of the orbit, have been drilled away. The tumor was found to be infiltrating into the cavernous sinus and orbit. Total removal was not possible without sacrifice of ocular nerve function. A small remaining area of tumor within the orbit and cavernous sinus can be seen in the postoperative CT scan image in Figure 28. Also seen is the temporal bone reconstruction with methyl methacrylate.

The frontal-orbital-zygomatic approach, as described in detail in Chapter 17, may be used as an alternative for removal of these types of meningiomas.

Meningiomas that originate in the middle fossa with involvement of Meckel's cave as well as the posterior portion of the cavernous sinus may be removed by the subtemporal approach. This approach is described in detail in Chapter 3. After a transbasal incision of the dura, the temporal lobe is carefully elevated. The middle fossa is exposed, and the meningioma gradually is resected while respecting the surrounding cranial nerves (oculomotor, trochlear, trigeminal). If the tumor involves the petrous bone, care must be exercised to avoid entry into the carotid artery in its intrapetrous course. The greater superficial petrosal nerve and geniculate ganglion must be protected to avoid facial nerve palsy. With more posterior extension of the tumor in the middle fossa, particularly when the tumor has reached the arcuate eminence, the surgeon should avoid opening the superior semicircular canal.

The approach to the cavernous sinus is determined by the extent of the tumor growth. The cavernous sinus can be opened dorsal to the entry zone of the trochlear nerve, respecting the trigeminal nerve (Parkinson's triangle). Because the tumor usually has obliterated the lumen of the cavernous sinus, it can be removed without major bleeding. Increased bleeding usually signals that the end of the tumor extension into the cavernous sinus has been reached. Hemostasis is now achieved with application of Surgicel gauze with gentle packing.

Figure 29 is a CT scan image of a meningioma with involvement of the middle fossa, sphenoid ridge, and cavernous sinus. The optic nerve, carotid artery, and oculomotor nerve were incased by the well-encapsulated tumor, which was completely removed. Figure 30 is a postoperative CT scan image showing complete removal of the well-encapsulated tumor.

REMOVAL OF MENINGIOMAS OF THE CLIVUS (UPPER, MIDDLE, LOWER), PETROCLIVUS, CEREBELLOPONTINE ANGLE, AND TENTORIUM

Meningiomas of the petroclivus region with extension into the cerebellopontine angle and some meningiomas of the tentorium are best removed through a retrosigmoid or presigmoid approach. The decision to use a presigmoid approach depends on involvement of the supratentorial region through the tentorial notch into the middle fossa and posterior portion of the cavernous sinus.

The complete transection of the tentorium extends the view to the middle fossa, Meckel's cave, and posterior aspect of the cavernous sinus. Figure 31 demonstrates a large parasellar, petroclival meningioma with infiltration of the cavernous sinus. With a presigmoid transtentorial approach, the tumor was exposed and the petroclival portion of the tumor was completely removed. Partial excision of the tumor within the cavernous sinus was possible. Total removal could not be accomplished without sacrifice of the ocular muscle nerves. In Figure 32, the postoperative CT scan shows subtotal tumor excision.

Figures 33 through 35 show MRI scan images and intraoperative photographs of another example of an infiltrating petroclival meningioma with involvement of the cavernous sinus. Figure 34 demonstrates the intraoperative exposure of the tumor by way of a presigmoid transtentorial approach with compression and displacement of cranial nerves V, VII, and VIII. Partial tumor removal is shown in Figure 35. The tumor is observed to be infiltrating the arachnoidal membrane, and for this reason total removal was not possible without traumatizing the important brain stem perforating arterial branches.

The next example is a petroclival meningioma with involvement of the cavernous sinus that was completely removed, preserving all cranial nerves and vessels as well as the brain stem by way of a presigmoid-transtentorial approach (Figures 36 through 43).

In our experience, even extended petroclival tumors in the cerebellopontine angle, with displacement of the brain stem to the contralateral side and with upward elevation, but without extension into the middle fossa, can be nicely removed with a simple retrosigmoid approach.

Tentorial meningiomas with supratentorial and/or infratentorial extensions are also removed through a lateral retrosigmoid approach. The dura is opened close to the transverse and sigmoid sinuses. Once cerebrospinal fluid drainage is achieved, the cerebellum is free to shift downward, thus exposing the supracerebellar space. The surgeon now has a view of the entire part of the involved tentorium. Without brain compression, the tentorium can be resected in a safe area and the tumor portion that extends into the supratentorial area can be safely removed.

For a tentorial meningioma that has extended into the pineal region we have two approach options. One is the same supracerebellar exposure, extending to the midline. The other option is a transparietal-occipital, parasagittal approach along the falx cerebri.

The disadvantage of the supracerebellar approach is that in some cases it is necessary to sacrifice bridging veins, risking venous compromise, and the matrix of tumor is located anteriorly along the tentorial edge. This area can be reached more easily by way of a parietal-occipital, parasagittal exposure. In a normal situation, when this approach is positioned posterior to the Rolandic vein, venous compromise is not a problem.

Using the retrosigmoid or the presigmoid approach to the cerebellopontine angle and the petroclival region, we distinguish different surgical "floors," which are determined by the location of the cranial nerves within the cerebellopontine angle. They create the surgical opening to tumor. When tumor is located and extends anterior to the internal auditory canal, jugular foramen, and Meckel's cave, all cranial nerves are displaced in different directions because of the growth of tumor. Once we reach the posterior aspect of the meningioma, we can enter between the nerve, or nerve groups, into the tumor.

One important opening that is available for removal of large cerebellopontine angle meningiomas or petroclival meningiomas is between the caudal cranial nerves and cranial nerves VII and VIII. Another available opening is between cranial nerves VII and VIII and the trigeminal nerve. For the supratentorial portion of the tumor, the opening is between the trigeminal nerve and the trochlear and oculomotor nerves. During resection of the tumor, it is recommended that these nerve groups be protected with moist cottonoids to avoid mechanical or thermal trauma.

Great attention must be paid to avoiding injury to the sixth cranial nerve, which is not in the field of vision until late in the procedure of tumor removal. Tumor coagulation in the area of the abducens nerve must be avoided. Once the tumor is reduced in size and the brain stem is decompressed, it is necessary to identify the abducens nerve at the brain stem and follow it along the tumor surface to its point of entry into Dorello's canal.

Figures 44 through 53 demonstrate the retrosigmoid approach for removal of a large cerebellopontine angle meningioma with displacement of the brain stem and cranial nerves. In Figure 44, the posterior aspect of the tumor is seen in the cerebellopontine angle, with the well-preserved arachnoidal membrane visible. Figure 45 shows the caudal aspect of the tumor with involvement of the lower cranial nerves. Debulking of the tumor with use of the ultrasonic aspirator is shown in Figure 46. In Figure 47, the posterior inferior cerebellar artery and caudal cranial nerves are shown freed from tumor tissue. Dissection of the tumor capsule from the brain stem is seen in Figure 48, and Figure 49 demonstrates the cranial nerves in the cerebellopontine angle, with the remaining tumor matrix between the porus acusticus and the jugular foramen. Figure 50 shows total removal of the tumor mass, but the site of tumor attachment to the dura is still present. Resection of the dura in the area of the tumor attachment is seen in Figure 51, and Figure 52 demonstrates drilling of bone at the site of tumor attachment just posterior to the porous. Complete radical tumor removal is seen in Figure 53.

In rare cases of meningiomas in the cerebellopontine angle, the tumor can extend into the internal auditory canal, sometimes reaching the fundus. When this occurs, complete opening of the internal auditory canal is necessary to achieve total tumor removal. Figures 54 through 57 show a cerebellopontine angle meningioma with extension into the internal auditory canal. Figure 54 shows the tumor within the cerebellopontine angle. After removal of the posterior lip of the internal auditory canal, tumor extension into the canal is demonstrated (Figure 55). Figure 56 shows complete tumor excision with preservation of cranial nerves VII and VIII within the internal auditory canal. Figure 57 shows the bone and dural defect filled with muscle and sealed with fibrin glue.

Preservation of the vertebral and basilar arteries and their branches is one of the points of major importance in cerebellopontine angle meningioma surgery. The perforators should not be coagulated. Only those pathological arteries that are definitely feeding the tumor should be coagulated and transected. A sensitive and fragile area is the entry zone of the trochlear nerve into the cavernous sinus. In case of infiltration of the dura in this region by tumor, there is a high risk of trochlear nerve damage, which is not a significant functional loss for the patient if radical excision is achieved.

If radical surgery is to be justified, the complete removal of tumor is essential. When the tumor has extended into the petrous carotid canal and into the cavernous sinus with involvement of the carotid artery and oculomotor nerves, a decision is made to perform a radical tumor excision only when tumor removal allows safe preservation of these structures.

Purely clival meningiomas are rare. For removal of these tumors, the presigmoid transpetrosal approach is the method of choice when most of the tumor is located along the upper and middle portions of the clivus. Meningiomas of the lower clivus, which reach the craniocervical junction, are removed by the lateral craniocervical approach to this area described later in this chapter.

REMOVAL OF MENINGIOMAS OF THE CRANIOCERVICAL JUNCTION (ANTERIOR, LATERAL, POSTERIOR)

Meningiomas or other tumors that arise from the inferior third of the clivus or along the anterior foramen magnum are best approached from a lateral craniocervical approach. The lower cranial nerves, vertebral artery, and posterior inferior cerebellar artery must be carefully protected.

Figure 58 shows MRI scan images of a meningioma that is located at the craniocervical junction in an anterior position. After a lateral approach to this area, as detailed in Chapter 12, the tumor can be visualized displacing the brain steam posteriorly (Figure 59). In Figure 60, partial tumor removal is observed, and in Figure 61, the tumor removal is complete. Figure 62 shows postoperative CT scan images confirming total tumor removal. In Figure 63, MRI scan images performed 6 months postoperatively are demonstrated, and no evidence of residual or recurrent tumor is seen.

The outcome of this rare but risky meningioma depends on the preservation of the perforating vessels to the brain stem and medulla oblongata. Vascular compromise to neural tissue that occurs in this area can lead to the catastrophic postoperative complications of respiratory impairment, difficulty with swallowing, and resultant aspiration pneumonia. The best advice we can give for surgical removal of this type of meningioma is to avoid blind coagulation of tumor tissue that may include perforating vessels to the brain stem.

In case the tumor infiltrates the wall of the vertebral artery, one should be as conservative as possible, and attempts at total removal should be avoided.

Tumors that arise in the lateral portion of the foramen magnum are removed by a lateral suboccipital retrosigmoid approach with the addition of the removal of the rim of the foramen magnum and the arch of C1. For the removal of craniocervical junction meningiomas located anterior and lateral, there is no necessity to mobilize the extradural portion of the vertebral artery from lateral to medial. In addition, there is no necessity to remove a portion of the condyle as has been recently recommended by some authors.

Posterior (midline) craniocervical junction meningiomas are removed by a midline suboccipital craniectomy approach (see Chapter 4) with removal of the arch of C1.

RECOMMENDED READING

Al-Mefty, O.: Clinoidal meningiomas. J. Neurosurg. 73:840–849, 1990.

Andrews, B., Wilson, C.: Suprasellar meningiomas: The effect of tumor location on postoperative visual outcome. J. Neurosurg. 69:523–528, 1988.

Bradac, G., Riva, A., Stura, G.: Cavernous sinus meningioma: An MRI study. Neuroradiology 29:578–581, 1987.

Brandis, A., Mirzai, S., Tatagiba, M., et al.: Immunohistochemical detection of female sex hormone receptors in meningiomas: Correlation with clinical and histological features. Neurosurgery 33:212–218, 1993.

Brihaye, J., Brihaye-Van Geertruyden, M.: Management and surgical outcome of suprasellar meningiomas. Acta Neurochir. Suppl. (Wien) 42:124–129, 1988.

Gabibov, G., Blinkov, S., Tcherekayev, V.: The management of optic nerve meningiomas and gliomas. J. Neurosurg. 68:889–893, 1988.

Hakuba, A., Nishimura, S.: Total removal of clivus meningiomas and the operative results. Neurol. Med. Chir. (Tokyo) 21:59–73, 1981.

Kondoh, T., Tamaki, N., Taomoto, K., et al.: Surgical approaches to foramen magnum meningioma. Report of three cases. Neurol. Med. Chir. (Tokyo) 30:163–168, 1990.

Leonetti, J., Reichman, H., Smith, P., et al.: Meningiomas of the lateral skull base: Neurorologic manifestations and patterns of recurrence. Otolaryngol. Head Neck Surg. 103:972–980, 1990.

Lesoin, F., Jomin, M., Bouchez, B., et al.: Management of cavernous sinus meningiomas. Neurochirurgia 28:195–198, 1985.

Probst, C.: Possibilities and limitations of microsurgery in patients with meningiomas of the sellar region. Acta Neurochir. (Wien) 84:99–102, 1987.

Rausing, A., Ybo, W., Stenflo, J.: Intracranial meningioma. A population study of ten years. Acta Neurol. Scand. 46:102–110, 1970.

Samii, M., Ammirati, M.: Surgery of Skull Base Meningiomas. New York: Springer-Verlag, 1992.

Sekhar, L., Jannetta, P., Burkhart, L., Janosky, J.: Meningiomas involving the clivus: A six-year experience with 41 patients. Neurosurgery 27:764–781, 1990.

Walker, A., Robins, M. Weinfeld, F.: Epidemiology of brain tumors: The national survey of intracranial neoplasms. Neurology 35:219–226, 1985.

Zülch, K.: Brain Tumors. Their Biology and Pathology. New York: Springer-Verlag, 1986.

Zülch, K. (ed.): Histological Typing of Tumours of the Central Nervous System. International Histological Classification of Tumors, no. 21. Geneva: World Health Organization, 1979.

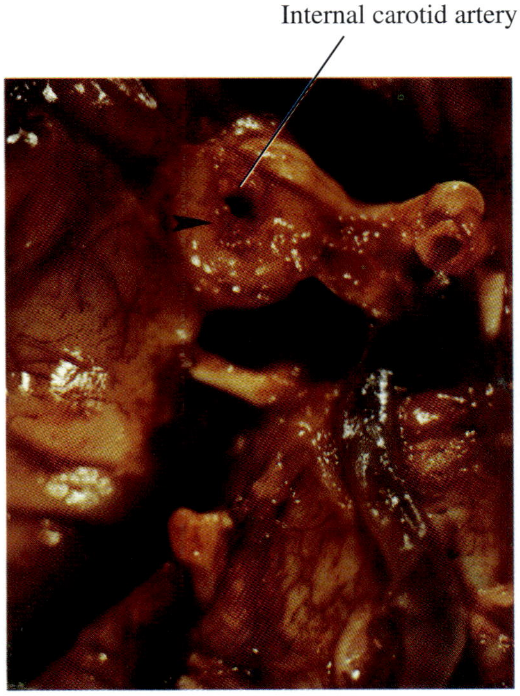

Figure 1. Globular meningioma *(arrowhead)* surrounding the right internal carotid artery.

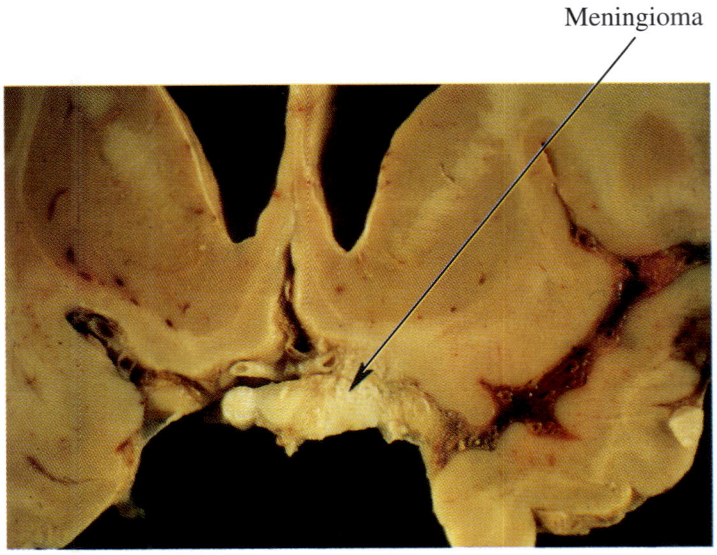

Figure 2. Meningioma en plaque *(arrowhead)* compressing the optic chiasm.

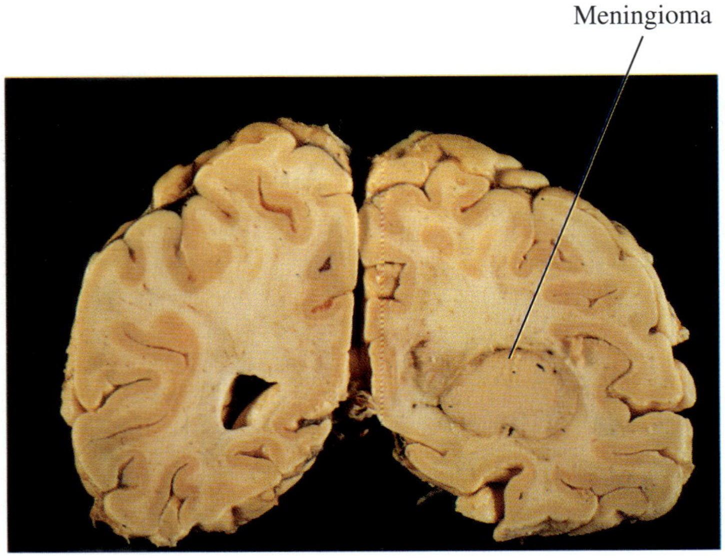

Figure 3. Intraventricular meningioma occluding the lateral ventricle.

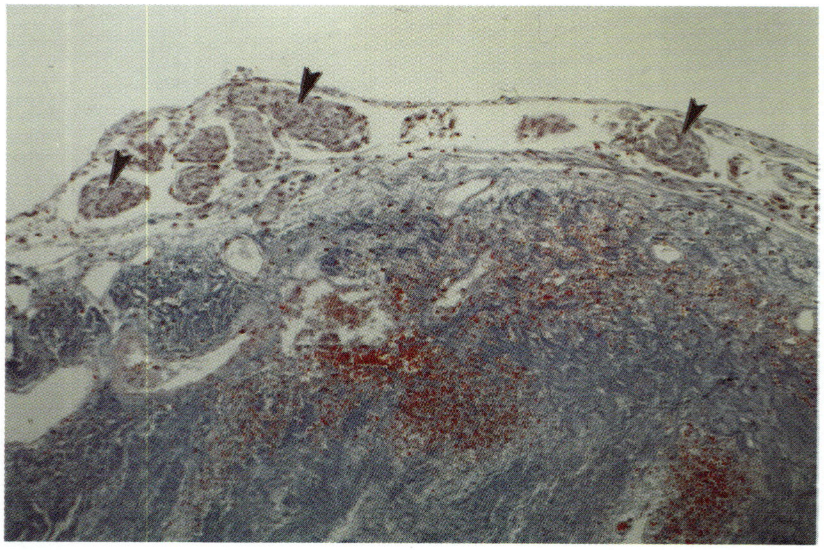

Figure 4. Small meningotheliomatous nodules *(arrowheads)* extending along the dura, eventually responsible for the meningeal sign in MRI. Masson-trichrome, 50×.

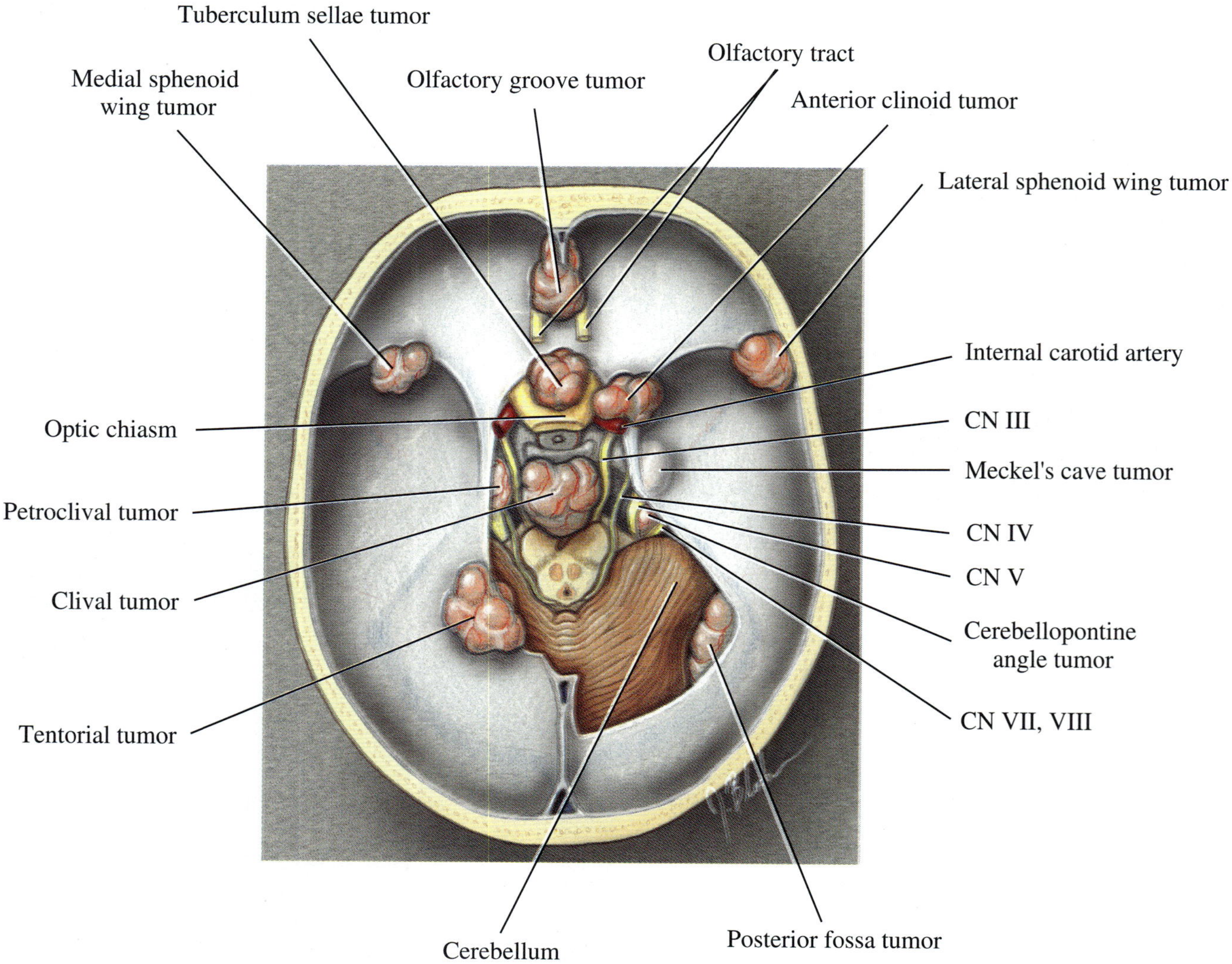

Figure 5. Common locations of cranial base meningiomas.

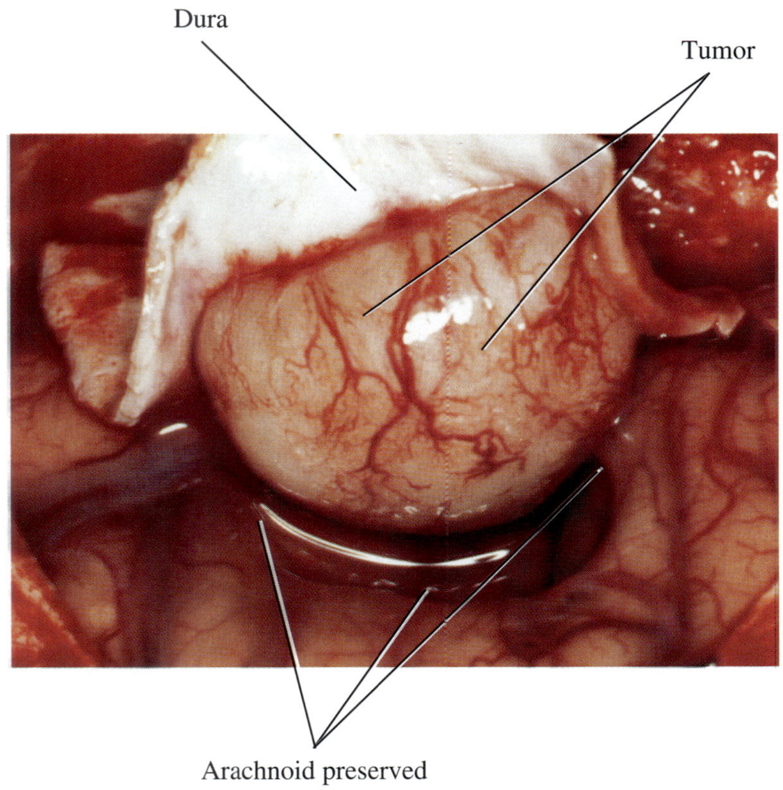

Figure 6. Dissection of the tumor capsule away from the neural tissue and vessels while staying within the arachnoid plane.

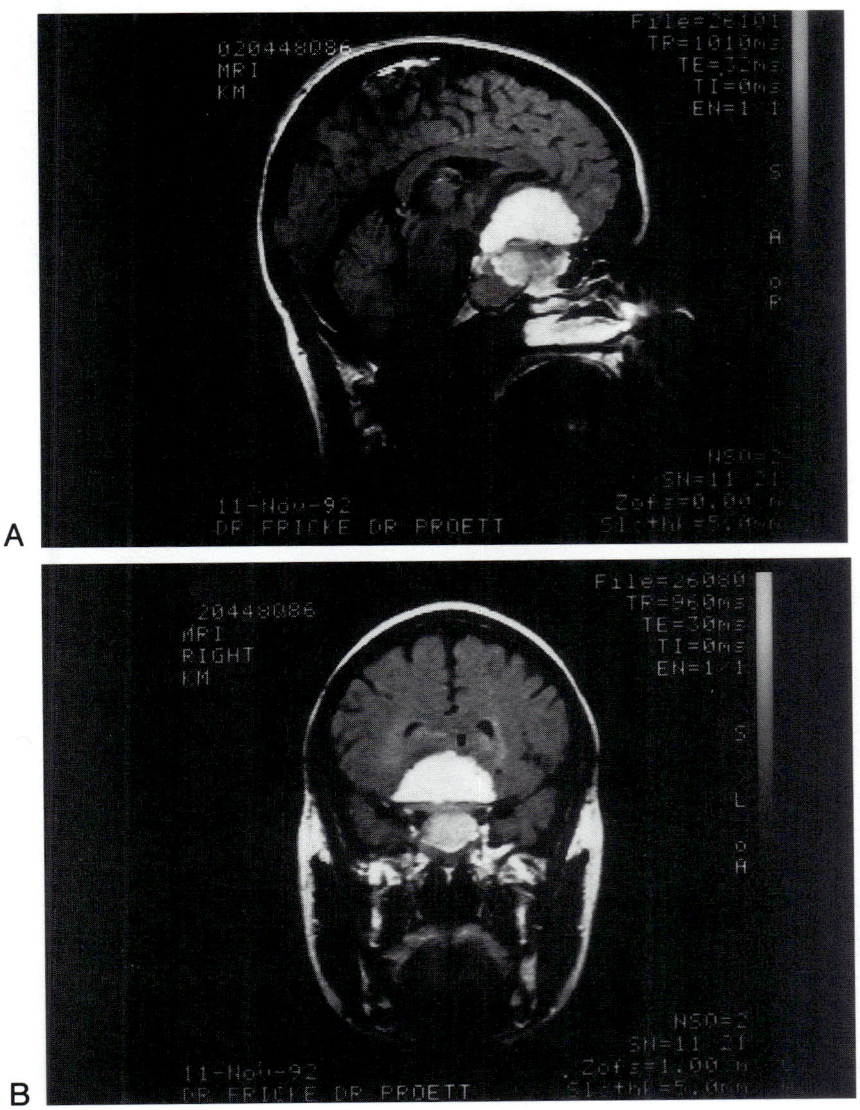

Figure 7. MRI scan showing a large subfrontal meningioma involving the planum sphenoidale, tuberculum sellae, olfactory groove, and ethmoid and sphenoid sinuses.

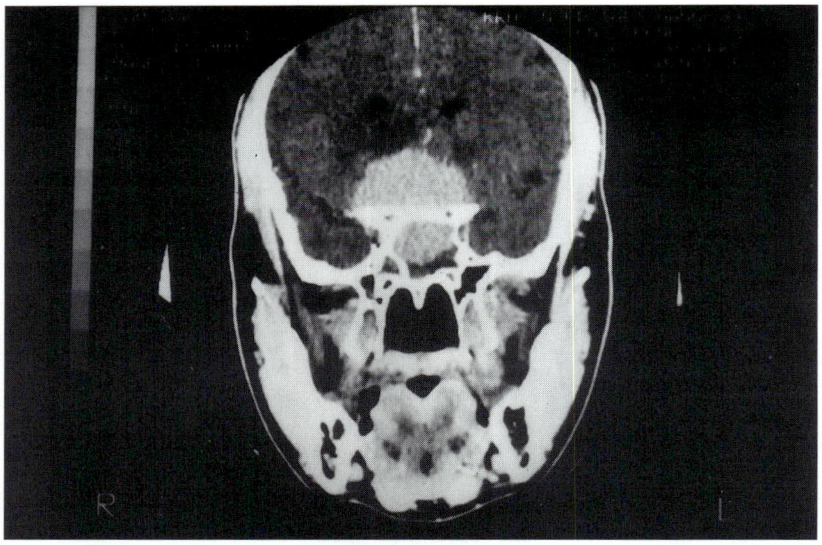

Figure 8. CT scan showing tumor extension into the sphenoid sinus.

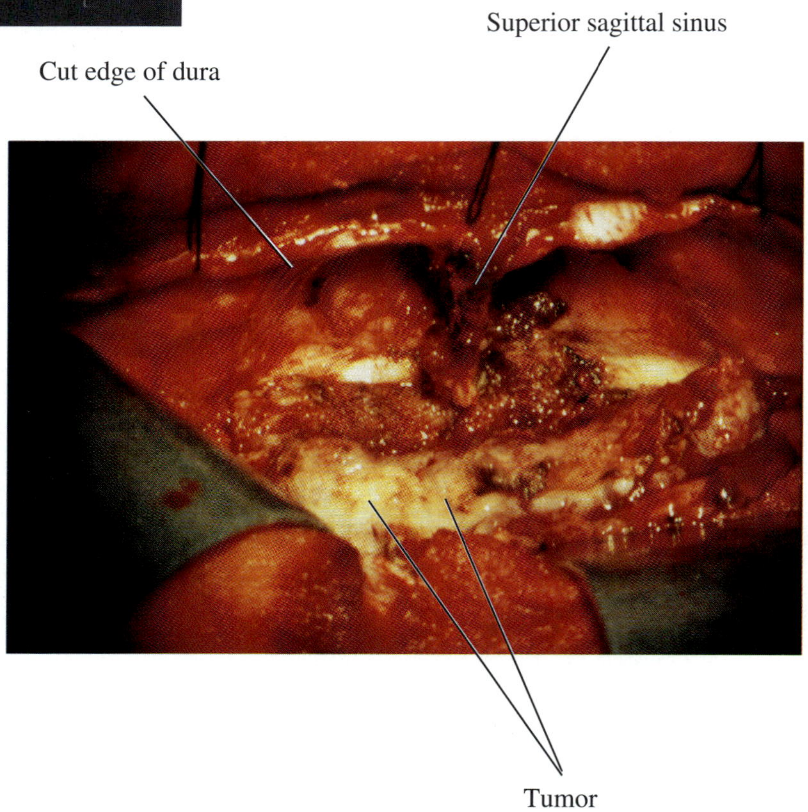

Figure 9. Bifrontal craniotomy with the dura opened and the superior sagittal sinus ligated and transected. The frontal lobes are gently retracted and the anterior aspect of the tumor is exposed.

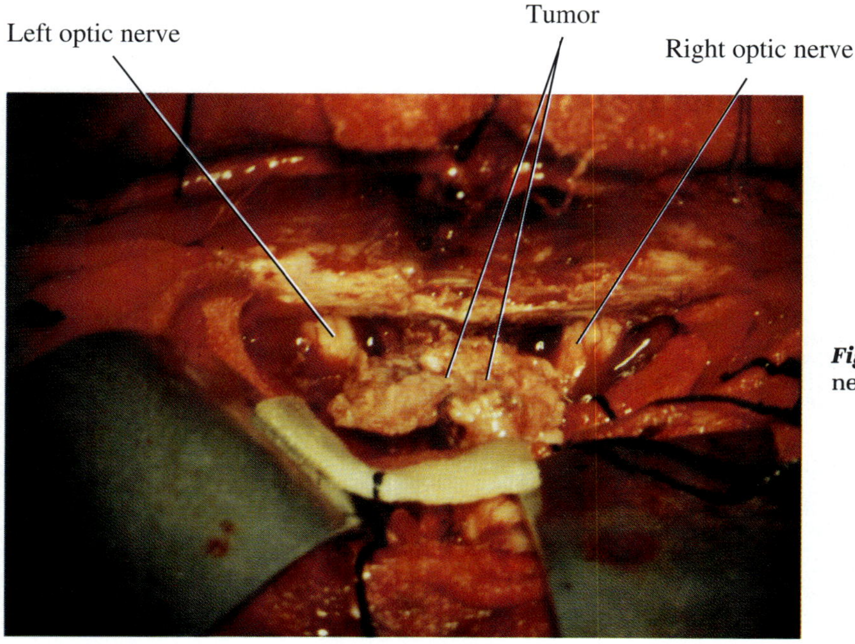

Figure 10. Partial tumor removal with both optic nerves visible.

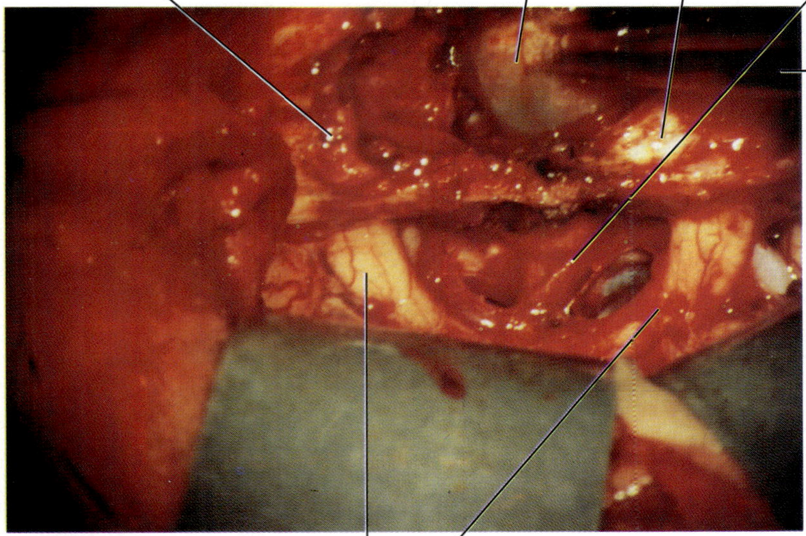

Figure 11. Total removal of the intracranial portion of the tumor with opening of the sphenoid sinus. The portion of the tumor in the sphenoid sinus is elevated with forceps. Both optic nerves and the infundibular stalk are seen.

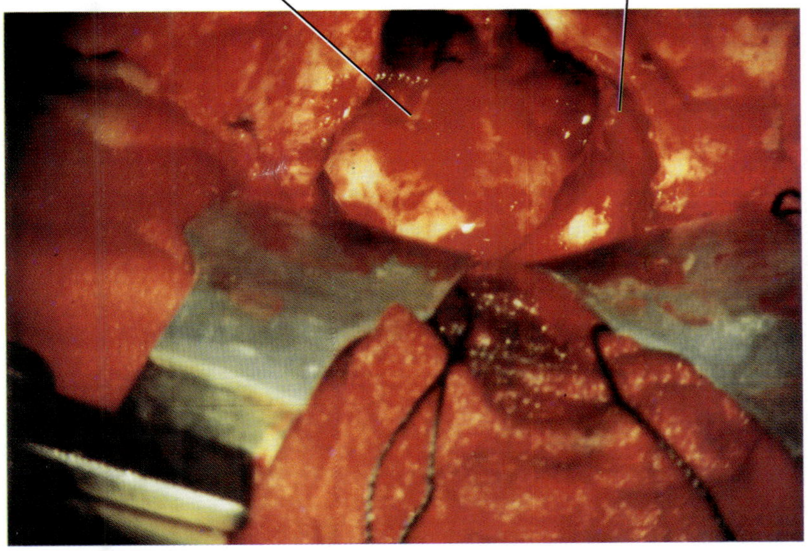

Figure 12. Complete removal of the tumor from the paranasal sinuses.

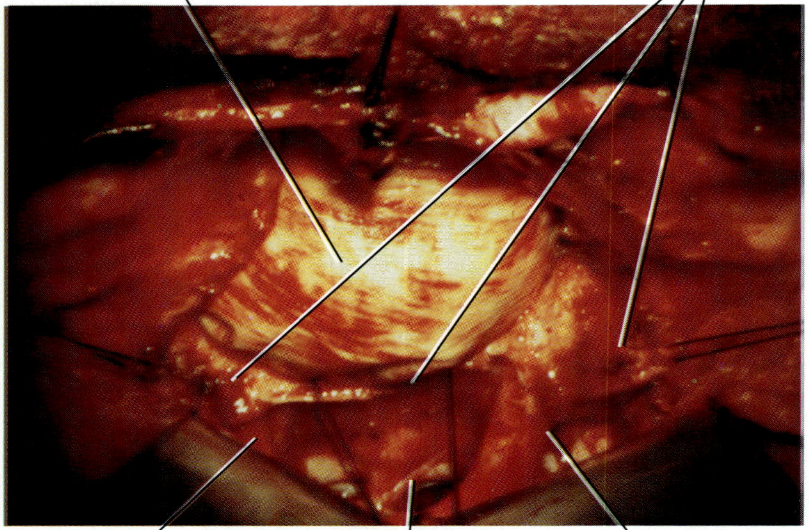

Figure 13. Paranasal sinuses after being packed with Xeroform gauze. The dural defect is covered by lyophilized dura. Several dural sutures will fix the pedicled pericranial flap.

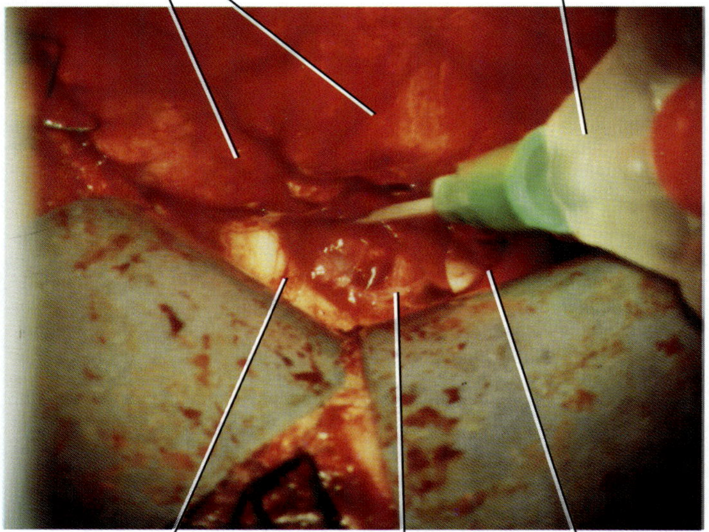

Figure 14. The entire anterior skull base is covered by pedicled pericranial flap. The suture line is sealed with fibrin glue.

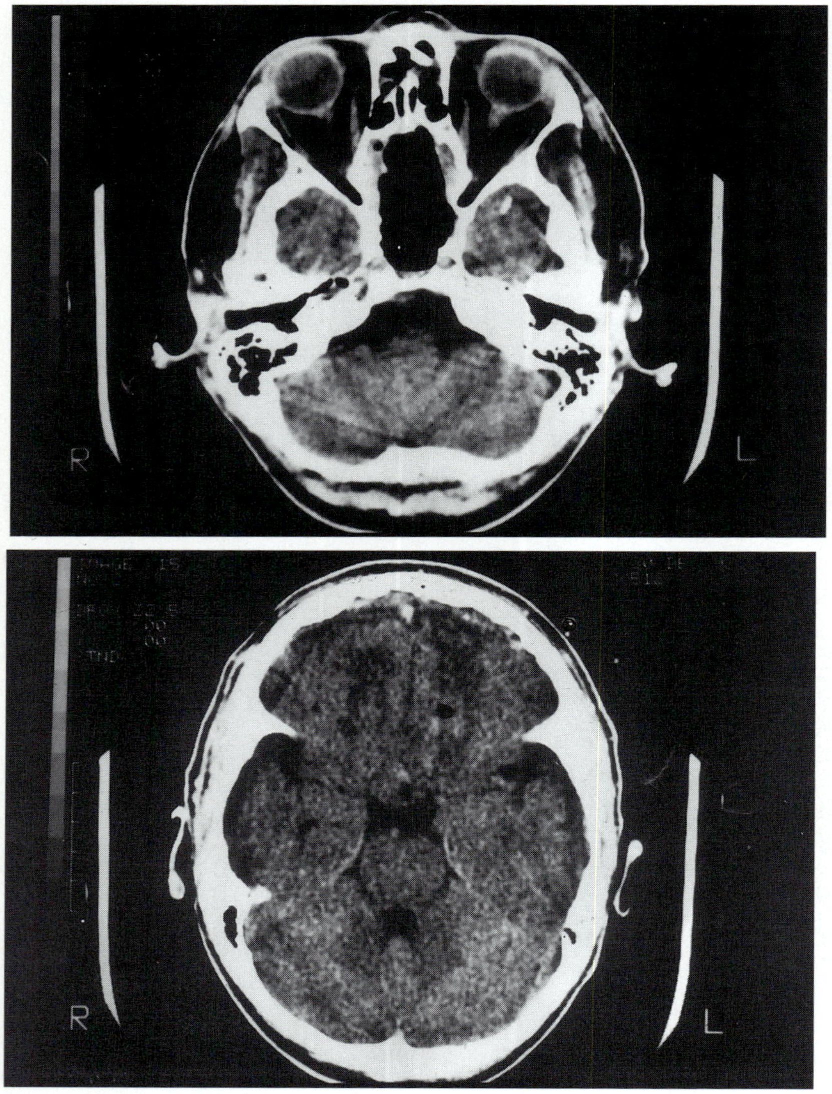

Figure 15. Postoperative CT scan demonstrating complete tumor removal.

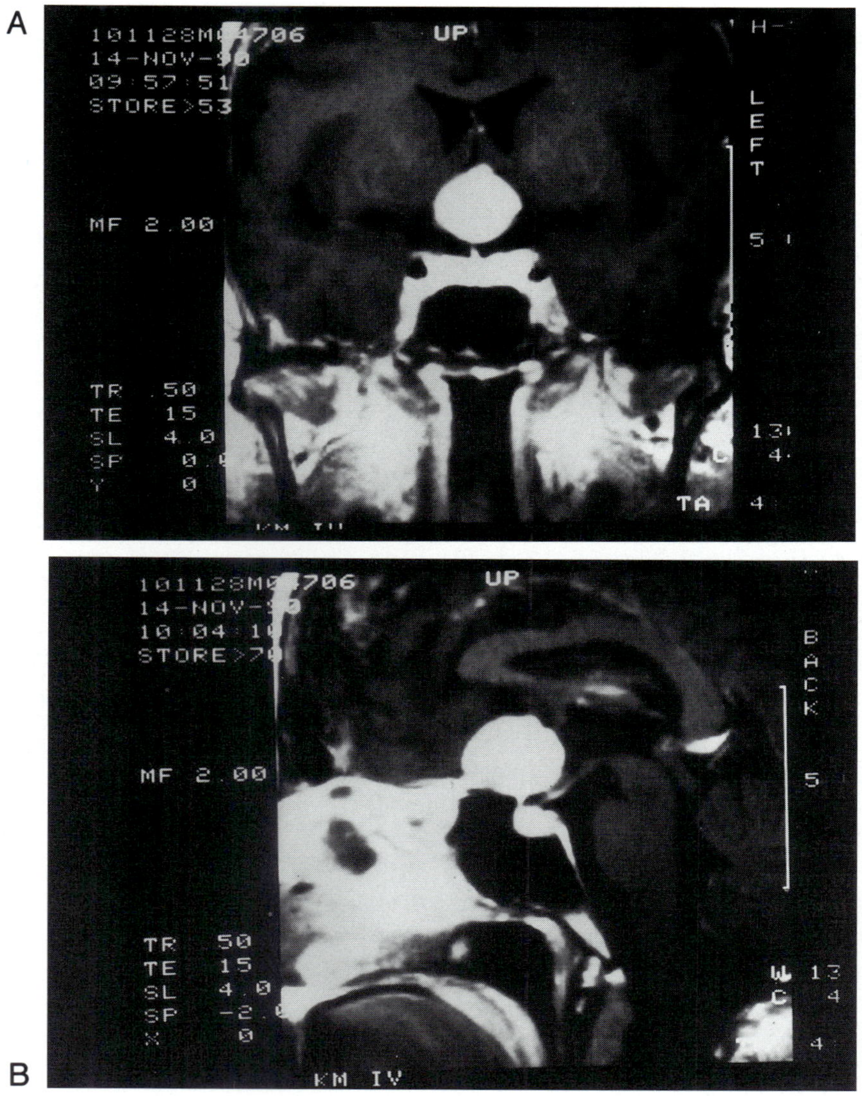

Figure 16. MRI scans showing tuberculum sella meningioma.

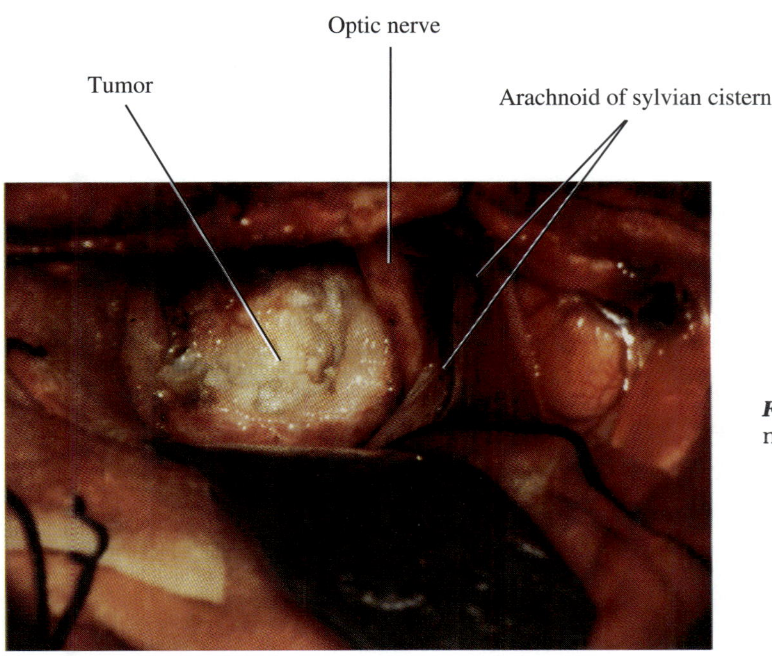

Figure 17. Pterional approach showing the meningioma compressing the right optic nerve.

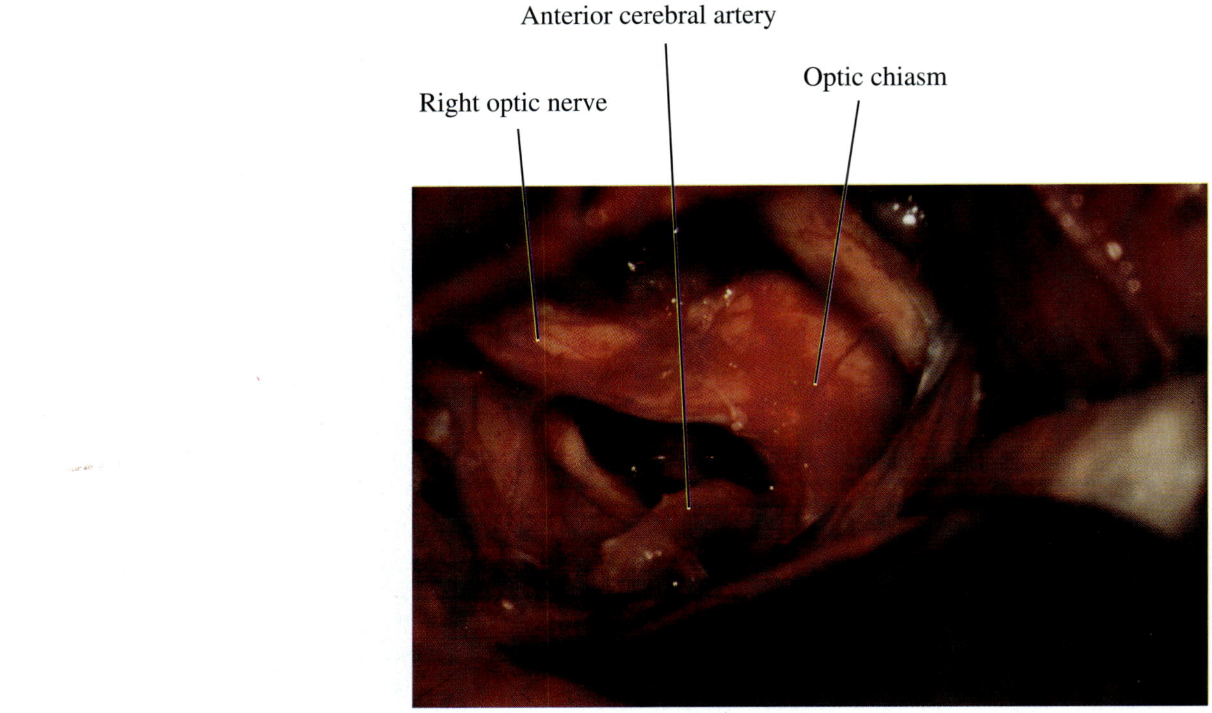

Figure 18. Total tumor removal with preservation of the optic nerve and chiasm as well as the anterior cerebral arteries, which were intimately attached to the tumor capsule.

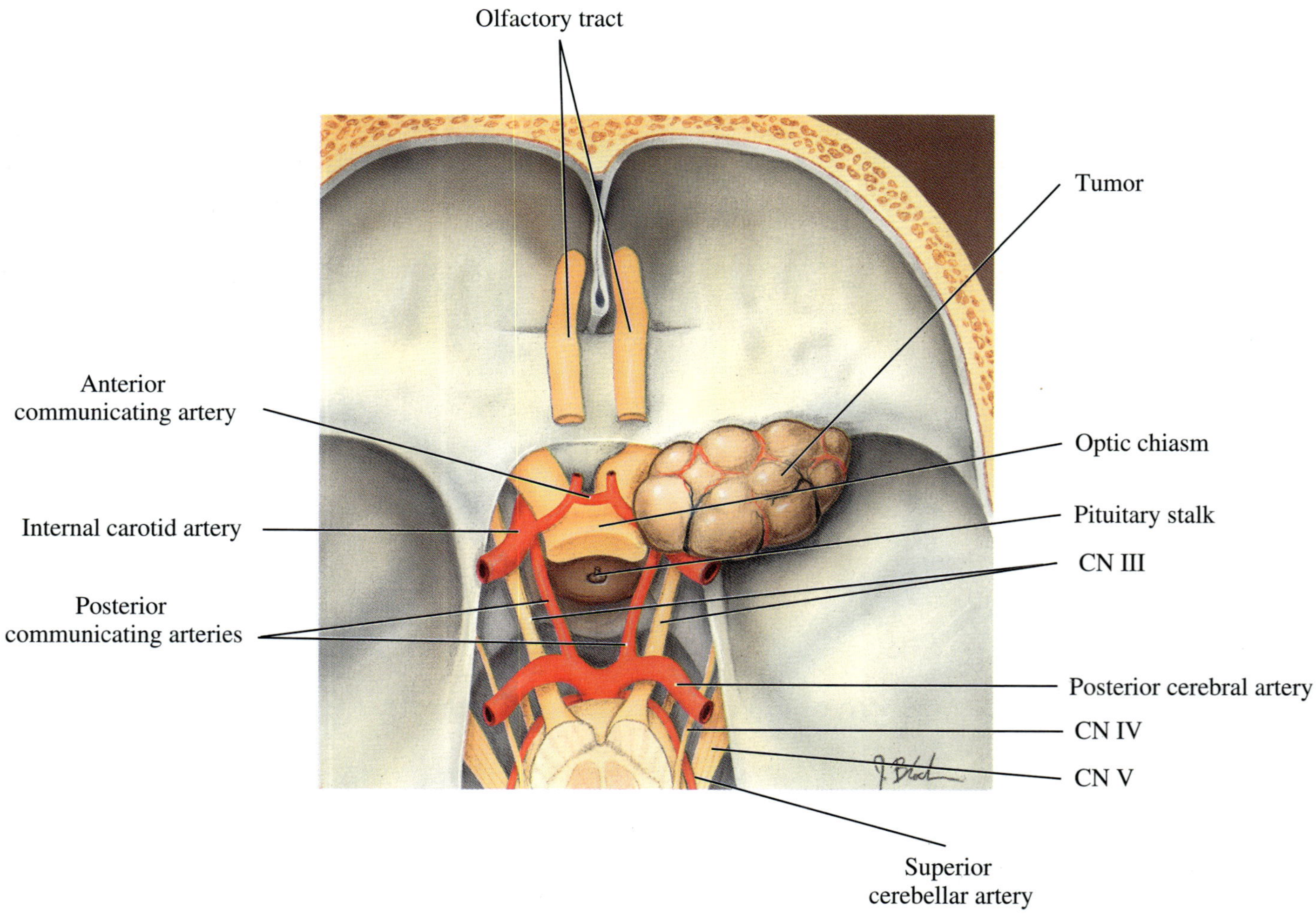

Figure 19. Meningioma of the medial third of the sphenoid ridge and anterior clinoid process.

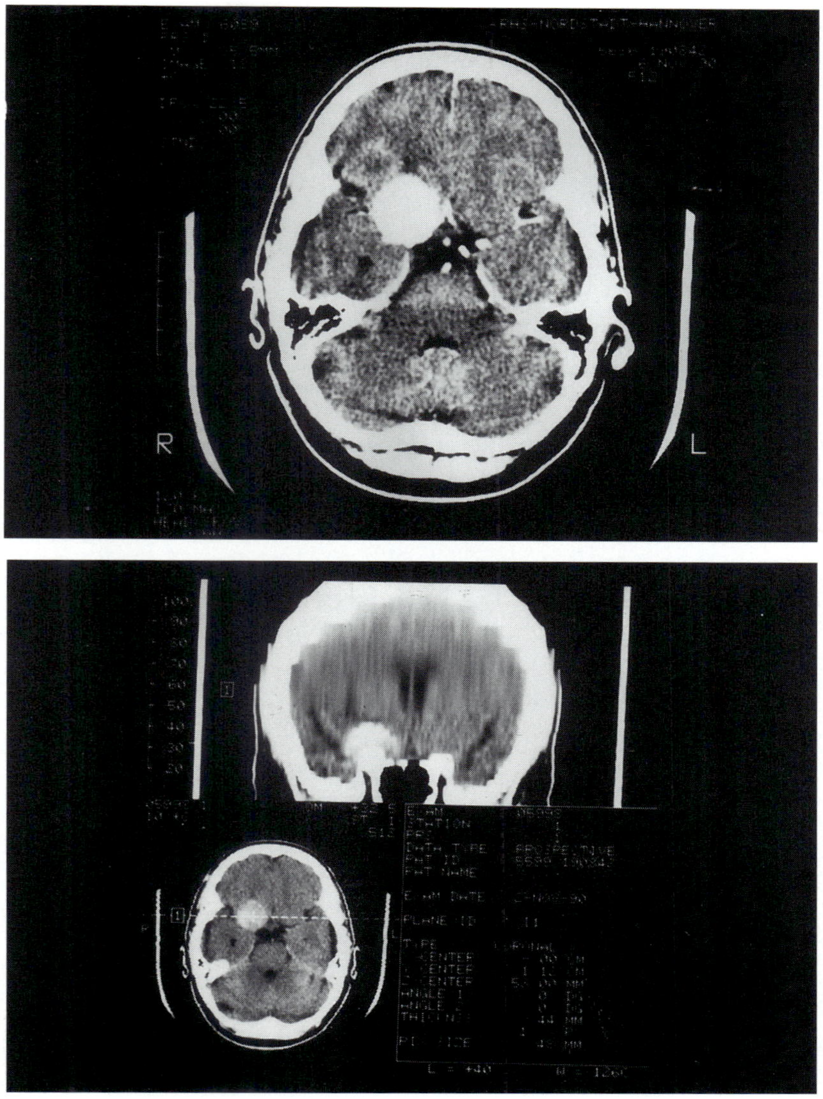

Figure 20. CT scan showing a right-sided meningioma of the anterior clinoid process.

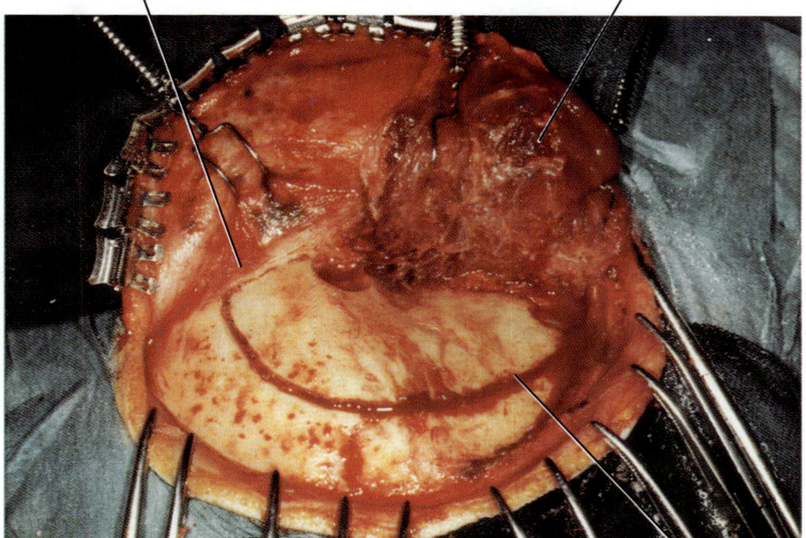

Figure 21. Placement of a frontotemporal craniotomy flap.

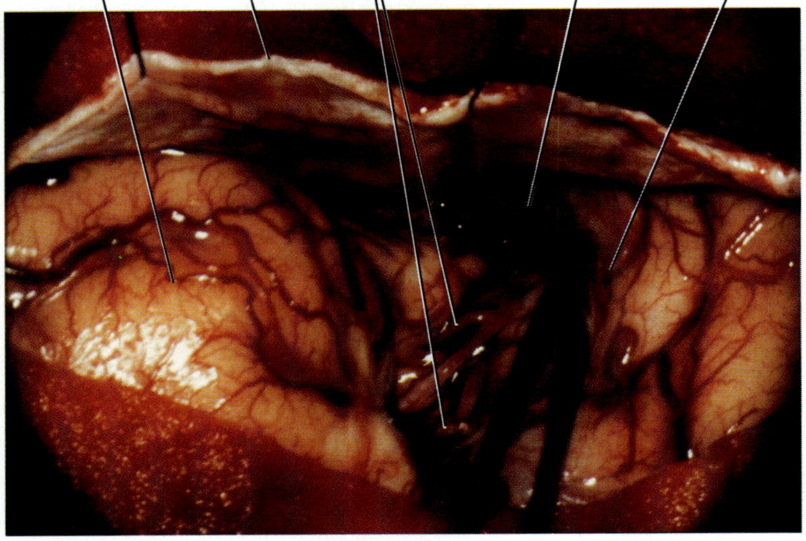

Figure 22. The dura has been opened and the sylvian fissure dissected.

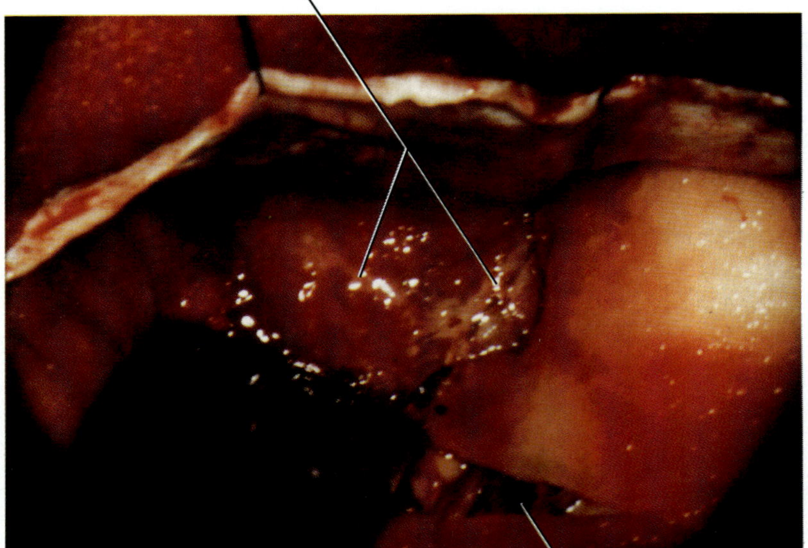

Figure 23. The sylvian fissure is open and the anterior clinoid meningioma exposed.

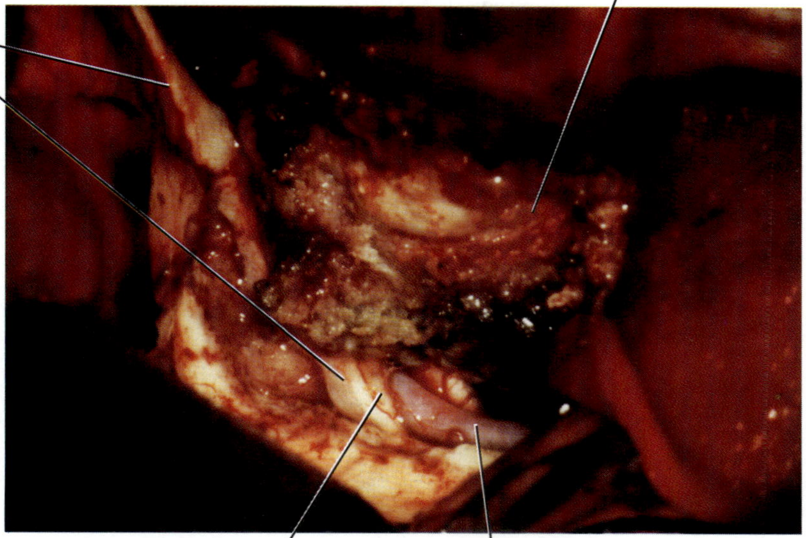

Figure 24. The tumor mass has been partially removed. The olfactory nerve and internal carotid artery are exposed.

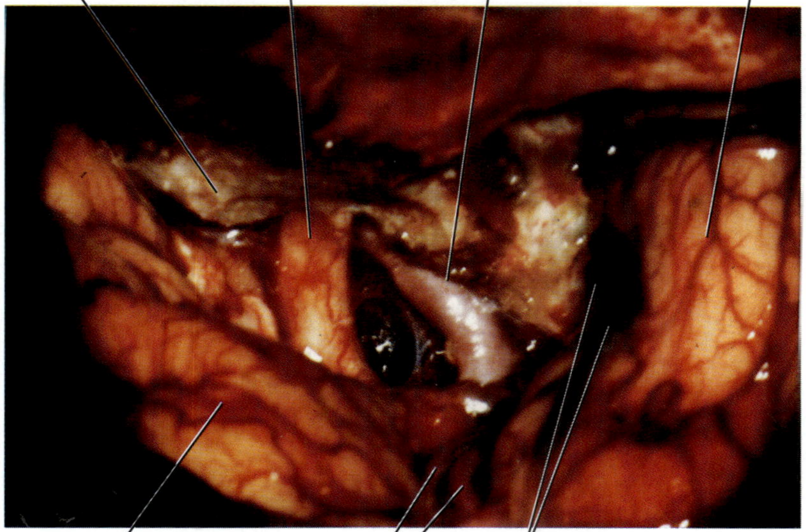

Figure 25. The tumor matrix, including the anterior clinoid process, has been removed using a diamond drill. The optic nerve canal is open. To achieve radical bony removal, the sphenoid sinus was opened.

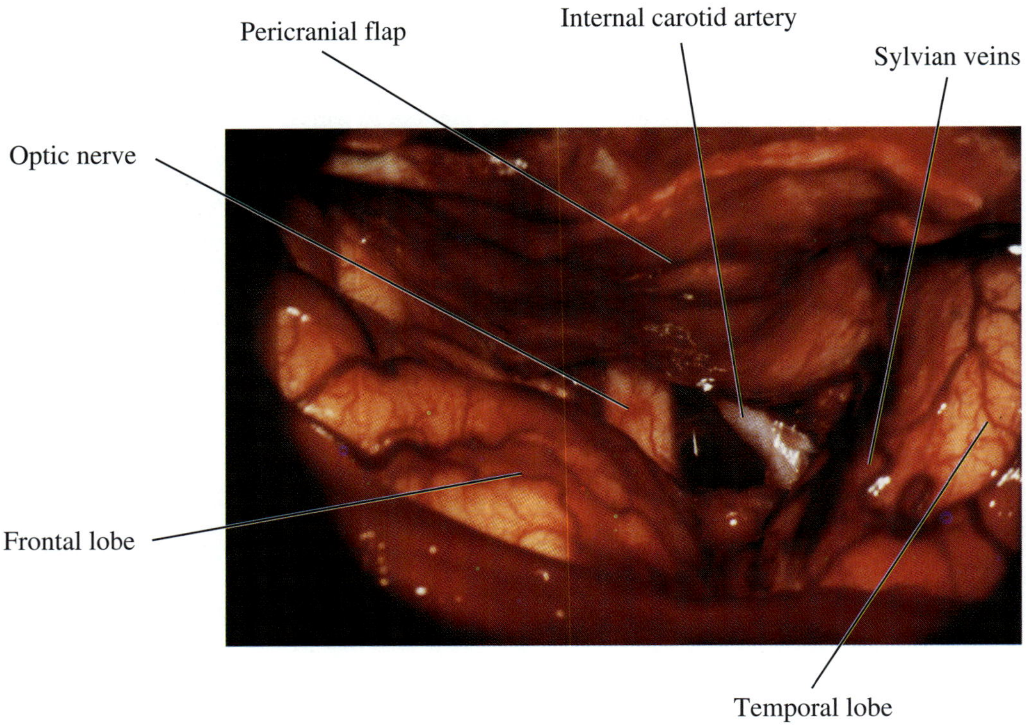

Figure 26. The dural defect around the optic canal and the clinoid process has been covered by a pericranial flap and sealed by fibrin glue.

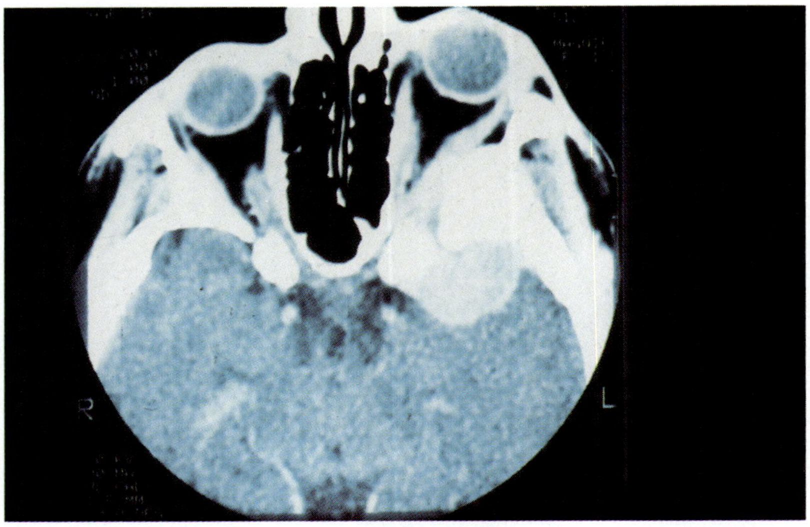

Figure 27. CT scan showing a meningioma of the sphenoid wing and orbit.

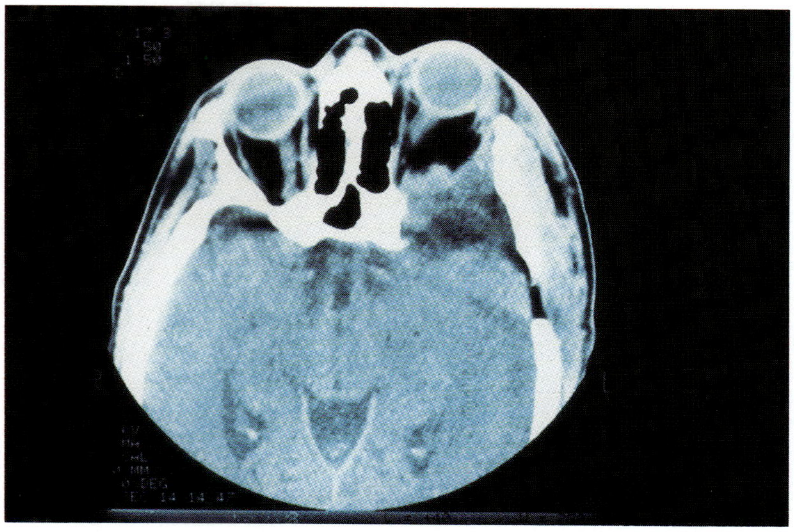

Figure 28. Postoperative CT scan showing partial removal of the meningioma with bony decompression of the orbit.

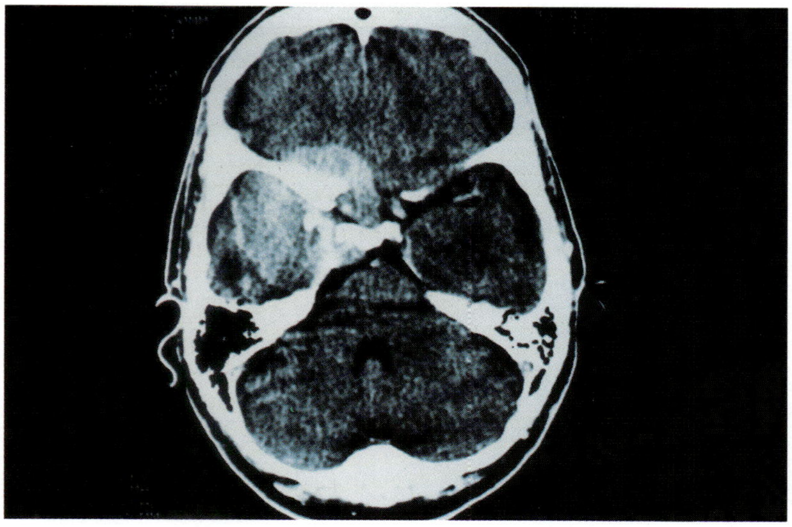

Figure 29. CT scan of a meningioma with involvement of the cavernous sinus, orbit, and sphenoid wing.

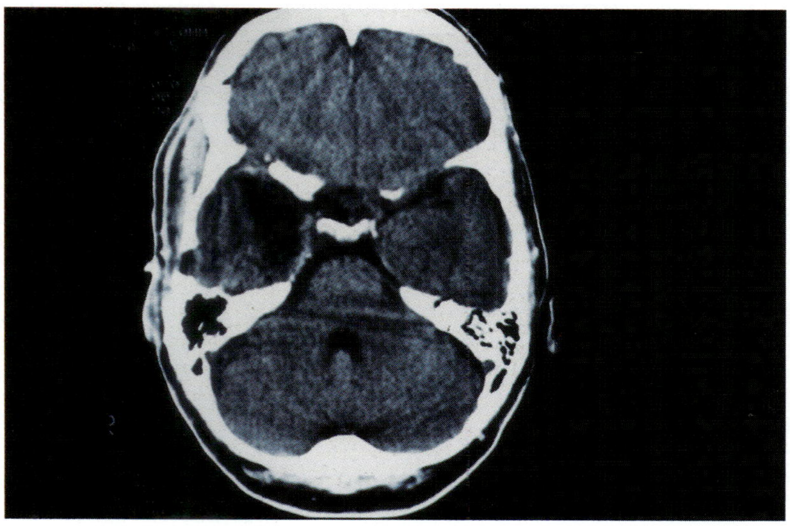

Figure 30. Postoperative CT scan showing removal of the well-encapsulated meningioma.

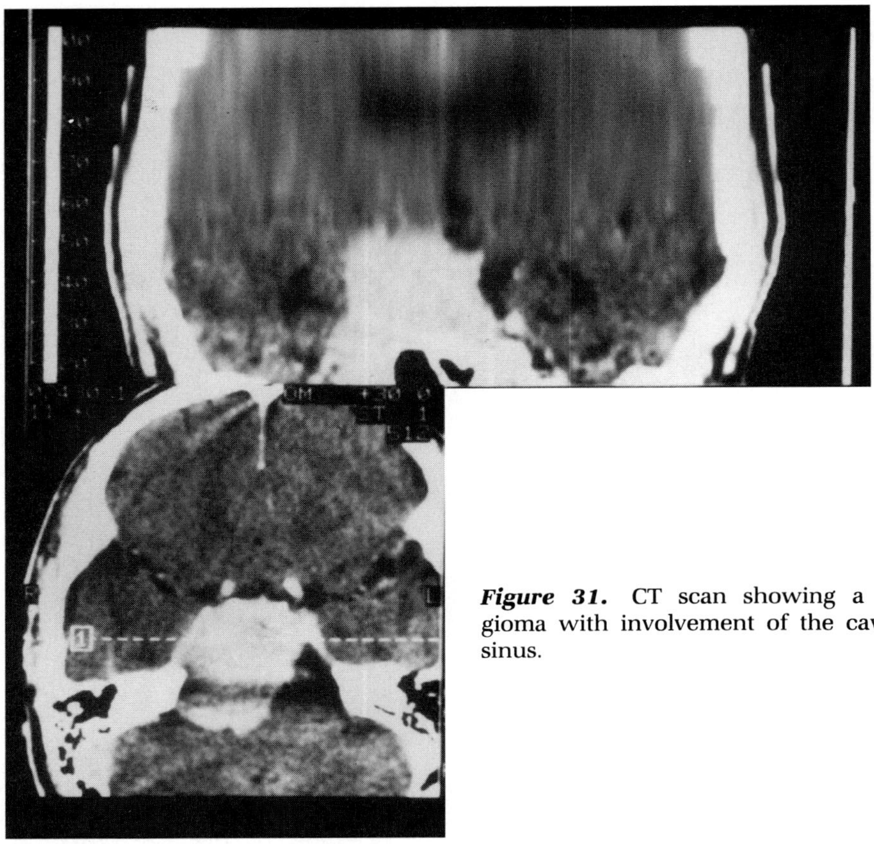

Figure 31. CT scan showing a meningioma with involvement of the cavernous sinus.

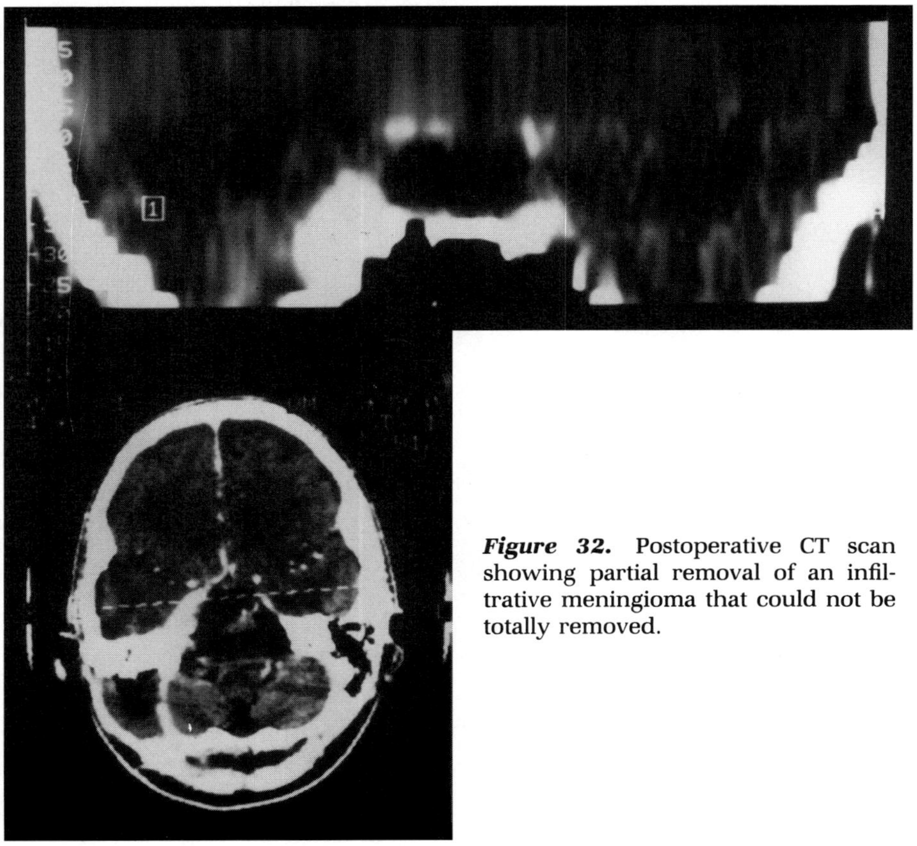

Figure 32. Postoperative CT scan showing partial removal of an infiltrative meningioma that could not be totally removed.

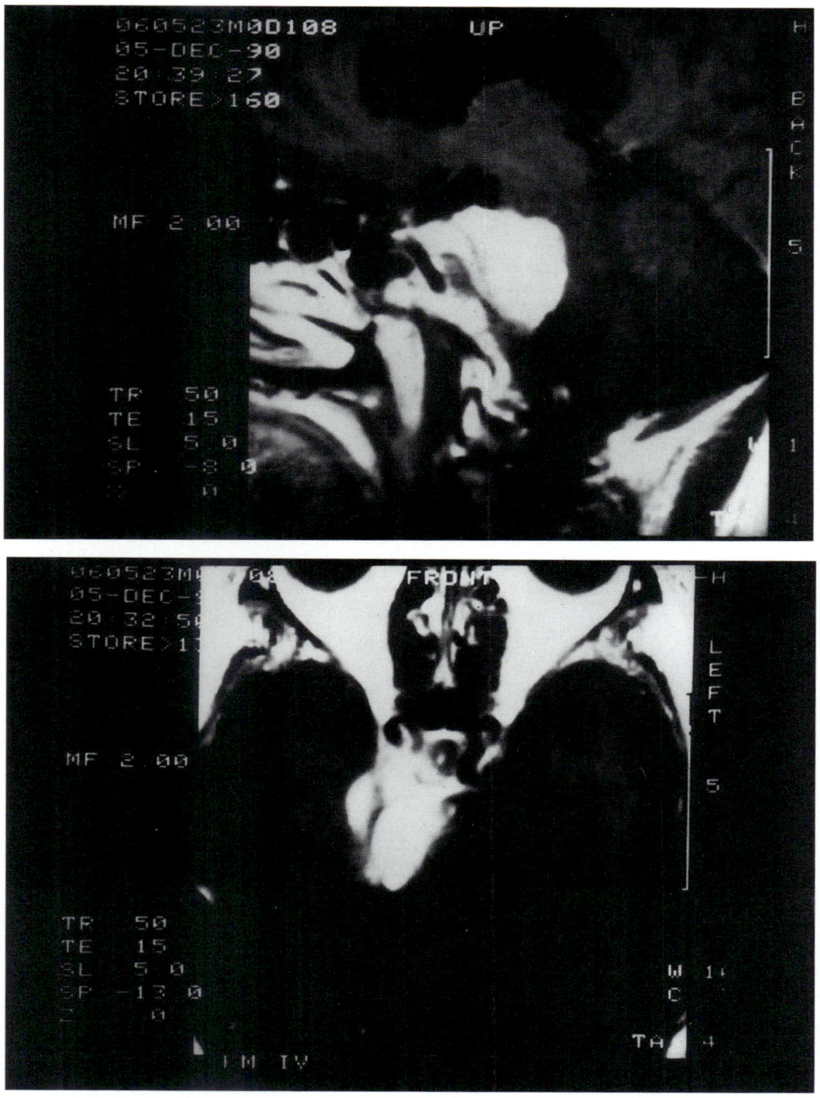

Figure 33. MRI scans demonstrating a petroclival meningioma with brain stem displacement.

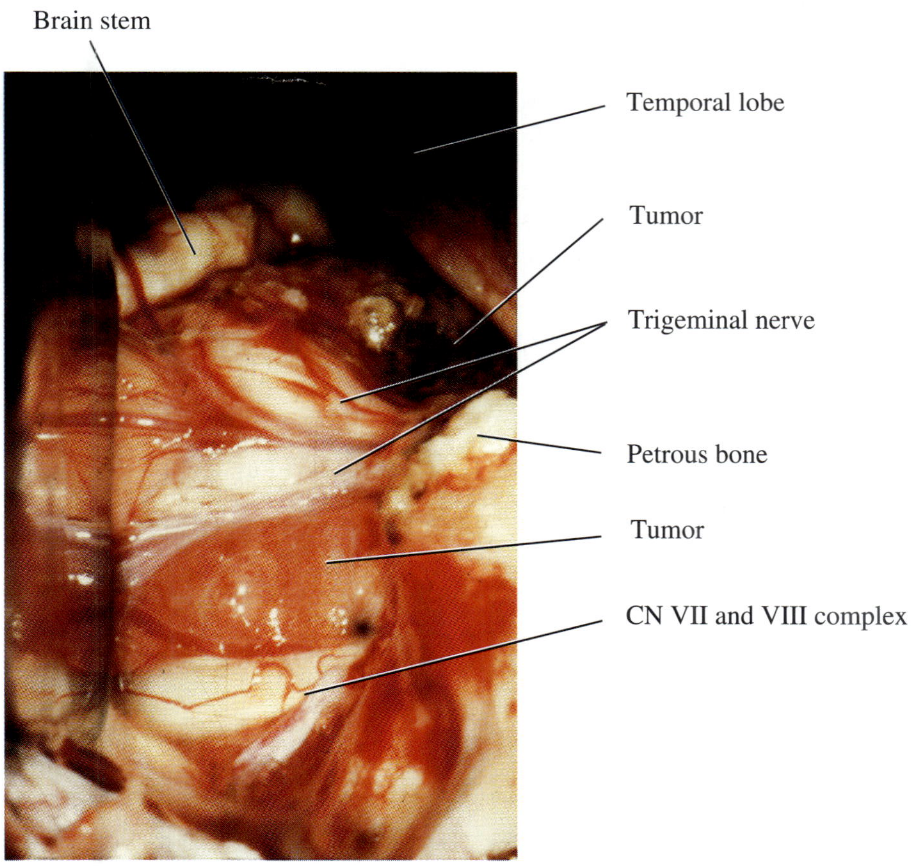

Figure 34. Transtentorial exposure of the petroclival meningioma. The trigeminal nerve and cranial nerves VII and VIII are shown compressed by tumor.

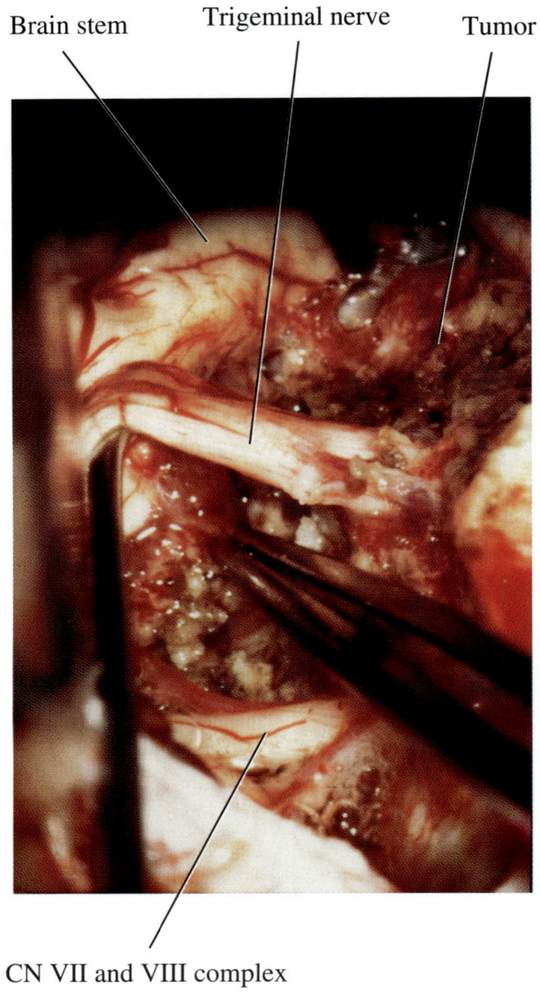

Figure 35. Partial tumor removal has been achieved. The infiltration of tumor tissue is visualized along the brain stem. The arachnoid membrane has been destroyed; therefore, total tumor removal is not possible.

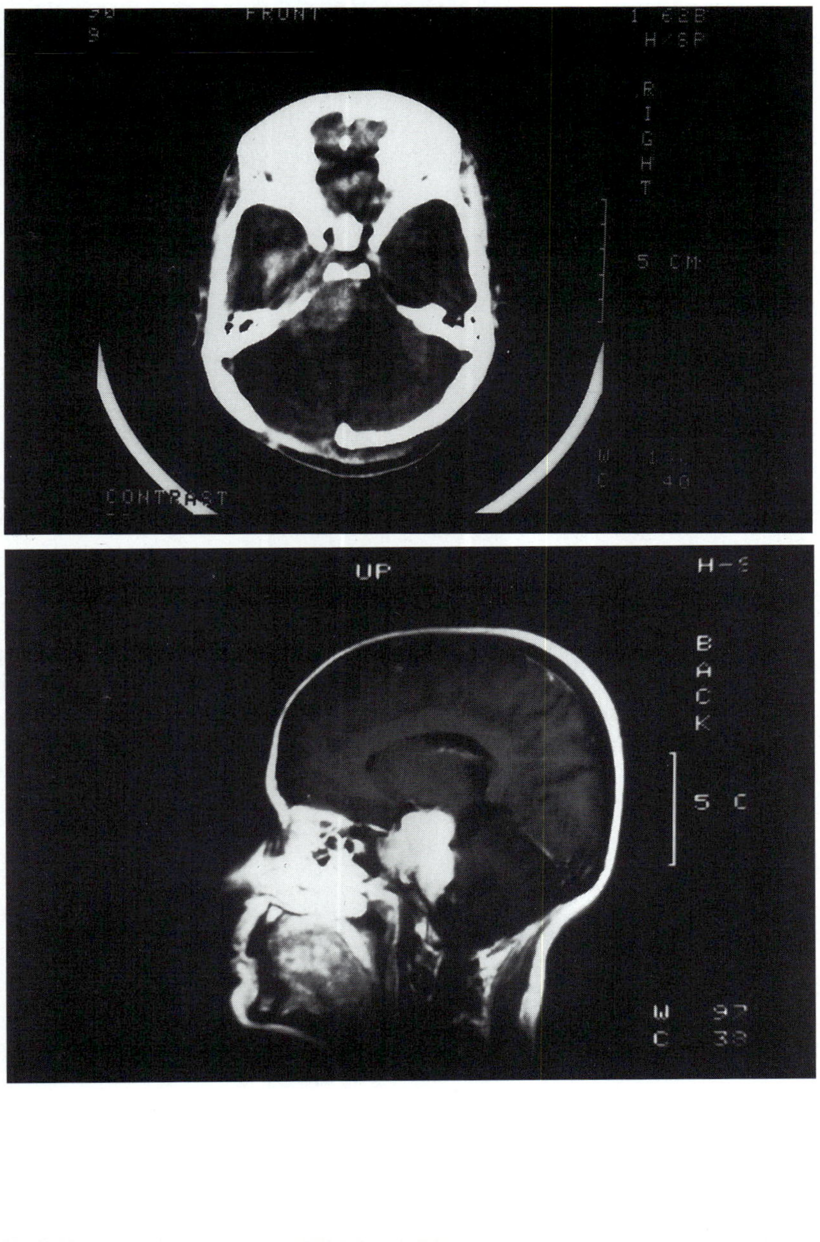

Figure 36. CT and MRI scans showing left-sided petroclival meningioma with involvement of the cavernous sinus. This 40-year-old female had undergone partial tumor removal elsewhere 2 years earlier by a subtemporal approach.

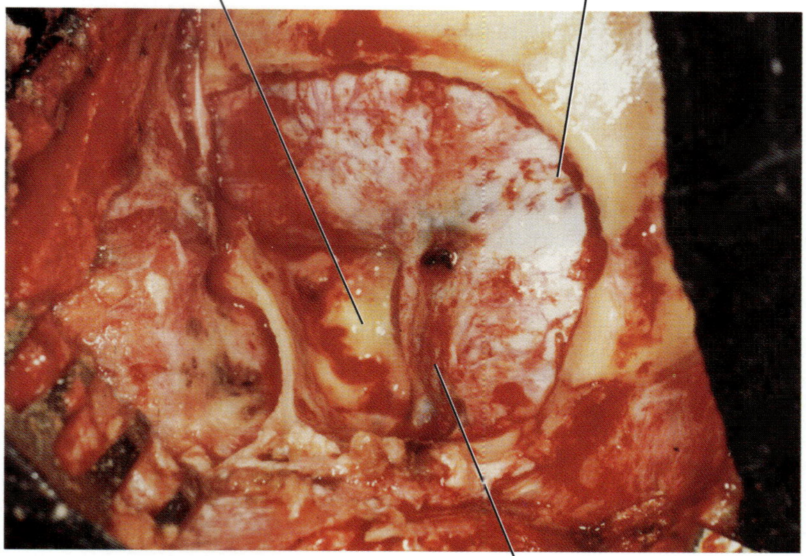

Figure 37. Combined temporal and lateral suboccipital craniotomy with exposure of the transverse and sigmoid sinuses.

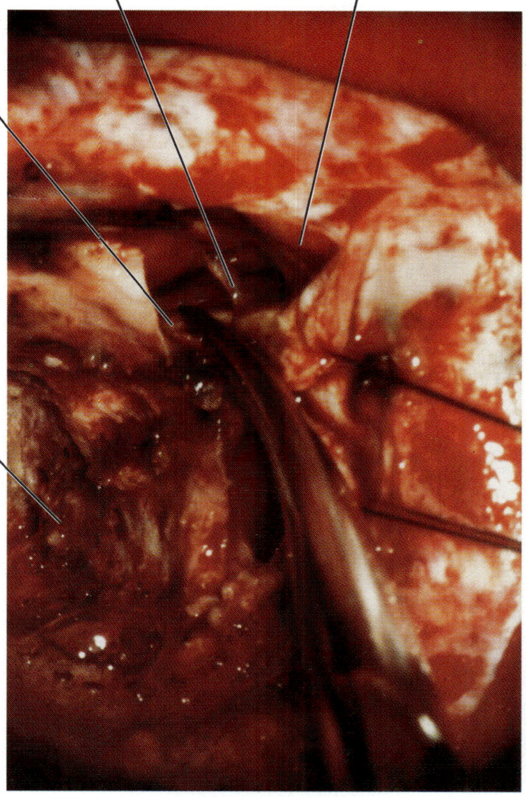

Figure 38. Presigmoid approach with transection of the tentorium.

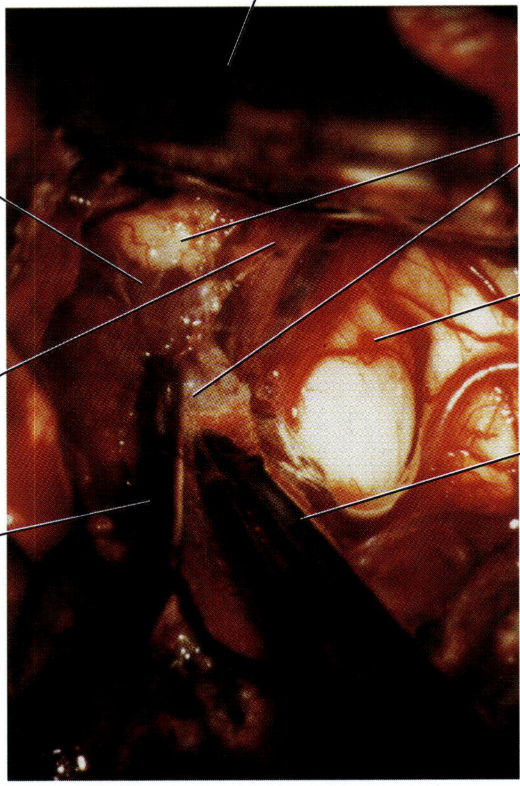

Figure 39. Tumor dissection from the brain stem showing well-preserved arachnoid membrane.

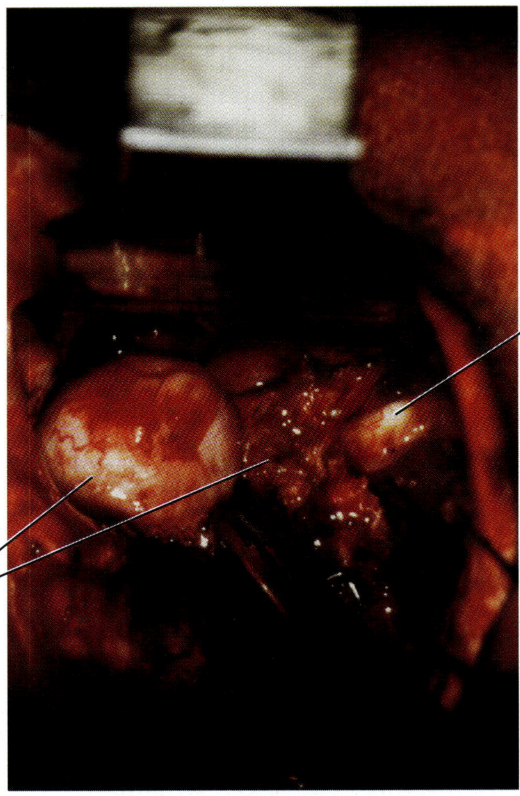

Figure 40. Meningioma in the middle fossa with demonstration of the well-developed tumor capsule.

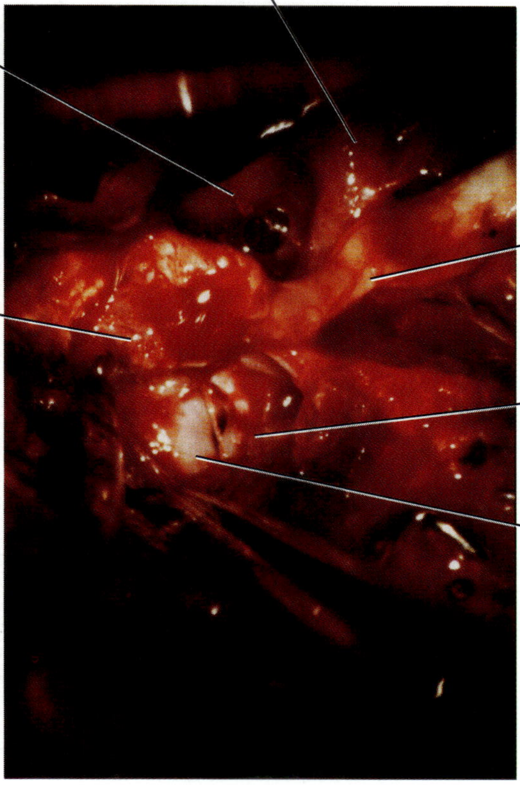

Figure 41. Removal of tumor tissue from the cavernous sinus. The carotid artery and abducent nerve can be seen within the sinus.

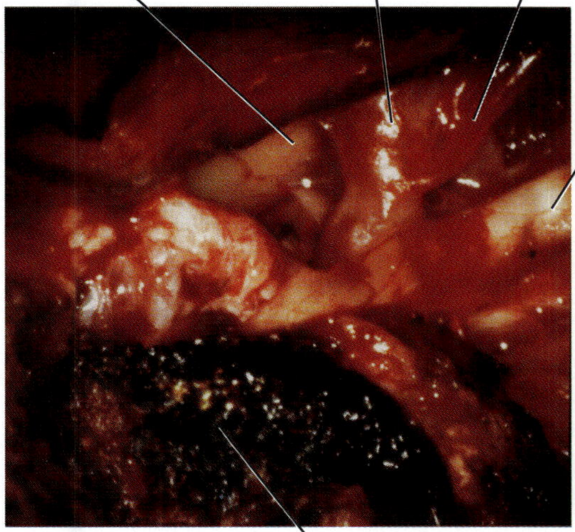

Figure 42. Hemostasis within the cavernous sinus has been achieved with the use of Surgicel. The internal carotid artery (supraclinoidal) and oculomotor nerve can be seen.

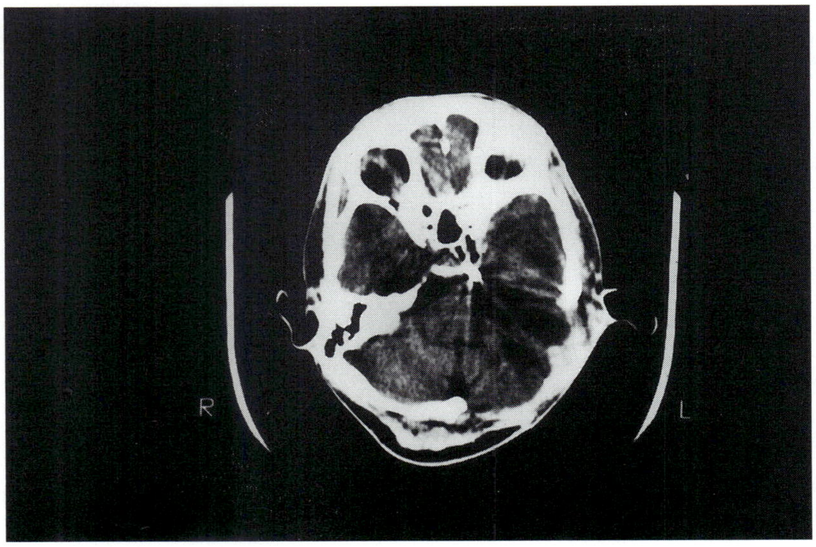

Figure 43. Postoperative CT scan showing total tumor removal.

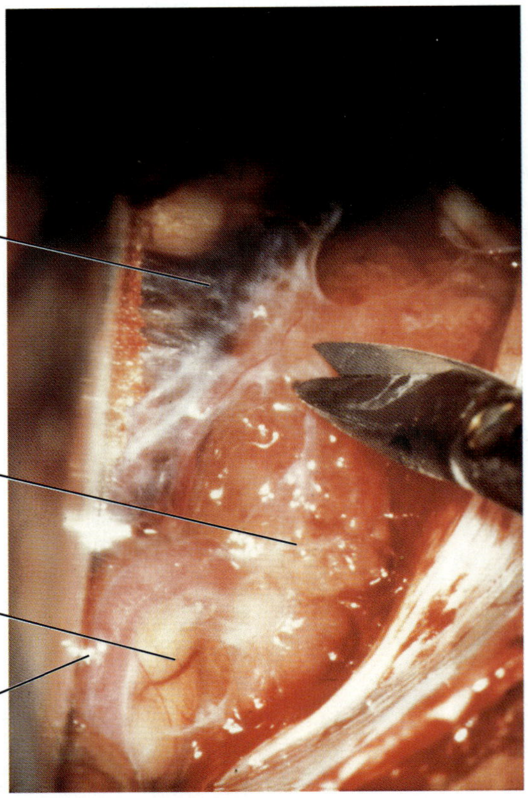

Figure 44. Large meningioma in cerebellopontine angle with well-preserved arachnoidal membrane.

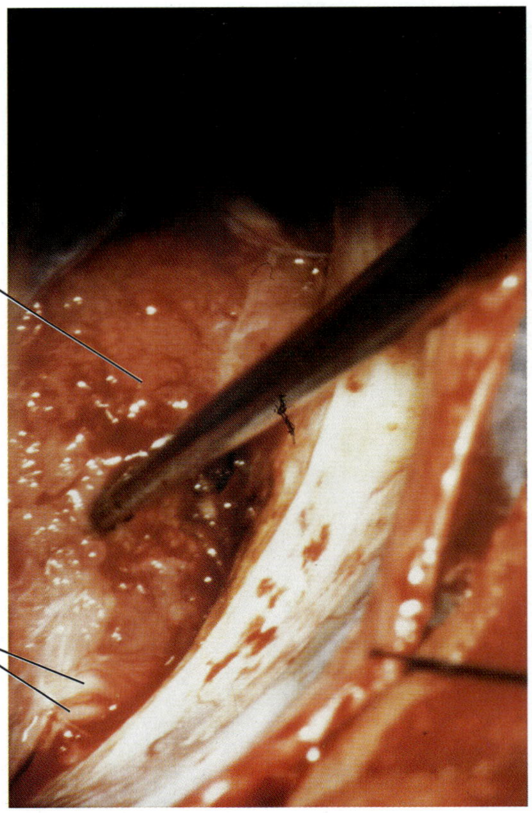

Figure 45. Caudal aspect of the tumor is shown with involvement of the lower cranial nerves.

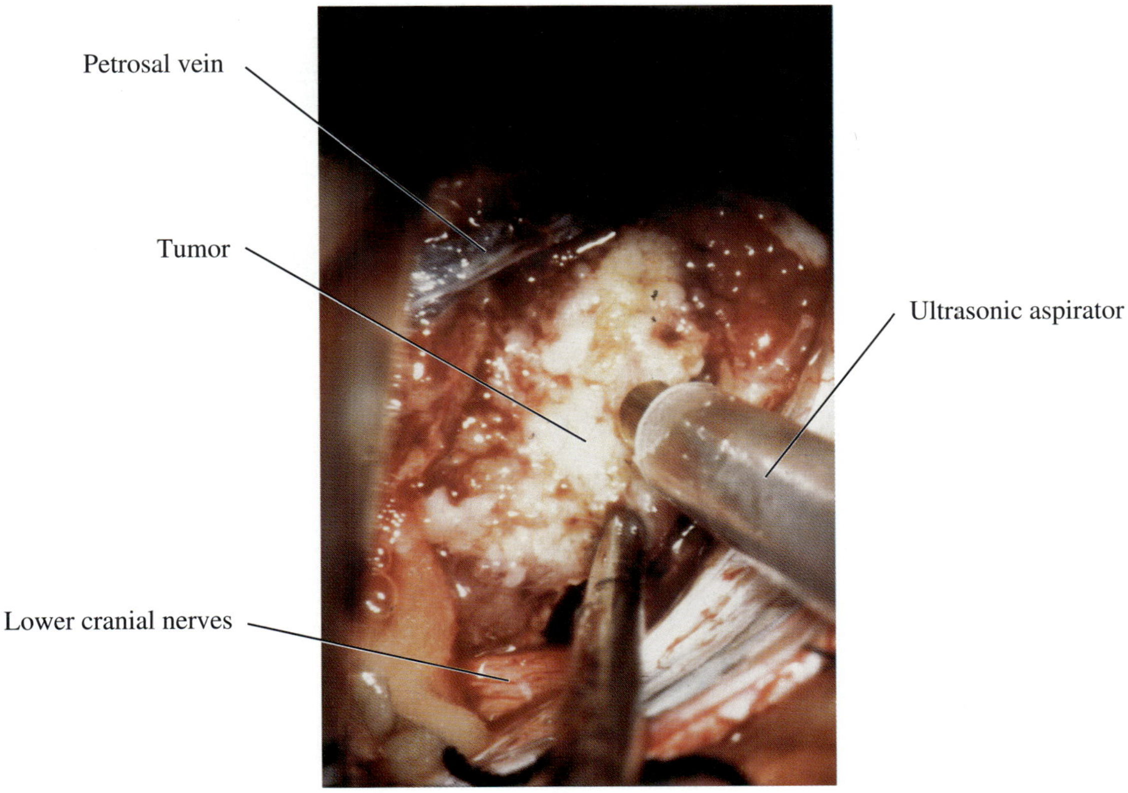

Figure 46. Lower cranial nerves are dissected. The ultrasonic aspirator is shown debulking the tumor.

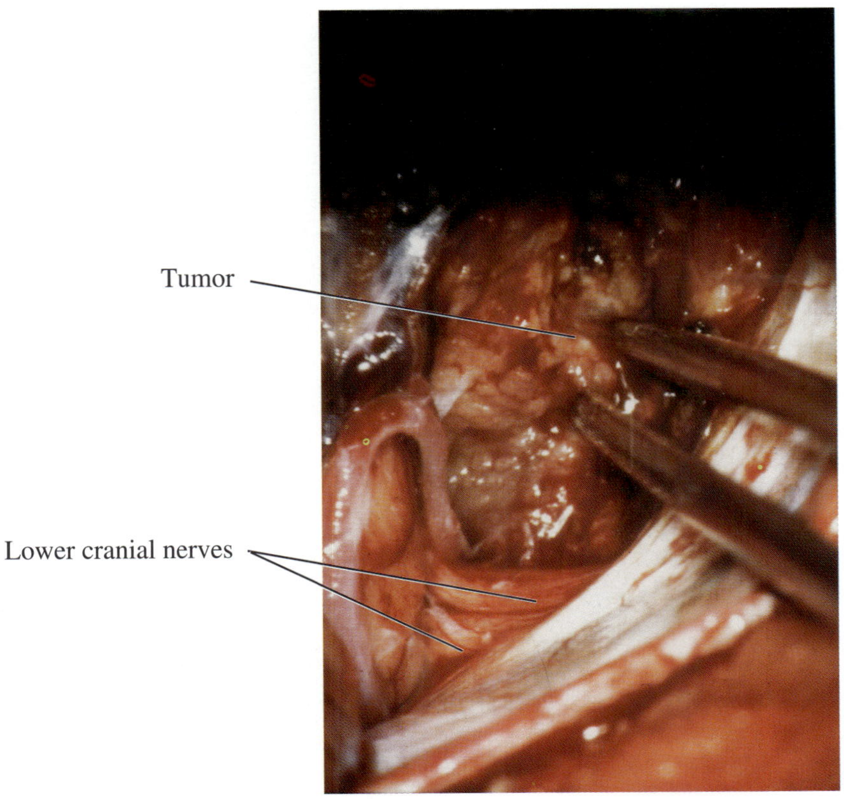

Figure 47. The anterior inferior cerebellar artery is shown dissected free from the tumor capsule.

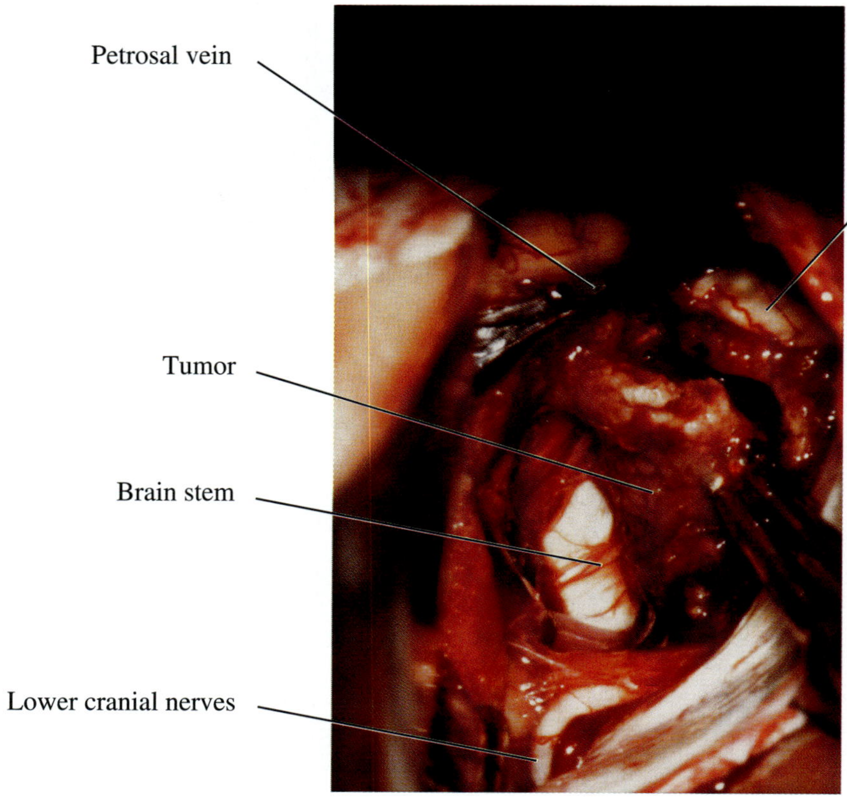

Figure 48. Dissection of the tumor capsule from the brain stem is shown. The lower cranial nerves are visible.

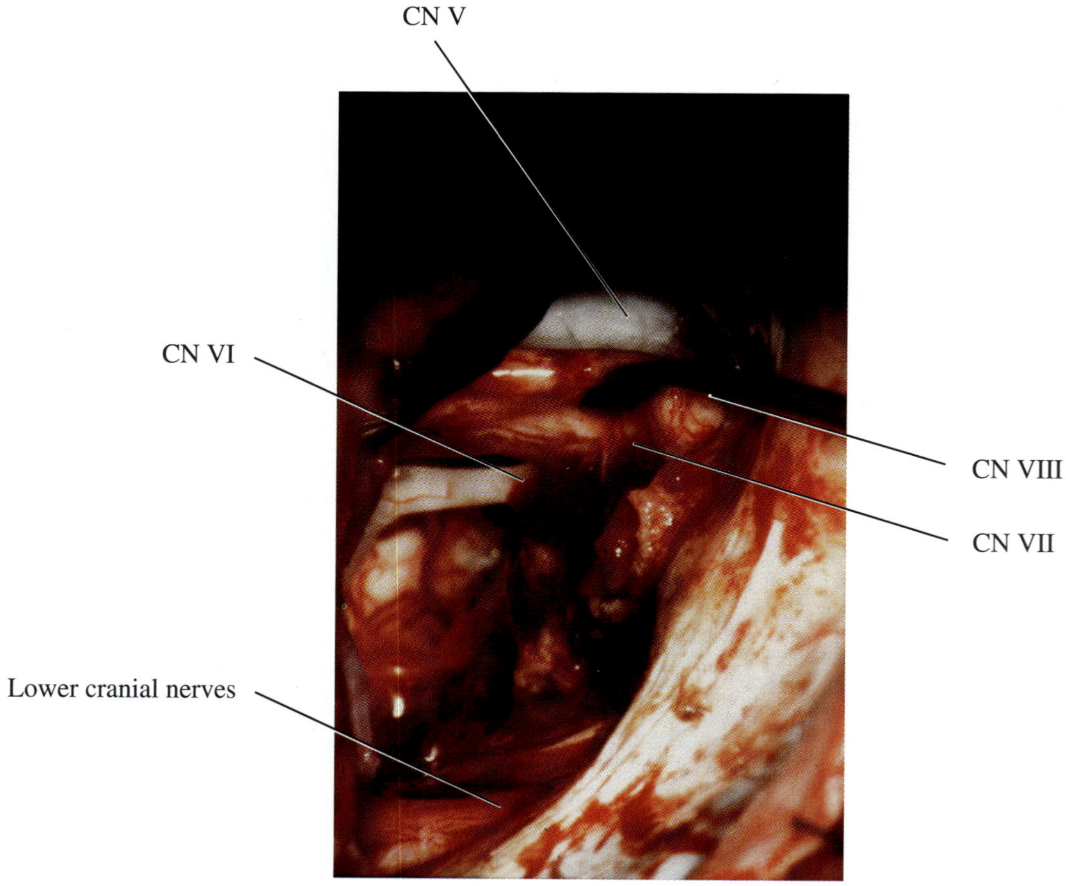

Figure 49. The tumor mass is removed from the cerebellopontine angle, and cranial nerves V, VII, and VIII are shown dissected free.

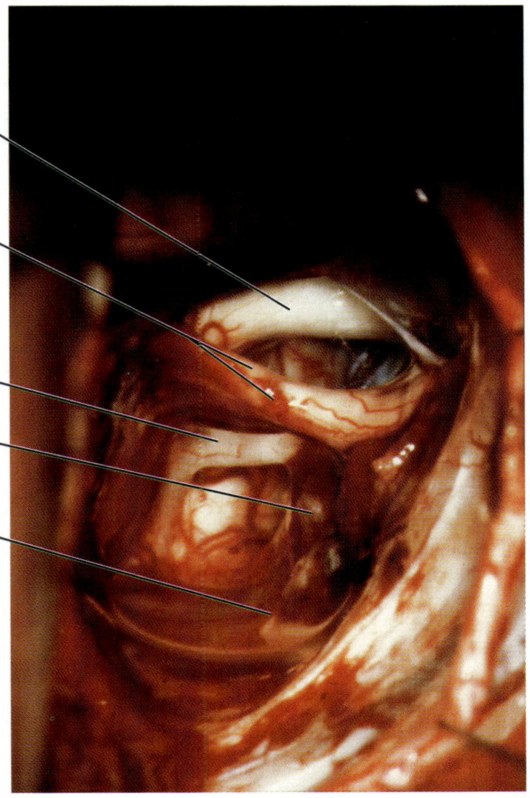

Figure 50. The tumor matrix is located just between the porus acusticus and the jugular foramen beneath cranial nerves VII and VIII.

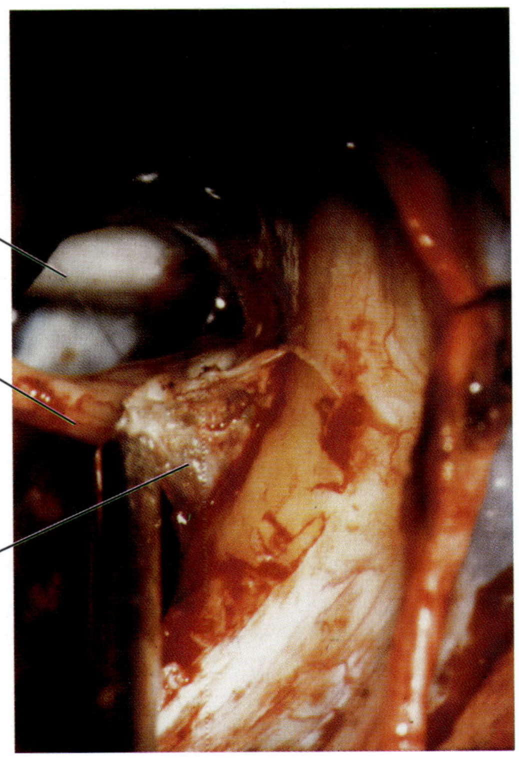

Figure 51. Resection of the dura in the area of the tumor attachment.

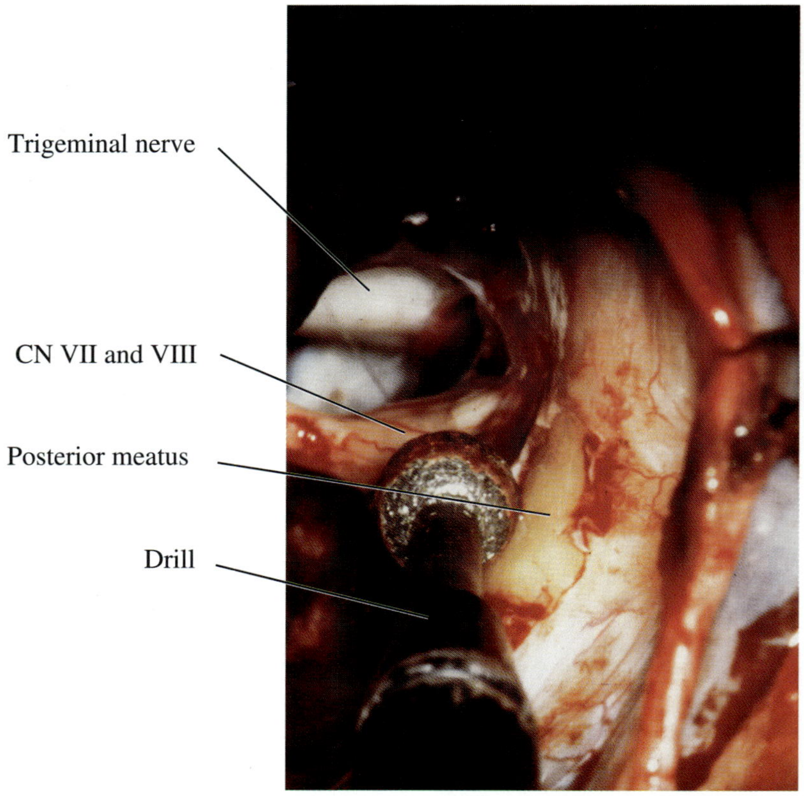

Figure 52. Drilling of bone at the site of tumor attachment.

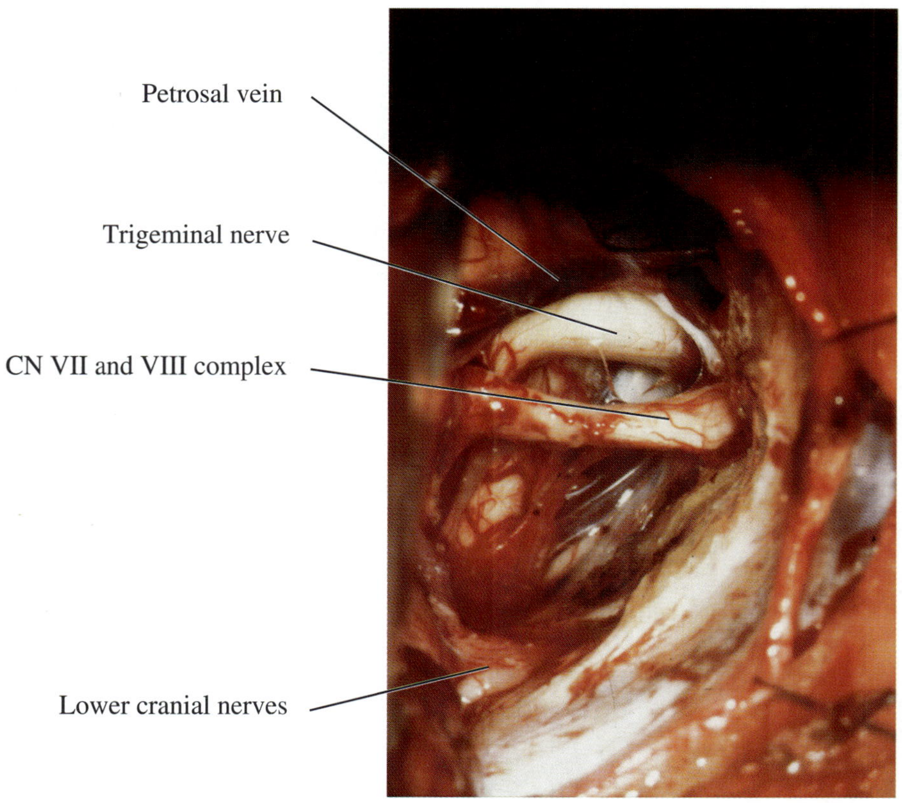

Figure 53. Total tumor removal with preservation of cranial nerves and vessels.

Figure 54. Cerebellopontine angle meningioma with extension into the internal auditory canal.

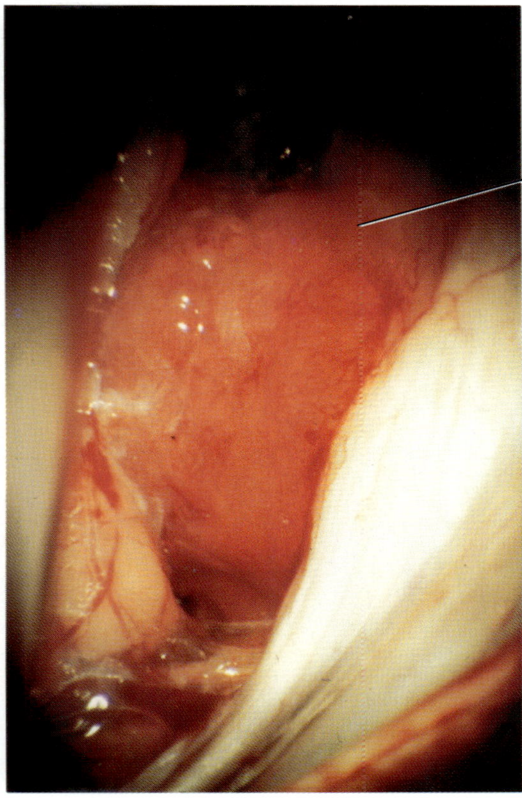

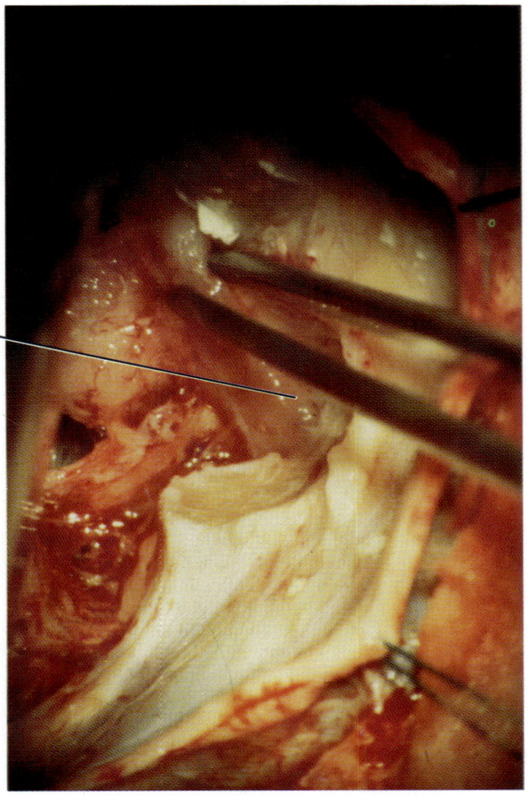

Figure 55. The internal auditory canal is opened, and tumor extension into the canal is shown exposed and partially dissected from cranial nerves VII and VIII.

Figure 56. The internal auditory canal is shown free of tumor tissue. Cranial nerves VII and VIII can be visualized up to the fundus.

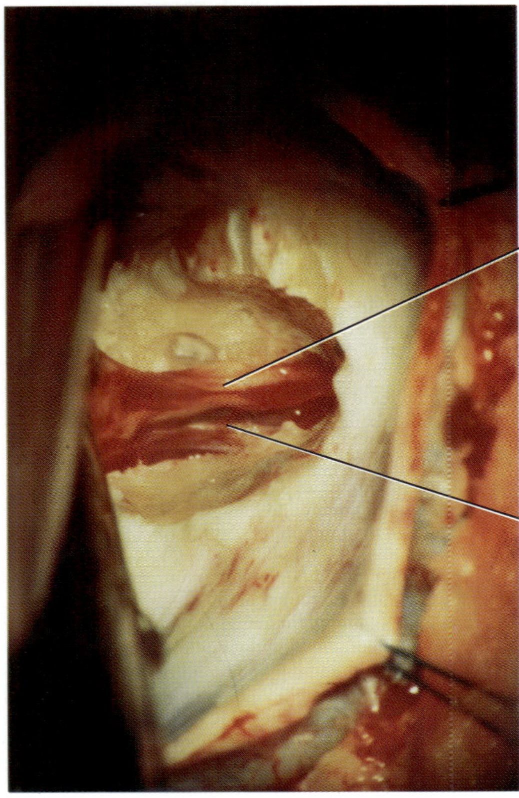

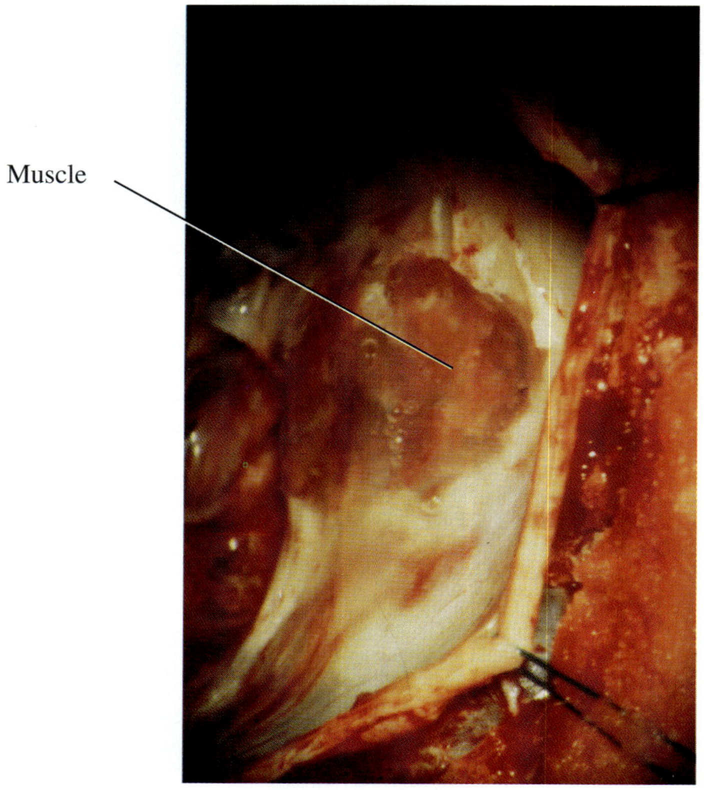

Figure 57. The dural and bony defects around the internal auditory canal are shown filled with muscle and sealed with fibrin glue.

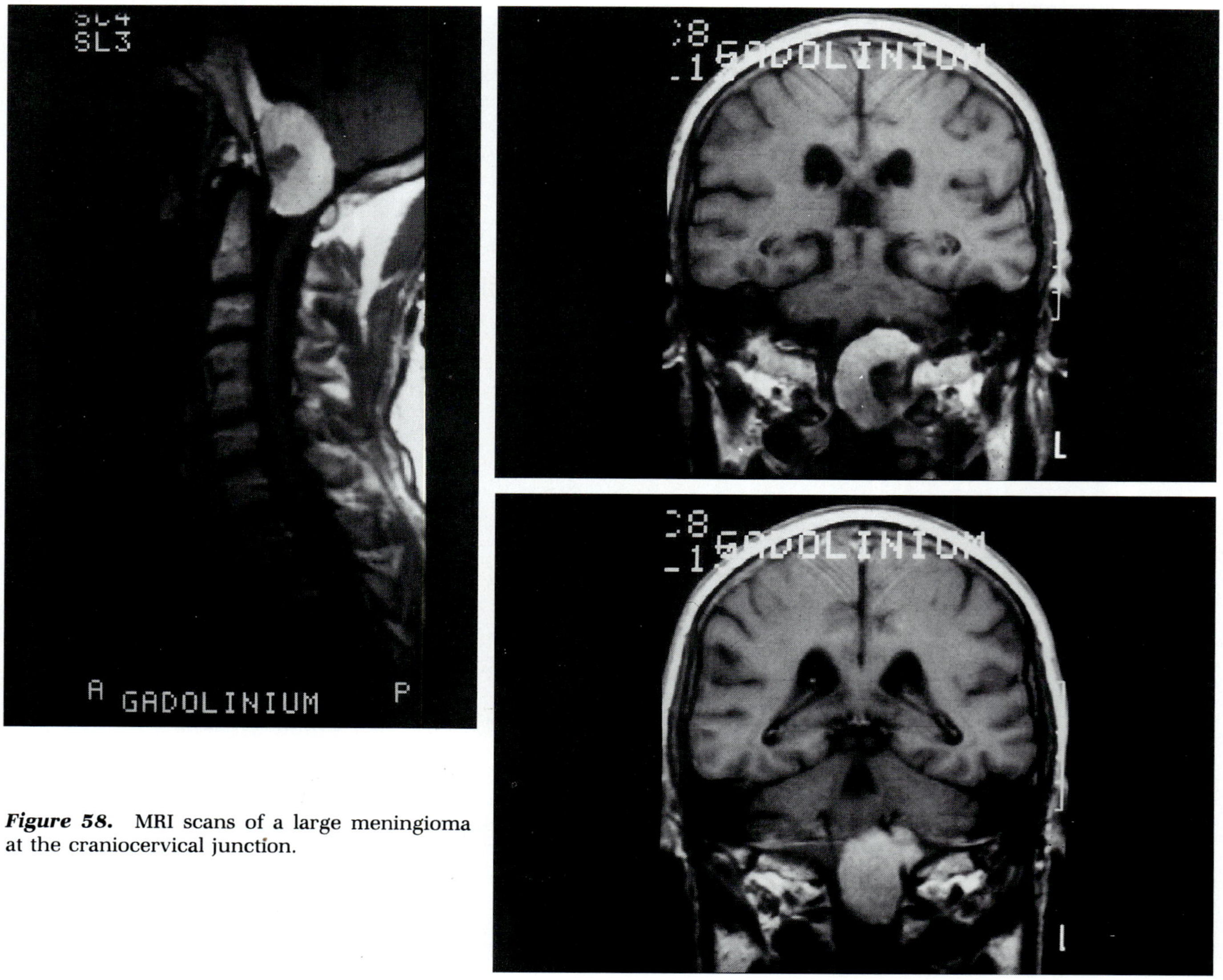

Figure 58. MRI scans of a large meningioma at the craniocervical junction.

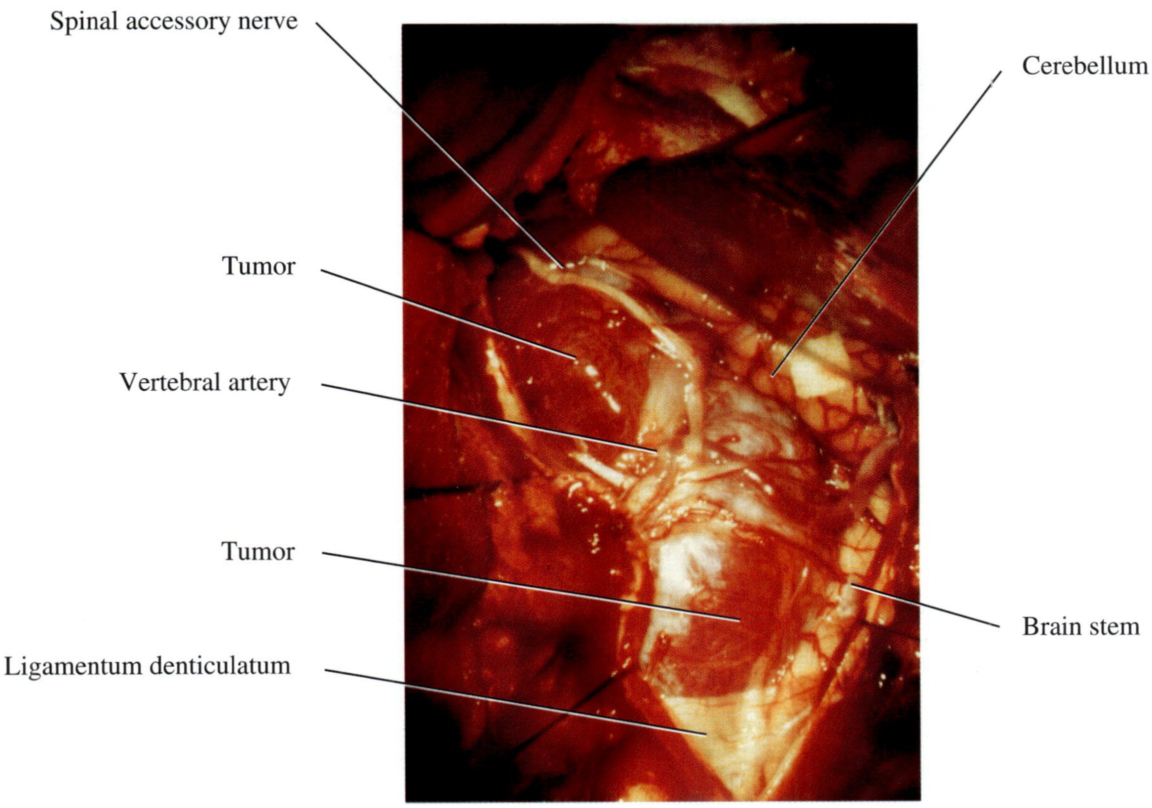

Figure 59. Meningioma at the craniocervical junction with displacement of the brain stem.

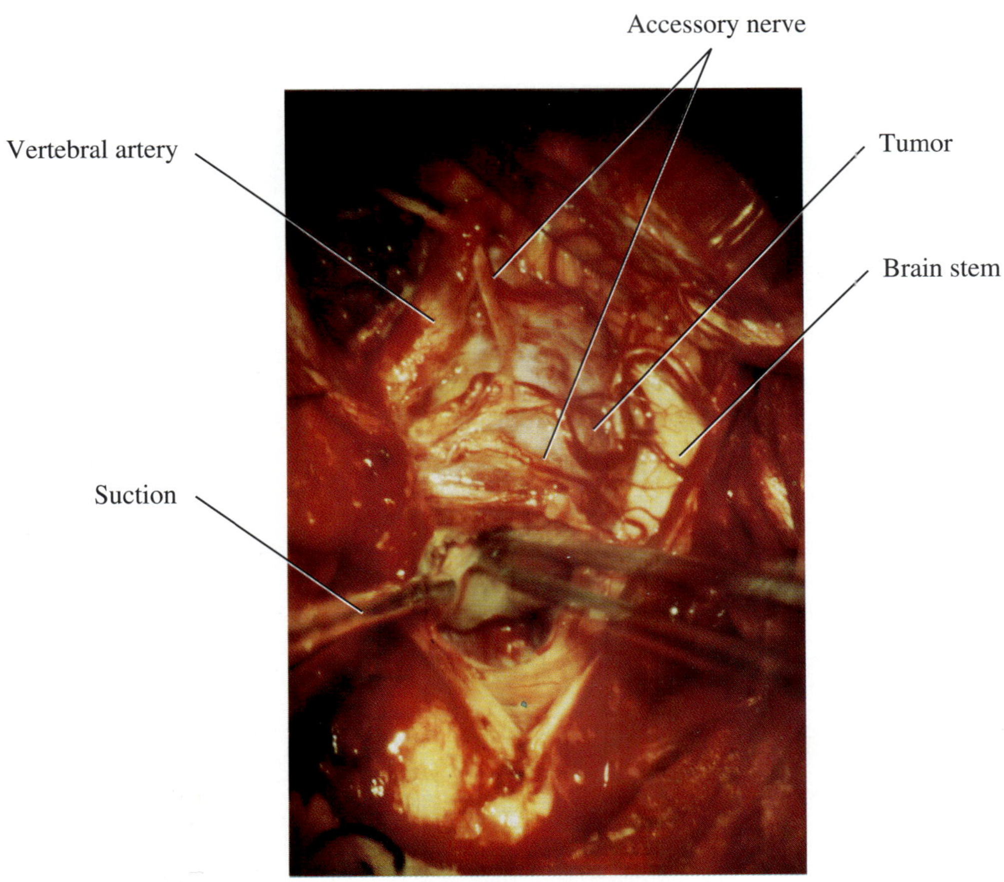

Figure 60. Tumor partially removed.

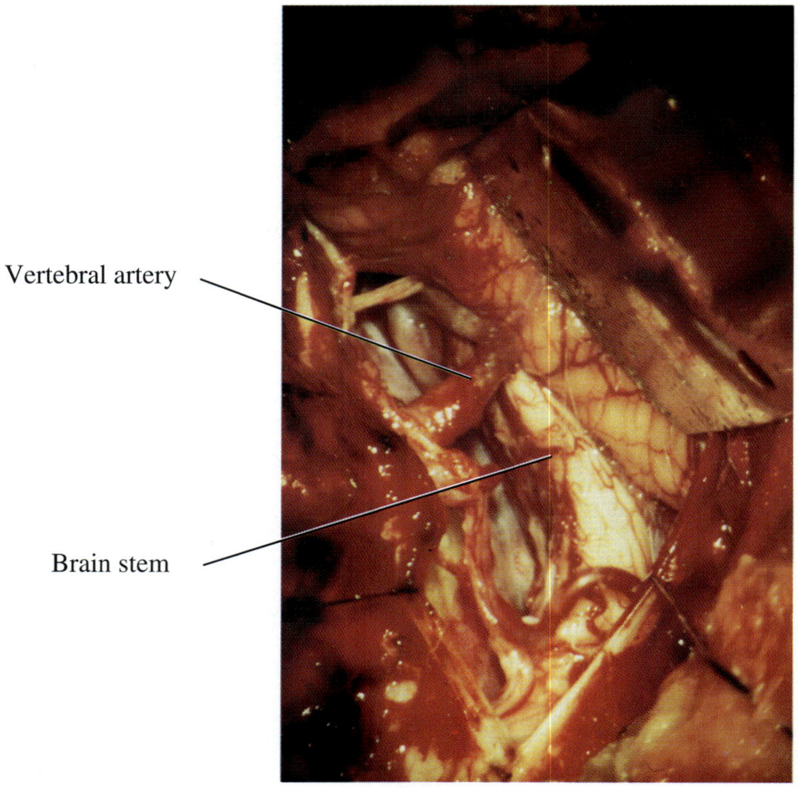

Figure 61. Total tumor removal with preservation of cranial nerves and vessels.

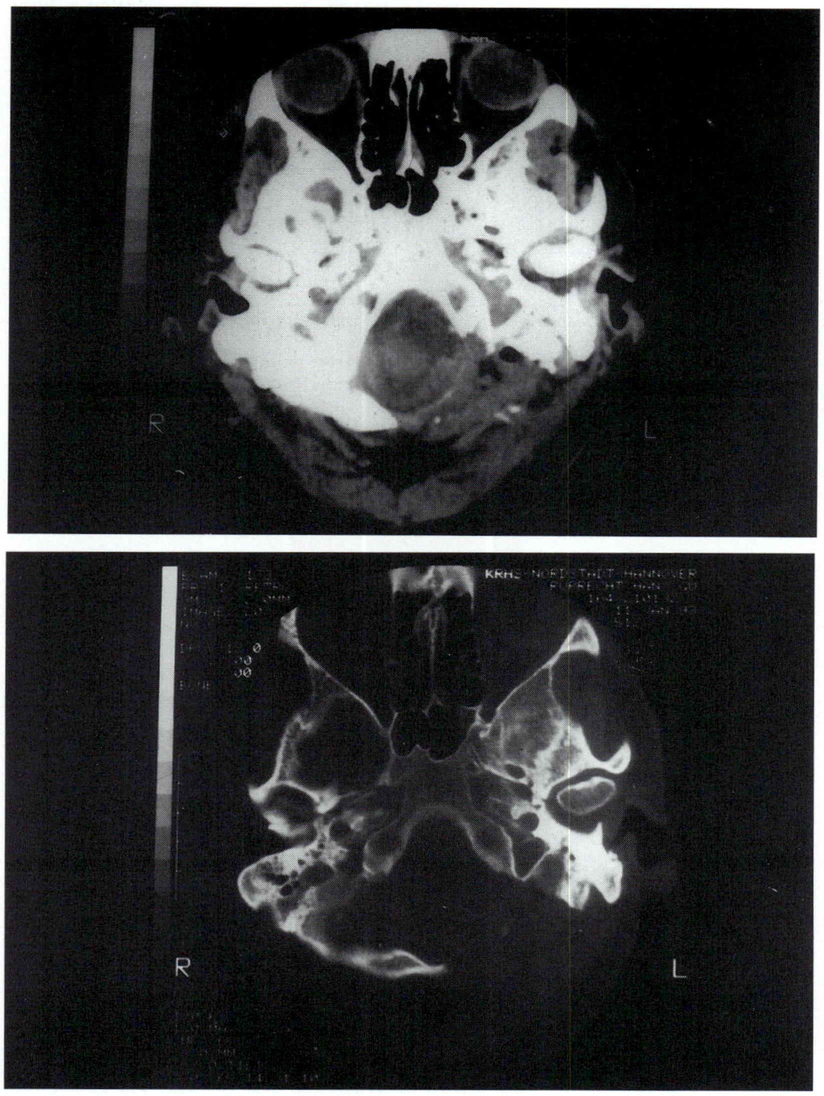

Figure 62. Postoperative CT scans showing total tumor removal.

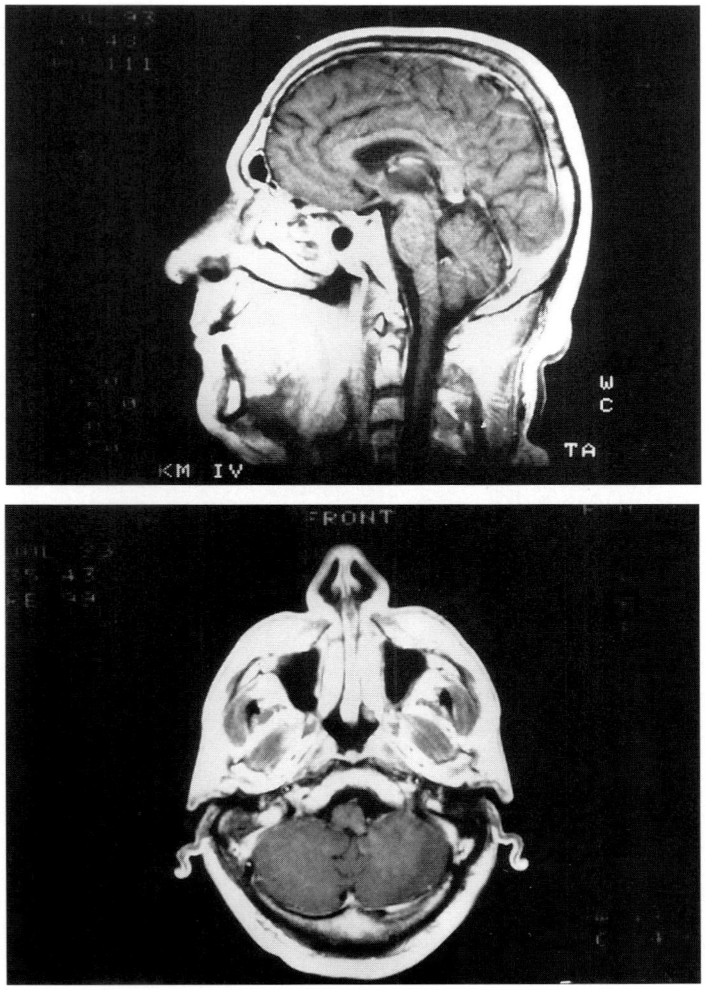

Figure 63. MRI scan images in axial and sagittal projections taken 6 months postoperatively showing complete tumor removal and no evidence of recurrence.

28 Acoustic Neurinoma

Acoustic neurinomas, or vestibular schwannomas, are benign tumors that arise from the vestibular portion of the eighth cranial nerve, most commonly the superior portion. They usually originate within the internal auditory canal and extend into the cerebellopontine angle (Figure 1). The eighth cranial nerve consists of a central portion with oligodendroglial cells forming the myelin and a peripheral portion with Schwann cells forming the myelin (Figure 2). The tumors arise from the Schwann cells of the peripheral portion. Therefore, in the recent literature, the term vestibular schwannoma replaces the classic term acoustic neurinoma with increasing frequency.

Bilateral acoustic neurinomas in combination with schwannomas of the spinal roots, meningeal and glial tumors, and ocular symptoms (juvenile cataracts, optic sheath meningiomas) are typical for neurofibromatosis type 2, a genetic disorder localized on chromosome 22. The genetic defect responsible for the formation of sporadic unilateral acoustic tumors may also be located on chromosome 22.

Acoustic neurinomas are slow-growing and initially produce tinnitus or vestibular dysfunction. Less than 20 per cent of patients experience true vertigo, but up to 50 per cent experience imbalance. Later, because of compression of the cochlear portion of the eighth cranial nerve, acoustic neurinomas produce progressive unilateral sensorineural hearing loss and tinnitus.

DIAGNOSTIC CONSIDERATIONS

Preoperative workup should include high-resolution computed tomography (CT) with thin cuts through the internal auditory canal, as well as magnetic resonance imaging (MRI). CT is most helpful in demonstrating bone erosion and showing the anatomical features and developmental variations of the petrous bone. MRI is a more sensitive test for demonstrating small tumors, especially those localized to the internal auditory canal, and showing the relations of larger tumors to vessels, cranial nerves, and the brain stem.

In Figure 3A, widening of the porus of the internal auditory canal in the case of an acoustic neurinoma is shown by axial 1.5-mm CT section. Figure 3B is a postcontrast CT scan of the same patient showing the acoustic neurinoma in the cerebellopontine angle cistern. The postgadolinium axial T_1-weighted MRI image in the same patient (Figure 3C) shows displacement of the brain stem by the acoustic neurinoma, which is also seen to enter the internal auditory canal. In Figure 3D, the tumor in the same patient is better appreciated within the internal auditory canal by coronal image.

Figure 4A and B are axial and coronal T_1-weighted MRI images with gadolinium showing a small enhancing acoustic neurinoma in the internal auditory canal and just emerging from the porus.

In Figure 5A and B, a small intracanalicular acoustic neurinoma is demonstrated by postgadolinium T_1-weighted coronal and axial images. Figure 5C shows a postcontrast CT scan in a different patient, demonstrating an enhancing intracanalicular acoustic neurinoma. CT cannot reliably demonstrate small tumors of this type.

ANATOMICAL CONSIDERATIONS

Acoustic neurinomas arise from the intracanalicular portion of the vestibular nerve, with initial growth within the internal auditory canal. As the neurinomas grow, they extend into the cerebellopontine angle, usually displacing the facial nerve anteriorly, superiorly, or inferiorly and the cochlear nerve posteriorly or caudally. They eventually may grow to sufficient size to compress the brain stem medially and the trigeminal nerve superiorly, or they may grow inferiorly to compress the lower cranial nerves.

The cerebellopontine angle is bordered anteriorly by the petrous ridge with the superior petrosal sinus running along its upper surface. Inferomedially, the inferior petrosal sinus extends downward, traversed in its anterior portion by the sixth cranial nerve as it enters Dorello's canal. Inferolaterally lie the ninth, tenth, and eleventh cranial nerves and the jugular foramen, through which the sigmoid sinus drains into the jugular bulb. The petrosal vein of Dandy enters the superior petrosal sinus at a point superior to the seventh and eighth cranial nerves as they enter the internal auditory canal. Figure 6 shows an acoustic neurinoma in the cerebellopontine angle, with important anatomical relations.

Within the temporal bone, the labyrinth extends posterolaterally and posterosuperiorly and the cochlea, anteromedially relative to the internal auditory canal (Figure 7). Of importance to the surgeon is awareness of the anteromedial extension of the greater superficial petrosal nerve from the geniculate ganglion of the seventh nerve, and the carotid artery, which enters the cranial cavity just inferior to this nerve and anterior to the cochlea.

Of special anatomical importance in surgery for acoustic neurinomas is the anterior inferior cerebellar artery. This artery gives rise to the internal auditory (labyrinthine) artery, which provides the blood supply to the inner ear. As the anterior inferior cerebellar artery courses from the basilar artery, it passes in proximity to the seventh and eighth cranial nerves and frequently forms a loop that extends into the internal auditory canal. Disturbance of the anterior inferior cerebellar artery can result in infarction of the lateral brain stem with catastrophic consequences. Small perforating branches pass from the anterior inferior cerebellar artery as well as from the basilar artery and superior cerebellar artery to give blood supply to the midbrain and the brain stem.

The facial nerve exits the brain stem at the pontomedullary fissure and then courses laterally in the cerebellopontine angle to enter the internal auditory canal.

Within the internal auditory canal, the facial nerve lies in the anterior superior quadrant; the cochlear nerve, in the anterior inferior quadrant; and the superior and inferior vestibular nerves, in the posterior quadrants. The vertical crest (Bill's bar) separates the superior vestibular nerve from the facial nerve and serves as an important surgical landmark in the translabyrinthine approach to the cerebellopontine angle. The facial nerve enters the fallopian canal at the fundus of the internal auditory canal.

The labyrinthine segment of the facial nerve is its shortest segment (about 4 mm), extending from the meatal foramen to the geniculate ganglion. This segment travels anterior, superior, and lateral, forming an anterior medial angle of 120 degrees with the internal auditory canal portion, an important relation to understand to avoid surgical trauma to the facial nerve during the middle cranial fossa approach for resection of acoustic neurinomas.

At the geniculate ganglion, the facial nerve assumes a posterolateral course and passes horizontally through the middle ear before curving sharply downward at the second genu within the fallopian canal. It then passes vertically through the temporal bone until it exits from the cranium at the stylomastoid foramen. Posterior to the fallopian canal and the semicircular canals lie the mastoid air cells and the sigmoid sinus.

SURGICAL APPROACHES

There are four principal surgical approaches for removal of acoustic neurinomas: retrosigmoid lateral suboccipital transmeatal approach, middle fossa approach, translabyrinthine approach, and transcochlear approach.

Retrosigmoid Lateral Suboccipital Transmeatal Approach

The procedure for the retrosigmoid lateral suboccipital transmeatal approach is explained in Chapter 4. Continuous brain stem evoked potentials monitoring and facial nerve monitoring are carried out throughout the operation.

Figure 5 shows CT and MRI scans of a small intracanalicular acoustic neurinoma, which was removed through this approach. After completion of the craniectomy, with exposure of the transverse and sigmoid sinuses, the dura is opened in a curved manner with the convexity laterally placed and with dural relaxing incisions superolaterally and inferolaterally. Beginning with the opening of the dura, the entire operative procedure is done with the use of the operating microscope.

A retractor is placed to gently elevate the cerebellar hemisphere, exposing the cerebellomedullary cistern. The cistern is opened to allow drainage of cerebrospinal fluid. The cerebellum is covered with a moist cottonoid and a brain retractor placed to offer support and provide exposure but with care exercised to avoid compression or trauma to the cerebellar tissue.

In this approach, cranial nerves IX, X, and XI are identified and protected with a wet cottonoid. The portion of the acoustic neurinoma within the cerebellopontine angle is now visualized. In this operative case of a small intracanalicular acoustic neurinoma, no tumor could be seen in the cerebellopontine angle (Figure 8). With medium-sized tumors, the flocculus and the origin of the seventh and eighth nerves at the pontomedullary junction are visualized at this point.

Other than in the case of large acoustic neurinomas that cover the posterior surface of the petrous bone, the internal auditory canal is opened as a first step to establish the lateral tumor extension. This procedure is begun with the circular excision of dura from the petrous bone posterior to the internal auditory canal followed by drilling of the posterior wall of the meatus with a high-speed diamond burr, as seen in Figure 9. This drilling initially is done using a 4- to 5-mm burr; as the fundus is approached, progressively smaller diamond burrs are used. All drilling is done under continuous saline solution irrigation.

In Figure 10, the internal auditory canal is seen to be open and the intracanalicular acoustic neurinoma is exposed. Figure 11 shows the tumor to be partially dissected and gently elevated with a microforceps, exposing CN VII and VIII as they pass from the brain stem to the internal auditory canal.

The tumor is seen in Figure 12 to be originating from a fascicle of the superior vestibular nerve, which will be transected. The preserved facial, cochlear, and inferior vestibular nerves are visualized. Figure 13 shows these nerves intact and the tumor totally removed.

It is important to know the position of the jugular bulb before drilling the porus, and this can be determined from review of preoperative high-resolution CT scans. During drilling, the roof of the internal auditory canal is used as a landmark, and as the posterior wall is removed, drilling is done cautiously to avoid entry into the jugular bulb. In such a case, the highly positioned jugular bulb is skeletonized by gentle drilling of the posterior wall of the internal auditory canal. Now the jugular bulb can be displaced downward and the remaining bone of the posterior wall of the internal auditory canal can be drilled away and the tumor in the internal canal exposed.

To avoid injury to or opening of the semicircular canal and vestibule, the last part of the bony plate next to the fundus is left intact during drilling. The remaining distance to the fundus can be continuously assessed by using an angulated microinstrument. If one of the semicircular canals should become fenestrated, suctioning of the perilymph and endolymph must be avoided, and the fenestration should be closed with fascia sealed with fibrin glue immediately to preserve cochlear function. Careful study of preoperative high-resolution CT scans is helpful in knowing the relation of these important structures to the internal auditory canal and the tumor.

As the fundus is approached, the bone drilling should proceed in a medial-to-lateral direction to preserve the bone plate between the internal auditory canal, the ampulla of the semicircular canal, and the jugular bulb. The depth of the remaining internal auditory canal can be palpated with a micro nerve hook, and drilling should leave at least 2 mm of bony distance from the fundus of the internal auditory canal to avoid entering the labyrinth.

Once the posterior wall of the porus has been drilled, the decision regarding the procedure for tumor removal depends on tumor size. As discussed earlier, with small, primarily intracanalicular tumors, the next step is to identify the facial and vestibulocochlear nerves medially near the brain stem. The position and extent of tumor feeding vessels must also be considered.

Figure 14 shows a medium-sized acoustic neurinoma that is growing into the right cerebellopontine angle. As described for removal of smaller intracanalicular acoustic tumors, the first step is incision of the dura posteriorly followed by drilling of the posterior lip of the internal auditory canal, as seen in Figure 15. With the internal auditory canal open, the tumor can be well visualized (Figure 16). Figure 17 shows the cerebellopontine angle and internal auditory canal to be free of tumor after complete removal. The facial and cochlear nerves are seen to be intact, and the superior petrosal vein and trigeminal nerve are well demonstrated. In Figure 18, the facial and cochlear nerves are gently elevated with a microdissector for better identification.

Figure 19 shows the proper closure of the internal auditory canal after tumor removal by placement of a piece of muscle, sealed with fibrin glue to avoid a cerebrospinal fluid leak.

A slightly larger but still middle-sized acoustic neurinoma is shown in Figure 20. The lower cranial nerves can be seen inferiorly as well as some of the fascicles of the vestibular nerve. The overlying arachnoid sheath is also well visualized. CN IX, X, and XI should be covered with a wet cottonoid to avoid injury. The anterior inferior cerebellar artery is identified and protected as well. Again, the first step in tumor removal is the drilling of the posterior wall of the internal auditory canal to enable identification of the lateral extent of the tumor in the fundus (Figure 21). In Figure 22, the tumor has been partially debulked.

Figure 23 shows the tumor capsule being held with forceps in the surgeon's right hand as the facial and cochlear nerves are identified at the brain stem. The same gentle medial-to-lateral dissection is continued (as shown in Figure 24), with the surgeon grasping the tumor with the right hand and using the microforceps in his left hand to "push" the arachnoid away. This maneuver progressively separates the tumor capsule from the facial nerve.

In Figure 25, the facial nerve can be seen laterally within the internal auditory canal, having been carefully dissected free from the tumor capsule. Figure 26 shows the critical final step in removal of the tumor as its last area of attachment is gently and sharply, if necessary, dissected free from the facial nerve. This is the point of greatest concern in avoiding traction or other injury to the facial nerve. Figure 27 shows complete tumor removal with preservation of both the facial and the cochlear nerves.

For larger acoustic neurinomas, such as the one shown in the MRI scans in Figure 28, partial debulking of the tumor is necessary before beginning further lateral or medial dissection. In such a case, the first step is to identify a part of the tumor capsule that can be entered without traction or potential injury to CN VII or VIII. Exposure of the tumor capsule surface is seen in Figure 29. After entering the tumor, an intracapsular debulking is carried out. The cavitron is useful in achieving this debulking (Figure 30). It is important to exercise great care not to penetrate through the anterior wall of the tumor capsule. It is also extremely important not to cause traction pressure on the nerves because this may result in nerve deficit.

As the intracapsular decompression progresses, the tumor capsule becomes lax. It is then possible to proceed with drilling of the posterior lip of the internal auditory canal and to identify the lateral extent of tumor (Figure 31) as well as those points at which the capsule is especially adherent to CN VII and VIII and the brain stem medially. The tumor capsule can then be gently dissected from the nerves and brain stem. As previously discussed, it is critical to stay within the arachnoid plane, grasping the tumor capsule with microforceps held in the surgeon's right hand and "pushing" the arachnoid away to separate it from the tumor capsule with forceps held in the left hand. Finally, as the tumor mass becomes reduced in size, the intercanalicular portion of the tumor is carefully dissected from the facial and cochlear nerves within the internal auditory canal and the cerebellopontine angle, and the final remnant of tumor is removed. During tumor removal, bipolar cautery is used sparingly. The operative field is irrigated continuously with sterile saline solution to wash away bleeding and to maintain good visualization. Figure 32 shows complete tumor removal and good visualization of the cranial nerves and other structures in the cerebellopontine angle. The facial nerve is intact.

For removal of even larger (giant) acoustic neurinomas, the procedure is the same as described for large acoustic tumors, but additional intracapsular debulking is necessary before the internal auditory canal is opened or dissection is performed medially. Additional care is also necessary in avoiding injury to CN IX, X, and XI inferiorly and to CN V and the petrosal vein and anterior inferior cerebellar artery superiorly.

KEY POINTS: To achieve total removal of an acoustic neurinoma, regardless of size, with the highest percentage of facial and cochlear nerve preservation, certain principles need to be considered. Careful opening of the internal auditory canal, primary debulking of the tumor mass, identification of the facial and cochlear nerves at the brain stem and at the fundus of the internal auditory canal, and continuous respect for the arachnoid plane are key factors in successful removal of acoustic neurinomas. The most adherent point of the tumor capsule to the facial nerve should be dissected at the very end of the tumor removal. Sometimes sharp dissection at this point is necessary to avoid traction injury to the facial nerve.

FACIAL NERVE RECONSTRUCTION: In case of facial nerve interruption, end-to-end suture or direct nerve grafting should be accomplished immediately. The nerve of choice for grafting is the sural nerve. In rare cases of giant acoustic neurinoma, the central stump of the facial nerve is damaged or thinned in such a way that primary reconstruction is not possible. Hypoglossal-facial anastomosis should then be done within 2 to 6 weeks.

CLOSURE: For closure, multiple jugular compressions (three times) should help to identify a venous opening. After copious saline solution irrigation and after achieving meticulous hemostasis with bipolar cautery, the bone surface that was drilled along the posterior meatus is sealed with bone wax. It is then covered with muscle and sealed with fibrin glue. After removing all cottonoids and retractors, the dura is closed in a watertight manner using a continuous 4-0 suture and fibrin glue. Final inspection of the cranial defect surface to assure complete sealing with muscle and fibrin glue is followed by multiple-layer closure, as described in Chapter 4.

Middle Fossa Approach

The middle fossa approach is for removal of acoustic neurinomas that are within the internal auditory canal. This approach is described in Chapter 8. Operative dissection from this point is done with the operating microscope using 12- to 20-power magnification. With a 3- to 4-mm diamond burr, the superior semicircular canal is identified and the roof of the internal auditory canal is removed from the fundus to the cerebellopontine angle. All drilling is done with continuous saline solution irrigation. As this drilling is done, care is taken to preserve a thin shell of bone to avoid tearing of the dura with injury to the facial nerve, which lies immediately below. The internal auditory canal is exposed as widely as possible, being careful to avoid entering the superior semicircular canal posteriorly and the cochlea anterolaterally. Bone removal is progressively widened as drilling is carried medially because maximum exposure at the porus is necessary for tumor removal and a 270-degree arc of bone can be safely removed at the level of the porus.

The thin remaining shell of bone is then lifted away using a small nerve hook or a Fisch microraspatory, and the dura is opened over the internal auditory canal. By placing this dural incision as posteriorly as possible over the internal auditory canal, injury to the facial nerve is avoided. The tumor is now visualized within the internal auditory canal, and the vertical crest is identified laterally. Anterior to the vertical crest (Bill's bar) the facial nerve is seen. Posterior to the vertical crest the superior vestibular nerve and, extending medially from it, the tumor can be identified.

Meticulous dissection with microdissectors and microforceps is used to separate the facial nerve from the superior vestibular nerve and acoustic tumor. Intraoperative facial nerve electromyographic monitoring facilitates this dissection. The tumor is then gently displaced posteriorly, away from the facial nerve, which lies anteriorly within the canal. With a nerve hook, the lateral end of the internal auditory canal, behind the vertical crest, is palpated, and the distal ends of both vestibular nerves are sharply sectioned, allowing the distal extent of the acoustic tumor to be delivered from the canal in a posterior plane.

With elevation of the tumor, the line of cleavage between the facial and cochlear nerves and the tumor capsule can be developed using fine microdissectors. As the tumor is removed in a posteromedial direction toward the internal auditory canal, the anterior inferior cerebellar artery is identified because it often loops into the porus. It is important to avoid injury to this artery and its brain stem–perforating branches. Uncontrolled bleeding or injury to the anterior inferior cerebellar artery poses the most serious complication during the operation. After dissection from the anterior inferior cerebellar artery, the tumor can be lifted from the internal auditory canal and removed.

CLOSURE: After achieving careful hemostasis, the wound is irrigated with saline solution, the dural flap is laid back in place, and the internal auditory canal is covered with a pad of temporalis muscle. A free bone graft is placed perpendicular to the internal auditory canal on the floor of the middle fossa, and this is covered with a temporalis fascia graft. The free bone flap is sutured in place, and the galea is closed with 3-0 Vicryl. Skin closure is with 4-0 nylon.

Translabyrinthine Approach

The translabyrinthine approach is outlined in Chapter 6. After drilling of the temporal bone and exposure of the dura and the facial, cochlear, and vestibular nerves at the internal auditory canal, exposure of the tumor is carried out. The dura is opened in a stellate manner to expose the cerebellopontine angle and posterior fossa and to visualize the superior and inferior vestibular nerves. This is carefully done to avoid injury to the facial nerve in those infrequent cases in which it emerges from the internal auditory canal to pass around the posterior surface of the acoustic tumor. The removal of the tumor begins with identification of the facial nerve at the meatal foramen. With the translabyrinthine approach, the facial nerve has been skeletonized throughout the vertical and horizontal segments. The fibers of the superior and inferior vestibular nerves are avulsed, and just anteriorly, the grayish facial nerve is seen in front of the vertical crest (Bill's bar).

With medium-sized or large tumors, the mass fills the entire area of dural exposure by the translabyrinthine approach. Continuous facial nerve monitoring is carried out throughout the operative procedure. With smaller acoustic tumors in those patients with no useful hearing who are undergoing the translabyrinthine approach, it often is possible to open the arachnoidal cistern that surrounds the tumor. This allows drainage of cerebrospinal fluid to assist in decompressing the cerebellopontine angle. The presenting surface of the tumor capsule is opened, and gentle intercapsular tumor removal is carried out piecemeal. Care is taken to avoid any traction of the tumor mass or capsule that might cause stress injury to the facial nerve or pressure against the brain stem.

Removal of even large acoustic neurinomas is possible through this approach by using the technique of intracapsular debulking of the tumor mass, as described earlier in this chapter. It is important to avoid penetration of the tumor capsule, especially anterosuperiorly, where injury to the facial nerve or the anterior inferior cerebellar artery might occur.

After completion of most of the internal tumor removal, the tumor capsule begins to infold, allowing visualization of the brain stem and cranial nerves IX, X, and XI. Attention is now turned to the internal auditory canal, where the intracanalicular portion of the tumor is carefully dissected away from the facial nerve with a small 1-mm right-angled hook using constant suction irrigation with a Brackmann fenestrated neuro-otologic suction. The dissection of the facial nerve must be gentle, and mechanical stimulation of the nerve can be monitored with intraoperative electromyographic recording. The facial nerve tends to be most adherent to the tumor capsule in this area near the porus, and it is important to avoid any manipulation of the tumor that may result in traction injury to the facial nerve or its anatomical disruption.

When the dissection reaches the internal auditory canal, the facial nerve courses anteriorly, away from view. To visualize the nerve again, it is necessary to remove all the anterior parts of the tumor. Care is exercised to avoid injury to the anterior inferior cerebellar artery and its perforating branches. All dissection is done while staying in the arachnoidal plane, gently pushing the arachnoid sheath away. Only those arterial branches that are definitely entering the tumor are cauterized with bipolar cautery and then sharply divided with microscissors. During this phase of tumor removal, care is also exercised to avoid injury to the fifth cranial nerve and the superior petrosal vein, which may be stretched over the superior pole of the mass. The anterior pole and the center of the neuroma are debulked. Then, the anterior pole of the tumor can be retracted and the dissection of the seventh nerve continued until the brain stem is reached. There often are adhesions medial to the porus, and the nerve is not visible. In such cases, the part that is adherent to the seventh nerve is removed at the end of the dissection. The inferior pole is then removed. Around the inferior pole, great care is necessary to avoid injury to the anterior inferior cerebellar artery, which often loops over the eighth nerve complex. Its preservation is essential because its interruption could produce a catastrophic brain stem infarction.

After the facial nerve is free in its entirety, the inferior pole has been debulked, and the capsule has been separated completely from the brain stem, the remaining tumor and capsule can be removed. The dissection of the seventh nerve is then followed in a medial-to-lateral direction until the portion of the nerve that had previously been dissected is reached. The last part of the dissection can be more difficult because of the thinning of the facial nerve over the tumor capsule or an intimate involvement of the facial nerve and the tumor capsule. It is there that the nerve is most vulnerable to transection. Cable grafting of the facial nerve at primary operation using either a sural nerve or greater auricular nerve should be performed if the nerve is transected. The entire operative field is irrigated with saline solution, and careful hemostasis is obtained by use of bipolar cautery in a continuously saline solution–irrigated field.

CLOSURE: A single sheet of rectus abdominis fascia is draped over the translabyrinthine defect in the temporal bone and filled with strips of abdominal fat. The pericranium is closed with 3-0 Vicryl, and the subcutaneous layer is closed with inverted interrupted 3-0 Vicryl. A running, locked 3-0 nylon suture in the skin follows to achieve a watertight closure. No drain is placed.

Transcochlear (Transotic) Approach

The transcochlear approach represents a forward extension of the translabyrinthine exposure. It is outlined in Chapter 7 and represents an anterior extension of the translabyrinthine approach. After drilling of the cochlea is completed and the facial nerve has been exposed from the geniculate ganglion medially into the internal auditory canal, the dura is opened and the tumor is exposed.

The tumor capsule is opened and an intracapsular debulking is carried out. Care is exercised to avoid injury to the facial nerve, which usually is displaced anteriorly and superiorly.

After the tumor mass has been substantially reduced in size, it is dissected away from the cerebellum and from the anterior inferior cerebellar artery. Small tumor feeding branches from the anterior inferior cerebellar artery are coagulated with the bipolar cautery and sectioned but with care exercised to avoid injury to the main arterial trunk.

The medial extent of the tumor is dissected from the brain stem, staying within the arachnoidal plane and pushing the arachnoid away as the tumor capsule is freed. The final step in tumor removal is careful sharp dissection of the adherent tumor capsule and remaining tumor mass from the facial nerve. Care is taken to avoid traction against the facial nerve as this is done.

A description of the technique of closure can be found in Chapters 6 and 7.

COMPLICATIONS

Complications of acoustic neurinoma removal include facial nerve palsy, hearing loss, cerebrospinal fluid leak, air embolism, and infarction of the brain stem or cerebellum.

RECOMMENDED READING

Brackmann, D.E.: Middle Cranial Fossa Approach. Acoustic Tumors. Vol. II: Management. Baltimore: University Park Press, 1979, pp. 15–41.

Camins, M.B., Oppenheim, J.S.: Anatomy and surgical techniques in the suboccipital transmeatal approach to acoustic neurinomas. Clin. Neurosurg. 38:567–588, 1990.

Dutton, J.E.M., Ramsden, R.T., Lye, R.H., et al.: Acoustic neurinoma (schwannoma) surgery 1978–1990. J. Laryngol. Otol. 105:165–173, 1991.

House, W.F.: The transcochlear approach to the skull base. Arch. Otolaryngol. 102:334–342, 1976.

Koos, W.T., Perneczky, A.: Suboccipital approach to acoustic neurinomas with emphasis on preservation of facial nerve and cochlear nerve function. Acta Neurochir (Wien) 92(1–4):55–66, 1988.

Rhoton, A.L.: Microsurgical anatomy of the cerebellopontine angle in acoustic neurinoma and hemifacial spasm. Neurosurgery 6:483–507, 1980.

Samii, M.: Operative treatment of cerebellopontine angle tumors with special consideration of facial and acoustic nerve. Adv. Neurosurg. 7:138–145, 1979.

Samii, M., Draf, W.: Surgery of the Skull Base: An Interdisciplinary Approach. New York: Springer-Verlag, 1989.

Shao, K.N., Tatagiba, M., Samii, M.: Surgical management of high jugular bulb in acoustic neurinoma via retrosigmoid approach. Neurosurgery 32:32–37, 1993.

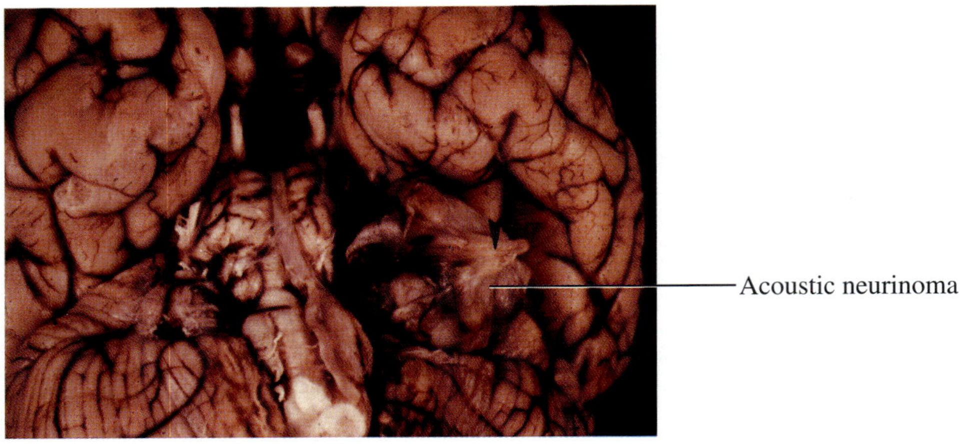

Figure 1. Acoustic neurinoma of the cerebellopontine angle with a stalk *(arrowhead)* reaching into the internal auditory canal.

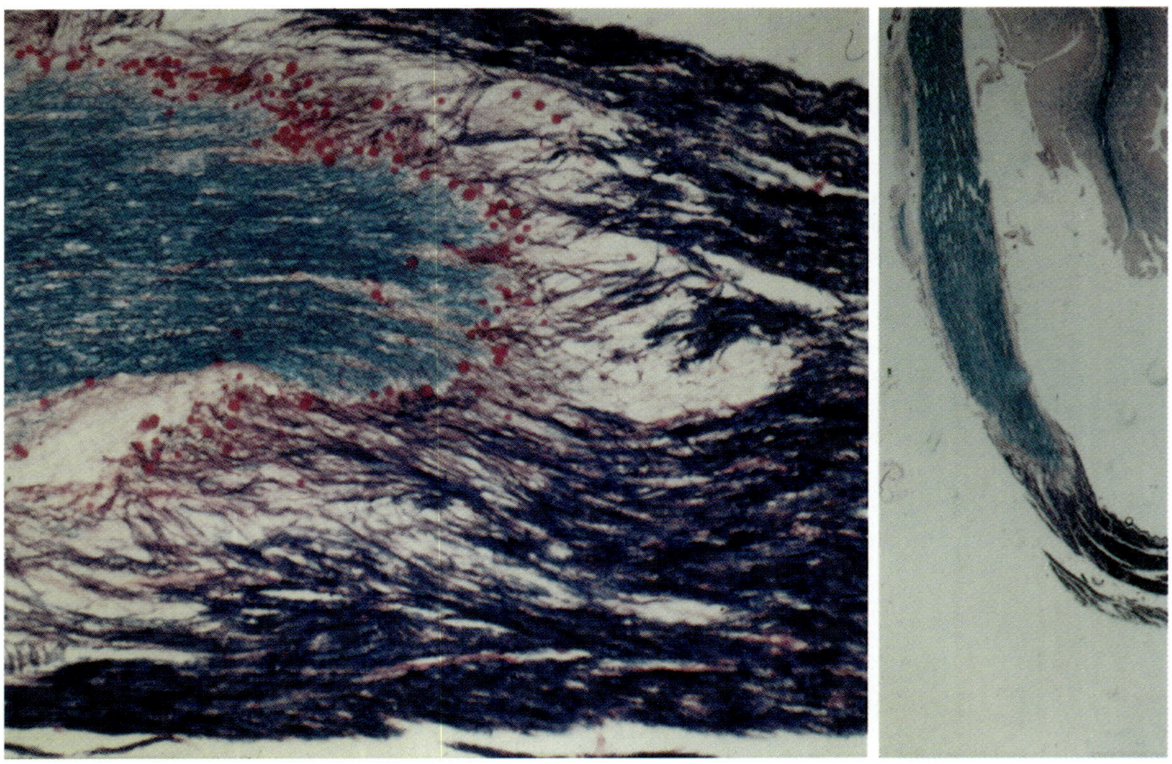

Figure 2. Eighth cranial nerve (vestibulocochlear of statoacoustic nerve) with histological demonstration of the central (light blue) and peripheral (dark blue) portions. Luxol fast blue–periodic acid–Schiff's reagent, 150×; *inset;* overview.

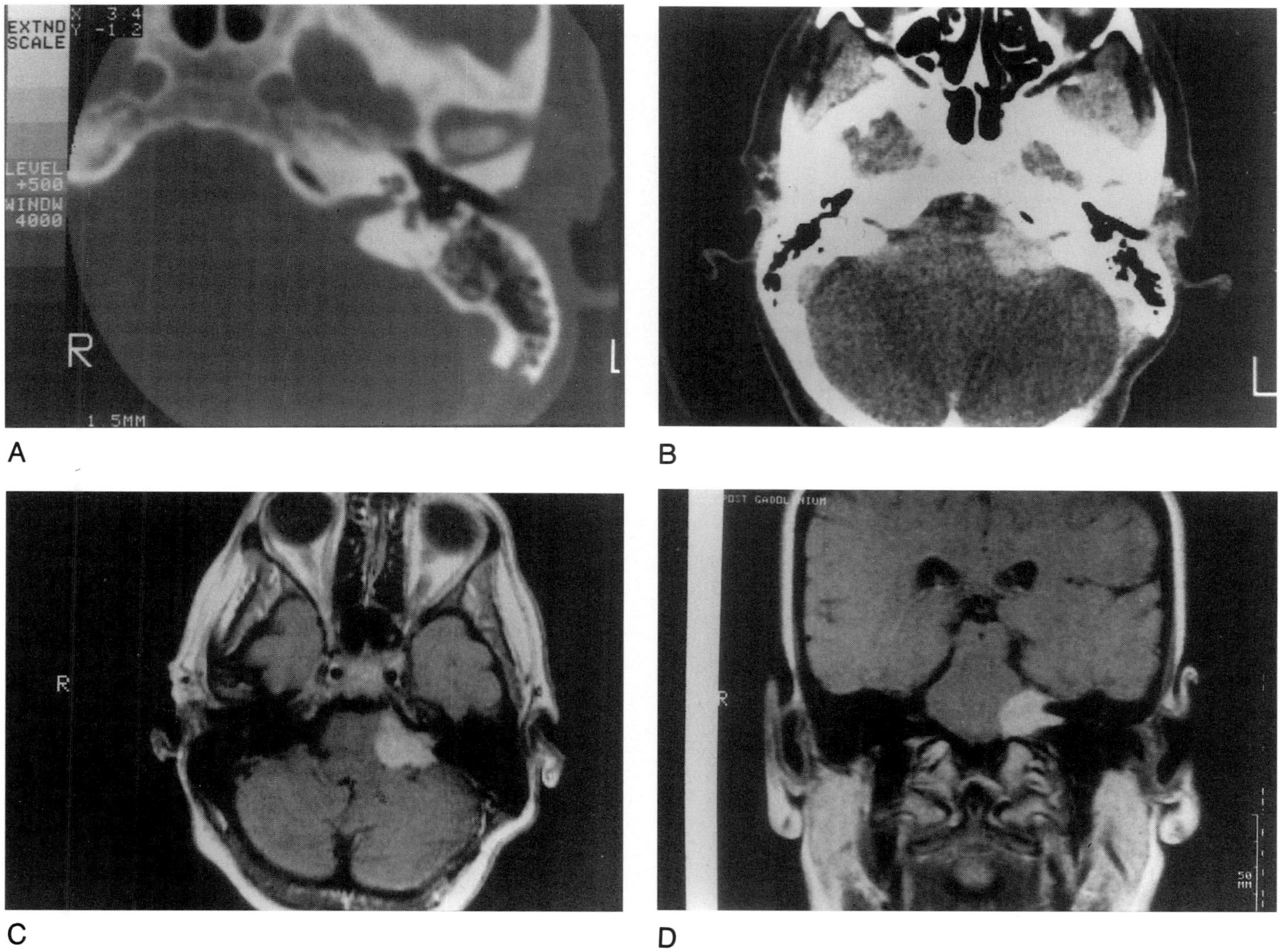

Figure 3. A. Axial 1.5-mm CT section showing widening of porus of internal auditory canal caused by acoustic neurinoma.

B. Postcontrast CT scan of same patient showing the neurinoma in the cerebellopontine angle cistern.

C. Same patient with postgadolinium axial T_1-weighted image showing displacement of brain stem by acoustic neurinoma, which also enters the internal auditory canal.

D. Same patient. The tumor in the internal auditory canal is better appreciated on coronal image in this case.

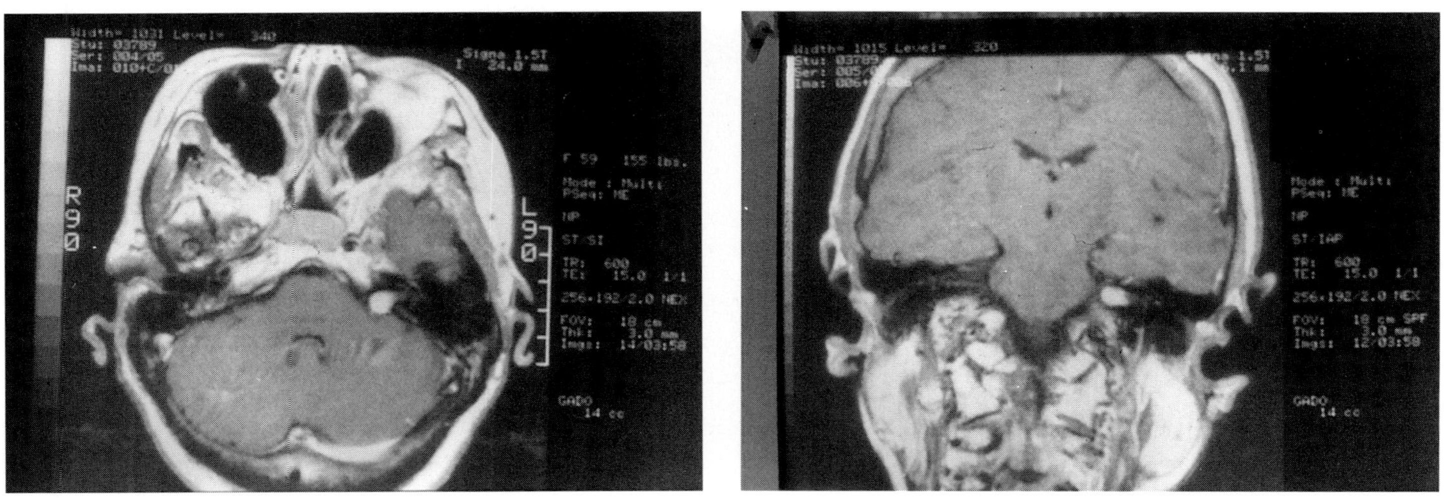

Figure 4. Axial and coronal T_1-weighted MRI images with gadolinium showing small enhancing acoustic neurinoma in the internal auditory canal and just emerging from the porus.

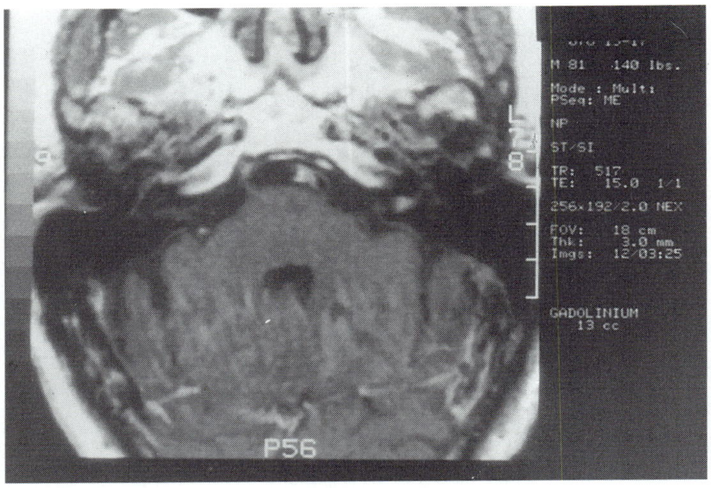

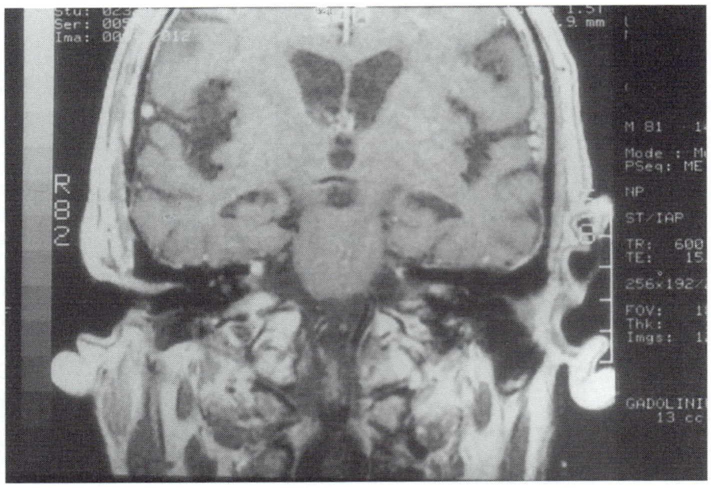

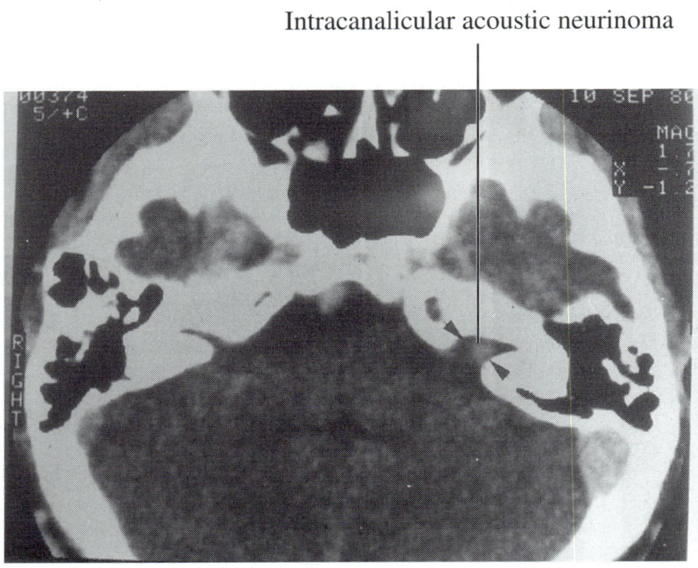

Figure 5. A, B. Postgadolinium T_1-weighted coronal and axial images showing a small intracanalicular acoustic neurinoma.

C. Postcontrast CT scan showing an enhancing intracanalicular acoustic neurinoma. CT does not reliably demonstrate these lesions.

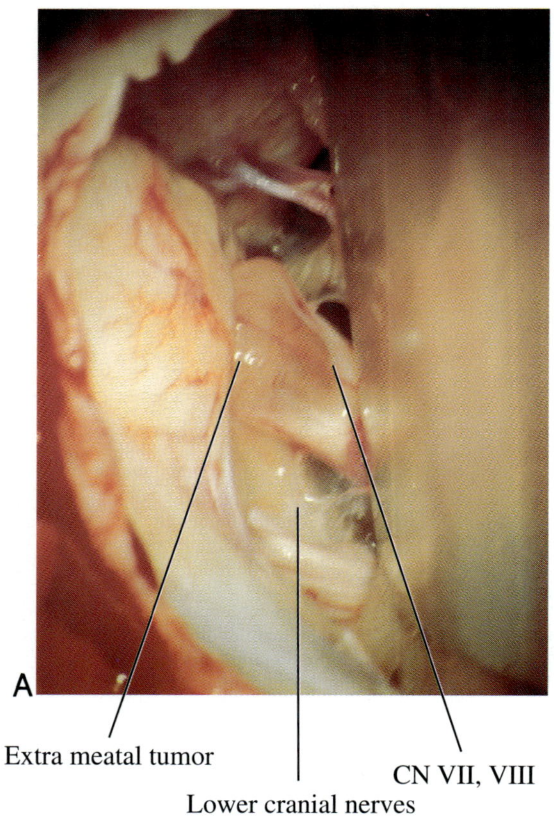

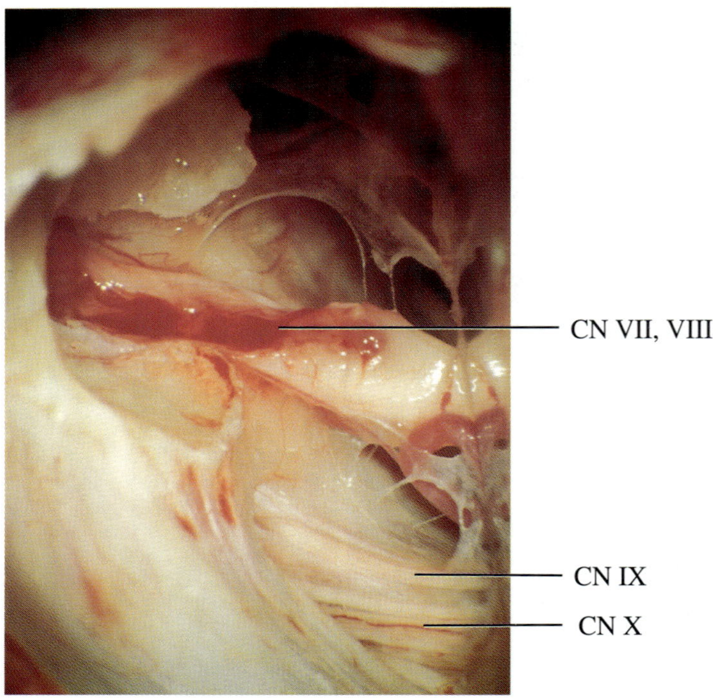

Figure 6. A. Acoustic neurinoma in the cerebellopontine angle showing anatomical relations.

B. Same patient after removal of tumor.

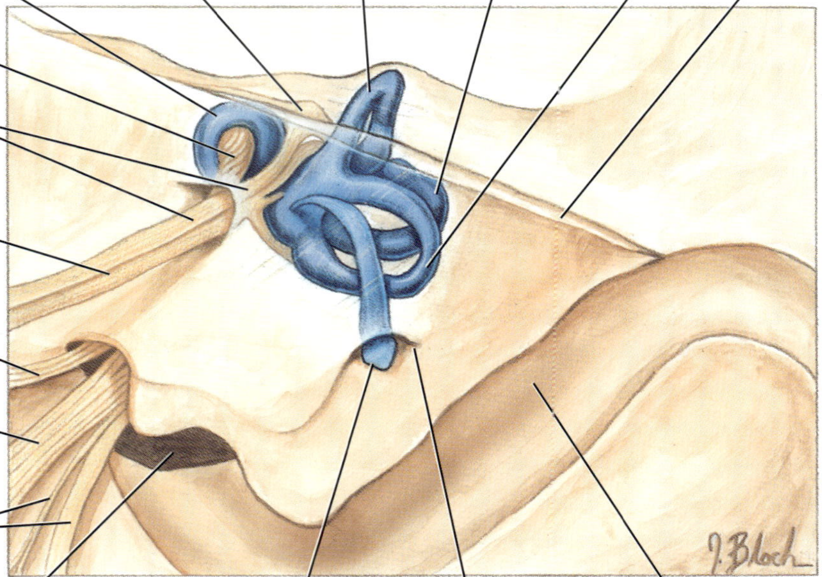

Figure 7. Cochlear, vestibular, and facial nerve relationships within the petrous bone.

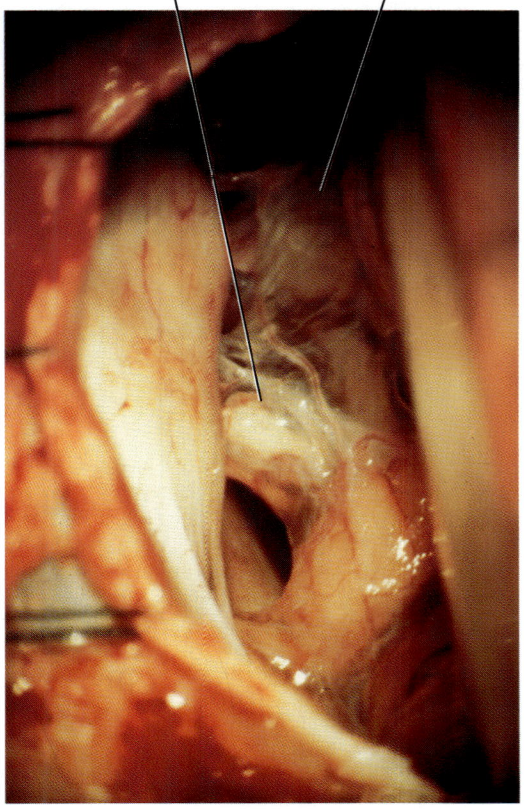

Figure 8. Exposure of the cerebellopontine angle in a case of intracanalicular acoustic neurinoma.

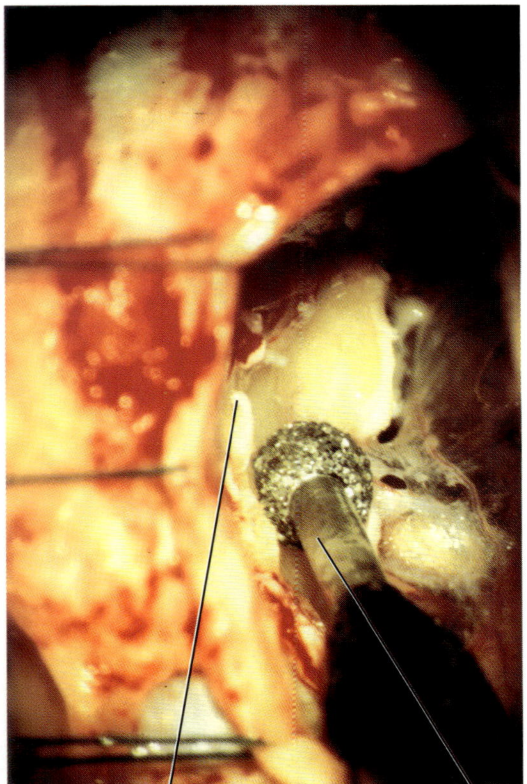

Figure 9. Drilling of the posterior lip of the internal auditory canal.

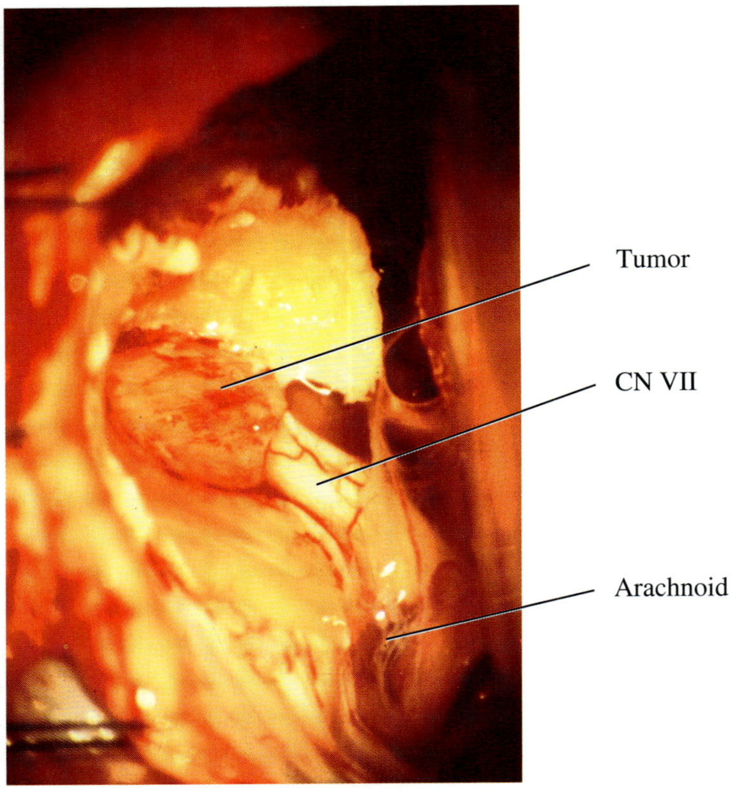

Figure 10. The internal auditory canal is open, and the acoustic neurinoma is exposed.

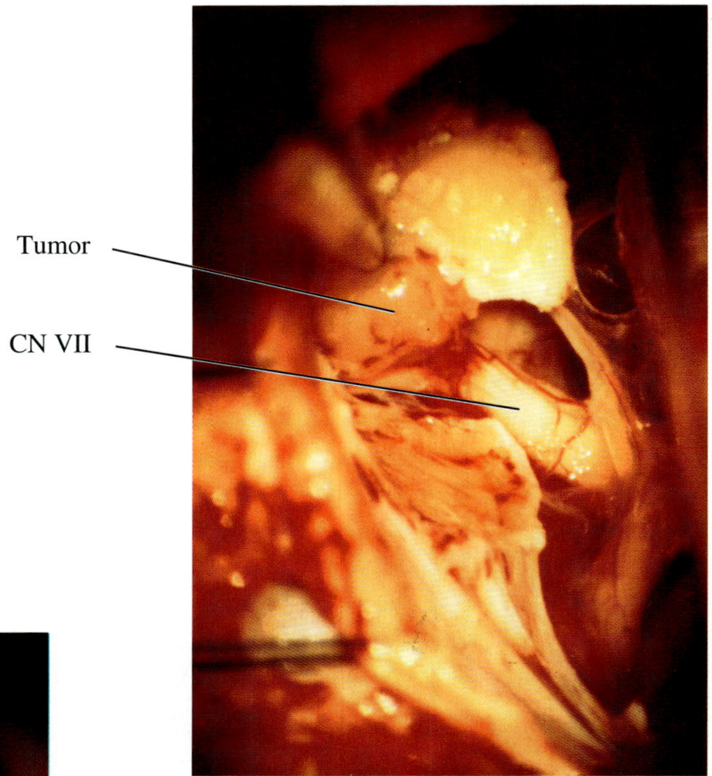

Figure 11. The tumor is partially dissected and elevated.

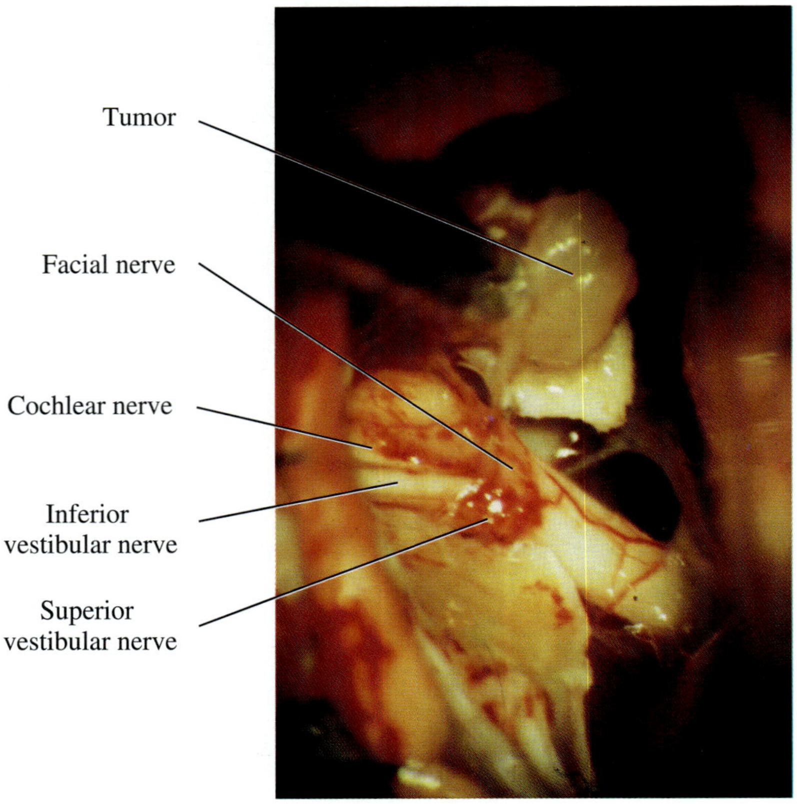

Figure 12. The tumor originates from a fascicle of the superior vestibular nerve, which will be transected. The preserved facial, cochlear, and pars inferior vestibular nerves can be seen.

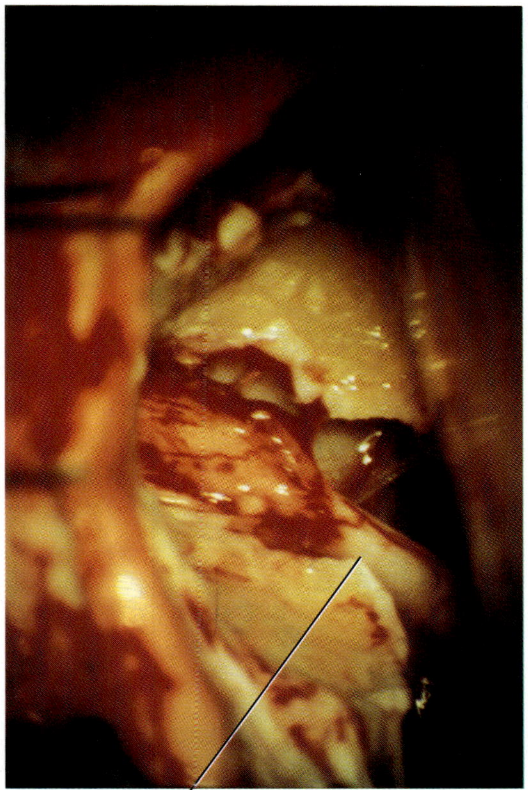

Figure 13. Complete tumor removal.

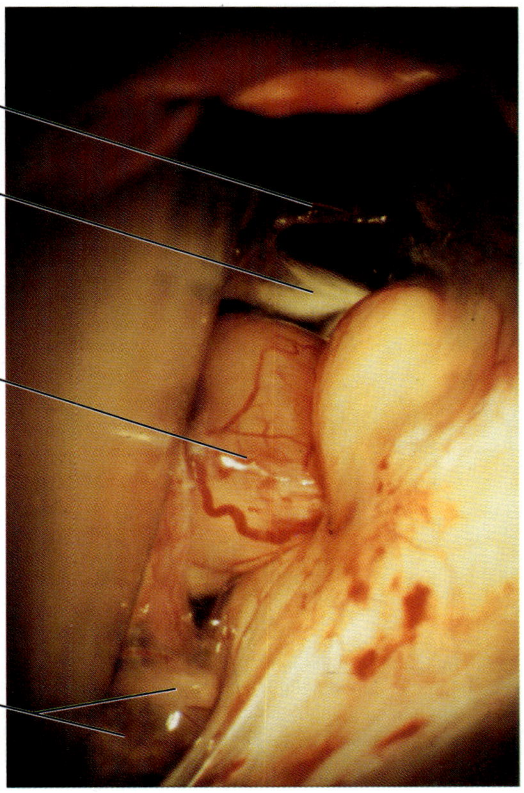

Figure 14. Small acoustic neurinoma in the cerebellopontine angle and internal auditory canal, right side.

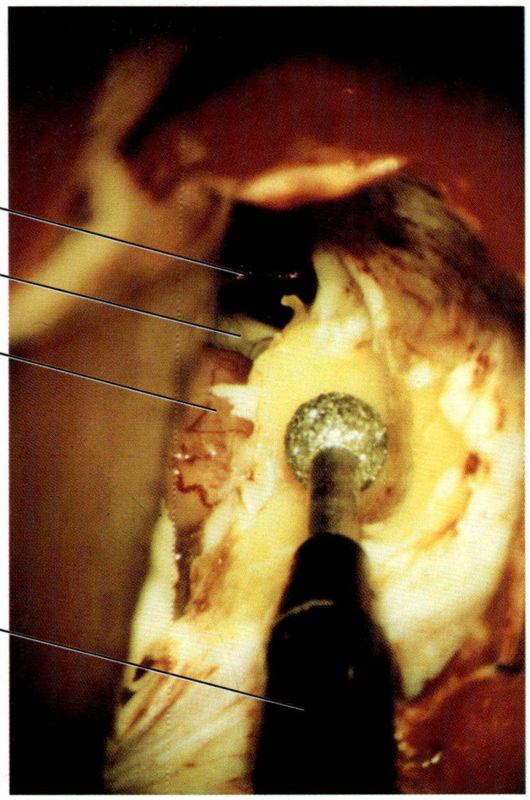

Figure 15. Drilling of the posterior lip of the internal auditory canal.

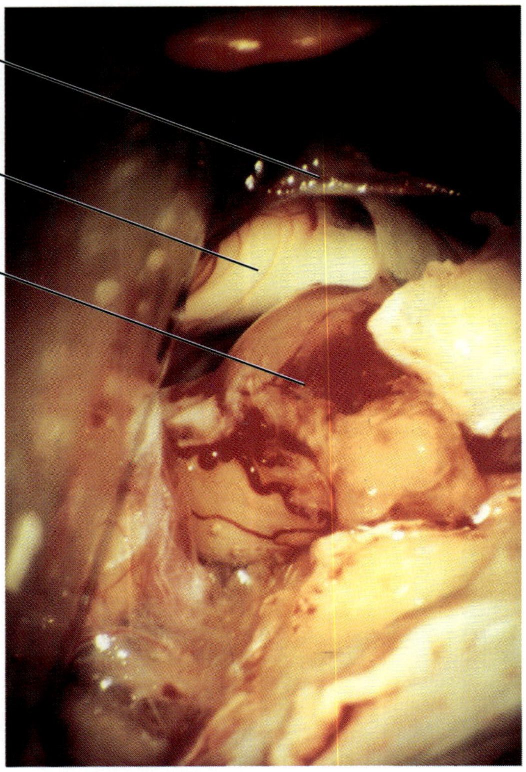

Figure 16. The internal auditory canal is open, and the entire tumor is exposed.

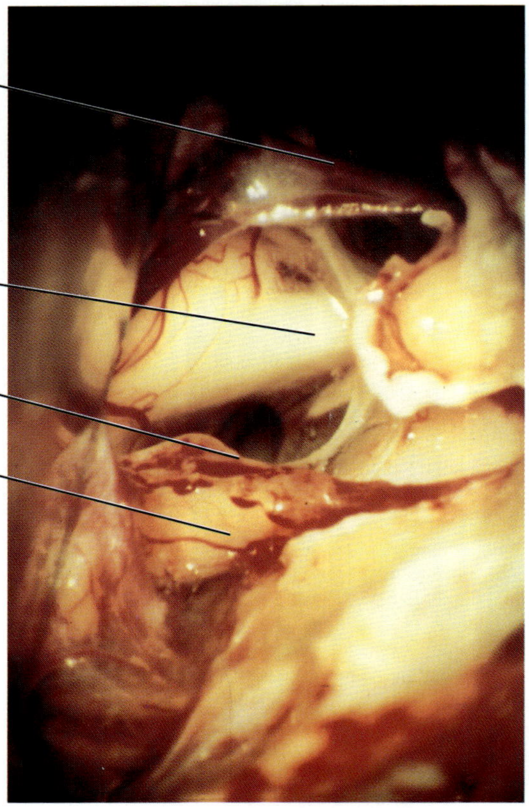

Figure 17. Total removal of the acoustic neurinoma with preservation of facial and cochlear nerves. The trigeminal nerve and petrosal vein are visible.

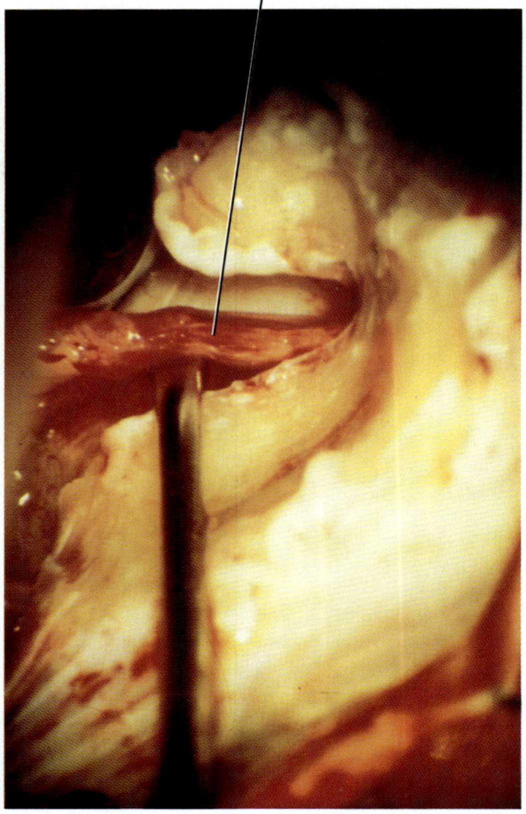

Figure 18. Facial and cochlear nerves are shown elevated in the internal auditory canal for better identification.

Figure 19. The bone and dural defect at the internal auditory canal is filled with muscle and sealed with fibrin glue.

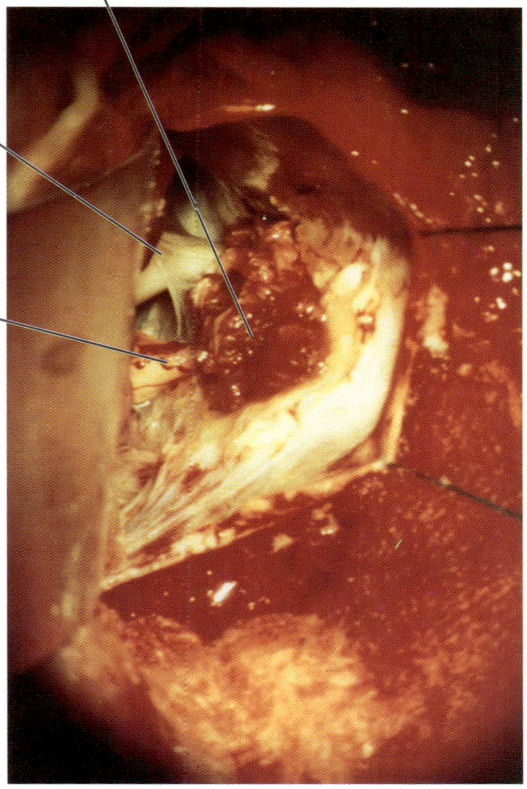

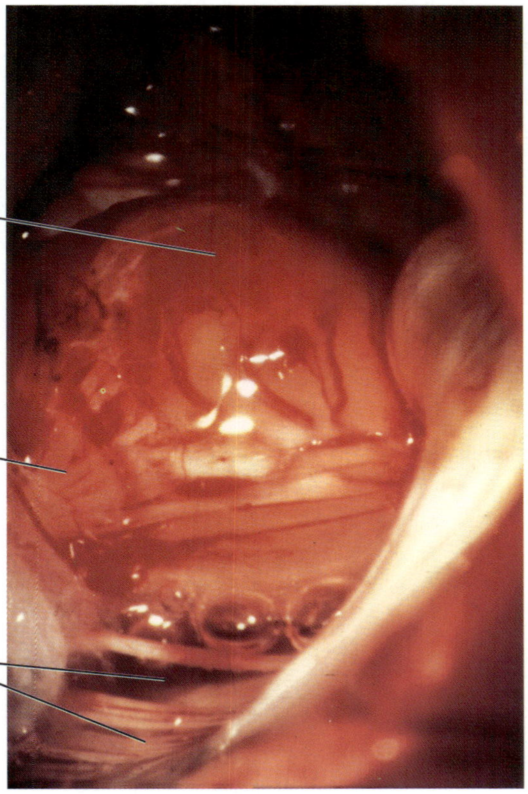

Figure 20. Middle-sized acoustic neurinoma. Lower cranial nerves are visualized as well as different fascicles of the vestibular nerve.

Figure 21. The internal auditory canal is open.

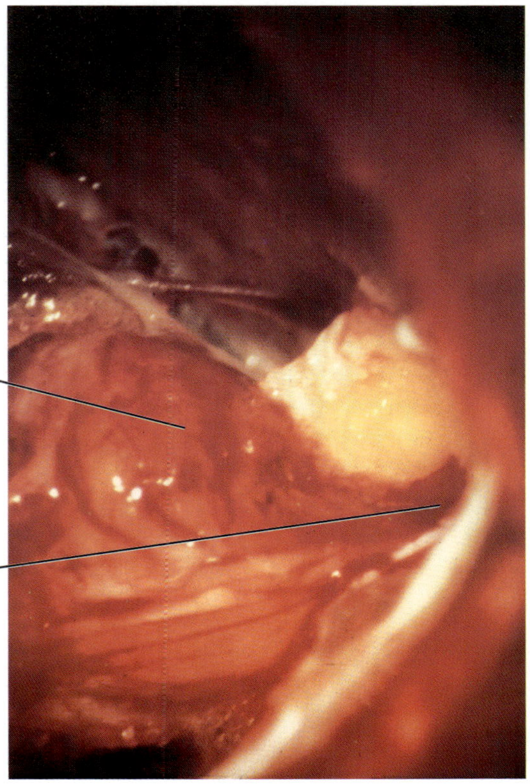

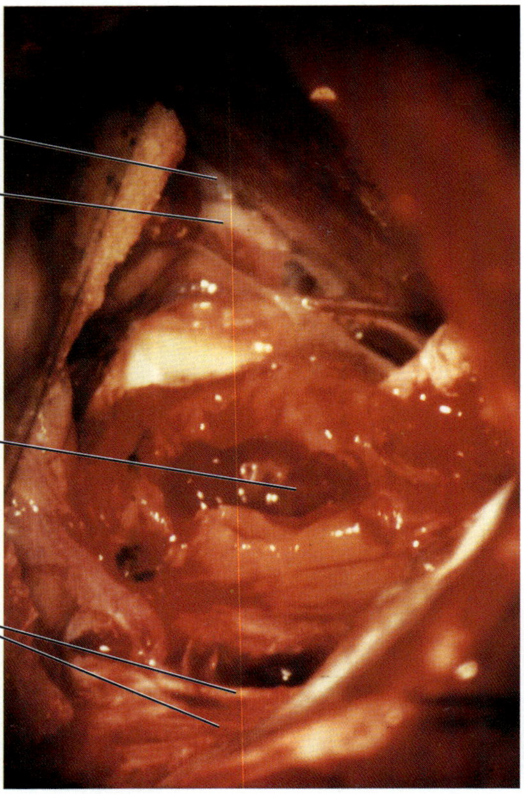

Figure 22. The tumor has been debulked.

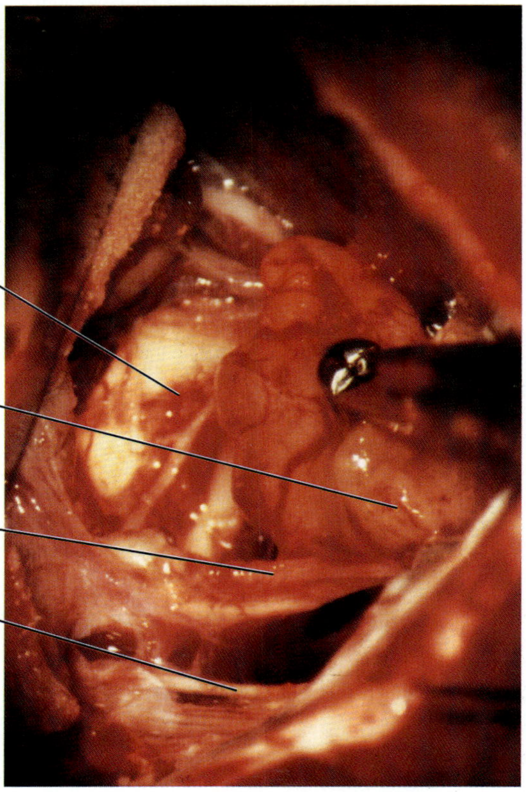

Figure 23. Tumor dissection from the facial and cochlear nerves at the brain stem.

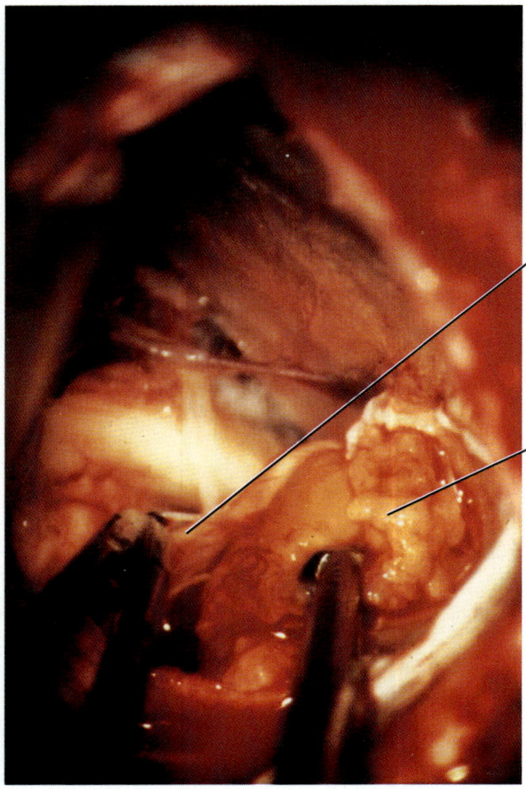

Figure 24. The tumor is held with forceps in the surgeon's right hand. With microforceps held in the left hand, the surgeon dissects the arachnoid along the facial nerve.

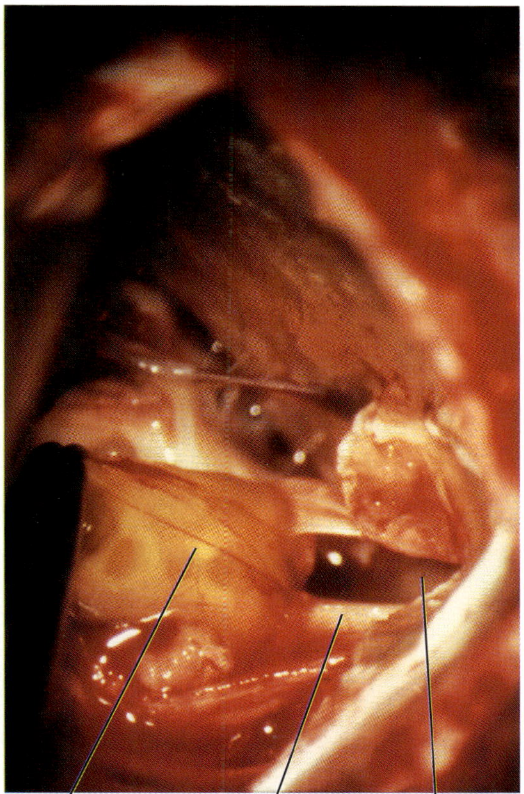

Figure 25. The facial nerve has been dissected free from the tumor capsule within the internal auditory canal.

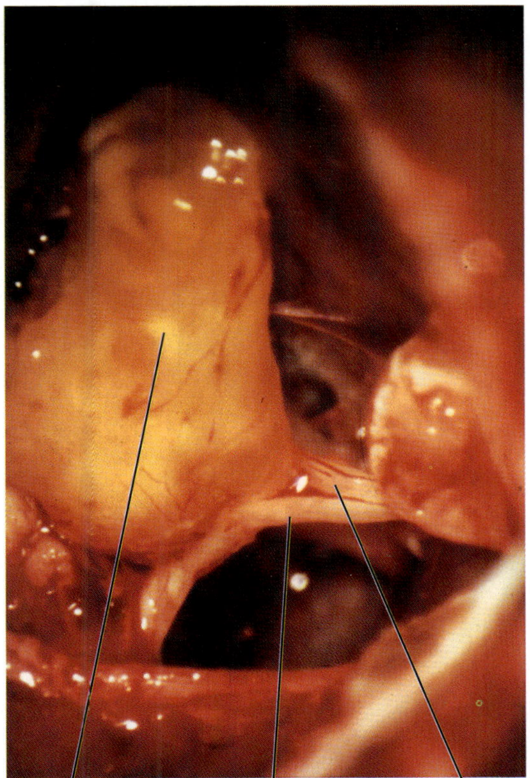

Figure 26. The cochlear nerve is dissected free. The tumor rest, which is severely adherent to the facial nerve, is elevated and can now be partially sharply dissected from the facial nerve.

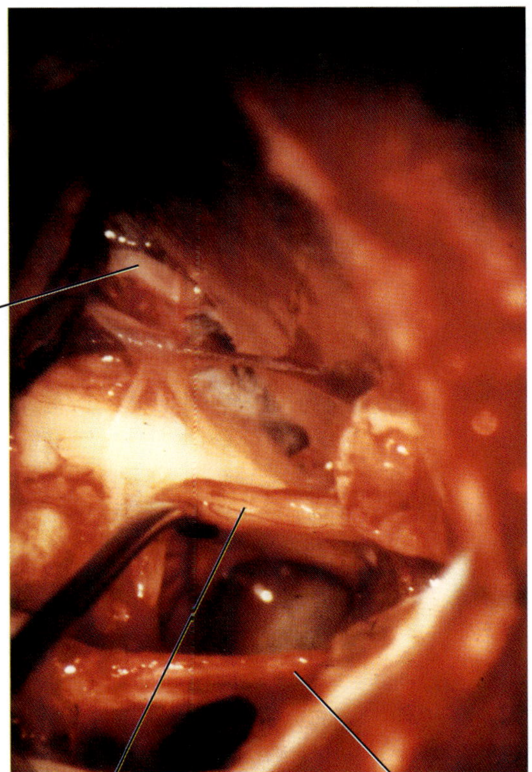

Figure 27. Complete tumor removal with preservation of the facial and cochlear nerves. The facial nerve is shown elevated by a microdissector. The trigeminal nerve can also be identified.

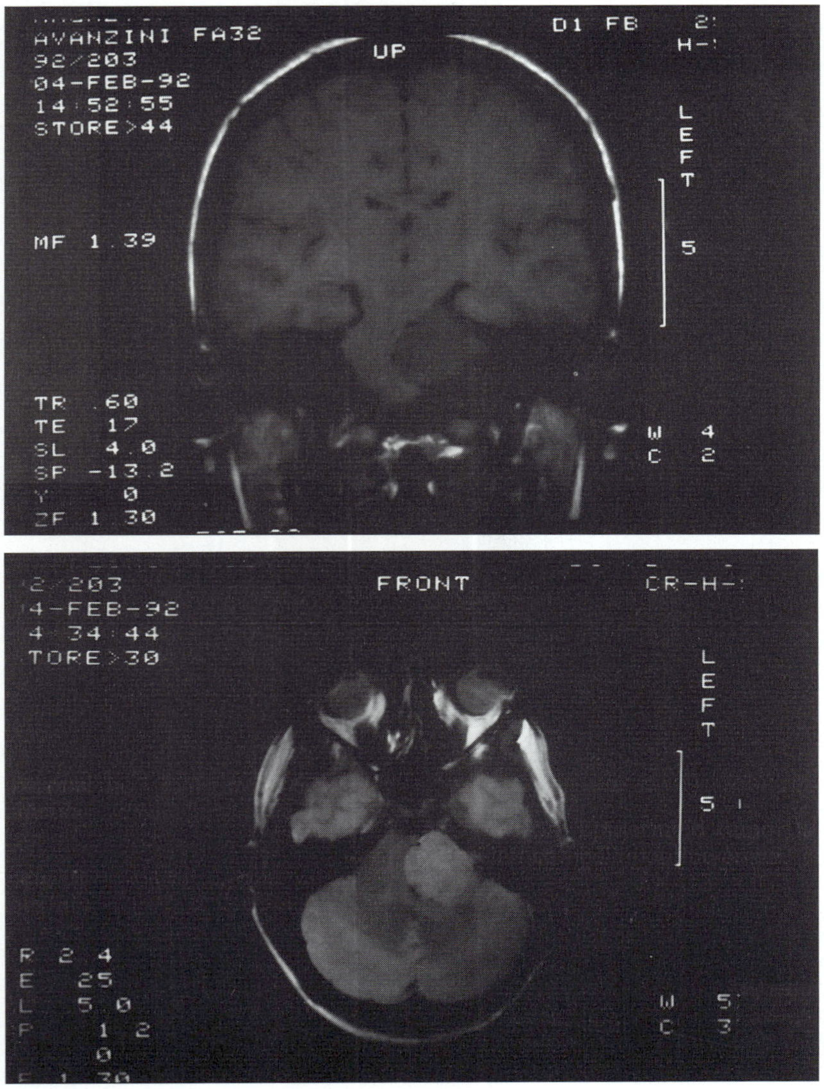

Figure 28. MRI scan images demonstrating a large left acoustic neurinoma.

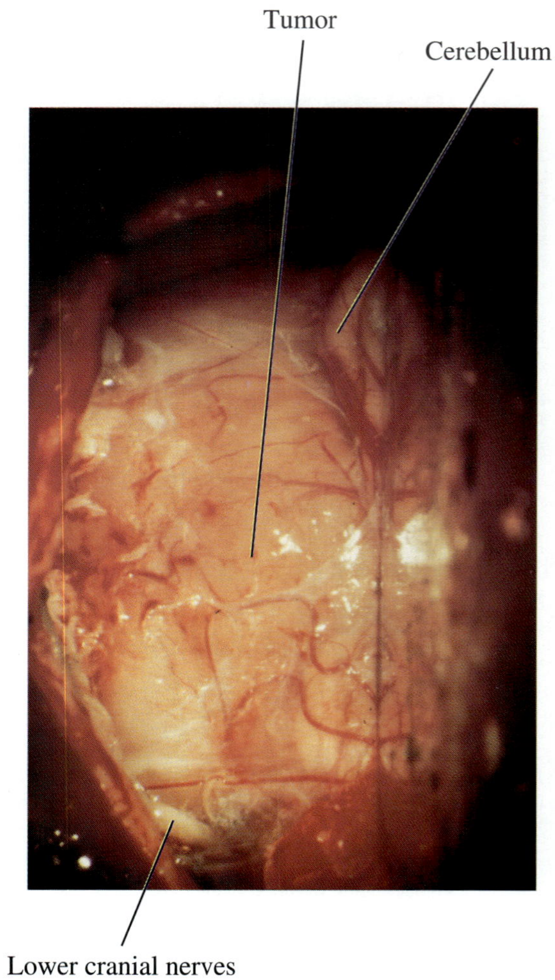

Figure 29. Exposure of a large acoustic neurinoma in the cerebellopontine angle.

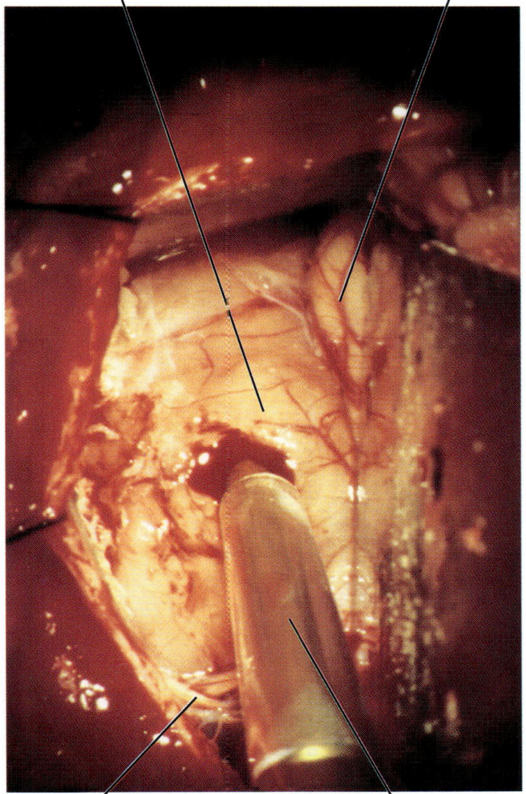

Figure 30. Cavitron is used to debulk the tumor mass.

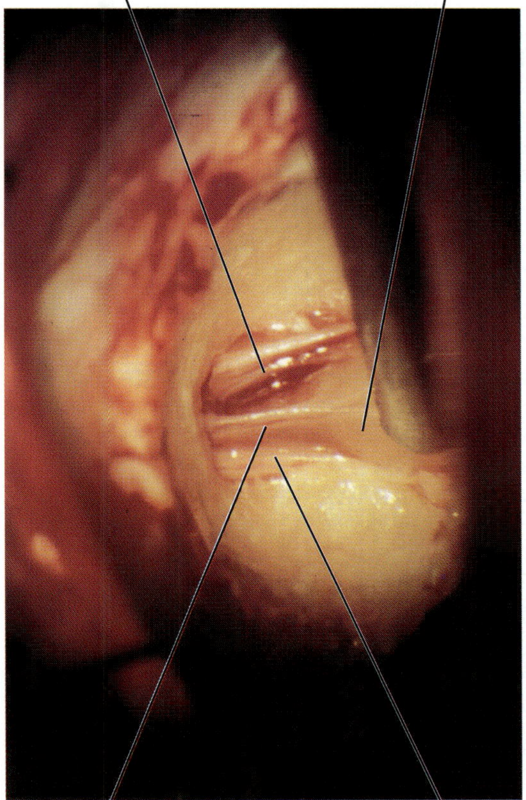

Figure 31. Opening of the internal auditory canal up to the fundus with exposure of CN VII and VIII.

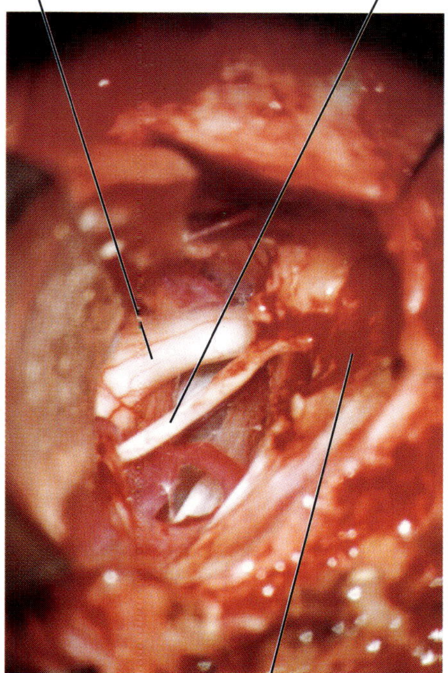

Figure 32. Total removal of a large acoustic neurinoma with preservation of the facial nerve.

29 Epidermoids and Dermoids

Epidermoid cysts are relatively uncommon, constituting less than 1 per cent of all space-occupying lesions of the brain. As is true of dermoid cysts, they are congenital, tumor-like malformations that are thought to arise from inclusion of cells of squamous epithelium during the time of closure of the primitive neural tube. Dermoids occur even less commonly than do epidermoids.

Epidermoid cysts most frequently are located at the skull base and constitute 4 to 6 per cent of all cerebellopontine angle tumors. Removal of these lesions can be difficult because of their tendency to adhere tenaciously to blood vessels, cranial nerves, and other structures. Dermoids can also be especially adherent to adjacent tissues.

Epidermoids are also referred to as cholesteatomas because of their content of cholesterol crystals, or as pearly tumors because of their characteristic appearance caused by epidermal squamous scaling off into the inside of the cyst (Figure 1).

These cysts may grow either intradurally or extradurally, the former occurring much more frequently. They often grow to a large size before being diagnosed clinically because of their tendency to spread out within the subarachnoid space, growing into cisterns and insinuating into crevasses of the cerebellopontine angle (Figure 2) or the parasellar or suprasellar area. Those tumors that arise within the third or fourth ventricle of the brain are also capable of slowly growing to relatively large size.

Epidermoid cysts that grow extradurally do so within the bone of the skull or orbit or within the soft tissues of the anterior fontanelle.

Dermoid cysts are also slowly growing tumors composed not only of epidermal squamous epithelium but also of dermal fibrous stroma with skin appendages (e.g., sebaceous glands, hair follicles). For this reason, these cysts contain a yellowish fatty mass with hairs, lacking the whitish appearance of epidermoids (Figure 3). Dermoid tumors usually are located near the midline. They are encapsulated in a way similar to that of epidermoids and are more firm in consistency.

CLINICAL PRESENTATION

A distinct tendency to occur more often in men than in women has been noted for epidermoids and dermoids. Because of their very slow growth, especially when located intradurally, symptoms may be present for 5 to 10 years before becoming prominent enough to lead to diagnosis. The average age of patients at the time of first operation for these tumors has been reported to be in the 30s or 40s. With availability of computed tomography (CT) and magnetic resonance imaging (MRI), earlier diagnosis and treatment may occur.

Most patients with epidermoid cysts in the cerebellopontine angle present with a history of progressive hearing loss and tinnitus, followed by gait disturbance, and with signs of trigeminal neuralgia. The latter features are thought to be related to displacement of the fifth nerve against vascular structures within the cerebellopontine angle. As the tumors enlarge even further, involvement of the lower cranial nerves can occur.

In patients in whom the tumor arises in a parasellar location, headache is frequent, and fourth and sixth nerve paresis or palsy, long tract signs, and homonymous hemianopia caused by optic tract compression may occur. Suprasellar tumors may compress the optic nerves or chiasm, producing visual difficulty.

Epidermoid cysts present with characteristic x-ray, CT, and MRI findings. Those that present within the diploë of the skull have a punched-out appearance on plain x-ray films and CT scans, usually with clear-cut and often sclerotic margins. Intradural skull base epidermoids are characteristically uniformly hypodense on CT scans, having a density similar to that of cerebrospinal fluid. They do not enhance with contrast administration, and do not show signs of peritumoral edema.

On MRI, epidermoid cysts are decreased in signal intensity on T_1-weighted images as compared with brain tissue and usually have signal intensity identical to that of cerebrospinal fluid. On T_2-weighted images, they are hyperintense compared with brain tissue and isointense compared with cerebrospinal fluid. The irregular cauliflower-shaped configuration that is characteristic of epidermoids can be readily appreciated on MRI. It is necessary to distinguish cholesterol granulomas, which show increased signal intensity on T_1-weighted images, and dermoids, which are more midline in location than epidermoids, hyperintense on T_1-weighted images, and hypointense on T_2-weighted images.

OPERATIVE CONSIDERATIONS

Epidermoid cysts are histologically benign. Sometimes complete removal may not be possible because of their tendency to invade the available spaces in their pathway and to adhere tightly to important structures. Total removal is the goal in surgical treatment because tumor tissue left in place continues to grow, resulting in subsequent tumor recurrence. From a practical point of view, subtotal excision of epidermoid cysts is often necessary to avoid significant neurological deficit or even catastrophic surgical outcome. Because of the slow-growth characteristics of these tumors, it is feasible in a case of severe adherence of tumor capsule to cranial nerves and vessels to leave tissue and anticipate reoperation at some future time if significant regrowth should occur. The availability of CT and MRI has helped a great deal in following residual tumor growth and timing future surgery.

Procedures for surgical access to the skull base, commonly used in the removal of epidermoid and dermoid tumors, include the medial and lateral suboccipital, presigmoid, subtemporal, and pterional approaches. These approaches have been presented earlier in this atlas.

Figure 4 shows a CT scan image of a left cerebellopontine angle epidermoid tumor. In Figure 5, the characteristic tumor appearance is demonstrated by a lesion that fills the cerebellopontine angle. Partial removal is in evidence in Figure 6. In Figure 7, the trigeminal nerve has been dissected free, but tumor is still attached to the brain stem. In Figure 8, complete excision of the epidermoid tumor, with decompression of the trigeminal nerve, is demonstrated. The anterior inferior cerebellar artery can be seen, having been dissected free from the tumor mass without injury.

An example of a large dermoid tumor in the temporal area is shown by postcontrast MRI scan images in Figure 9. Its appearance characteristics are seen in Figure 10.

Figure 11 shows complete removal of this large dermoid tumor, including the area of involved skull base. Postoperative CT scans show no sign of residual tumor (Figure 12), and an MRI scan done 6 months postoperatively shows no evidence of tumor mass (Figure 13).

COMMON COMPLICATIONS

The most frequent complications after removal of epidermoid cysts are those that arise because of injury to cranial nerves or vascular structures to which the tumor is adherent or in proximity. Depending on tumor location, this may mean visual loss; extraocular nerve paresis or palsy; facial pain, numbness, or paralysis; and deafness. Deficits involving lower cranial nerves, such as dysarthria, and difficulty swallowing may also occur. Cerebellar disturbance, long tract signs, and brain stem injury caused by direct trauma, vascular impairment, or major infarction can constitute major complications.

Chemical meningitis may occur after surgery for removal of epidermoid cysts. A later sequela of this may be formation of dense adhesions. This complication has become less common with magnification and microsurgical techniques, which have resulted in more complete tumor removal. Irrigation to remove tumor debris intraoperatively and the use of steroids intraoperatively and postoperatively have helped to reduce the occurrence of these complications.

RECOMMENDED READING

Conley, F.: Epidermoid and dermoid tumors: Clinical features and surgical management. *In* Wilkins, R.H., Rengachary, S.S. (eds.): Neurosurgery. Vol. 1. New York, Williams & Wilkins, 1985, pp. 668–673.

Netsky, M.: Epidermoid tumors. Surg. Neurol. 29:477–483, 1988.

Rubin, G., Scienza, R., Pasqualin, A., et al.: Craniocerebral epidermoids and dermoids. Acta Neurochir. (Wien) 97:1–16, 1989.

Sabin, H., Bordi, L., Symon, L.: Epidermoid cysts and cholesterol granulomas centered on the posterior fossa: Twenty years of diagnosis and management. Neurosurgery 21:798–805, 1987.

Wasenko, J., Rosenblood, S., Estes, M., et al.: Magnetic resonance of intracranial epidermoids. Eur. J. Radiol. 13:103–106, 1991.

Yamakawa, K., Shitara, N., Genka, S., et al.: Clinical course and surgical prognosis of 33 cases of intracranial epidermoid tumors. Neurosurgery 24:568–573, 1989.

Yasargil, M., Abernathey, C., Sarioglu, A.: Microneurosurgical treatment of intracranial dermoid and epidermoid tumors. Neurosurgery 24:561–567, 1989.

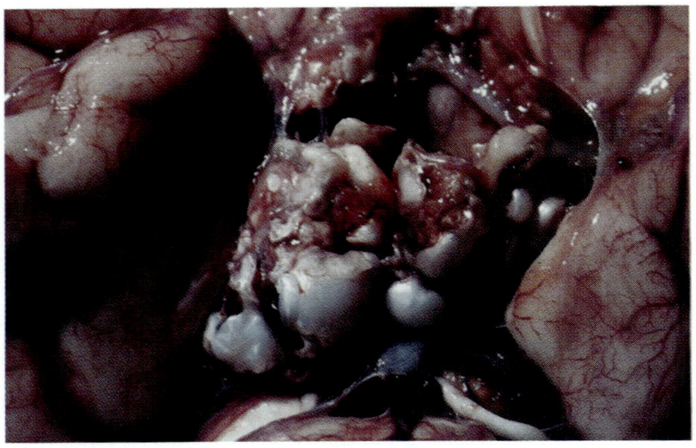

Figure 1. Suprasellar epidermoid cyst with the typical appearance of a pearly tumor and irregular cauliflower-shaped configuration.

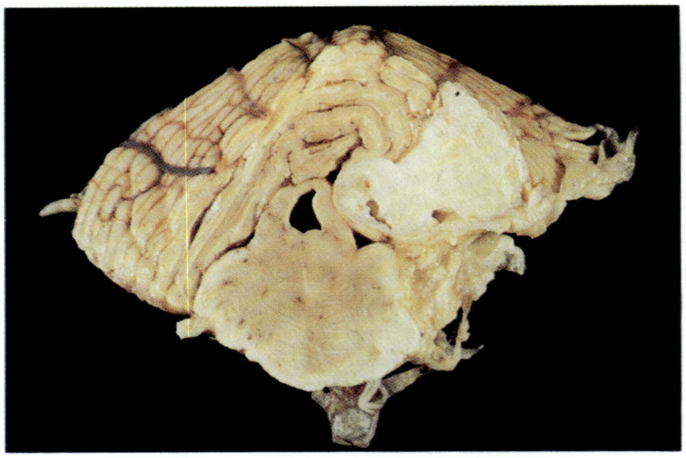

Figure 2. Epidermoid cyst with typical whitish appearance insinuating into crevasses of the cerebellopontine angle.

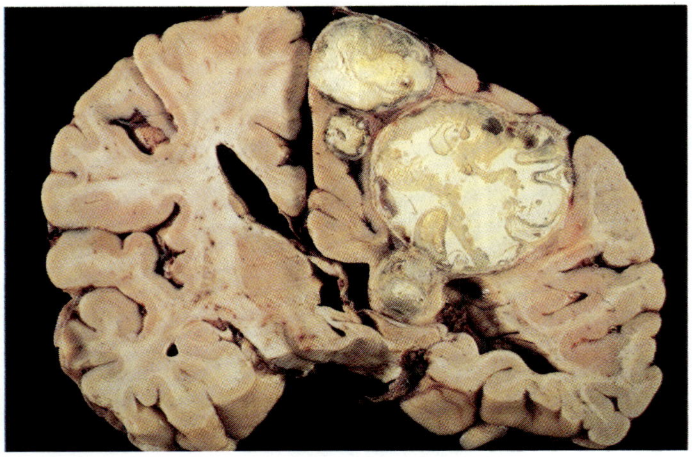

Figure 3. Large yellowish dermoid cysts that contain fatty masses with hairs.

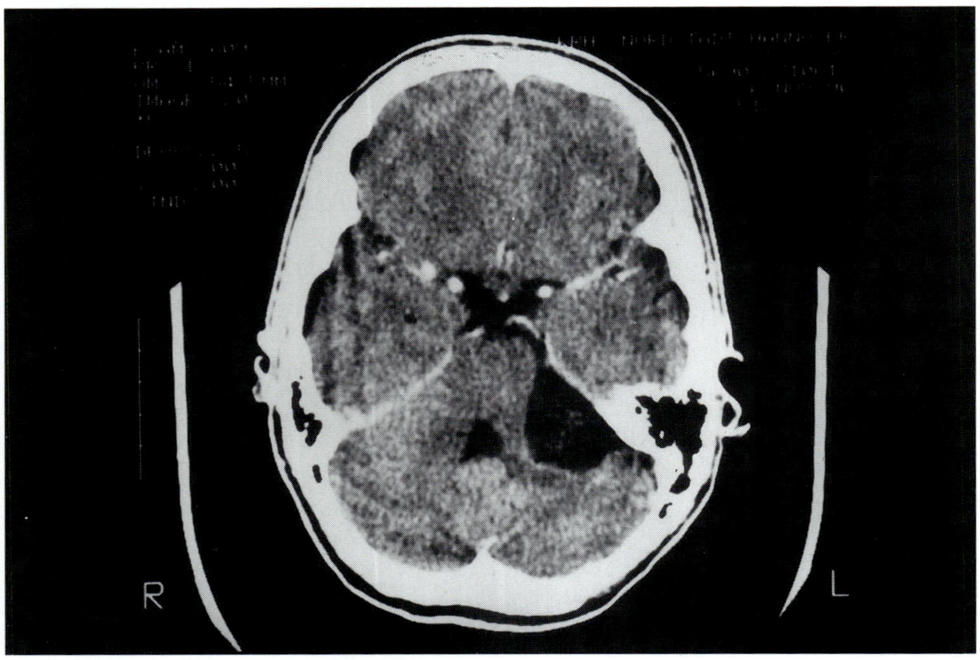

Figure 4. Left cerebellopontine angle epidermoid tumor.

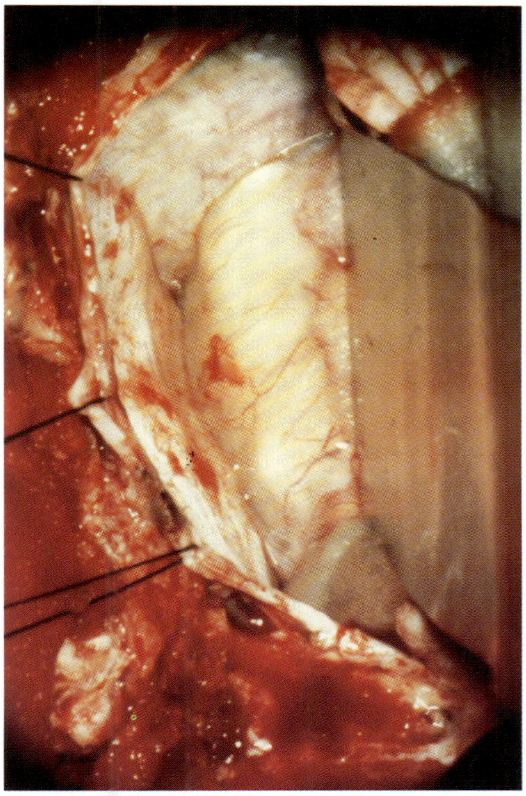

Figure 5. Epidermoid tumor is shown filling the left cerebellopontine angle.

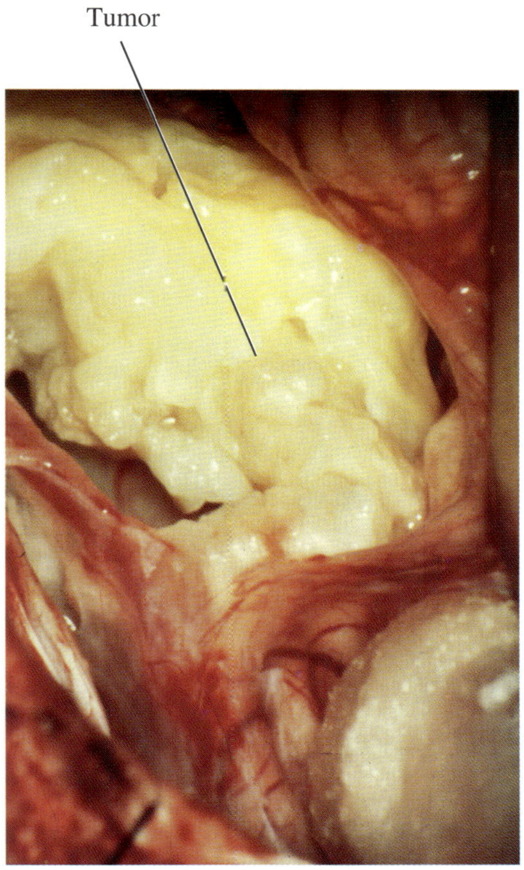

Figure 6. Partial removal of epidermoid tumor.

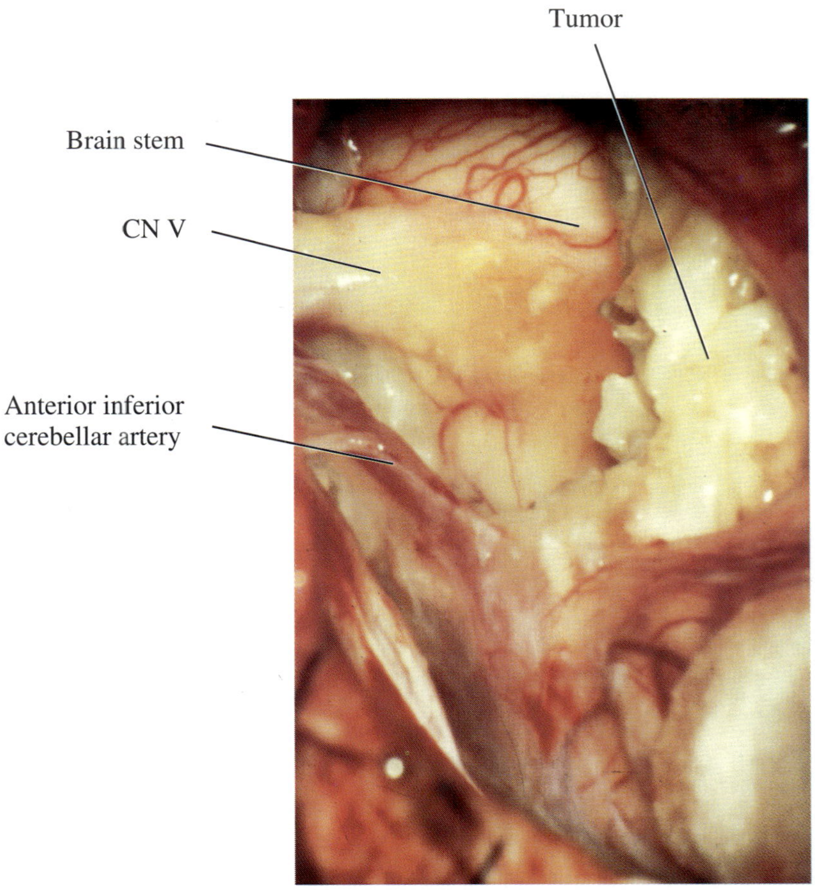

Figure 7. Fifth cranial nerve is dissected free. The remaining tumor is attached to the brain stem.

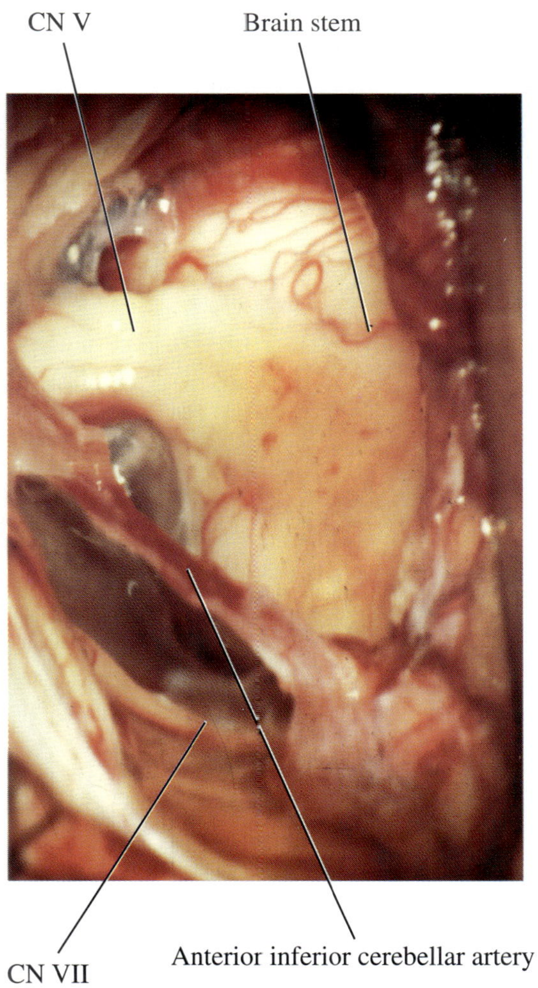

Figure 8. Complete removal of an epidermoid tumor, with cranial nerve V exposed and decompressed. The anterior inferior cerebellar artery is dissected free.

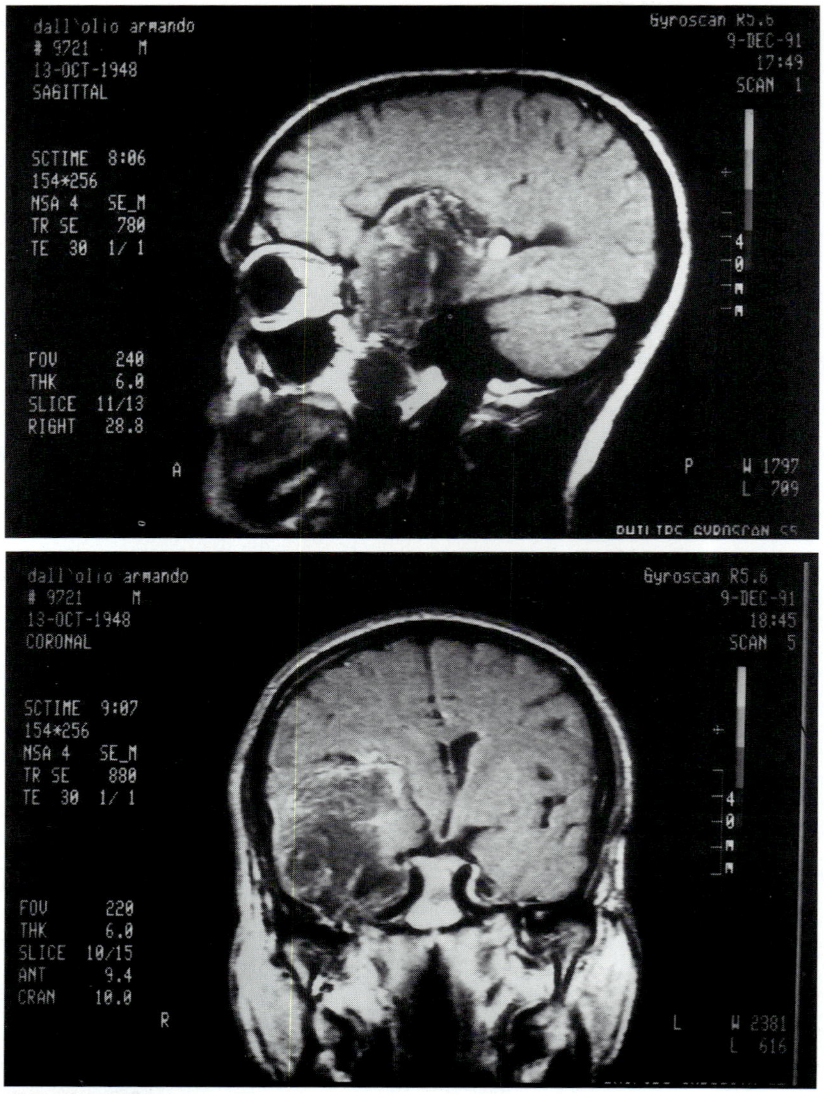

Figure 9. MRI scan showing a large dermoid tumor in the temporal area.

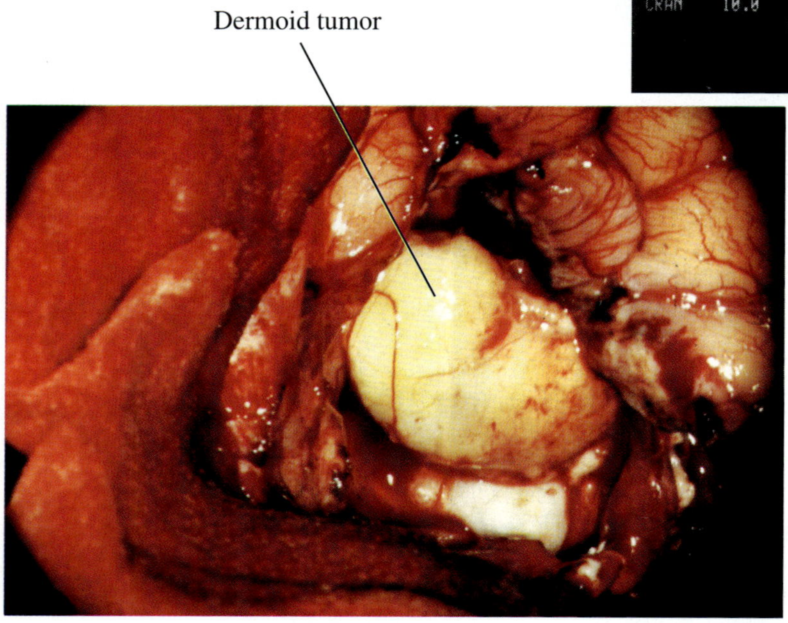

Figure 10. Dermoid tumor involvement in the temporal region.

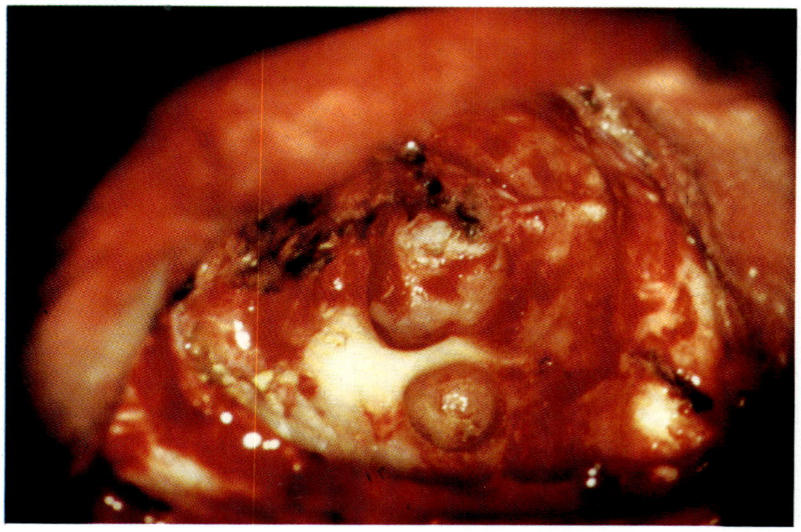

Figure 11. Complete removal of tumor, including the involved skull base compartment.

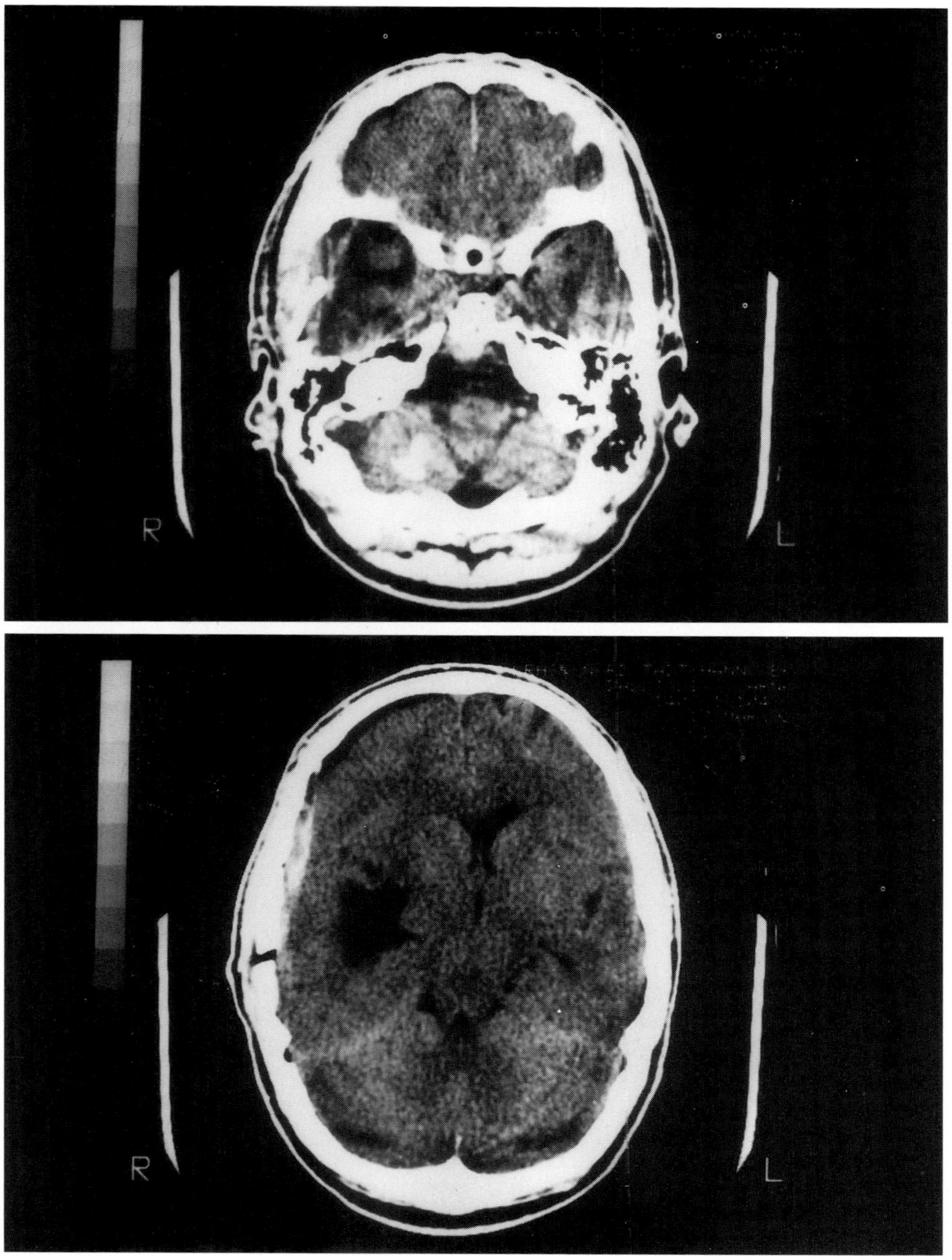

Figure 12. Postoperative CT scans demonstrating complete tumor removal.

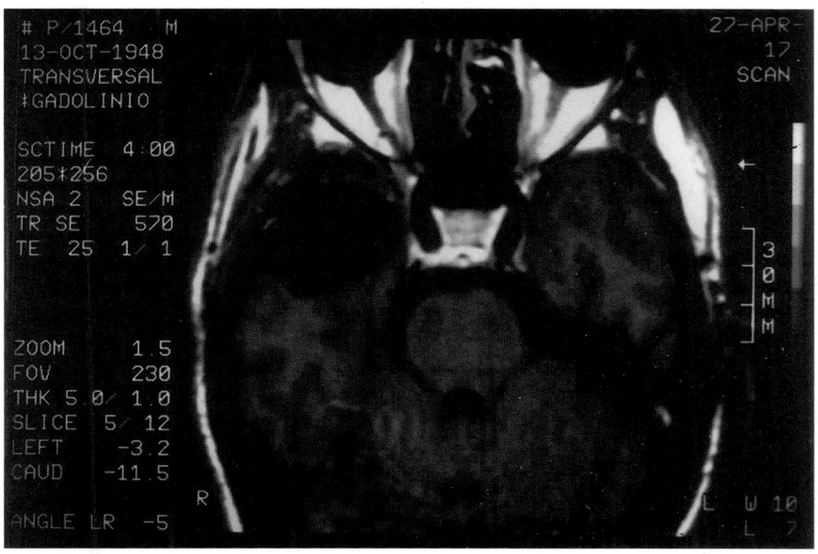

Figure 13. MRI scan done 6 months postoperatively showing no tumor mass.

30 Craniopharyngiomas

Craniopharyngiomas are congenital midline tumors that are histologically benign but often result in death or great disability because of location. They can be one of the most difficult of cranial base tumors to remove. Craniopharyngiomas arise from epithelial cell rests deriving from the primitive pharyngeal Rathke's pouch and usually are in association with the infundibular stalk. For this reason, they may be intrasellar, suprasellar, or both. These tumors may be solid histologically with an adamantinomatous pattern (Figure 1), or partially cystic. At times, they may have large cystic components (Figure 2). They may be partially calcified (Figure 3).

Craniopharyngiomas have been considered by some to be infiltrative with a tendency to grow into the hypothalamus (Figure 4). This has led neurosurgeons to stop at partial removal. On histological sections, finger-like interdigitations of tumor may be seen extending into the hypothalamus. Because craniopharyngiomas are encapsulated tumors, it appears that infiltration does not occur, but that capsule-covered extensions of tumor do spread into adjacent neural tissue (Figure 5).

Craniopharyngiomas can be classified in terms of their relation to the third ventricle (Figure 6). They can also be distinguished as prechiasmatic, intrasellar, and retrochiasmatic. If they arise below the diaphragma sellae, the sella turcica usually is enlarged. Those tumors that arise above the diaphragma sellae compress the infundibulum and hypothalamus early as well as the optic nerves and chiasm. Even those craniopharyngiomas that arise below the diaphragm grow upward, causing similar compression. Craniopharyngiomas eventually invaginate the hypothalamus and extend into the third ventricle and may grow into the anterior, middle, or posterior fossae. They occasionally arise entirely within the third ventricle.

The most difficult craniopharyngiomas to remove often are those that are retrochiasmal with vertical extension. The degree of vertical extension can be classified into five grades (see Figure 6). Grade I tumors are intrasellar or infradiaphragmatic, whereas grade II tumors are localized to the suprasellar cistern. Grade III craniopharyngiomas extend into the lower third ventricle, and grade IV extend into the upper third ventricle. Grade V tumors reach the septum pellucidum or lateral ventricle. Figure 7 shows various sites of origin of craniopharyngiomas in relation to the infundibular stalk. Atypical craniopharyngiomas may occur in other locations distant to the infundibular stalk, including the sphenoid sinus, pineal region, and pharynx.

Viewed in the horizontal sense, craniopharyngiomas may rarely extend into the sphenoid sinus or interhemispheric fissure anteriorly, into the middle fossa laterally, or into the posterior fossa posteriorly. In the coronal section shown in Figure 8, the vertical and horizontal growth patterns of these tumors can be seen.

INCIDENCE

Craniopharyngiomas constitute about 1.2 to 4 per cent of intracranial tumors and often present in childhood but may not present until well into adult life. Overall, the most common presenting complaint is visual impairment. In childhood, the most frequent presenting sign is growth retardation; in adults, it is sexual dysfunction. In men, the dysfunction is in the form of impotence or reduced libido with changes in secondary sexual characteristics. In women, amenorrhea occurs, often with associated galactorrhea. Headache is a presenting complaint in about one-half of patients with craniopharyngiomas. There is a male predominance of 3 : 2.

TREATMENT

Complete surgical excision is the treatment goal. If tumor tissue is left in place, the tumor mass will recur. A second surgery for these tumors usually is difficult because of scar tissue formation, which makes identification of tumor margins impossible. With computed tomography (CT) and magnetic resonance imaging (MRI), earlier diagnosis of these tumors has become possible. The operating microscope, modern anesthesia, and endocrine replacement therapy have made definitive surgery more successful.

The preoperative workup should include plain skull radiographs, CT scan with thin cuts through the sella and suprasellar area, and MRI. MRI angiography should be done rather than cerebral angiography. If the MRI angiogram does not show enough detail concerning location of the carotid artery and its branches relative to the tumor, cerebral angiography should also be done.

One of the most serious and potentially life-threatening complications after surgery for craniopharyngiomas is hormonal disturbance with associated fluid and electrolyte imbalance. For this reason, a complete preoperative workup by an endocrinologist, precise monitoring, and immediate treatment response are mandatory. Fluid, electrolyte, and hormonal replacement therapy are especially critical during the initial 48 hours after surgery.

SURGICAL ANATOMY

Knowledge of the surrounding anatomy, including the microvascular circulation, is extremely important in the surgical excision of craniopharyngiomas. This is true because of the intimate association with the hypothalamus and the infundibular stalk as well as the optic nerves and chiasm and the major vessels in the suprasellar area. In addition, disturbance of the small perforating vessels in this area can yield catastrophic results.

Most of these tumors are separated from adjacent structures by a subarachnoid plane, although they may invaginate the hypothalamus in such a way that dissection to separate them from neural tissue is difficult or impossible.

PREOPERATIVE CONSIDERATIONS

If the patient has hydrocephalus, it is important to perform a shunting procedure preoperatively. Those patients who present with hormonal imbalance should be treated medically to correct this problem before scheduling for surgery.

CHOICE OF SURGICAL APPROACH

The location and size of the tumor determine the optimal surgical approach. To achieve total excision, it is important to plan a multidirectional approach. The approach chosen should also offer the least trauma, the shortest route to the tumor, and a necessary overview of important structures.

Tumors that are totally or substantially within the sella (grade I) can best be treated by a transsphenoidal approach. This is especially true in the case of cystic intrasellar lesions. Craniopharyngiomas of this type are rare.

Craniopharyngiomas that are primarily suprasellar, displacing the optic nerves and chiasm upward and invaginating the hypothalamus (Figure 9), are best approached by a pterional or subfrontal approach. Figure 10 shows the anatomical relations after excision of a tumor in this location via subfrontal approach.

Craniopharyngiomas that are small and retrochiasmatic or that extend primarily laterally into the middle fossa can be operated on from a subtemporal approach or a combined pterional and subtemporal approach.

Those tumors that are spilling into the posterior fossa or extending down the clivus may be approached by a transpetrosal-transtentorial route.

Craniopharyngiomas that are totally or largely growing within the third ventricle are still technically skull base tumors. They can be approached by the interhemispheric, transcallosal approach, removing the tumor through the foramen of Monro or through a transfrontal approach through the lamina terminalis.

For removal of craniopharyngiomas that are grade III to grade V, a subfrontal unilateral or bilateral approach is preferred. The reason for this is that because these tumors arise from remnants of Rathke's pouch, they are initially midline tumors. They grow by expansion in different directions, but a midline operative approach to the suprasellar area remains most optimal for their total removal. The choice of whether to do a unilateral or a bilateral approach depends on the extent and direction of tumor expansion.

SPECIFIC OPERATIVE CONSIDERATIONS

Transsphenoidal Approach

The description of patient positioning and operative technique for the transsphenoidal approach are outlined in Chapter 9. This approach can be used for removal of tumors within the sella or suprasellar tumors that do not engulf the optic chiasm or invaginate the hypothalamus.

Once the transsphenoidal approach has been made and the sphenoid sinus opened, an enlarged sellar floor often is encountered in those cases of primarily intrasellar craniopharyngioma. Extensive removal of the floor of the sella is then carried out to maximize the exposure. This is followed by opening of the dura as widely as possible without entering the cavernous sinus laterally or the circular sinus anteriorly.

The capsule of the tumor usually can be dissected free from the dura and from the medial dural layer of the cavernous sinus without great difficulty. To remove the superior portion of the tumor, which is adherent to the diaphragma sellae and often extends into the suprasellar area, the diaphragm must be removed. At this point, the intracranial portion of the tumor may be progressively "delivered" downward by the pulsation of the brain, and traction on the tumor is not necessary and should be avoided.

As more of the tumor mass is removed, the infundibular stalk should be identified and preserved along with any identifiable anterior pituitary lobe tissue.

It is critical to avoid coagulation or tearing of small perforating branches from the circle of Willis as they enter the hypothalamus and to avoid trauma to the optic nerves and chiasm.

Craniopharyngiomas with suprasellar extension should not be approached transsphenoidally if they involve or are attached to the optic chiasm or are likely to involve the hypothalamus or important vascular structures in this area.

Subfrontal Approach

In those patients with a primarily suprasellar craniopharyngioma, the subfrontal approach, with entry through the lamina terminalis if needed, is the approach of choice. An example of this type of craniopharyngioma is shown in the preoperative CT scan in Figure 11. The basic procedural description of the subfrontal approach is described in Chapter 1. A bitemporal coronal incision is made. For a unilateral exposure, three burr holes are made, with the lateral burr hole placed in the keyhole position at the root of the zygomatic process of the frontal bone. The medial burr hole is placed at the midline, as low as possible. If the frontal sinus is entered in doing this, the mucosal lining is stripped away and displaced downward toward the ostia.

For a bifrontal approach, burr holes are placed bilaterally in the keyhole position, a third burr hole is placed low in the midline, and a fourth is made several centimeters above the glabella overlying the sagittal sinus. This approach offers the advantage of a direct view of the craniopharyngioma anteriorly or anterolaterally, with good visualization of both optic nerves as well as the chiasm. In those patients who have a prefixed chiasm, the tumor is entered through the lamina terminalis, which has been rendered an inert structure by the expansion of the tumor. If additional exposure is needed anteriorly, the tuberculum sellae can be removed.

After turning the craniotomy flap, the dura is opened frontobasally and the arachnoidal cisterns are opened progressively as the frontal lobes are elevated. The olfactory tracts are spared by carefully dissecting them away from the subfrontal cortical surface. In giant craniopharyngiomas, the lesser sphenoid ridge is used as a landmark as dissection is continued to expose both optic nerves. The basal cisterns are then opened to drain cerebrospinal fluid and gain additional exposure. If a postfixed optic chiasm is encountered, the approach to the tumor is subchiasmatic, and if prefixed, it is through the lamina terminalis.

It is necessary to visualize both anterior cerebral arteries and the anterior communicating artery. It usually is not possible to distinguish the posterior border of the optic chiasm. The lamina terminalis should be entered close to the anterior communicating artery.

From the multidirectional vantage point of the subfrontal approach, it usually is possible to remove even large suprasellar craniopharyngiomas while preserving vital neural and vascular structures, including small perforating branches. Good visualization of the tumor attachment to the hypothalamus is also possible. After removal of the bulk of the tumor, it is possible to visualize and remove tumor that may be extending posteriorly over the dorsum sellae.

The operative removal of the craniopharyngioma shown in the CT scan in Figure 11 is shown in Figures 12 through 15. In Figure 12, the frontal lobes can be seen as they are being gently retracted to expose the craniopharyngioma that is presenting between the optic nerves. Figure 13 shows partial removal of the tumor with both optic nerves and the right anterior cerebral artery exposed. In Figure 14, the total removal of the tumor can be seen. The optic nerves have been decompressed, and the basilar and vertebral arteries and brain stem are visualized after removal of the part of the tumor that was projecting over the dorsum sellae. The same operative exposure is shown in Figure 15 by a higher magnification. Figure 16 shows a postoperative CT scan image that confirms total tumor removal.

In doing the dissection of craniopharyngiomas from this approach, it is important to stay within the arachnoid tissue plane to avoid trauma to important structures. Because of the close adherence of tumor to the hypothalamus, this arachnoidal plane is missing, and careful direct dissection from the neural tissue is required in this area. This may also be necessary in dissecting tumor from the optic nerves and chiasm. No attempt to remove calcified portions of the tumor that are attached to the optic nerves or chiasm should be attempted until the mass has been thoroughly enucleated. Only then will the calcified portion fall away sufficiently from the optic nerves to allow complete removal. If there is tumor involvement of the infundibular stalk, the involved portion should be removed and the stalk sectioned above to assure complete tumor removal.

In cases of large craniopharyngiomas, the surgeon should again remember that the lamina terminalis is not a living tissue, but only a membrane without function. It is safe to go through the lamina terminalis and debulk the tumor between the optic chiasm and carotid arteries to allow a frontolateral approach for removal of remaining tumor.

Frontotemporal (Pterional) Approach

Many neurosurgeons prefer the pterional approach to the suprasellar area for the removal of craniopharyngiomas. The basic technical aspects of this approach can be found in Chapter 2.

Although not offering a directly anterior view of the suprasellar area, the pterional approach is primarily anterior with the added advantage of an anterior temporal approach. The technique of tumor removal by this approach is the same as that described for the subfrontal approach. Every effort is made to stay within the arachnoidal plane with avoidance of unnecessary trauma to perforating vessels or important anatomical structures.

Transcallosal Approach

Craniopharyngiomas that are midline and extend primarily into the third ventricle, causing hydrocephalus, can be approached transcallosally. This is done through a 5-cm-diameter free craniotomy bone flap with its medial border along the midline and its posterior limb just behind the coronal suture line. The exposure is made along the falx with gentle retraction of the frontal lobe laterally and with exposure of the corpus callosum within the interhemispheric fissure. A 3-cm transcallosal incision is made just lateral to the pericallosal arteries, providing entrance into the lateral ventricle at the location of the dilated foramen of Monro.

Craniopharyngioma tumor capsule usually can be easily seen through the dilated foramen of Monro, and the tumor mass can be removed from this vantage point. Care must be exercised to avoid trauma to the fornix and to the hypothalamus as it forms the walls and floor of the third ventricle.

At times, a pterional approach to the suprasellar tumor mass is combined with a transcallosal approach for removal of the intraventricular tumor.

Subtemporal Approach

The subtemporal approach to the base of the brain has been described in detail in Chapter 3.

Craniopharyngiomas that extend laterally from the suprasellar area to underlie the temporal lobe can be removed from a subtemporal approach. If a slightly lower exposure is desired, this may be converted to a subtemporal-transzygomatic approach (see Chapter 10).

Rarely, in cases in which craniopharyngiomas extend into the posterior cranial fossa or along the clivus, a presigmoid approach to this area is needed (see Chapter 13). The presigmoid approach should not be used for removal of calcified craniopharyngiomas with adherence to the carotid arteries and optic nerves.

Successful removal of a craniopharyngioma depends on planning an approach that will offer multiple options for removal.

In the microsurgical era, two general strategies have been used by neurosurgeons for radical removal of large craniopharyngiomas with extension into the suprasellar and third ventricle areas. Some surgeons, such as Yasargil and Konovalov, prefer to combine the pterional approach with the transcallosal approach. Others, such as Samii, Hoffman, and Chaux, have had more successful results with bifrontal exposure, including the translamina terminalis option.

COMMON COMPLICATIONS AFTER SURGERY

1. Fluid, electrolyte, and hormonal imbalance
2. Olfactory nerve damage
3. Optic nerve or optic pathway damage
4. Diabetes insipidus
5. Thalamic and/or hypothalamic infarction caused by disturbance of perforating vessels
6. Subdural hygroma
7. Cerebrospinal fluid fistula

RECOMMENDED READING

Baskin, D.S., Wilson, C.B.: Surgical management of craniopharyngiomas. J. Neurosurg. 65:22–27, 1986.

Laws, E.R., Jr.: Transsphenoidal microsurgery in the management of craniopharyngiomas. J. Neurosurg. 52:661–666, 1980.

Patterson, R.H., Danylevich, A.: Surgical removal of craniopharyngiomas by a transcranial approach through the lamina terminalis and sphenoid sinus. Neurosurgery 7:111–117, 1980.

Samii, M., Draf, W.: Surgery of the Skull Base: An Interdisciplinary Approach. New York: Springer-Verlag, 1989.

Symon, L., Sprich, W.: Radical excision of craniopharyngioma. J. Neurosurg. 62:174–181, 1985.

Walter, G.F., Kleinert, R.: Dysontogenetic brain tumors—proposal for an improved classification. Neuropathol. Appl. Neurobiol. 13:273–287, 1987.

Yasargil, M.G., Curcic, M., Kis, M., et al.: Total removal of craniopharyngiomas: Approaches and long-term results in 144 patients. J. Neurosurg. 73:3–11, 1990.

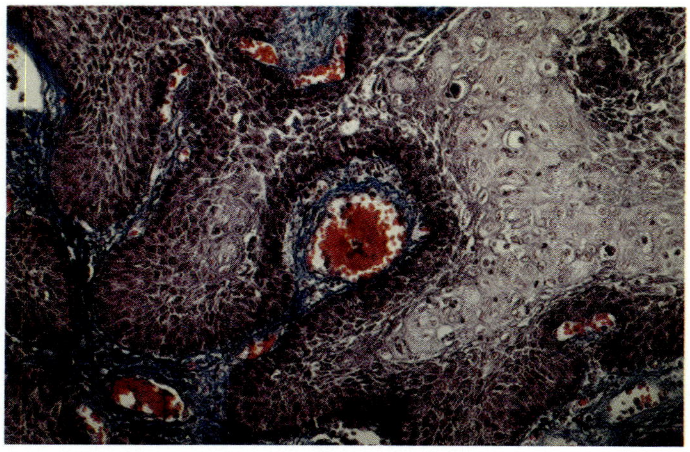

Figure 1. Adamantinomatous pattern of a solid part of a craniopharyngioma. Masson-trichrome, 150×.

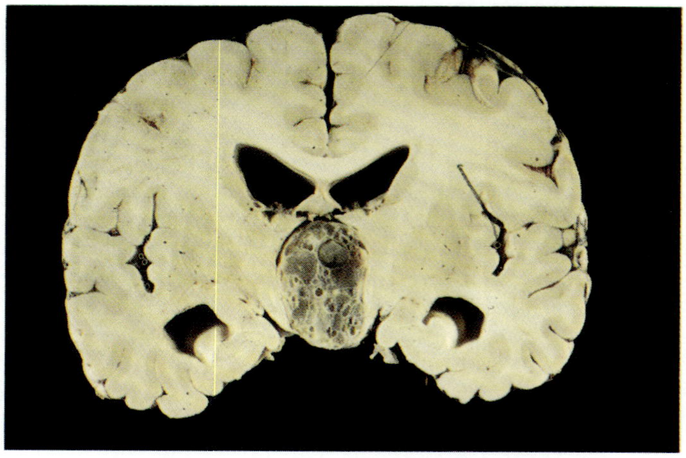

Figure 2. Well-encapsulated cystic craniopharyngioma.

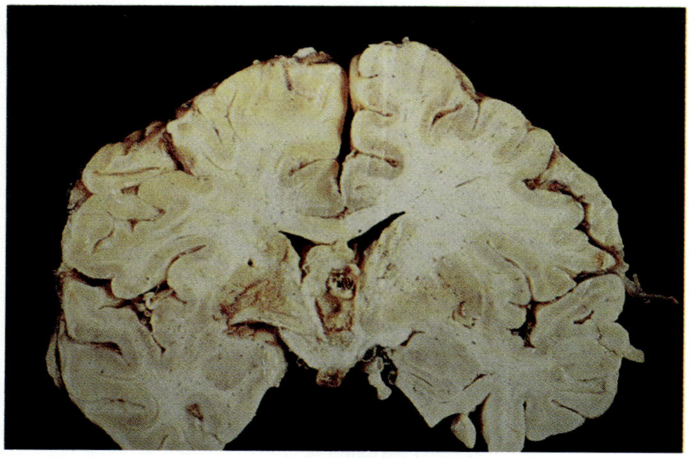

Figure 3. Heavily calcified craniopharyngioma.

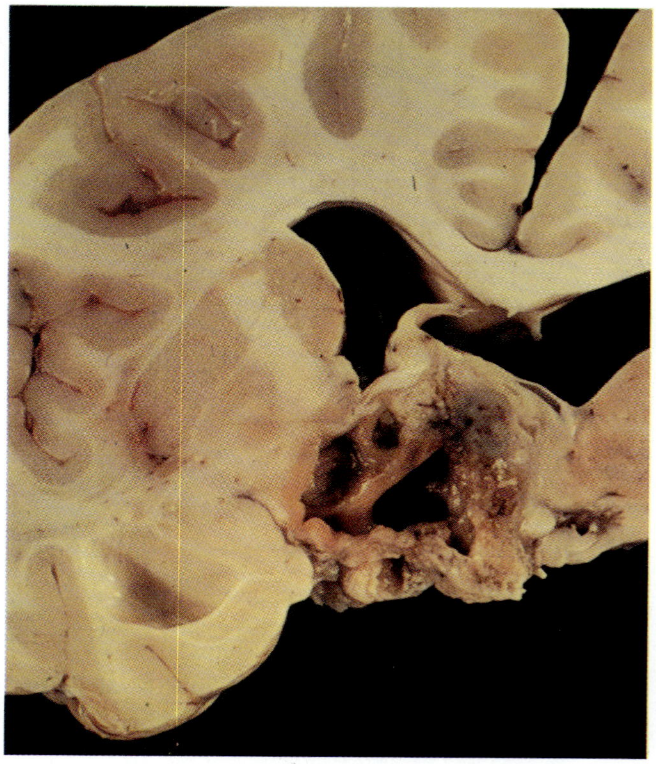

Figure 4. Craniopharyngioma grossly appearing as an infiltrative tumor.

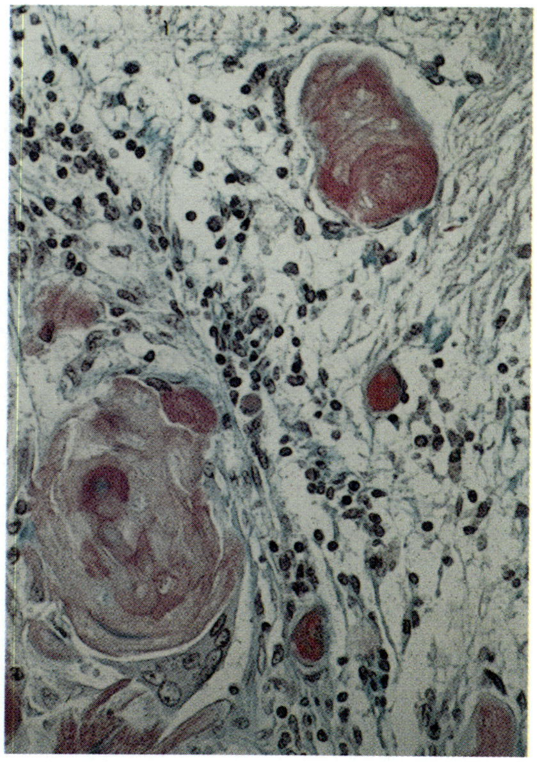

Figure 5. Finger-like interdigitation of craniopharyngioma into adjacent neural tissue. Masson-trichrome, 150×.

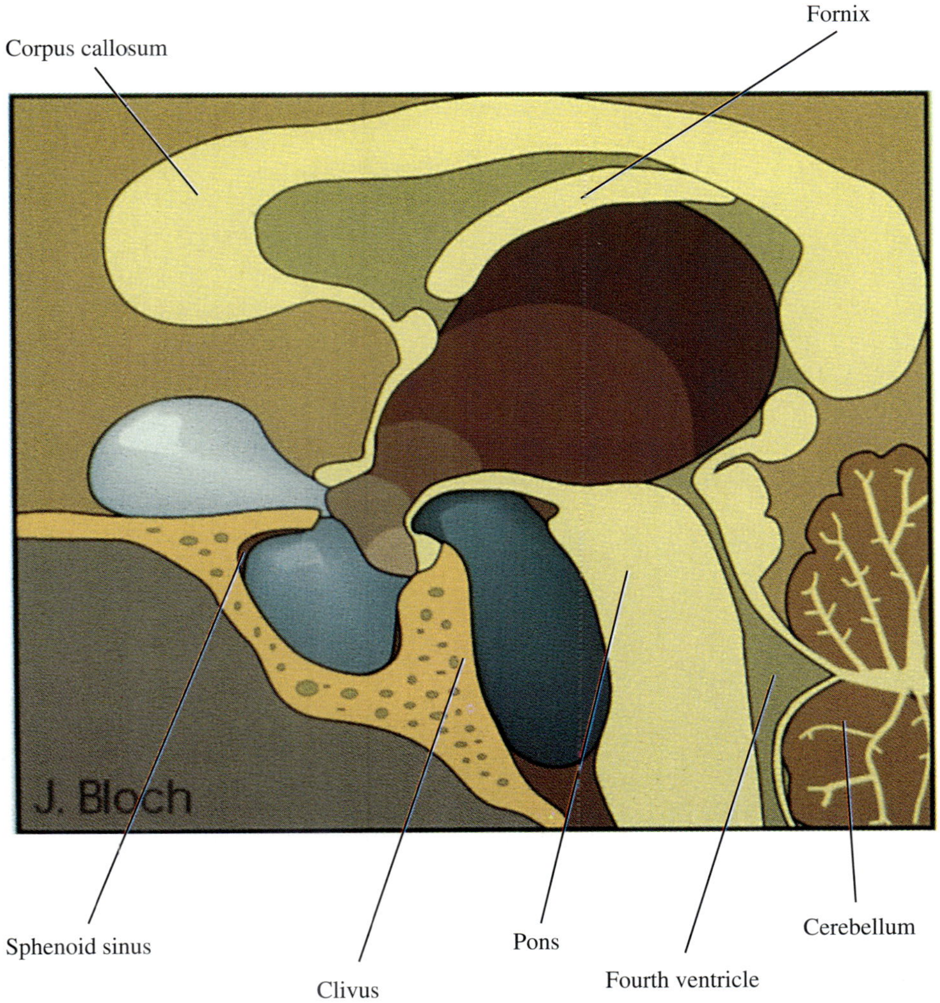

Figure 6. Five grades of craniopharyngioma classification based on vertical extension of tumor mass.

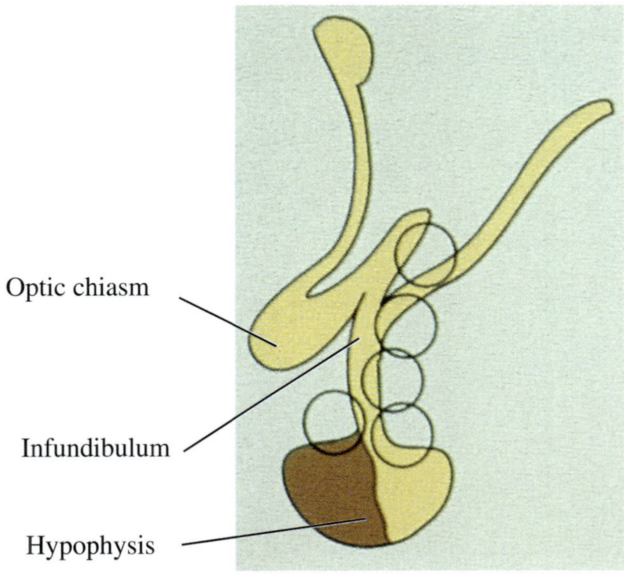

Figure 7. Sites of origin of craniopharyngiomas in relation to infundibular stalk.

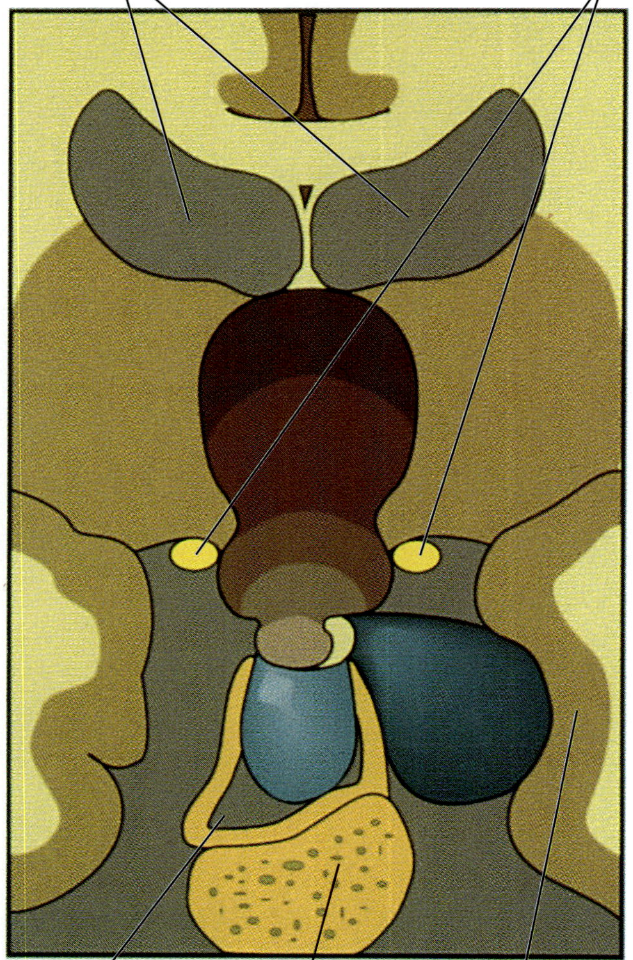

Figure 8. Coronal section showing vertical and horizontal growth patterns of craniopharyngiomas.

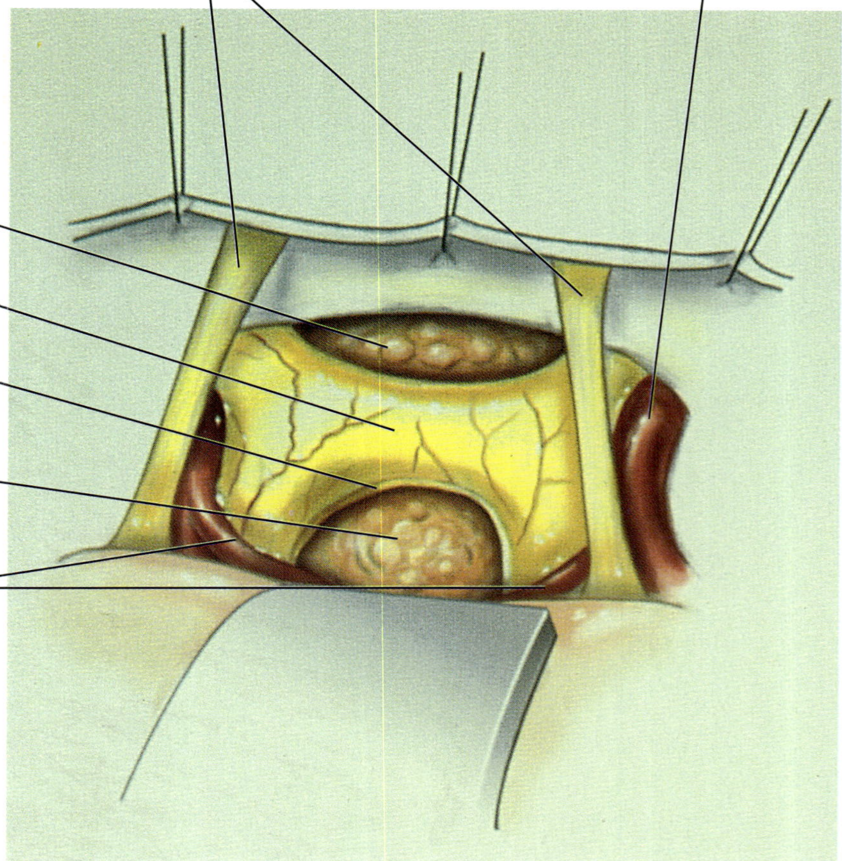

Figure 9. Upward displacement of the optic nerves and chiasm by suprasellar craniopharyngioma.

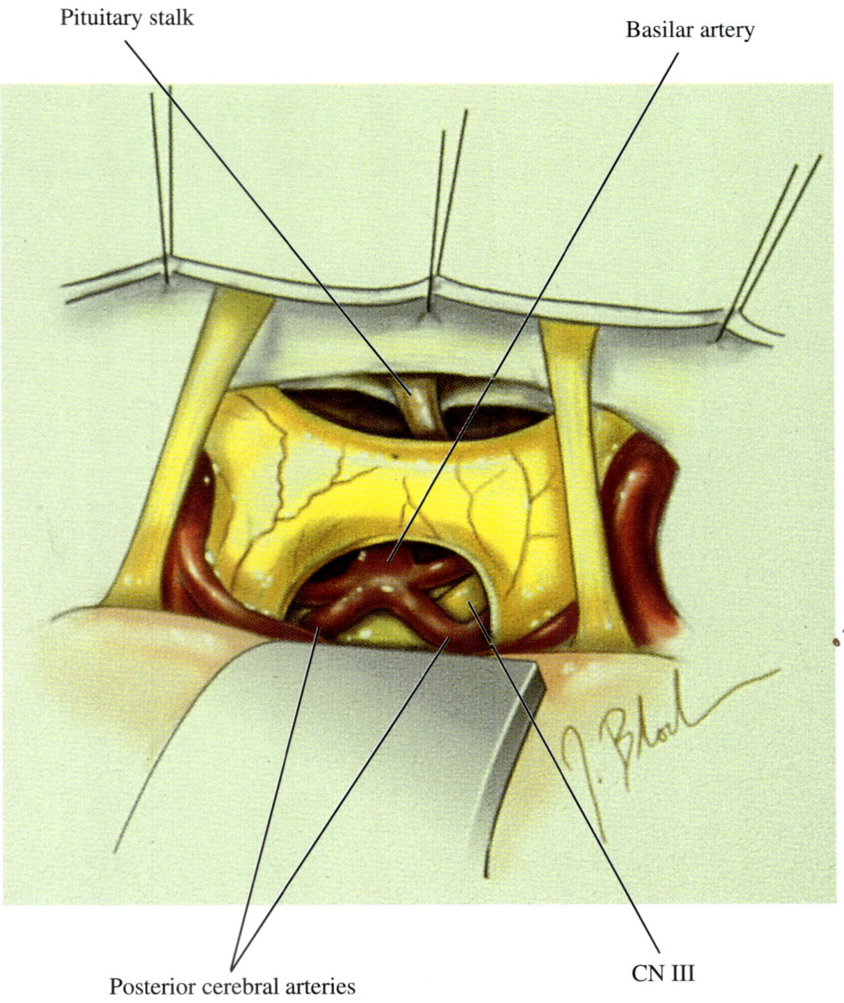

Figure 10. Anatomical relations after removal of suprasellar craniopharyngioma by subfrontal or pterional approach.

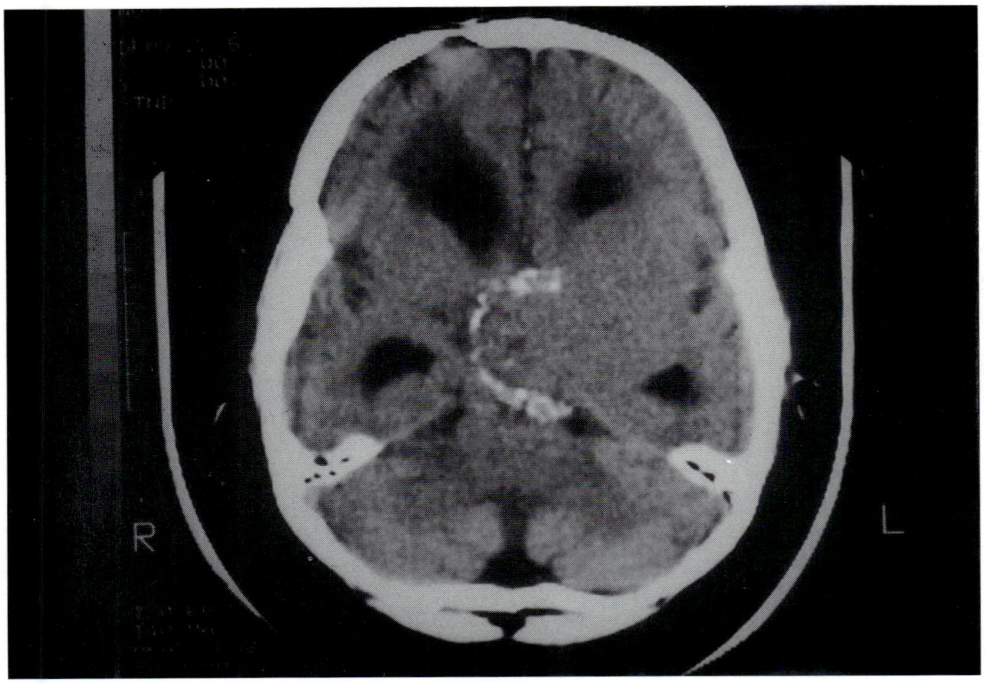

Figure 11. Preoperative CT scan showing a large suprasellar craniopharyngioma with calcification in the capsule and with obliteration of the third ventricle and early hydrocephalus.

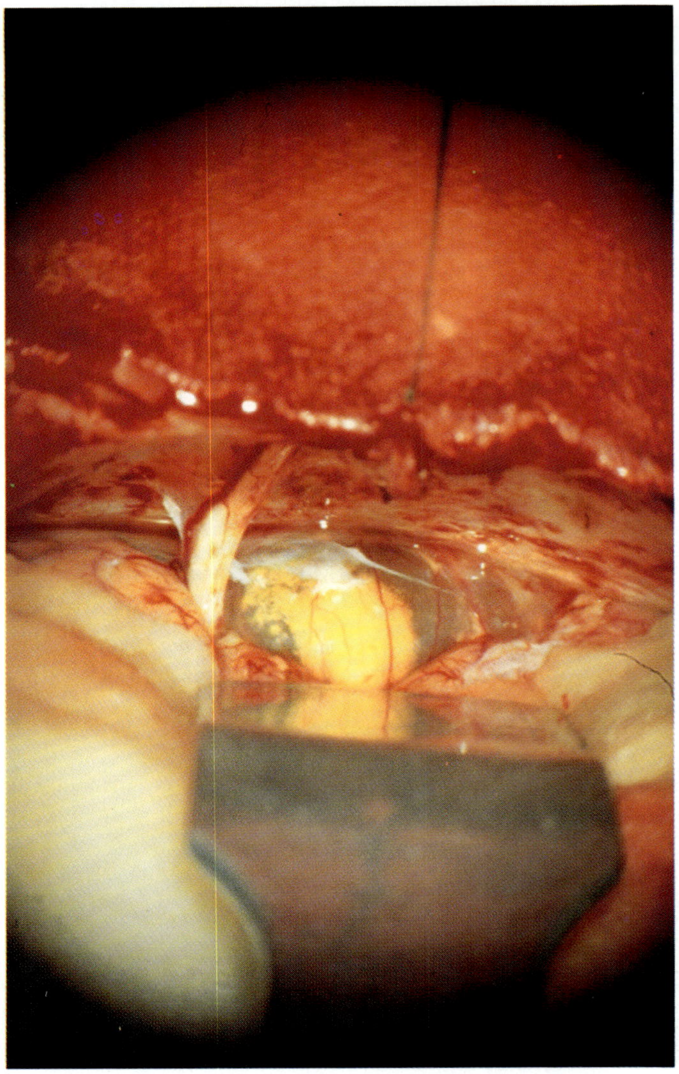

Figure 12. Frontal lobes retracted to expose the optic nerves with the craniopharyngioma visualized in the suprasellar area.

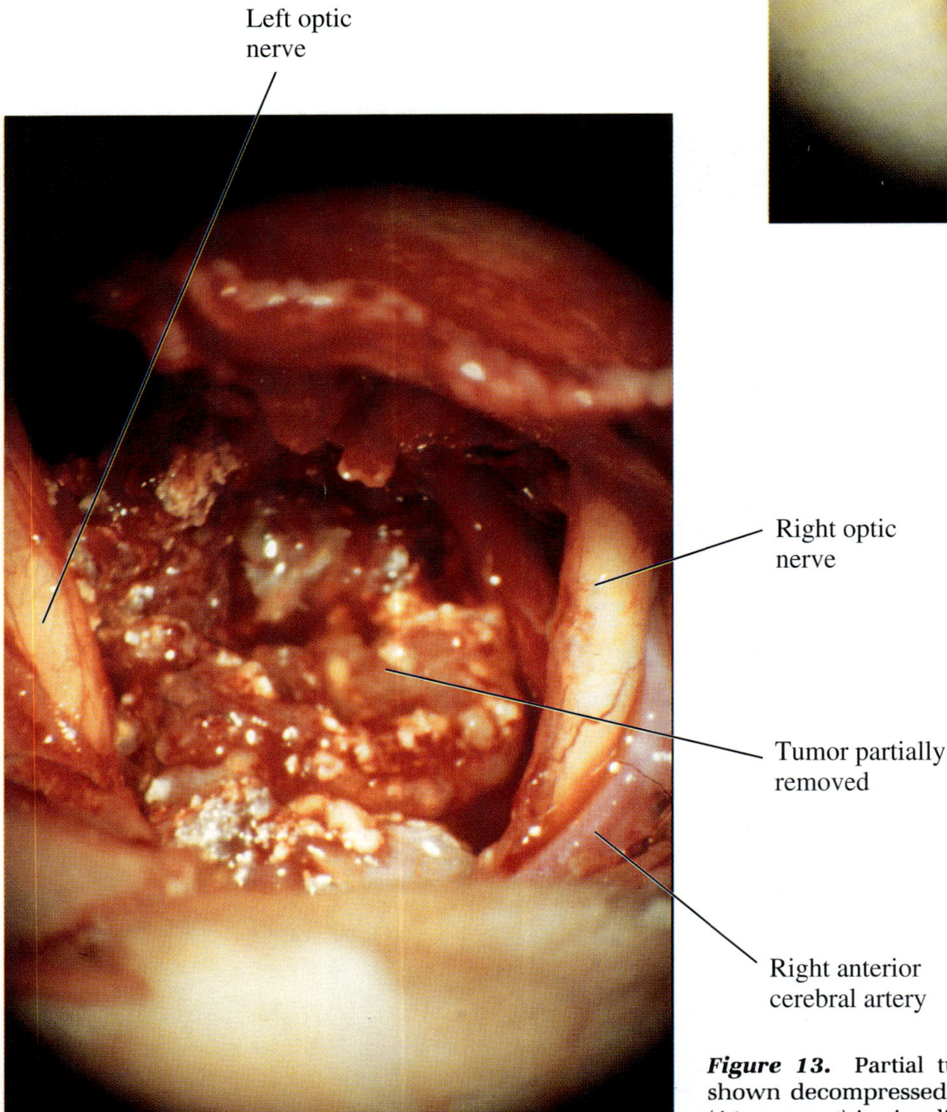

Figure 13. Partial tumor removal. Both optic nerves are shown decompressed and the right anterior cerebral artery (A1 segment) is visualized.

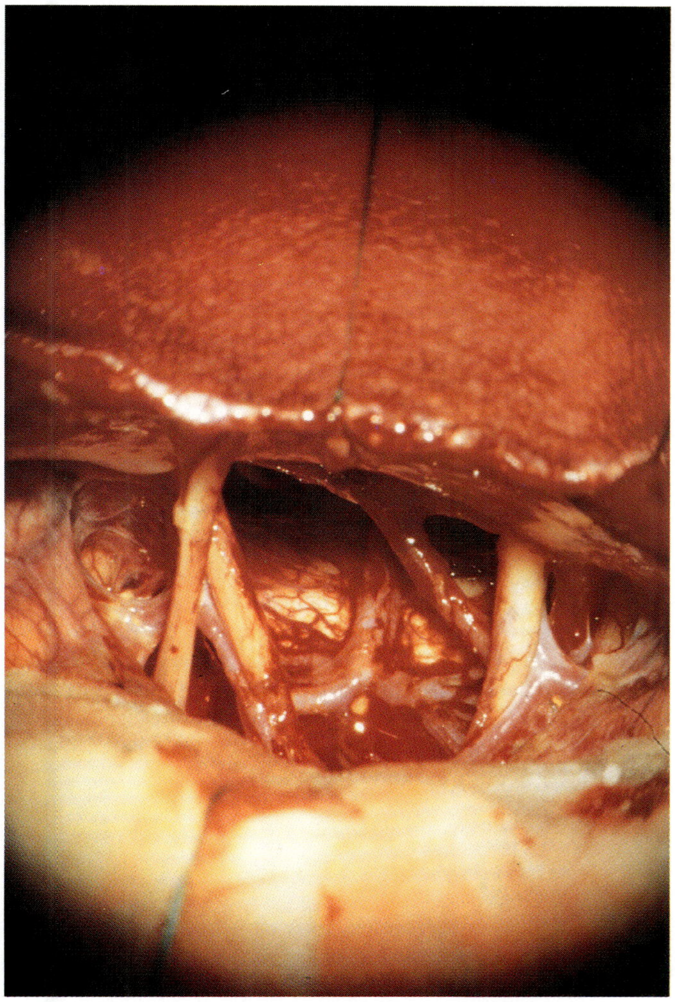

Figure 14. Total tumor removal has been achieved. The optic nerves are shown decompressed. The basilar and vertebral arteries and brain stem are visualized.

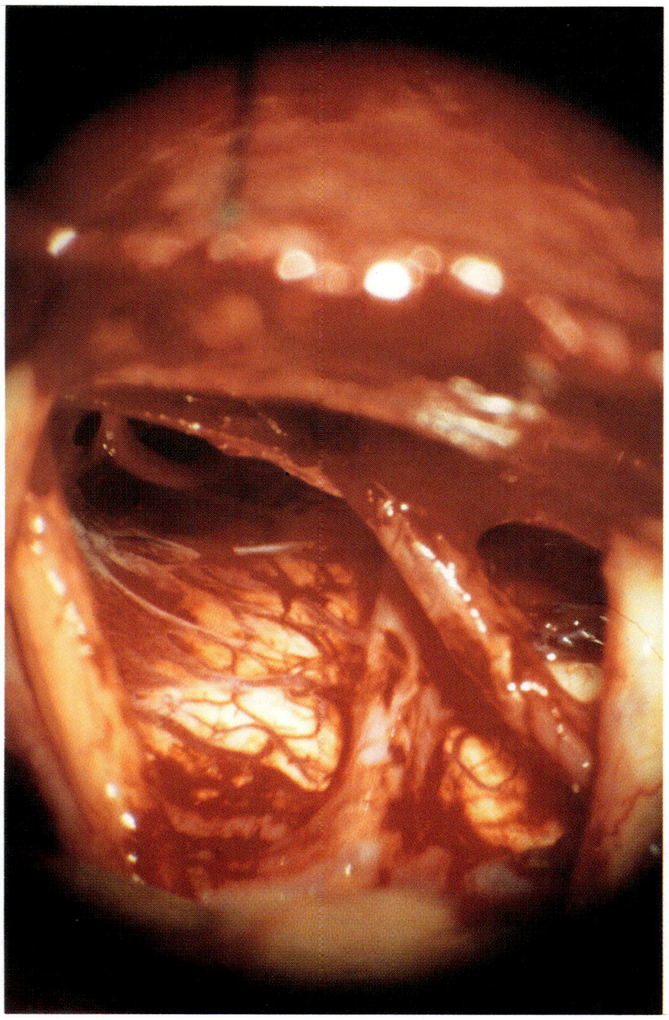

Figure 15. Same operative photograph as shown in Figure 14 but with higher magnification.

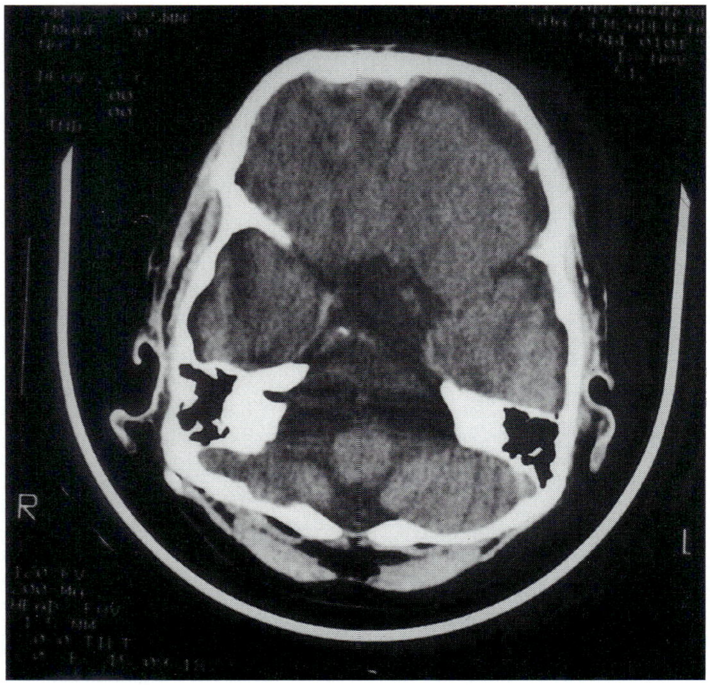

Figure 16. Postoperative CT scan showing total tumor removal.

31 Chordomas, Chondromas, and Chondrosarcomas

Chordomas, chondromas, and chondrosarcomas are tumors that are similar in terms of origin, location, pathological cell type, and behavior. Chordomas arise from remnants of the notochord, the primitive axial organ of the embryo. In contrast, chondromas and chondrosarcomas arise from cartilage. They most commonly are at the skull base and extradural in location (Figure 1). These tumors will recur unless they are totally removed along with involved bone or other structures. They are difficult to approach because of their deep location and involvement of cranial nerves, brain stem, and vital vascular structures, especially in the case of large tumors (Figure 2).

TUMOR CLASSIFICATION

Certain features of each of these tumors are similar, yet distinct classification according to cell type is possible. Chondromas and chordomas are benign but tend to recur locally. In contrast to chondromas and chondrosarcomas, chordomas show a distinct immunostaining with antibodies against cytokeratin (Figure 3). This possibility for a clear differentiation is worthwhile because chondrosarcomas may behave in a malignant manner, although they most commonly belong to the less malignant, low-grade type of chondrosarcoma. However, transformation into a metastasizing high-grade tumor is possible.

INCIDENCE

Chordomas, chondromas, and chondrosarcomas are rare and constitute less than 1 per cent of intracranial tumors. They are twice as common in men as in women and most frequently occur in the fourth through sixth decades of life.

SYMPTOMS

Due to their slow growth, symptoms may be present for several years before a diagnosis is made. On occasion, these tumors are identified in symptom-free patients who undergo brain scans for reasons other than the tumor.

Because of their location in the midline, at the skull base, single or multiple cranial nerve palsies are common presenting signs with these tumors. They frequently cause headache and diplopia or other visual symptoms. With growth into the middle and anterior skull base, they may cause proptosis, visual loss, nasal obstruction, and even epistaxis.

TREATMENT

The primary treatment of these tumors is surgical removal, and the goal of surgery must be total excision. This often is not possible because of their involvement of important structures. Another reason total removal sometimes is not possible is their large size at the time of diagnosis and the limited amount of exposure available for their removal. In cases in which surgical treatment is not possible, chordomas, chondromas, and chondrosarcomas may be treated with radiation therapy. This can offer some palliation, but tumors of this type usually are radioresistant and continue to grow despite radiation therapy. Surgery of these tumors after radiotherapy has been given is with high risk of morbidity and mortality.

SURGICAL ANATOMY

The most common site of origin of these tumors is along the clivus and the petrous portion of the temporal bone. They most commonly are extradural, but with time, they may invade the dura and then grow intradurally as well as extradurally. Their location leads to involvement of the cranial nerves, brain stem, cavernous sinus, and vascular network at the skull base. They may extend to the suprasellar area intracranially and may invade the soft tissues of the neck and pharynx extracranially.

Chordomas appear as multilobulated, grayish, gelatinous semitranslucent tumors. They have well-demarcated boundaries except in those areas in which the tumor involves bone, where they may appear invasive. An arachnoid plane usually is maintained between tumor and neurovascular structures, and it is possible to separate tumor from them with careful, meticulous dissection.

PREOPERATIVE CONSIDERATIONS

If gross total excision of chordomas, chondromas, and chondrosarcomas is to be achieved, careful preoperative planning is essential. Second operations are much less successful because postoperative scar tissue obliterates margins between tumor and normal tissues.

Most of these tumors can be approached extradurally. In case of dural invasion, intradural tumor resection can follow. To properly plan the most optimal approach, the workup must include high-resolution computed tomographic scans as well as magnetic resonance imaging (MRI) and MRI angiography. Contrast arteriography is indicated in those cases in which MRI angiography does not offer detailed enough information or when major vessel involvement by tumor is suspected.

SURGICAL APPROACH OPTIONS

Important in tumor removal is the option to approach the pathology in its entire extent. Sometimes this requires a combination of operative approaches.

The subfrontal approach offers access to the suprasellar area (see Chapter 1). For tumors that are midline and located in the sphenoid and ethmoid sinuses or along the clivus, the transfrontal basal approach can be used (see Chapter 15).

One of the simplest and most successful approaches for clivus chordomas with intracranial and extracranial extensions is the modification of the transethmoidal-transsphenoidal approach (see Chapter 19).

In Figure 4, an MRI scan shows a clivus chordoma with dorsal displacement of the pons. This tumor was approached transethmoidally, and the operative exposure of the tumor is shown in Figure 5. The operative photograph shown in Figure 6 demonstrates complete tumor removal. The decompressed brain stem, the left abducent nerve, and a portion of the basilar artery are seen. The dural reconstruction using lyophilized dura, sealed with fibrin glue, is shown in Figure 7. The postoperative MRI scan demonstrates complete removal of the chordoma (Figure 8).

The pterional and subtemporal approaches offer more lateral access to the middle fossa and the cavernous sinus (see Chapters 2 and 3).

The subtemporal-transzygomatic transtentorial approach offers a more basal, lateral approach to the cavernous sinus and the petroclival area with control of the petrous portion of the internal carotid artery (see Chapter 10).

The temporal and infratemporal approaches afford a lower, more extensive exposure of the petrous bone, clivus, and extradural tissues of the deep medial skull base (see Chapter 11).

The presigmoid extended retrolabyrinthine approach offers access to the extradural and intradural petroclival area (see Chapter 13).

The transoral approach to the clivus may be used for removal of chordomas that are extradural along the clivus (see Chapter 20). This approach does not afford access to tumor that may be extending laterally along the clivus or petroclival area.

The sublabial transnasal transmaxillary approach (modified midface degloving) is detailed in Chapter 18. This approach is useful in the removal of larger clival chordomas.

SPECIAL OPERATIVE CONSIDERATIONS

Every effort is made to achieve total tumor removal. Excision of involved dura followed by dural grafting with pericranium or temporalis muscle fascia or fascia lata is indicated. It is important to achieve a watertight dural closure followed by a skull base reconstruction of temporalis muscle and fascia as a vascularized flap.

These tumors may invade adjacent bone. Drilling away such bone is continued to a point where uninvolved bone can be identified under the microscope.

When possible, chordomas should be removed through an extradural approach to maintain the dural barrier, thus avoiding intracranial growth of recurrent tumor. In those cases in which chordomas have already extended through the dura, a primarily intradural approach may be necessary to afford the exposure needed to dissect tumor free from important neural and vascular structures.

RADIATION THERAPY

Even though this group of tumors is considered to be radioresistant, sometimes radiation therapy is used for treatment of tumor tissue that cannot be surgically removed. The response to this is variable.

COMPLICATIONS

1. Injury to neural and/or vascular structures
2. Cerebrospinal fluid leak
3. Meningitis

RECOMMENDED READING

Black, K.L.: Chordomas of the clival region. Contemp. Neurosurg. 12, 1990.

Brandis, A., Tatagiba, M., Samii, M., Ostertag, H.: Tumors and tumor-like lesions of the osseous skull base: An experience of 10 years. J Cancer Res. Clin. Oncol. 116(Suppl):234, 1990.

Kevton, J.F., Brackmann, D.E., Glasscock, M.E., et al.: Chondrosarcoma of the skull base. Otolaryngol. Head, Neck Surg. 94:23–32, 1986.

Pardo-Mindan, F.J., Guillen, F.J., Villas, C., Vasquez, J.J.: A comparative ultrastructural study of chondrosarcoma, chondroid sarcoma and chordoma. Cancer 47:2611–2619, 1981.

Raffel, C., Wright, D.C., Gutin, P.H., Wilson, C.B.: Cranial chordomas: Clinical presentation and results of operative and radiation therapy in twenty-six patients. Neurosurgery 17:703–710, 1985.

Samii, M., Draf, W.: Surgery of the skull base: An Interdisciplinary Approach. New York: Springer-Verlag, 1989.

Sekhar, L.N., Janecka, I.P., Jones, N.F.: Subtemporal-infratemporal and basal subfrontal approach to extensive cranial base tumors. Acta Neurochir. (Wien) 92:83–92, 1988.

Sen, C.N., Sekhar, L.N., Schramm, V.L., Janecka, I.P.: Chordoma and chondrosarcoma of the cranial base: An 8-year experience. Neurosurgery 25:931–941, 1989.

Stapleton, S.R., Wilkins, P.R., Archer, D.J., Uttley, D.: Chondrosarcoma of the skull base: A series of eight cases. Neurosurgery 32:348–356, 1993.

Volpe, R., Mazubraud, A.: A clinicopathologic review of 25 cases of chordoma. Am. J. Surg. Pathol. 7:161–170, 1983.

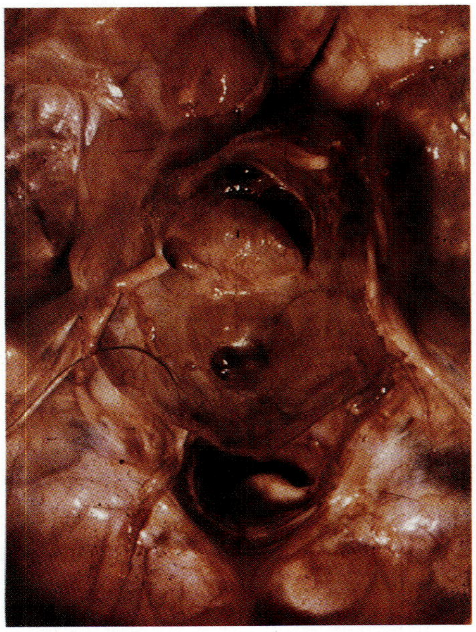

Figure 1. Extradural chordoma of the clivus narrowing the foramen magnum.

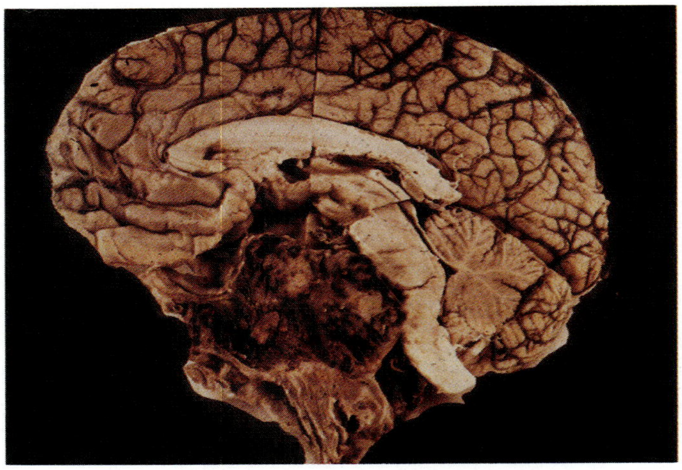

Figure 2. Large chordoma compressing central brain structures.

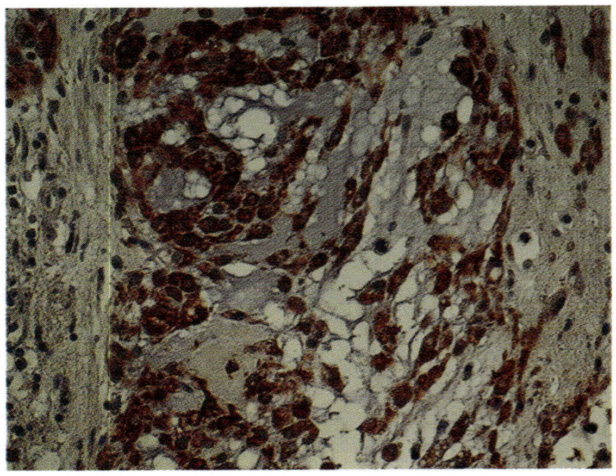

Figure 3. Strong positivity of chordoma cells for cytokeratin. PAP-pancytokeratin, 150×.

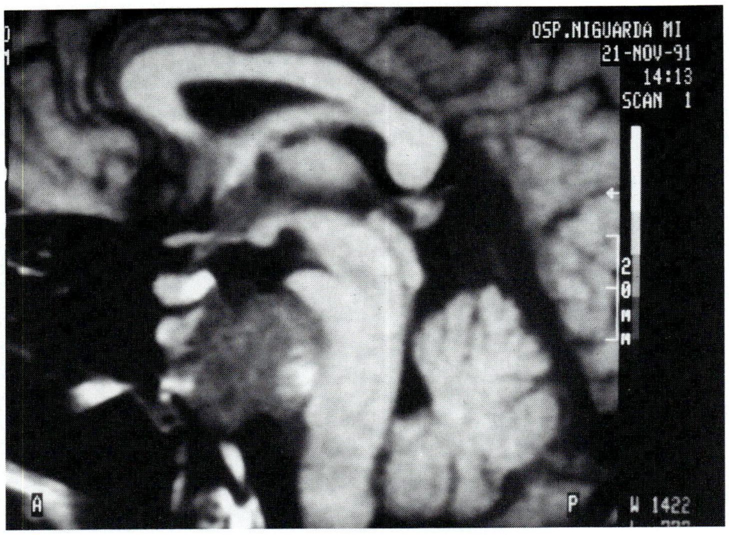

Figure 4. MRI scan showing clivus chordoma with dorsal displacement of pons.

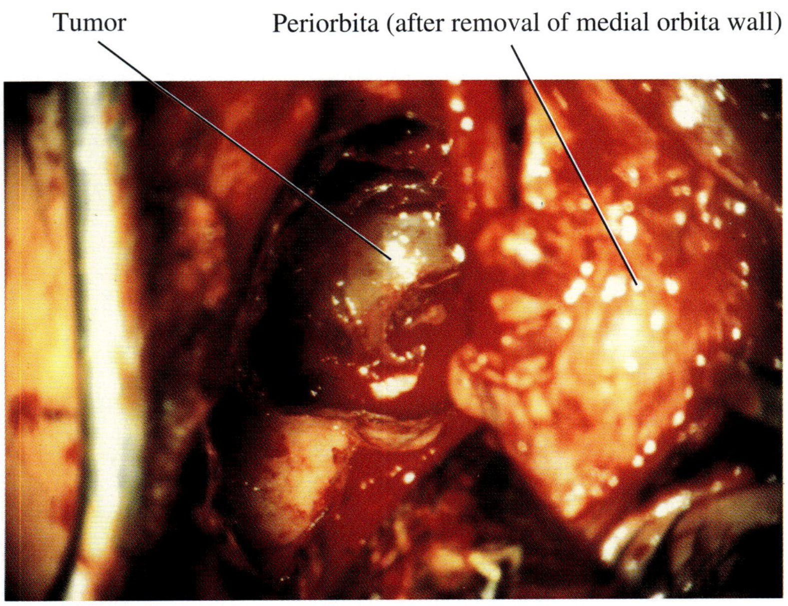

Figure 5. Transethmoidal approach demonstrating the tumor exposure.

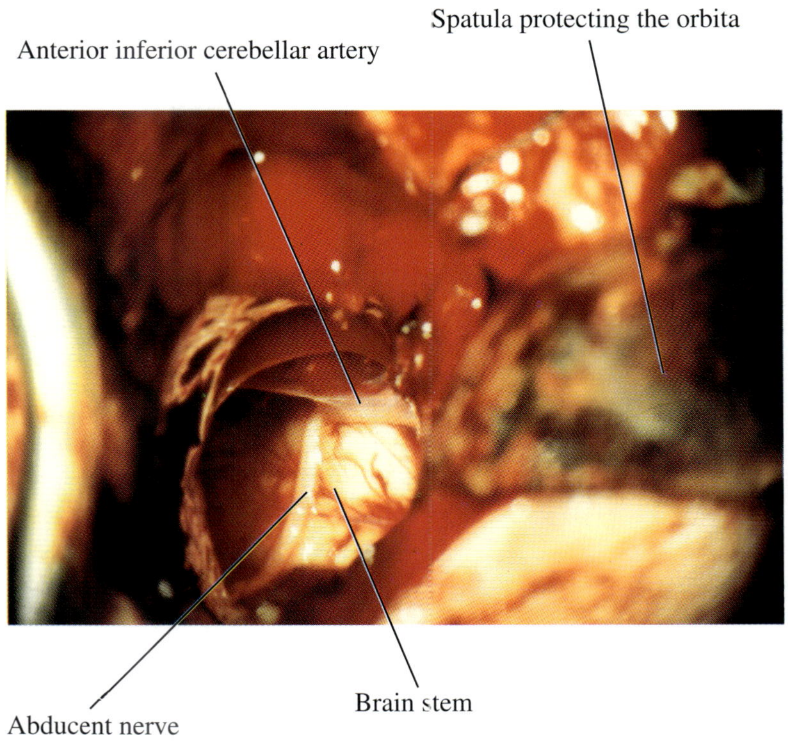

Figure 6. Complete tumor removal. The decompressed brain stem, left abducent nerve, and part of the basilar artery are visible.

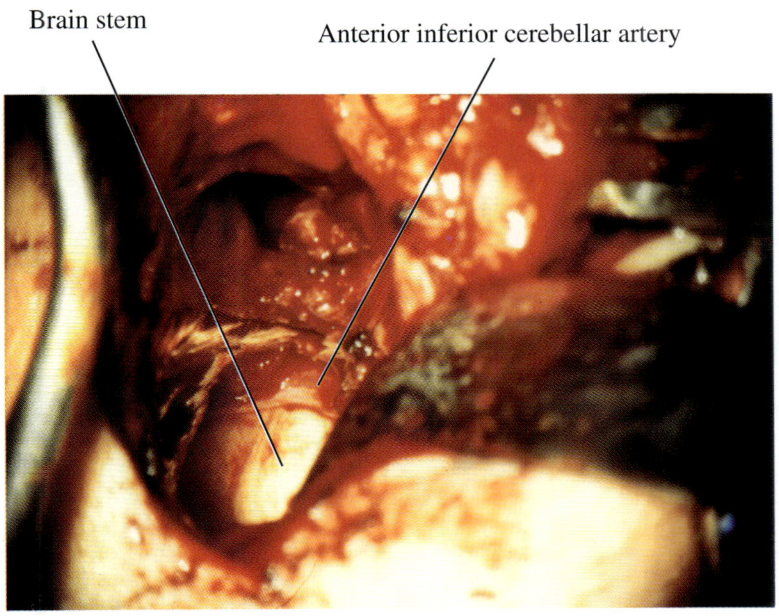

Figure 7. Dural reconstruction at the cranial base with lyophilized dura, sealed with fibrin glue.

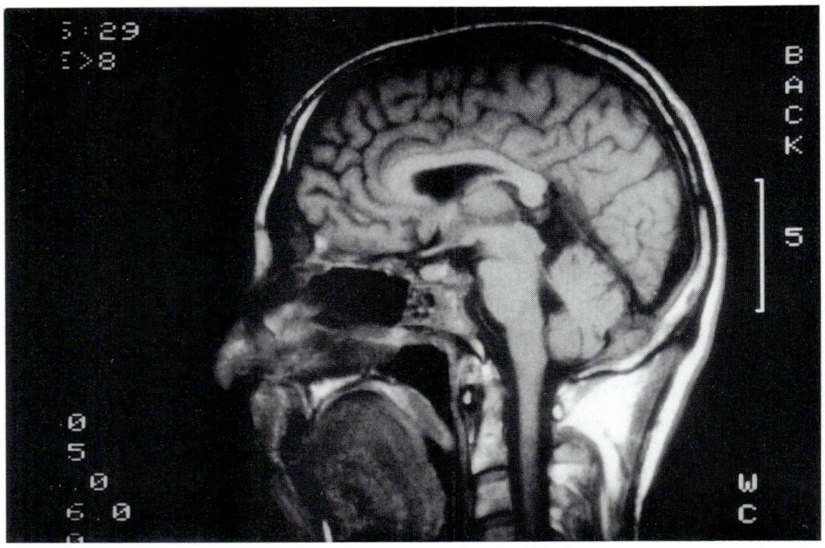

Figure 8. Postoperative MRI scan demonstrating complete tumor removal.

32 Chemodectomas (Paraganglioma)

Glomus jugulare and glomus tympanicum tumors (chemodectomas or paragangliomas) are not common. They tend to be slow growing and most often are seen in elderly people. Even though benign in more than 90 per cent of cases, they present a formidable challenge to the skull base surgeon because of their location, tendency to invade adjacent bone, and high vascularity. Major vessels may be totally surrounded by the tumor. In addition to involvement of cranial nerves, brain stem, and major vessels, they often extend into the various cisterns and fissures of the posterior fossa skull base, making surgical removal difficult.

Chemodectomas arise from nonchromaffin paraganglia tissue of the chemoreceptor system (Figures 1 and 2). This extra-adrenal paraganglia tissue is widely distributed in the head, neck, and mediastinal regions of the body. This tissue is of neural crest embryologic origin and considered part of the autonomic parasympathetic nervous system.

Paraganglia tissue in the temporal bone, termed glomus bodies, is distributed along Jacobson's and Arnold's nerves. In about 50 per cent of temporal bone studies, glomus bodies have been found in the adventitia of the jugular bulb. Other sites of predilection include the mucosa of the cochlear promontory, the tympanic canaliculus, and the vertical portion of the facial canal.

The site of origin of chemodectomas may be along cranial nerve IX or X or from cells in the adventitia of the jugular bulb. These tumors are referred to as glomus jugularae tumors, and they often grow to large size before causing enough symptoms to lead to clinical diagnosis. Common presenting symptoms include recurrent laryngeal nerve palsy, accessory nerve palsy, hypoglossal nerve palsy, headache, and, eventually, cerebellar and other cerebellopontine angle tumor signs. With erosion through the cranial base, these tumors may present as retropharyngeal masses. They may also have intracranial extension to lie intradurally as well as extradurally.

Glomus tumors that arise from glomus bodies in the middle ear are referred to as glomus tympanicum tumors. Paragangliomas constitute the most common neoplasm of the middle ear and are second only to acoustic neurinomas in their incidence of temporal bone involvement. By the time a patient presents with a paraganglioma in this area, it often is difficult to assess the region of origin.

Fisch has offered a classification of glomus tumors based on location and size. Glomus tympanicum tumors are referred to as type A when they are confined to the middle ear. With extension into the mastoid, they are classified as type B. With erosion through the infralabyrinthine bone structure into the petrous apex, tumors are called type C, and with intracranial extension, type D.

Glasscock and Jackson have classified glomus tumors as shown in Table 1.

ANATOMICAL CONSIDERATIONS

Glomus jugulare tumors may grow predominantly in one of several directions. Their growth determines their clinical presentation. They may extend into the cerebellopontine angle. They may grow more superiorly and laterally to involve the tympanic cavity, or their growth may be posteriorly to involve cranial nerves IX through XII.

The major arterial supply to glomus jugulare tumors is through the ascending pharyngeal artery. Additional blood supply from adjacent vessels contributes to the highly vascular nature of these tumors, making surgical removal difficult and challenging.

DIAGNOSTIC CONSIDERATIONS

High-resolution computed tomography (CT), coupled with magnetic resonance imaging (MRI) and cerebral angiography with selective catheterization of internal and external carotid arteries and vertebral arteries bilaterally, represents the minimum in preoperative evaluation of these tumors. CT can show tumor size, extent of growth, and degree of bone erosion. It is important to search for other chemodectomas because these tumors often are multicentric.

All glomus jugulare tumors show some enhancement with gadolinium. Although the extent of bone erosion may be best imaged with thin-cut CT images, it is with enhanced MRI that the degree of intracranial extension of these tumors can best be seen.

OPERATIVE APPROACHES

The operative approach of choice is dictated by the size and location of the tumor mass. The lateral approach to the middle fossa skull base lends itself well to removal of glomus jugulare tumors (see Chapter 11). Chemodectomas are highly vascular, and preoperative embolization may be beneficial in controlling bleeding during surgery.

For glomus tympanicum tumors that can be

TABLE 1. GLASSCOCK-JACKSON CLASSIFICATION OF GLOMUS TUMORS

Glomus tympanicum
I. Small mass limited to promontory
II. Tumor completely filling middle ear space
III. Tumor filling middle ear and extending into the mastoid
IV. Tumor filling middle ear, extending into the mastoid or through tympanic membrane to fill the external auditory canal; may extend anterior to carotid glomus jugulare
Glomus jugulare
I. Small tumor involving jugular bulb, middle ear, and mastoid
II. Tumor extending under internal auditory canal; may have intracranial canal extension (ICE)
III. Tumor extending into petrous apex; may have ICE
IV. Tumor extending beyond petrous apex into clivus or infratemporal fossa; may have ICE

classified as type A or B, a more limited otological approach is appropriate.

An example of the bony involvement of the jugular foramen and petrous bone in a case of chemodectoma is shown in the CT scan in Figure 3. Figure 4 shows three MRI scans demonstrating the entire extent of this glomus jugulare tumor and its relation to the brain stem in the cerebellopontine angle.

In Figure 5, the tumor blush and displacement of the carotid artery can be seen in the lateral projection of a carotid arteriogram. After preoperative embolization (Figure 6), much of the tumor blush has disappeared.

OPERATIVE PROCEDURE

The patient position and planned operative incision for removal of this chemodectoma at the jugular foramen is shown in Figure 7. After subcutaneous dissection, the mastoid tip is exposed as a point of reference. Figure 8 shows the parotid gland and sternocleidomastoid muscle dissected and the digastric muscle transected and reflected downward.

In Figure 9, the lateral suboccipital craniectomy is shown completed with the sigmoid sinus exposed and the facial nerve dissected at the stylomastoid foramen. In Figure 10, the sigmoid sinus is shown ligated and transected. Tumor can be seen within the sigmoid sinus, as is characteristic with glomus jugulare tumors.

In Figure 11, the tumor has been partially debulked and dissected from the carotid artery. The jugular vein is open with tumor exposed within. Figure 12 shows complete tumor removal accomplished, and in Figure 13, the dural defect of the posterior fossa has been reconstructed using lyophilized dura.

The postoperative CT scans in Figure 14 show complete removal of tumor with the resulting bony defect.

RADIATION THERAPY

Because of the high vascularity and slow growth of chemodectomas and the difficulties encountered in attempts to remove them surgically, radiation therapy has been advocated by some authors, especially in the case of massive tumors. Because of advances in diagnostic imaging, embolization, and surgical management, few patients are now treated primarily with radiation therapy. Favorable results have been reported in some studies with radiation therapy alone or with radiation therapy after partial operative tumor excision.

Therapeutic irradiation of paragangliomas of the temporal bone results in a number of histopathological effects. The neoplastic chief cells show a minimal reaction to radiation because they remain quite viable even though their nuclei show atypia. The surrounding stroma reacts to radiation by replacement of the reticulum with dense connective tissue. Vascular changes include myxoid degeneration of vessel walls, intimal proliferation, thrombosis, and, occasionally, revascularization. Control of some tumors by radiation has been hypothesized to occur secondary to the vascular effects of this therapy.

RECOMMENDED READING

Fisch, U.: Infratemporal fossa approach for glomus tumors of the temporal bone. Ann. Otol. Rhinol. Laryngol. 91:474–479, 1982.

Fisch, U., Fagan, P., Valvanis, A.: The infratemporal fossa approach for the lateral skull base. Otolaryngol. Clin. North Am. 17:413–552, 1984.

Jackson, C.G., Glasscock, M.E., Harris, P.F.: Glomus tumors: Diagnosis, classification and management of large lesions. Arch. Otolaryngol. 108:401–410, 1982.

Phelps, P.D., Cheesman, A.D.: Imaging jugulotympanic glomus tumors. Arch. Otolaryngol. Head Neck Surg. 116:940–945, 1990.

Pryzant, R.M., Chou, J.L., Easley, J.D.: Twenty year experience with radiation therapy for temporal bone chemodectomas. Int. J. Radiat. Oncol. Biol. Phys. 17:1303–1307, 1989.

Verniers, D.A., Keus, R.B., Schouwenburg, P.F., Bartelink, H.: Radiation therapy, an important mode of treatment for head and neck chemodectomas. Eur. J. Cancer 28A:1028–1033, 1992.

Wang, M.L., Hussey, D.H., Doornbos, J.F., et al.: Chemodectoma of the temporal bone: A comparison of surgical and radiotherapeutic results. Int. J. Radiat. Oncol. Biol. Phys. 14:643–648, 1988.

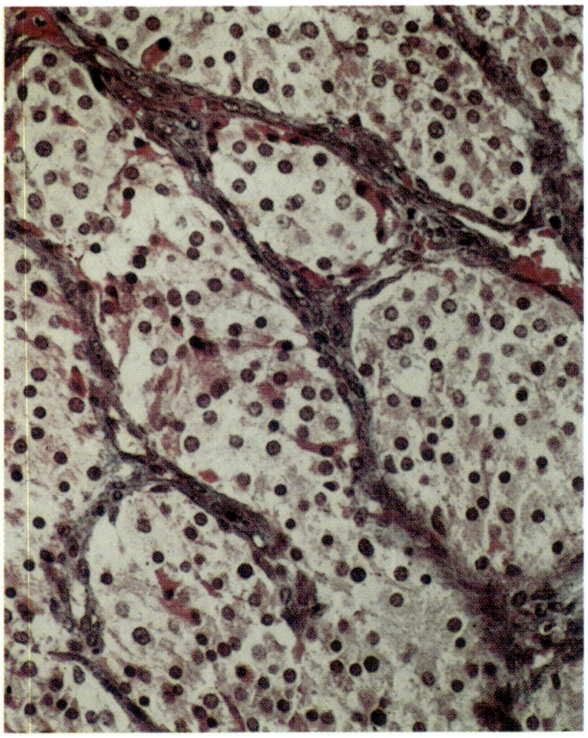

Figure 1. Lobular pattern ("Zellballen" configuration) of chemodectoma. Masson-trichrome, 150×.

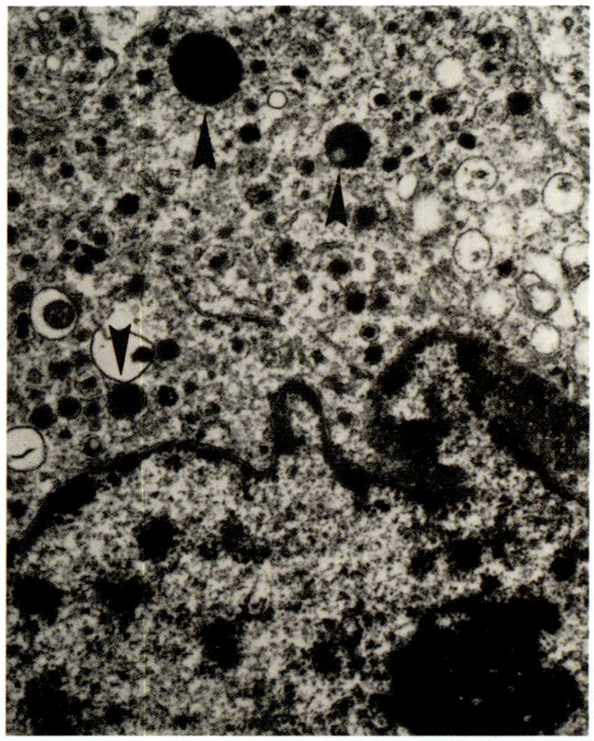

Figure 2. Electron microscopic demonstration of transmitter granules *(arrowheads)* in a chemodectoma cell. 20,000×.

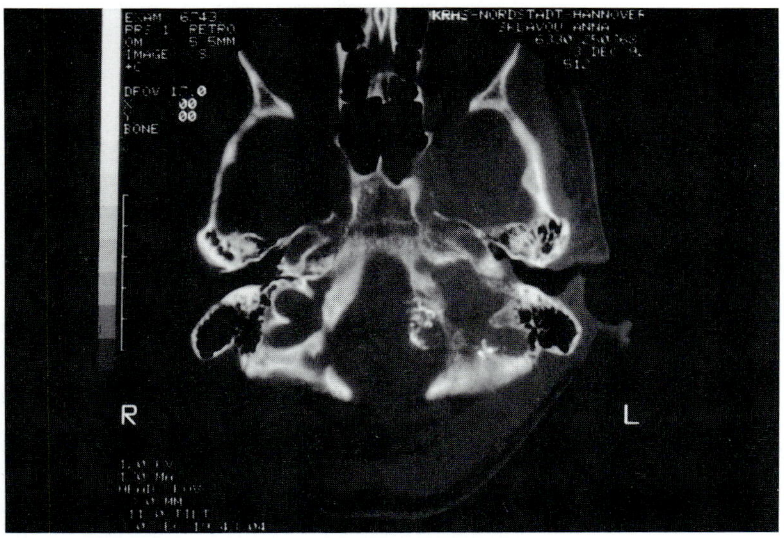

Figure 3. CT scan demonstrating bony involvement of jugular foramen and petrous bone.

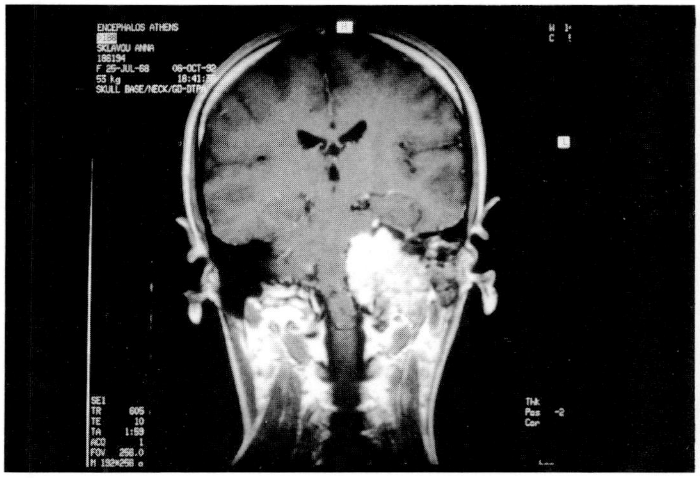

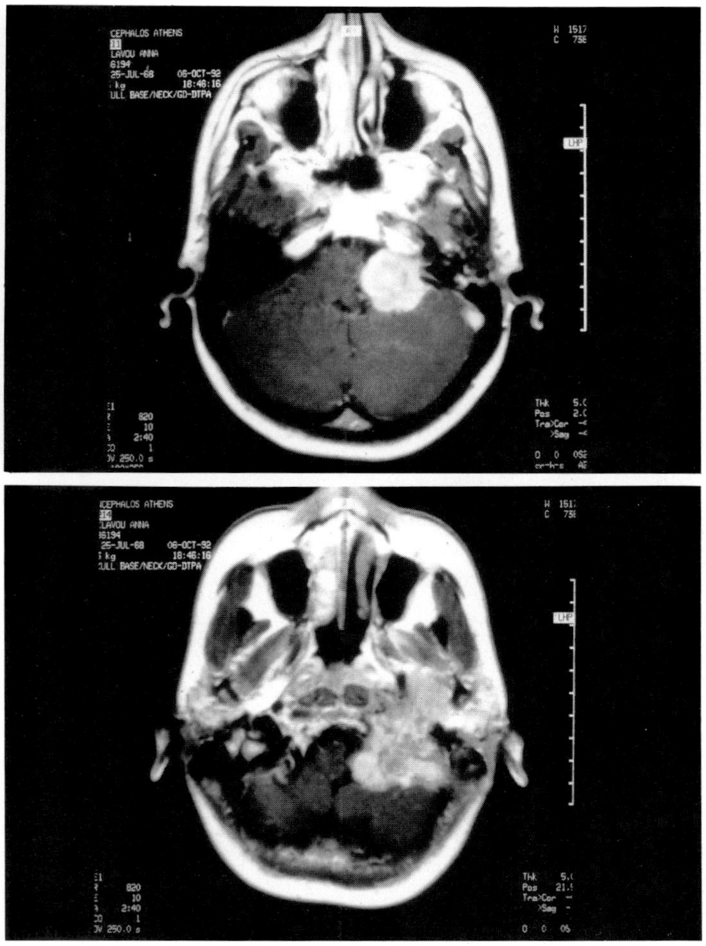

Figure 4. MRI scan images showing the entire extent of glomus jugulare tumor and its relation to the brain stem in the cerebellopontine angle.

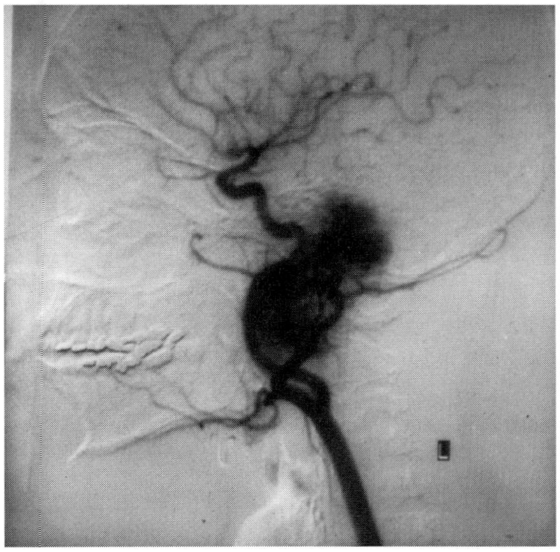

Figure 5. Carotid angiography showing tumor blush and displacement of the carotid artery.

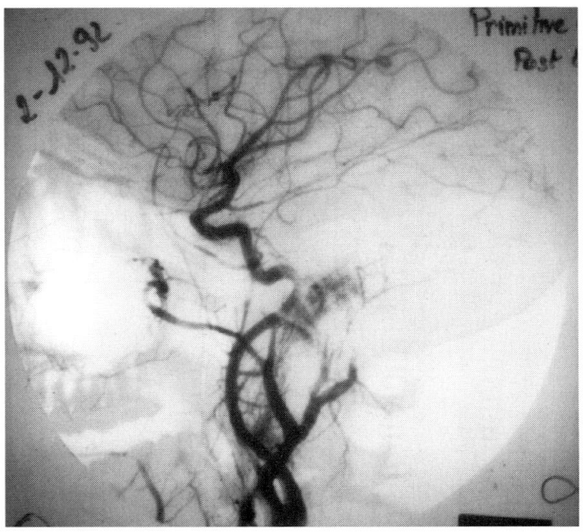

Figure 6. Carotid angiography after preoperative embolization of tumor.

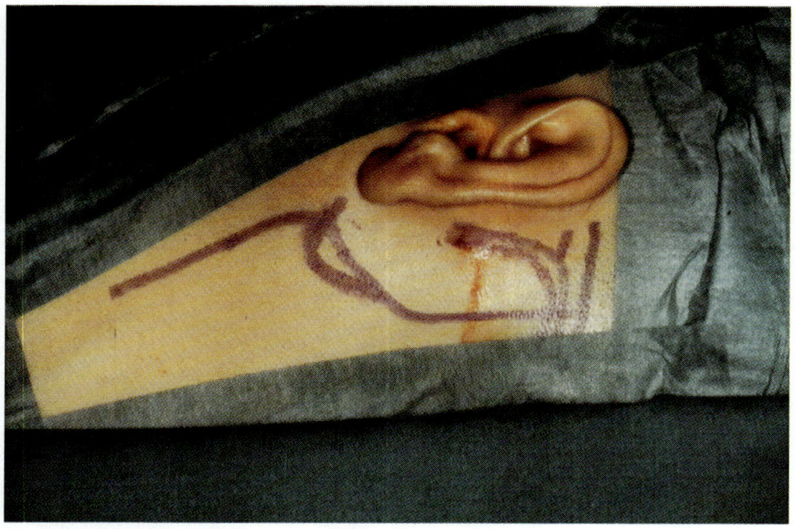

Figure 7. Outline of planned skin incision.

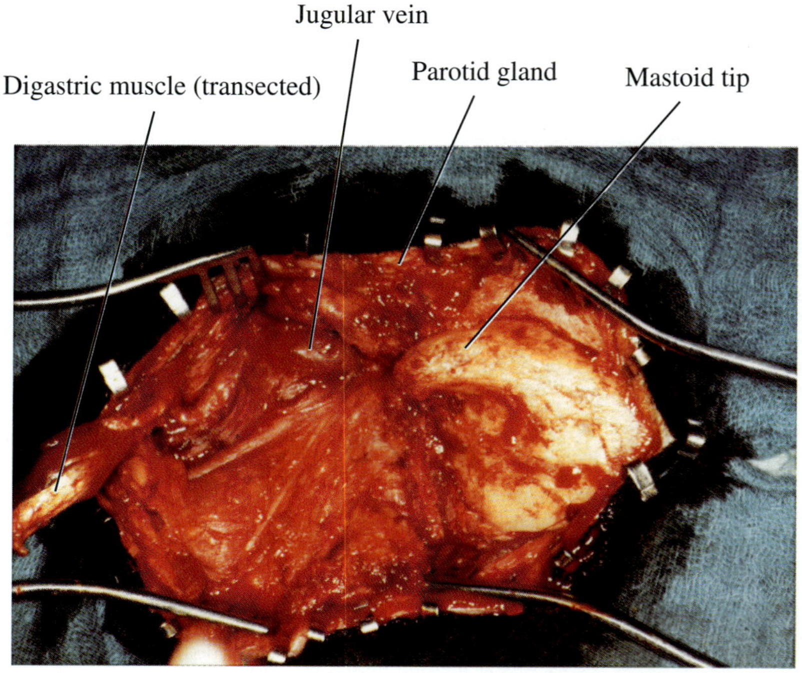

Figure 8. Mastoid tip exposed with parotid gland and sternocleidomastoid muscle dissected. Digastric muscle shown transected at the skull base and reflected downward.

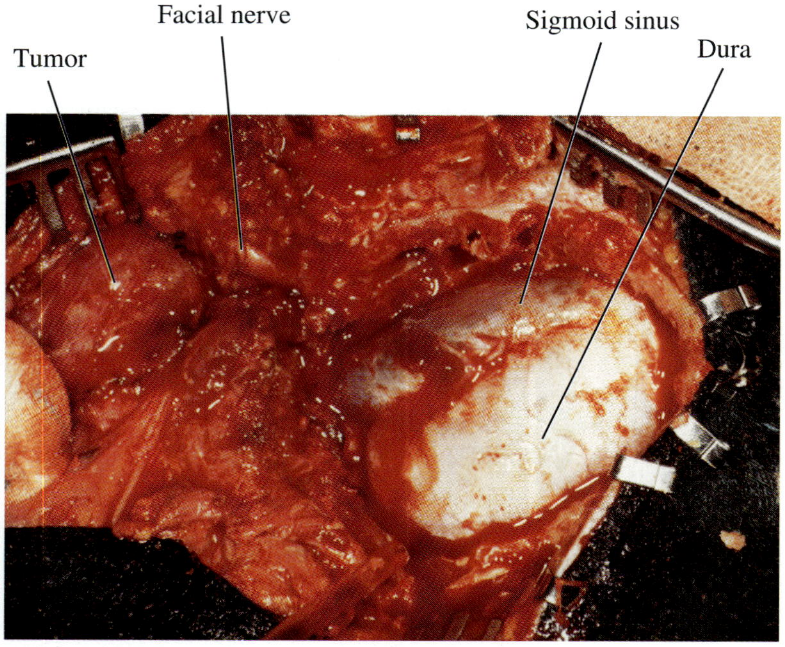

Figure 9. Lateral suboccipital craniectomy has been completed. The sigmoid sinus is completely exposed and the facial nerve is dissected at the stylomastoid foramen.

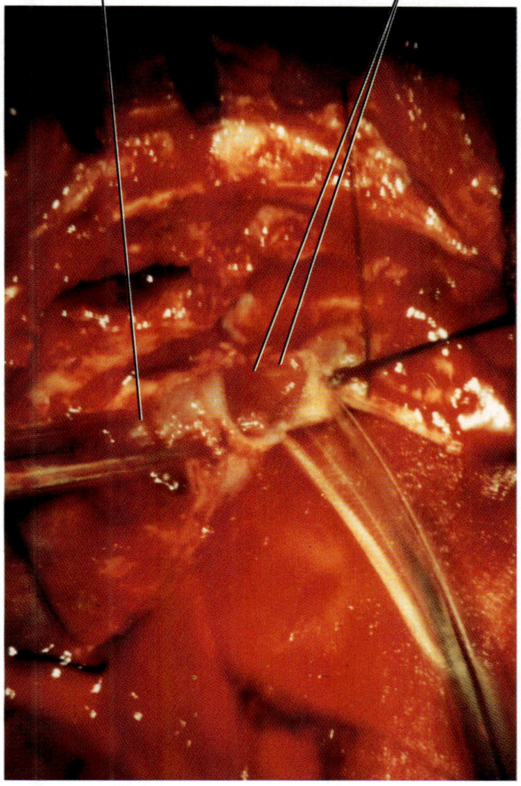

Figure 10. Sigmoid sinus is ligated and transected. Part of the tumor can be seen within the sigmoid sinus.

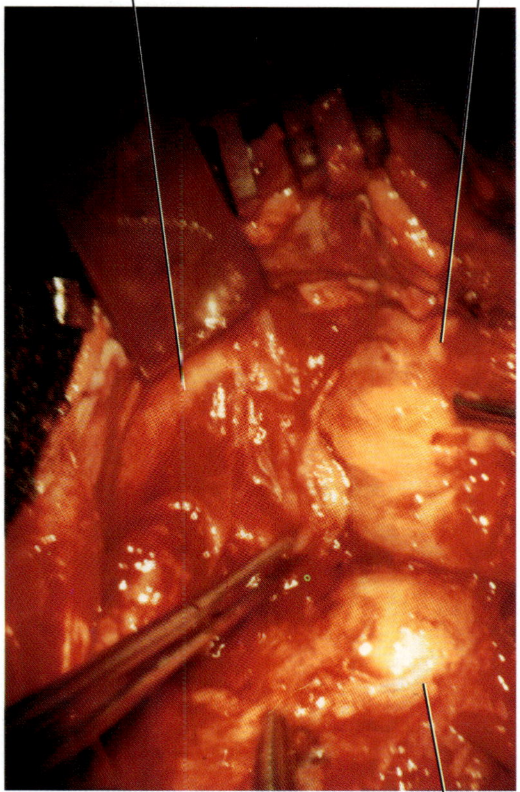

Figure 11. Tumor is partially debulked and has been partially dissected from the internal carotid artery.

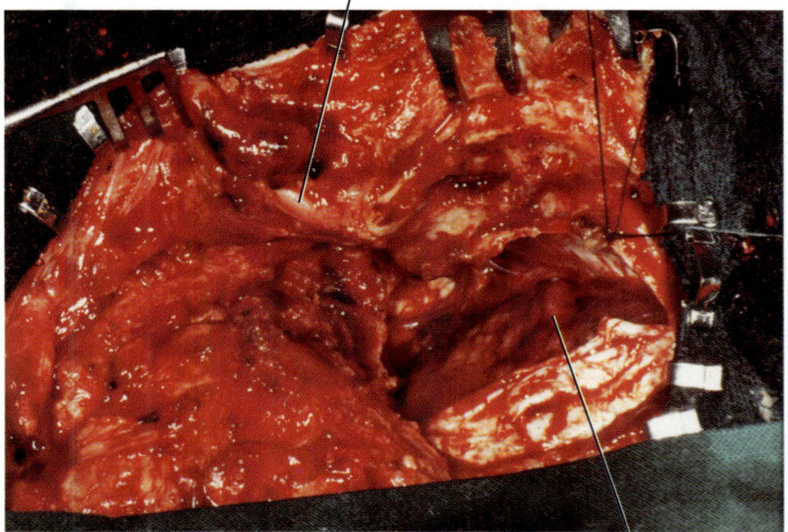

Figure 12. Complete tumor removal has been accomplished.

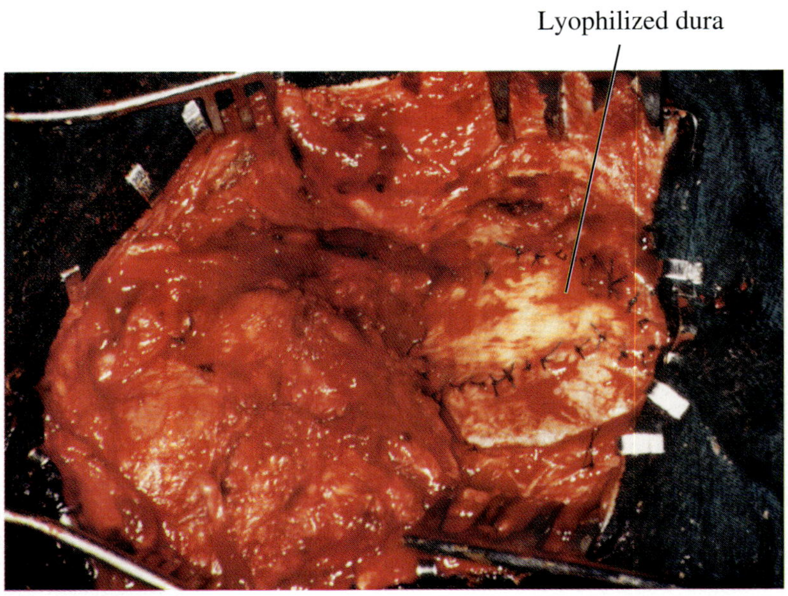

Figure 13. Dural defect of the posterior fossa has been reconstructed using lyophilized dura.

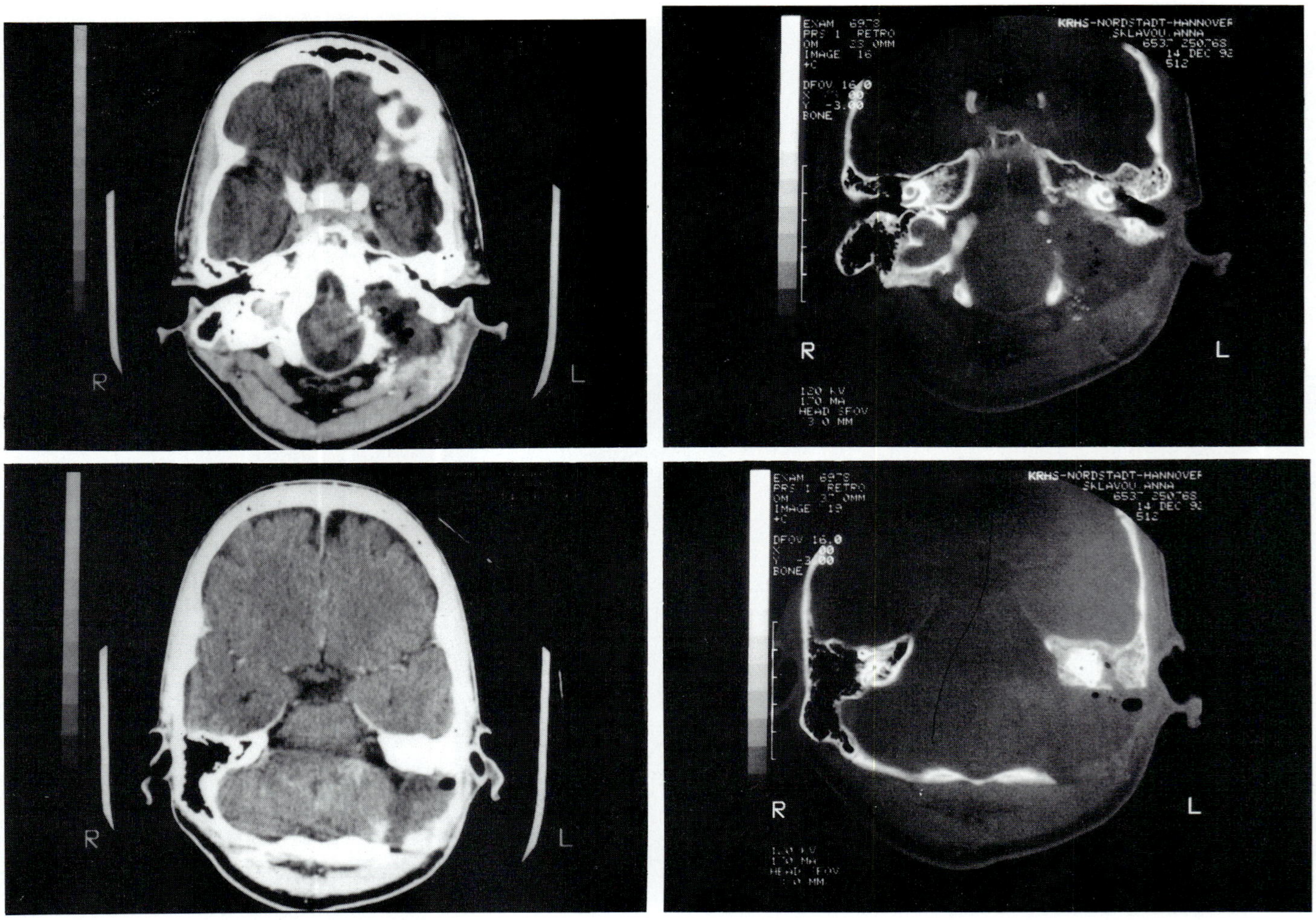

Figure 14. Postoperative CT scan images demonstrating total removal of tumor with resulting bone defect. Note the intact cochlea and labyrinth block.

Cholesterol Granuloma 33

Especially rare as cranial base tumors are cholesterol granulomas. The term "cholesteatoma" is widely used for these lesions for historical reasons, but this term is incorrect in a double sense. First, cholesterol inclusions are not obligatory and second, it is not a tumor.

A distinction must be made between those cholesterol granulomas which occur in the middle ear cavity and those which develop in the region of the petrous apex and are true skull base lesions. The former may occur as a result of primitive congenital inclusions or because of secondary (traumatic, inflammatory) inclusions of squamous epithelium. In this chapter, the discussion applies to cholesterol granulomas of the region of the petrous apex and not the middle ear cavity.

Congenital cholesterol granulomas may develop in the region of the petrous apex and need to be considered in the differential diagnosis of lesions in this location. In secondary lesions, invasion of squamous epithelium through inflammatory or traumatic defects of the tympanic membrane in combination with a small collection of static blood, coupled with lack of access for drainage and disturbance of aeration to the area, leads to granuloma formation. As the blood fractionates, the cholesterol crystals stimulate foreign-body giant cell reaction, and a cholesterol granuloma is the ultimate result (Figure 1).

Cholesterol granulomas found in the middle ear are associated with chronic otitis media. This is not necessarily the case with petrous apex lesions, which are believed to result from chronic obstruction of the outlets of air cells of the petrous bone with resultant cycles of bleeding and granulomatous formation. The lesion that results is a cyst that contains blood products and cholesterol crystals surrounded by a fibrous lining that contains cholesterol crystals, chronic inflammatory cells, and hemosiderin.

These cysts expand, causing smooth-bordered erosions of the petrous bone, as seen on the computed tomographic (CT) scans in Figure 2. The bone may be completely eroded in some cases, giving the false impression of a malignant process.

On CT, the contents of the cyst typically are isodense with brain and do not enhance. On magnetic resonance imaging (MRI), the T_1-weighted images show strong hyperintensity of the cyst because of the high lipid (cholesterol) content (Figure 3). These lesions do not enhance with gadolinium injection. Sometimes cyst rims are hypointense. Cholesterol granulomas or cysts are also hyperintense on T_2-weighted images.

ANATOMICAL CONSIDERATIONS

As these lesions enlarge within the region of the petrous apex, they eventually can compress cranial nerves V through VIII as well as the brain stem and cerebellum. Cholesterol granulomas may involve the intrapetrous carotid artery and obstruct the eustachian tube anterolaterally and cause erosion of the petrous bone.

CLINICAL PRESENTATION

The most common presenting symptoms of patients with petrous apex cholesterol granulomas are hearing loss, tinnitus, and hemifacial spasm. Signs related to dysfunction of cranial nerves V through XII may follow extension of the cholesterol granulomas beyond the petrous bone. The wall of the carotid canal may be eroded, but the artery should not be compromised by this lesion. Obstruction of the eustachian tube may produce serous otitis or mastoiditis. It is unusual to diagnose cholesterol granulomas before they reach a size of several centimeters in diameter, with considerable bone erosion.

TREATMENT OBJECTIVES

Lack of proper drainage of distintegrating blood elements (cholesterol crystals) leads to cholesterol granuloma formation. Therefore, instituting drainage should be the first objective in their treatment. This as well as necessary aeration can be achieved by the creation of a drainage fistula through the mastoid cavity by an infralabyrinthine approach between the facial canal and jugular bulb or through the eustachian tube by way of the middle ear. If the eustachian tube is not patent, placement of middle ear drainage tubes may be necessary. An infracochlear approach with transcanal drainage of cholesterol granulomas may be done.

The procedure of choice for individual cases of cholesterol granuloma is determined by the location of the lesion. When these lesions are confined to the petrous bone, they can be treated by way of anterior or posterior petrosal approaches. The most important principle is to first open the cyst and aspirate the contents and then clean the entire cavity.

If there is good hearing, it is necessary to be careful in sparing the cochlea and labyrinth.

Because cholesterol granulomas sometimes reach the fallopian canal, it is important to avoid operative trauma to the facial nerve. In those cases of extensive involvement of the petrous bone by cholesterol granuloma, the intrapetrous portion of the carotid artery must be protected.

Figure 4 shows a typical cholesterol granuloma as seen through a presigmoid exposure. In Figure 5, the tumor cavity is shown after drainage of the cyst fluid.

POSTOPERATIVE COMPLICATIONS

The contents of cholesterol granulomas are highly irritating to neural tissue and may cause an aseptic meningitis if spilled in the subarachnoid space during drainage.

Incomplete drainage and failure to create aeration of these lesions lead to reaccumulation and further mass effect.

RECOMMENDED READING

Lo, W.W.M., Solti-Buhman, L., Brackmann, D., Gruskin, P.: Cholesterol granuloma of the petrous apex: Computerized tomographic diagnosis. Radiology 153:705–711, 1984.

Latack, J.T.: Giant cholesterol cysts of the petrous apex: Radiologic features. AJNR 6:409–413, 1985.

Rosenberg, R.A., Hammerschlag, P.E., Cohen, N.L.: Cholesteatoma vs. cholesterol granuloma of the petrous apex. Otolaryngol. Head Neck Surg. 94:322–327, 1986.

Thedinger, B.A., Nadol, J.B., Montgomery, W.W., et al.: Radiographic diagnosis, surgical treatment, and long-term followup of cholesterol granulomas of the petrous apex. Laryngoscope 99:896–907, 1989.

Wyler, A.R., Leech, R.W., Reynolds, A.F., et al.: Cholesterol granuloma of the petrous apex. J. Neurosurg. 41:765–768, 1974.

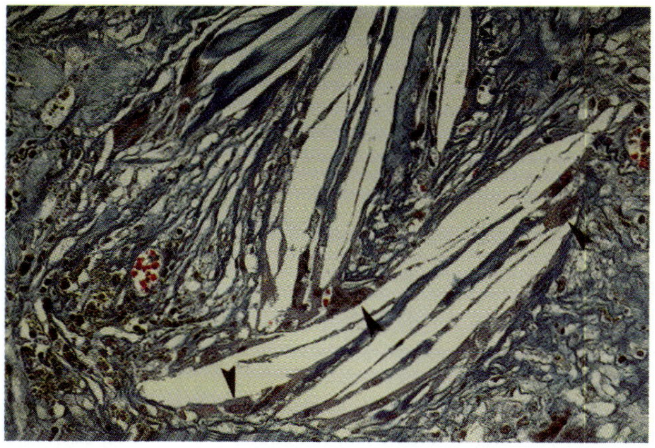

Figure 1. Whetstone-shaped cholesterol crystals surrounded by foreign-body giant cells *(arrowheads)* in a cholesterol granuloma. Note the brownish hemosiderin deposits as rest of the former small collection of static blood. Masson-trichrome, 75×.

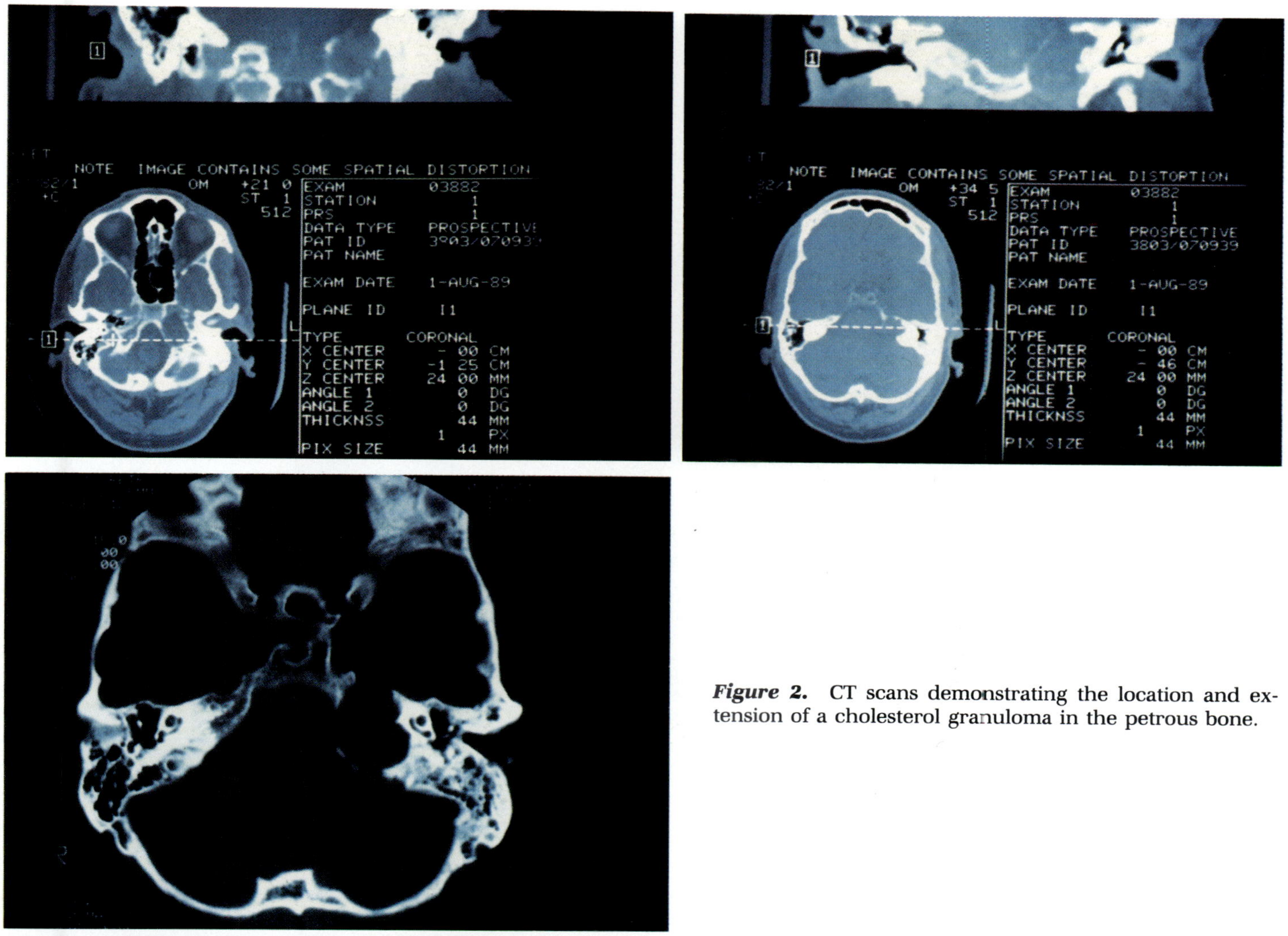

Figure 2. CT scans demonstrating the location and extension of a cholesterol granuloma in the petrous bone.

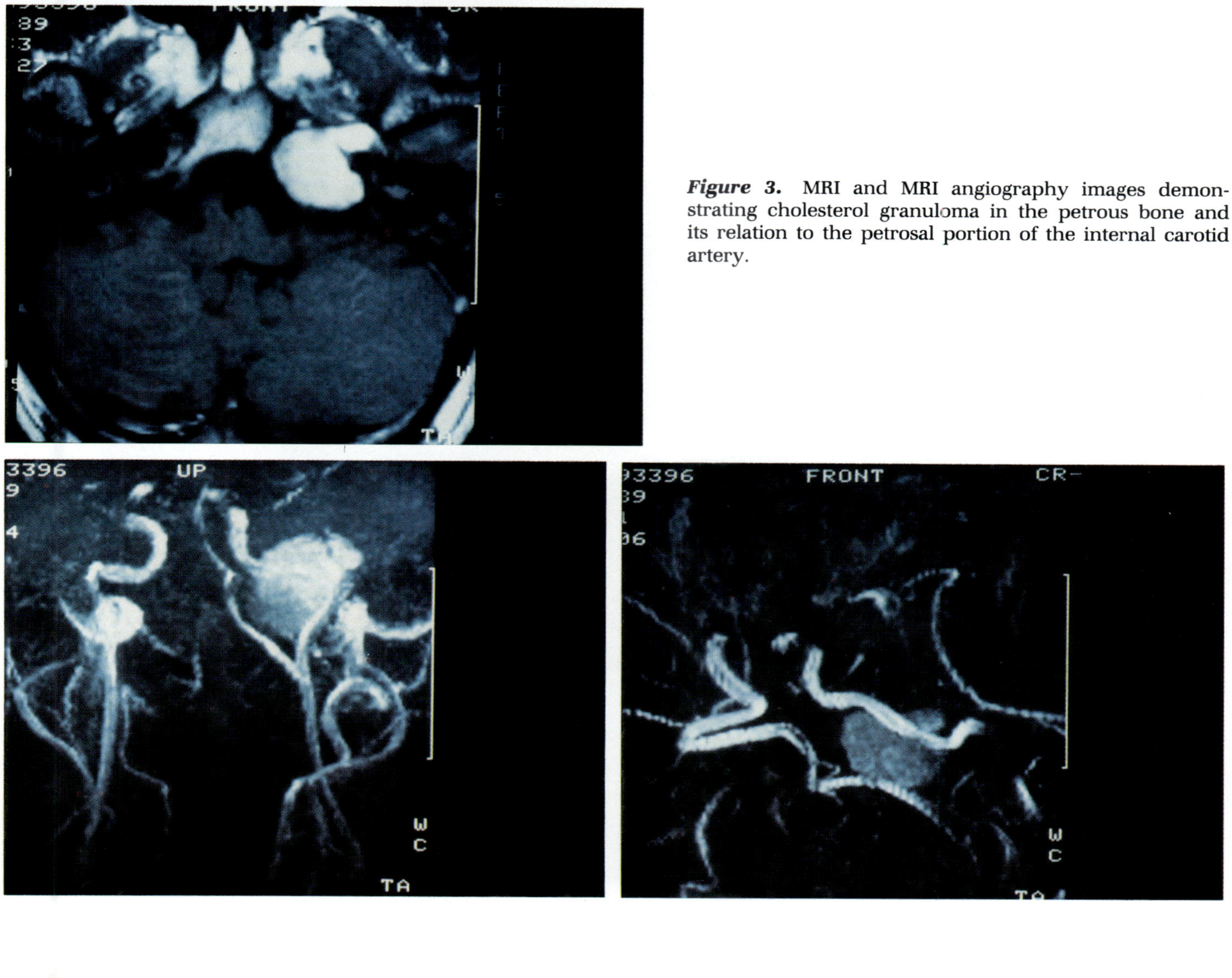

Figure 3. MRI and MRI angiography images demonstrating cholesterol granuloma in the petrous bone and its relation to the petrosal portion of the internal carotid artery.

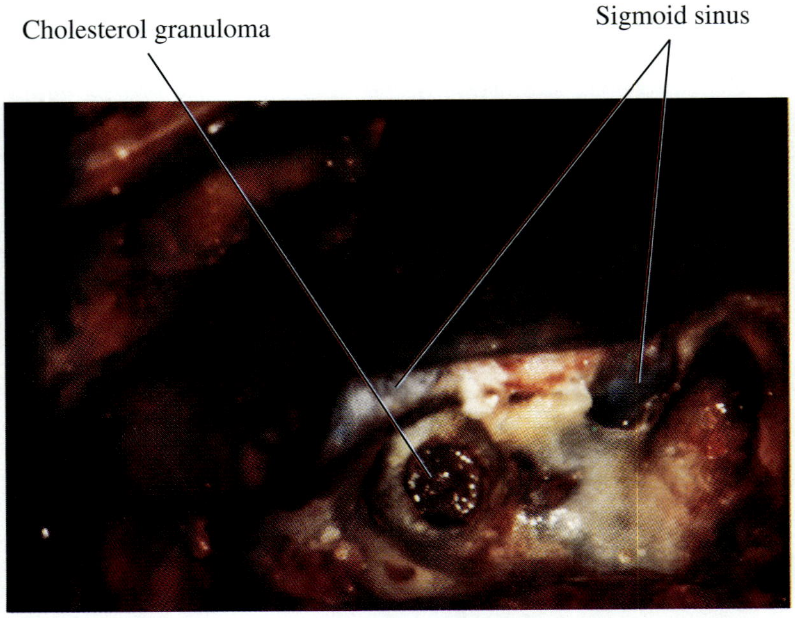

Figure 4. Cholesterol granuloma shown by a pre-sigmoid exposure.

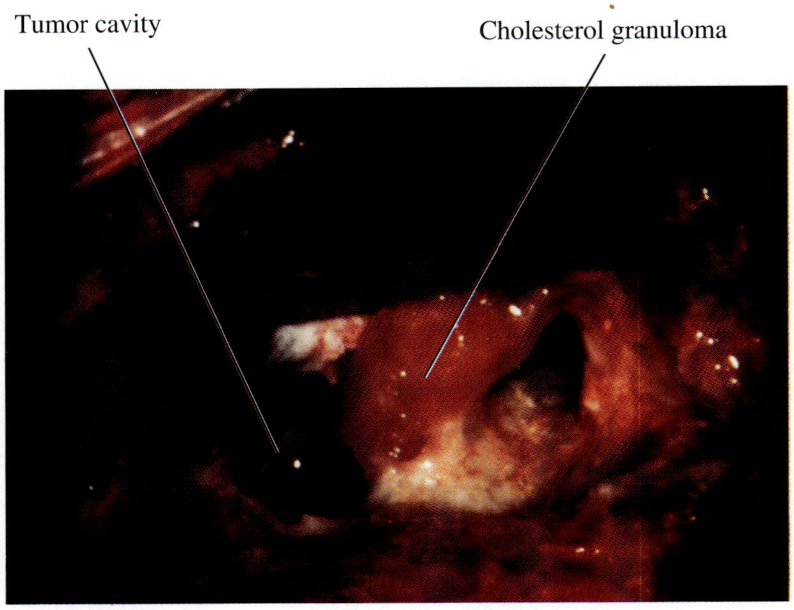

Figure 5. Tumor cavity after drainage of cyst fluid.

Vascular Lesions (Aneurysms and Skull Base Arterial Bypasses) 34

Neil Martin

INTRODUCTION

Arterial aneurysms have long been considered as inborn malformations of the vessel wall. In the recent literature, some evidence for an acquired pathogenesis caused by intra-arterial jet flow has been reported. Examples of ruptured arterial aneurysms are shown in Figures 1 and 2.

The application of skull base surgery principles has resulted in a major advance in the surgical management of intracranial aneurysms. This has been particularly true of carotid aneurysms located beneath or adjacent to the anterior clinoid process, basilar apex and basilar trunk aneurysms, and vertebral artery aneurysms. Skull base bypass procedures have evolved to provide vascular reconstruction after radical excision of lesions that involve the high cervical and petrous carotid artery.

SKULL BASE APPROACHES FOR ANEURYSMS

Exposure of the Carotid Artery in the Carotid Cave and the Anterior Cavernous Sinus: Removal of the Anterior Clinoid Process

The pterional approach (see Chapter 2) is used for carotid-ophthalmic, paraophthalmic, carotid cave, and anterior cavernous carotid aneurysms. It is used for those aneurysms that originate totally or in part from the segment of the carotid artery beneath the anterior clinoid process and within the anterior aspect of the cavernous sinus (Figures 3 through 6). This approach may also be used for neoplasms that involve the anterior aspect of the cavernous sinus or that invade the anterior clinoid process or optic canal.

OPERATIVE PROCEDURE

The patient is positioned supine with the head turned 45 degrees away from the side of the aneurysm. A standard pterional craniotomy is performed. The bone removal in the region of the anterior clinoid process and optic canal may be done extradurally or intradurally. We favor the extradural approach when the medial sphenoid ridge and region of the anterior clinoid process is involved by tumor (e.g., medial sphenoid ridge meningiomas). In these cases, the tumor may obscure the skull base bony anatomy when approached intradurally. The intradural approach is favored for proximal carotid aneurysms so that the aneurysm dome can be visualized and avoided during drilling and removal of the anterior clinoid process. When large or ruptured aneurysms are to be exposed, the internal carotid artery is exposed in the neck to provide proximal arterial control.

With the extradural approach, the dura is separated from the orbital roof medially as far as the superior orbital fissure. The sphenoid ridge, lateral and medial walls of the superior orbital fissure, anterior clinoid process, and roof and lateral wall of the optic canal are then removed with the high-speed drill under magnification. A diamond burr is used for removal of the bone immediately adjacent to the optic nerve and the carotid artery. During drilling of the anterior clinoid process, it is important to remember that the contents of the superior orbital fissure, particularly the third cranial nerve, lie in the dura immediately lateral to the clinoid.

Removal of the anterior clinoid process exposes the infraclinoid carotid artery in the region that has been termed by Ohmoto and others the "carotid cave." This segment of the carotid artery is defined proximally by the anteromedial wall of the cavernous sinus and distally by the dural ring, which separates the extradural from the intradural segments of the carotid artery. Although the cavernous sinus does not extend into this space, there may be bleeding from a venous plexus that surrounds the carotid. This bleeding can be easily controlled by packing with Surgicel or Oxycel.

After completing the extradural bone removal, the dura may be opened either deep within the exposure immediately adjacent to the carotid artery and optic nerve or in the routine manner. If the dura is opened in the routine manner, a second dural incision over the area of bone removal is required to expose the area of the carotid cave.

The dural optic nerve sheath may be incised to allow medial mobilization of the optic nerve. The distal dural ring is divided circumferentially to allow mobilization of the carotid artery. Laterally, this ring merges with the medial wall of the cavernous sinus. Cavernous sinus bleeding may also be controlled by packing with hemostatic material.

For the intradural drilling of the anterior clinoid and optic canal, the dura is opened in the routine manner. A rectangular dural flap is made over the bone of the anterior clinoid process and optic canal (Figure 3). Using the high-speed drill under magnification, the anterior clinoid process and the roof and lateral wall of the optic canal are removed (Figure 4). It is important to remove the optic strut, which is found between the optic nerve sheath and the medial aspect of the extradural carotid artery. The distal dural ring is incised as described previously (Figure 5). This allows mobilization of the carotid artery to expose and clip aneurysms arising from the carotid artery adjacent to the ophthalmic artery in the carotid cave (Figure 6). The cavernous sinus may be entered by making an incision along the roof of the cavernous sinus medial to cranial nerve III or by opening the lateral wall of the cavernous sinus immediately over the nerve.

It is important to recognize that the surgeon may enter the posterior ethmoid or sphenoid sinus. In some cases, the anterior clinoid process is pneumatized. If any of these air spaces are entered it is important to preserve the mucosal lining and to seal the opening into the sinus with muscle and fibrin glue.

In packing the carotid cave or cavernous sinus with hemostatic material, the surgeon must avoid compressing or occluding the carotid artery. We prefer to perform intraoperative angiography at the completion of surgery in such cases to ensure that the carotid artery has not been compromised. Alternatively, intraoperative Doppler may be used to assess flow in the internal carotid artery.

Approaches to the Upper Basilar Artery

A number of surgical approaches have been used for aneurysms that involve the basilar artery apex or the superior cerebellar artery origin. Although it provides a relatively narrow and deep field, the transsylvian approach medial or lateral to the carotid artery has been used effectively for basilar apex aneurysms (Figure 7). This approach is most suited for cases in which the basilar apex is situated above the level of the dorsum sellae and for smaller aneurysms. The pterional–anterior temporal (temporopolar) approach allows the surgeon to work from an anterolateral direction medially and laterally to the third cranial nerve.

The standard subtemporal approach is suitable for most aneurysms that arise from the upper basilar artery, but it provides a relatively narrow working space and requires extensive temporal lobe retraction if the basilar apex is high (Figure 8). This approach provides a rather limited segment of the basilar artery trunk below the superior cerebellar artery for temporary clipping, if this should be required.

For aneurysms that arise at or below the level of the dorsum sellae, the extended subtemporal approaches (subtemporal transzygomatic, described in Chapter 10, or subtemporal transtentorial, described in Chapter 14) provide a number of advantages. The transtentorial approach (with dissection of the trochlear nerve from the tentorial edge) affords a relatively wide working area that extends from above the oculomotor nerve to the level of the trigeminal nerve. This approach has the advantage of allowing both an anterolateral and a straight lateral approach to the basilar artery apex.

The wider exposure of the interpeduncular space provided by these extended subtemporal approaches provides improved illumination of this area. It also offers ample room for the application of proximal temporary clips. This exposure is suitable for approach to virtually all basilar apex aneurysms (with the exception of those that originate high above the dorsum sellae), superior cerebellar artery aneurysms, and upper basilar trunk aneurysms.

In addition to the subtemporal transtentorial approach, a transpetrous extension may be completed by drilling the petrous ridge, as outlined in Chapter 14. Removal of the petrous apex provides access to the basilar artery as far caudally as the anterior inferior cerebellar arteries (Figures 9 and 10).

Retrolabyrinthine Presigmoid Approach to Basilar Trunk and Anterior Inferior Cerebellar Artery Aneurysms

This approach has been used extensively for the exposure of cerebellopontine angle and petroclival neoplasms. It provides excellent visualization of the mid and lower basilar artery (from the vertebrobasilar junction to the basilar trunk above the anterior inferior cerebellar artery origins).

Drake and others have used a subtemporal transtentorial approach for midbasilar and anterior inferior cerebellar artery aneurysms with good results. As disadvantages, it requires a long reach, substantial temporal lobe retraction, and, occasionally, retraction of the brain stem. The retrolabyrinthine approach was initially combined by Giannotta with division of the sigmoid sinus for the approach of midbasilar aneurysms. This approach provides an excellent viewing angle to the basilar artery trunk without the need for brain stem retraction (Figure 11).

OPERATIVE PROCEDURE

We have used a variation of this approach (see Chapter 13), which includes division of the tentorium and retraction, rather than sacrifice, of the sigmoid sinus (Figure 11). The mid and lower basilar artery as well as the anterior inferior cerebellar artery and its origin are well seen. The surgeon works between the nerves of the jugular foramen and the seventh and eighth nerves or between the seventh and eighth nerves and the fifth nerve. There is ample room for temporary clipping if this should be required. This approach has also been used for pontine cavernous angiomas that are located beneath the pia of the ventrolateral surface of the pons (see Chapter 13, Figures 8 and 9).

Lateral Transcondylar Approach for Vertebral Artery Aneurysms

This approach was described by Heros in 1986 and is outlined in Chapter 12. It has also been used for the exposure of neoplasms that involve the hypoglossal foramen, jugular foramen, and lower clivus. This is the standard approach for aneurysms that arise from the vertebral artery at the origin of the posterior inferior cerebellar artery and is used for intradural vertebral microendarterectomy. In most patients, this approach provides access as far rostrally as the vertebrobasilar junction. The height of the vertebrobasilar junction and the specific anatomy of an individual aneurysm arising from this area determine whether it can best be approached in this way or, alternatively, from the retrolabyrinthine approach. With a minimal elevation of the cerebellar tonsil, vertebral–posterior inferior cerebellar artery aneurysms can be readily exposed.

The approach can be modified to allow isolation of the occipital artery, which can be used for arterial bypass. An upside-down L or J incision can be made that elevates a musculocutaneous flap on the side of the aneurysm. The occipital artery can be separated from the suboccipital musculature on the underside of this flap. This procedure has proved advantageous when treating fusiform aneurysms of the vertebral artery that include the posterior inferior cerebellar artery origin. Vertebral artery trapping and arterial bypass to the posterior inferior cerebellar artery have provided satisfactory treatment for such cases.

Operative Procedure

Once the operative exposure for this approach is completed (as outlined in Chapter 12), the arachnoid is opened and clipped to the dural margin (Figure 12). This exposes the upper cervical cord, cerebellar tonsil, and spinal root of cranial nerve XI. Elevation of the cerebellar tonsil exposes the vertebral artery, posterior inferior cerebellar artery origin, nerves that enter the jugular foramen, and cranial nerve XII. A slight superomedial retraction of the cerebellar hemisphere exposes completely the jugular foramen and allows visualization of the seventh and eighth nerve complex as well as the vertebrobasilar junction. The aneurysm can then be visualized and dissected for clipping.

SKULL BASE BYPASS PROCEDURES

Petrous-to-Supraclinoid Carotid Bypass

Indications

Skull base neoplasms may involve or invade the infratemporal, intrapetrous, or cavernous carotid artery. Definitive removal of such tumors may require excision or occlusion of the carotid artery. When a carotid artery balloon test occlusion before surgery has been associated with ischemic symptoms, arterial bypass must be performed if the carotid artery is to be sacrificed. The other option is to avoid carotid occlusion or sacrifice, realizing that, in some cases, this will require leaving a small amount of tumor attached to the vessel. Bypass is also required when trapping of intracavernous aneurysms is planned in patients who do not tolerate carotid occlusion.

The skull base bypass technique has certain advantages over other methods. Venous bypass from the external carotid artery to the middle cerebral artery requires a long graft that is subject to stress with head and neck movement. Bypass from the superficial temporal artery to the middle cerebral artery provides a relatively low initial flow, which may not be sufficient to support the circulation of the entire hemisphere. The petrous-to-supraclinoid carotid bypass provides a high-flow graft that is entirely within the cranium, minimizing the length of the graft and avoiding the stresses of head and neck rotation.

The primary disadvantage of this technique is that it requires a relatively prolonged period of occlusion of the carotid artery to construct the proximal and distal anastomoses. In patients who have not tolerated balloon test occlusion, this raises the possibility of permanent ischemic cerebral damage during the time the carotid artery is occluded intraoperatively. This disadvantage may outweigh the other advantages of this procedure. Because of this, extra-intracranial bypass to the middle cerebral artery may be safer than the skull base bypass. The precise indications, therefore, for petrous-to-supraclinoid carotid bypass remain uncertain.

Patient Position

The patient is positioned supine with the shoulder and hip slightly elevated on the side to be operated in order to minimize rotation of the head when placed in three-point fixation in a radiolucent head holder. The head is rotated away from the side of the craniotomy and the vertex is tilted downward to facilitate the subtemporal approach to the petrous carotid.

Operative Procedure

A pterional craniotomy is done (see Chapter 2). After elevating the bone flap, the sylvian fissure is opened. Drilling of the sphenoid ridge, anterior clinoid process, and roof and lateral wall of the optic canal is completed using a high-speed drill with diamond burr. The dural ring that surrounds the carotid artery beneath the anterior clinoid is divided. This allows clipping of the internal carotid artery proximal to the origin of the ophthalmic artery. Exposure of the intrapetrous portion of the carotid artery for the performance of the proximal anastomosis is carried out as described in Chapter 14 (see drilling of petrous ridge).

The saphenous vein graft is harvested. The segment of the saphenous vein in the upper thigh usually achieves a better match to the diameter of the internal carotid artery than does the vein in the lower leg.

Cerebral protection and cerebral monitoring are essential during carotid occlusion for the performance of the anastomoses. Barbiturates or etomidate is administered to reduce the cerebral metabolic rate and provide cerebral protection. Mild hypothermia may be used. Cerebral electrical function should be monitored using somatosensory evoked potentials, and electroencephalography is used to titrate the intravenous anesthetic agents to the correct level. Intravenous heparin (3000 units) is administered just before occlusion of the carotid artery. The exposed petrous segment of the internal carotid artery is isolated between aneurysm clips, and a linear arteriotomy is made.

The saphenous vein is positioned so that flow will occur in the proper direction related to the venous valves. The proximal anastomosis, which may be end to side or end to end, is made with continuous or interrupted sutures of 8-0 or 9-0 monofilament nylon. The distal end of the vein graft is connected to the supraclinoid internal carotid artery between the origin of the ophthalmic artery and the posterior communicating artery. The distal anastomosis is end to side in configuration. Permanent clips are left on the carotid artery distal to the petrous carotid anastomosis and proximal to the supraclinoid carotid anastomosis, thereby excluding the intracavernous carotid segment (Figure 13).

Cervical-to-Petrous Carotid Bypass

INDICATIONS

This bypass is used when the upper cervical or proximal intrapetrous carotid artery is involved by an invasive tumor, aneurysm, or occlusive lesion (e.g., dissection, atherosclerosis; Figures 14 and 15).

OPERATIVE PROCEDURE

The patient position and preparation are similar to those for the petrous-to-supraclinoid carotid bypass, with the addition that the cervical region is prepared to expose the carotid bifurcation. The craniotomy and exposure of the intrapetrous carotid artery are similar to those for the procedure described for petrous-to-supraclinoid carotid bypass (Figure 15*A*). The cervical carotid artery is exposed as for carotid endarterectomy.

A long curved clamp is passed from the inferior extent of the cranial incision into the cervical incision to make a tunnel for the saphenous vein graft. The clamp is used to grasp a large chest tube, which is then pulled through the tunnel. The trocar of the chest tube is used to pull a heavy silk suture through the tube. This is tied to the distal end of the saphenous vein graft, which is then passed through the tube from the cervical incision to the cranial exposure. Care is taken not to kink or twist the saphenous vein graft.

Before occluding the carotid artery for the performance of the anastomosis, barbiturates or edomidate and heparin are given as described for the procedure above.

The distal anastomosis to the petrous carotid is completed first; this allows the use of slack in the vein graft to expose the front and back walls of the anastomosis. The final interrupted suture is not tied so that the backbleeding can be performed before restoring circulation. An end-to-end or end-to-side anastomosis may be used (Figure 15*B*).

The proximal anastomosis may be made to either the internal carotid artery or the external carotid artery. Again, either an end-to-end or end-to-side anastomosis may be used.

Before restoring flow through the vein graft, the temporary clip distal to the petrous carotid anastomosis is removed to allow backbleeding through the distal anastomotic site. The clip is then replaced distal to the anastomosis, and the vein graft is flushed by opening the proximal anastomosis. The proximal clamp is replaced, and the final suture is tied at the distal anastomosis. At this point, flow is restored to the vein graft (Figure 15*C*). The cervical incision is closed in a routine manner. The temporal bone flap is trimmed to provide an opening for the saphenous vein graft. The remainder of the closure is routine.

RECOMMENDED READING

Andrews, J., Martin, N., Black, K., et al.: Middle cranial fossa transtemporal approach to the intrapetrous internal carotid artery. Skull Base Surgery 1:142–146, 1991.

Day, A.: Aneurysms of the ophthalmic segment. A clinical and anatomical analysis. J. Neurosurg. 72:677–691, 1990.

Dolenc, V.: A combined epi- and subdural approach to carotid-ophthalmic artery aneurysms. J. Neurosurg. 62:667–672, 1985.

Fitzpatrick, B., Spetzler, R., Ballard, J., Zimmerman, R.: Cervical-to-petrous carotid artery bypass procedure. J. Neurosurg. 79:138–141, 1993.

Giannotta, S., Maceri, D.: Retrolabyrinthine transsigmoid approach to basilar trunk and vertebrobasilar artery junction aneurysms. J. Neurosurg. 69:461–466, 1988.

Kobayashi, S., Kyoshima, K., Gibo, H., et al.: Carotid cave aneurysms of the internal carotid artery. J. Neurosurg. 70:216–221, 1989.

Ohmoto, T., Nagao, S., Mino, S., et al.: Exposure of the intracavernous carotid artery in aneurysm surgery. Neurosurgery 28:317–324, 1991.

Shikaw, Y., Saito, I., Aoki, N., Mizutani, H.: Zygomatic temporopolar approach for basilar artery aneurysms. Neurosurgery 25:793–797, 1989.

Spetzler, R., Fukushima, T., Martin, N., et al.: Petrous carotid-to-intradural carotid saphenous vein graft for intracavernous giant aneurysm, tumor, and occlusive cerebrovascular disease. J. Neurosurg. 73:496–501, 1990.

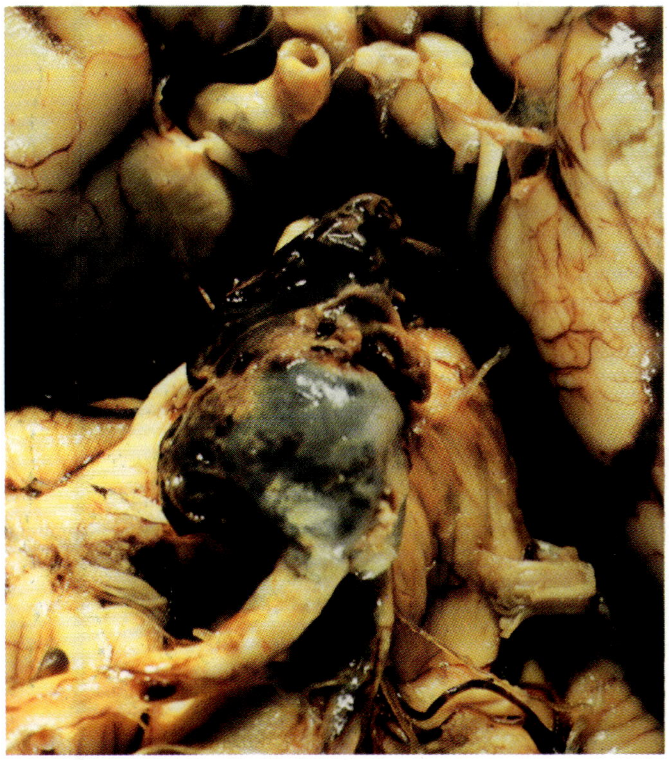

Figure 1. Ruptured arterial aneurysm of the trunk of the basilar artery next to the junction of the vertebral arteries.

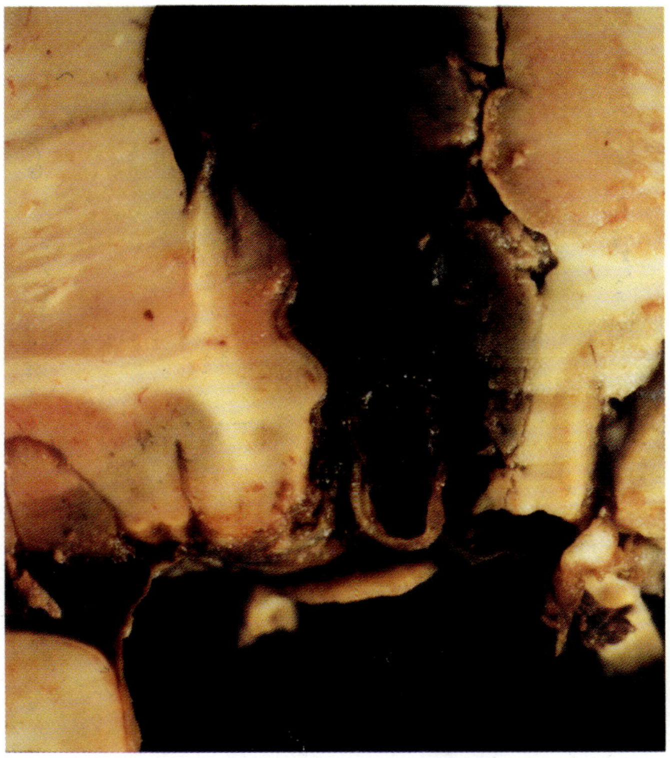

Figure 2. Ruptured arterial aneurysm of the anterior communicating artery with bleeding into the third ventricle.

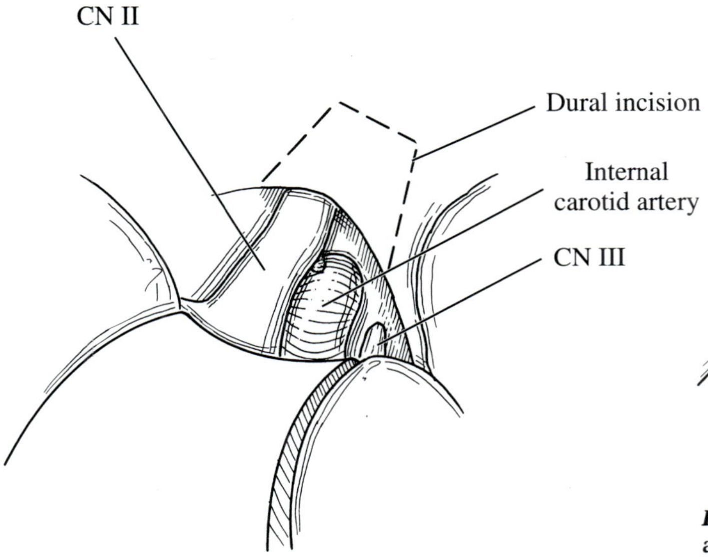

Figure 3. Incision *(dotted line)* in dura of anterior fossa floor used to expose the anterior clinoid process and optic foramen roof for drilling.

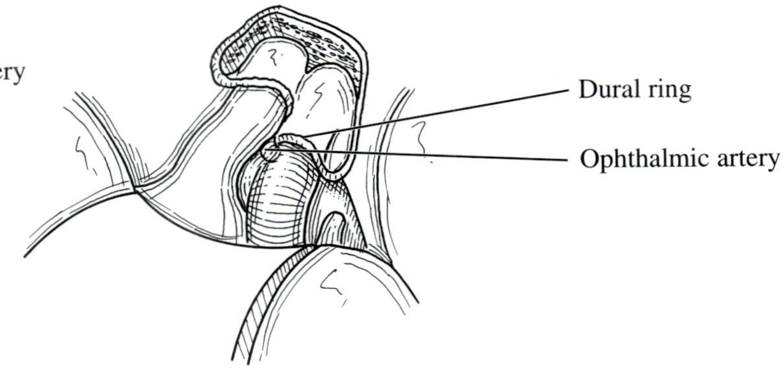

Figure 4. Drilling of bone to expose the infraclinoid carotid artery, carotid cave, and optic nerve sheath.

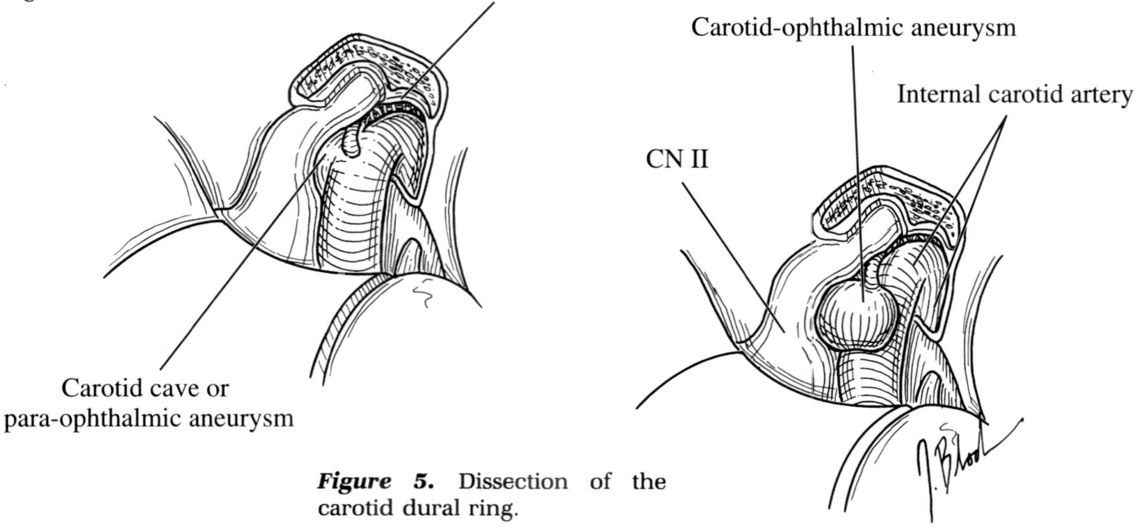

Figure 5. Dissection of the carotid dural ring.

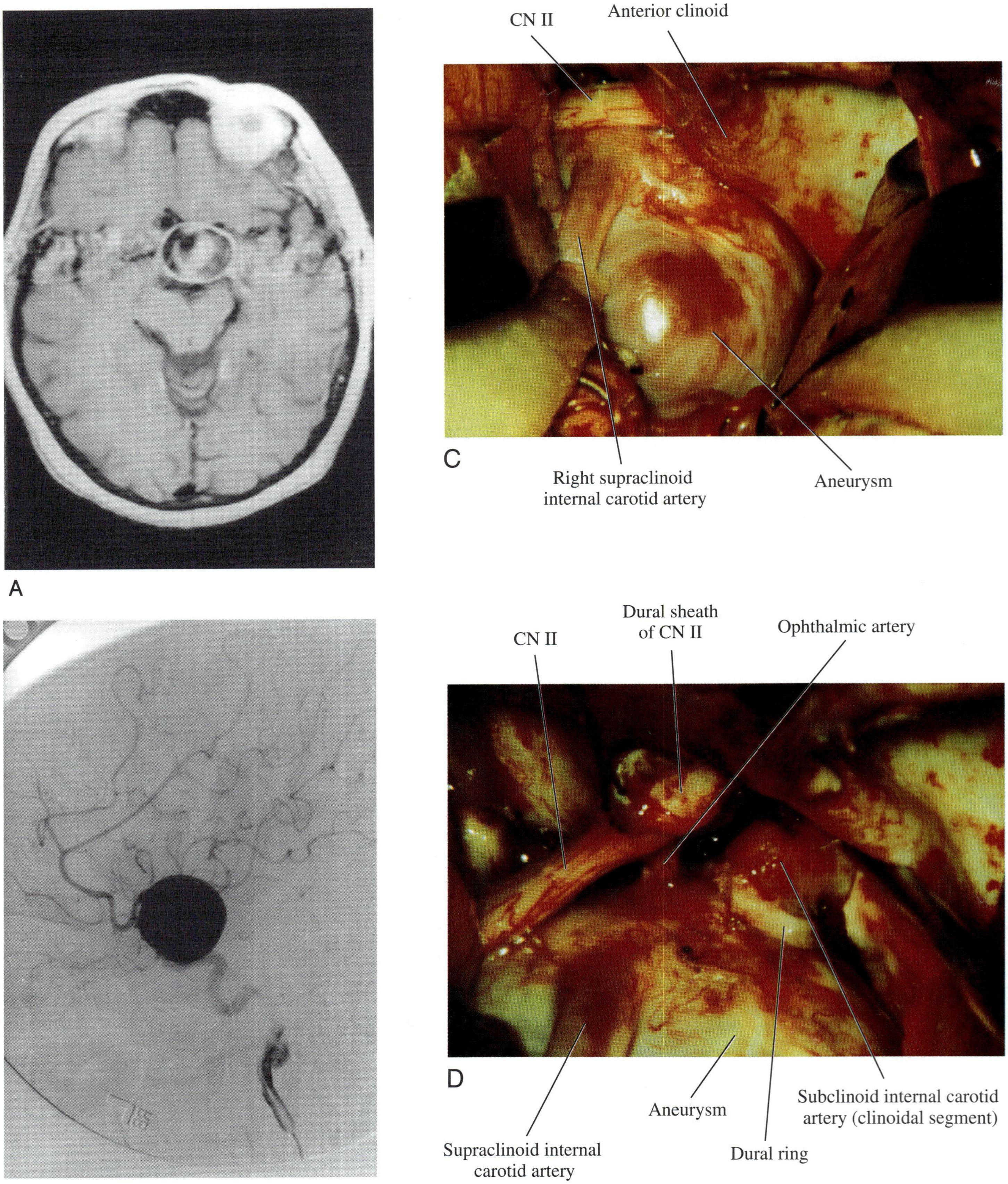

Figure 6. Giant paraclinoid (paraophthalmic) aneurysm.

A. MRI scan.

B. Lateral carotid angiogram.

C. Exposure of giant right internal carotid aneurysm through pterional craniotomy after opening of sylvian fissure.

D. Exposure of ophthalmic artery, infraclinoid carotid artery, and proximal aneurysm origin after drilling of anterior clinoid and optic foramen.

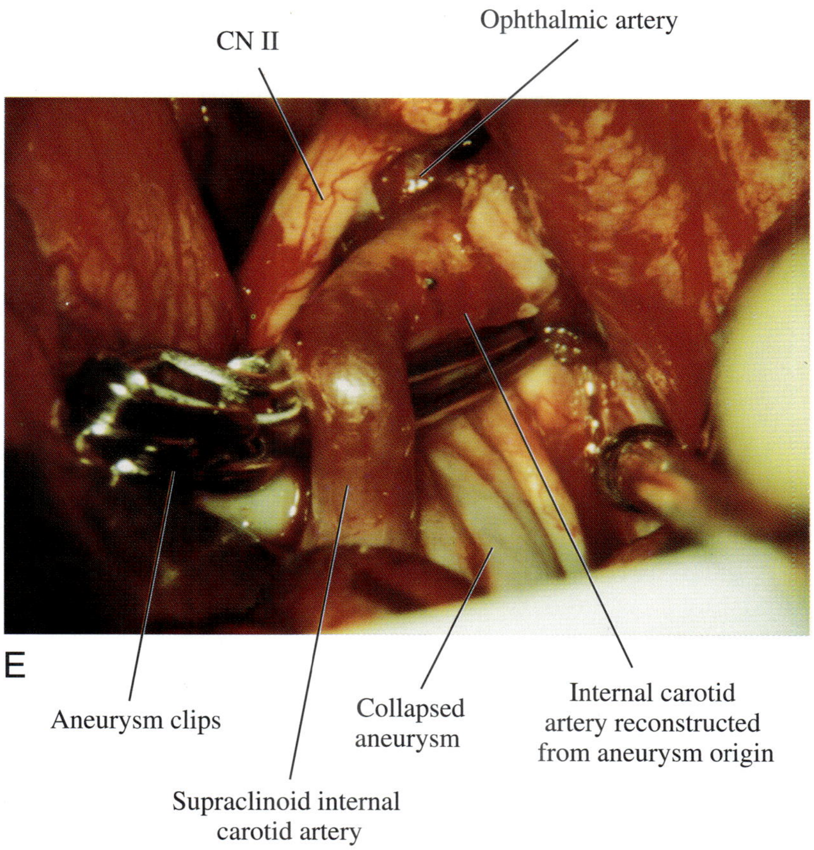

E

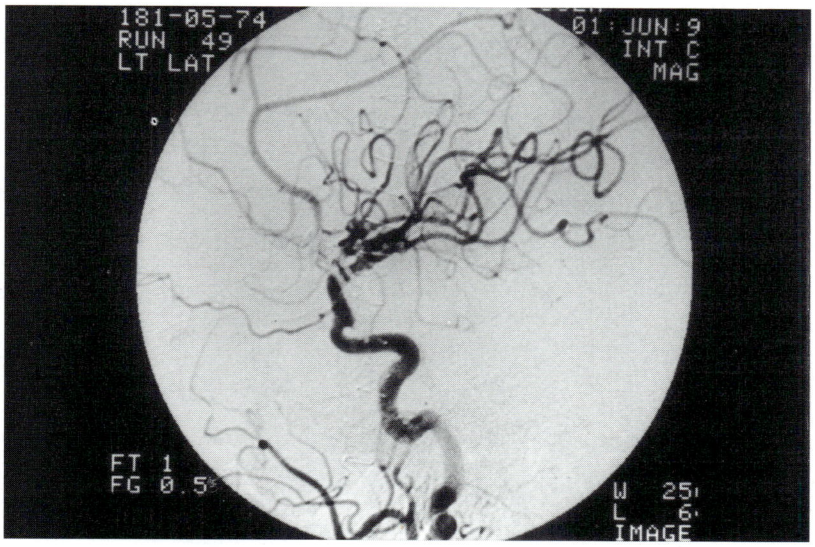

F

Figure 6. *Continued*

E. Clips occluding aneurysm and reconstructing carotid artery.

F. Postoperative angiogram.

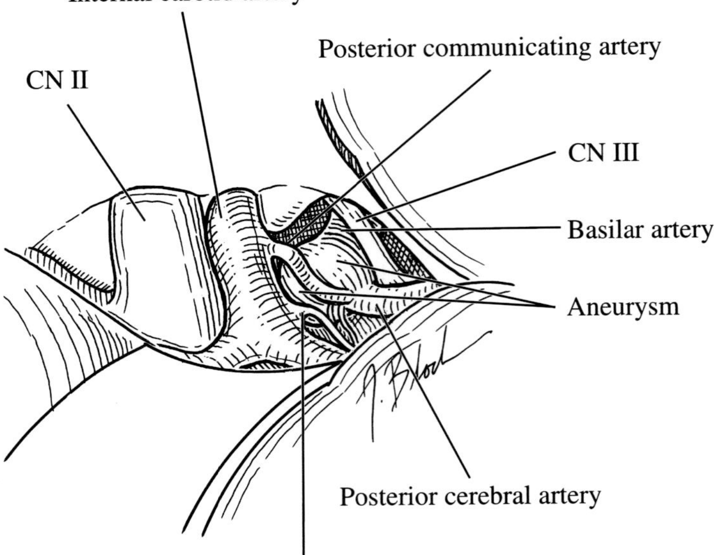

Figure 7. Pterional approach to basilar apex aneurysm.

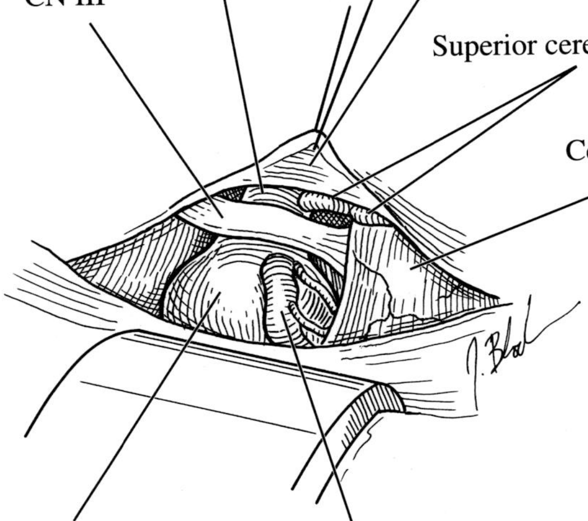

Figure 8. Standard subtemporal approach to basilar aneurysm.

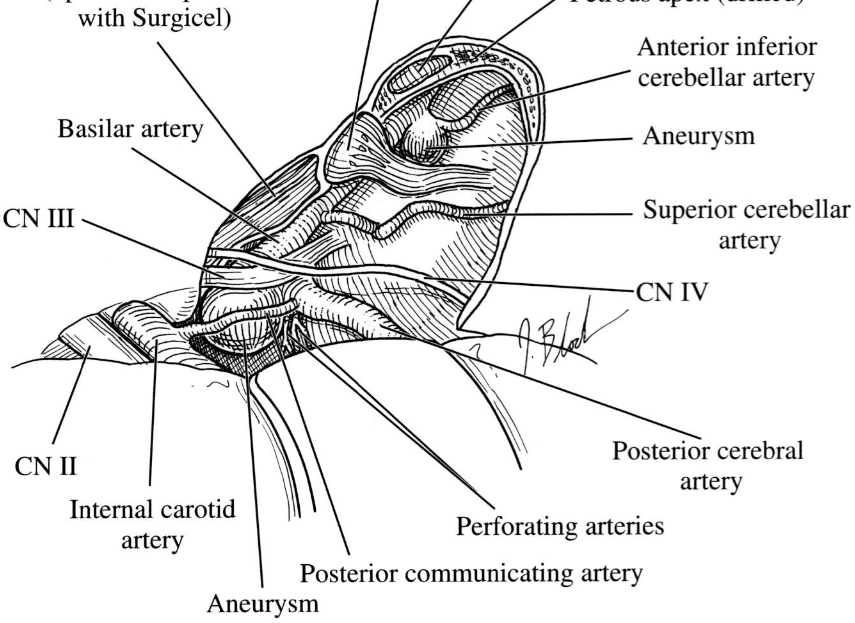

Figure 9. Transtentorial, transcavernous, transpetrous approach to upper and mid basilar artery.

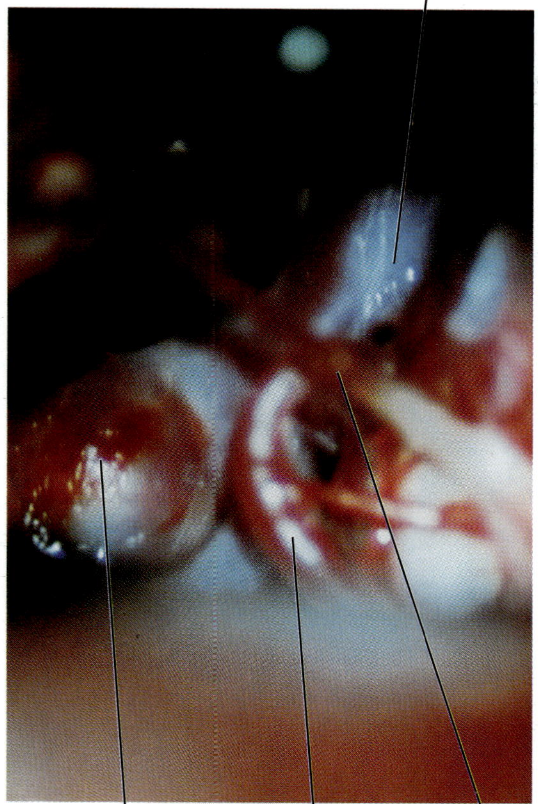

Figure 10. Operative view of basilar apex aneurysm through the left transtentorial exposure. The aneurysm can be seen above the fourth cranial nerve, and the basilar artery trunk can be seen and temporarily clipped below the nerve.

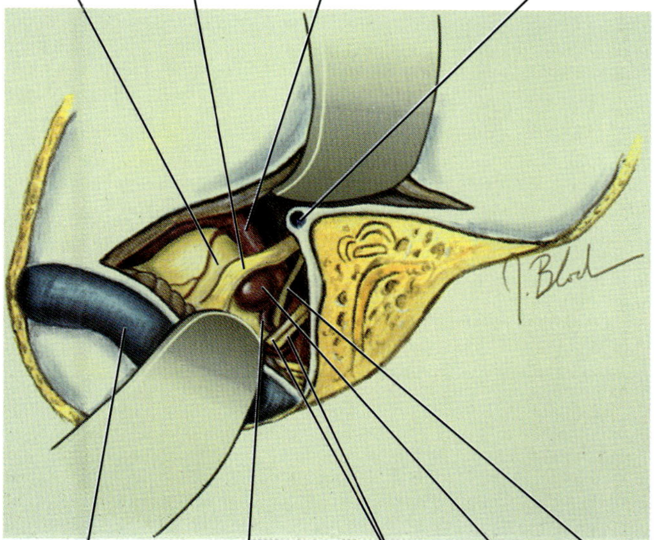

Figure 11. Presigmoid approach to the mid basilar artery and anterior inferior cerebellar artery aneurysms. Exposure of anterior inferior cerebellar artery aneurysm.

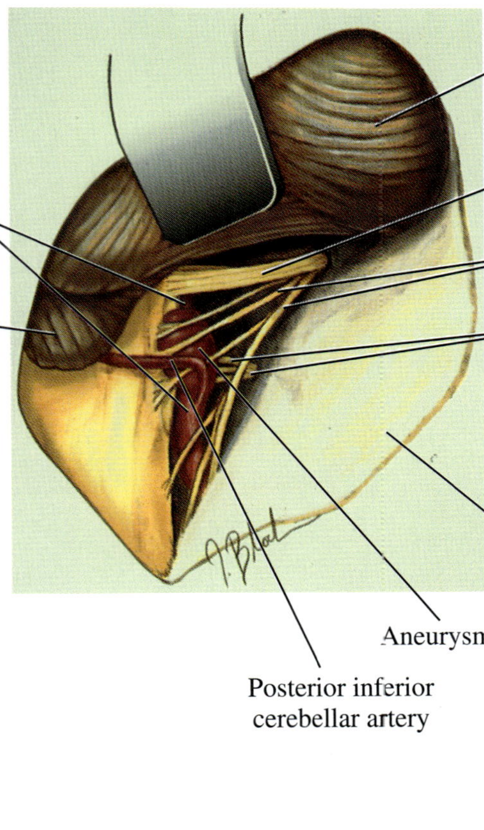

Figure 12. Far lateral suboccipital approach to the vertebral artery and posterior inferior cerebellar artery aneurysms. Exposure of posterior inferior cerebellar artery aneurysm.

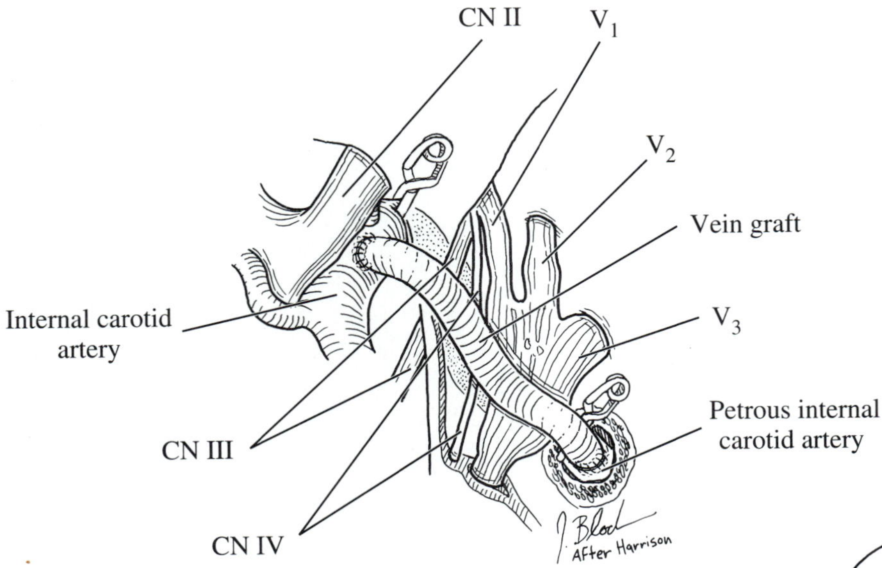

Figure 13. Petrous-to-supraclinoid carotid bypass.

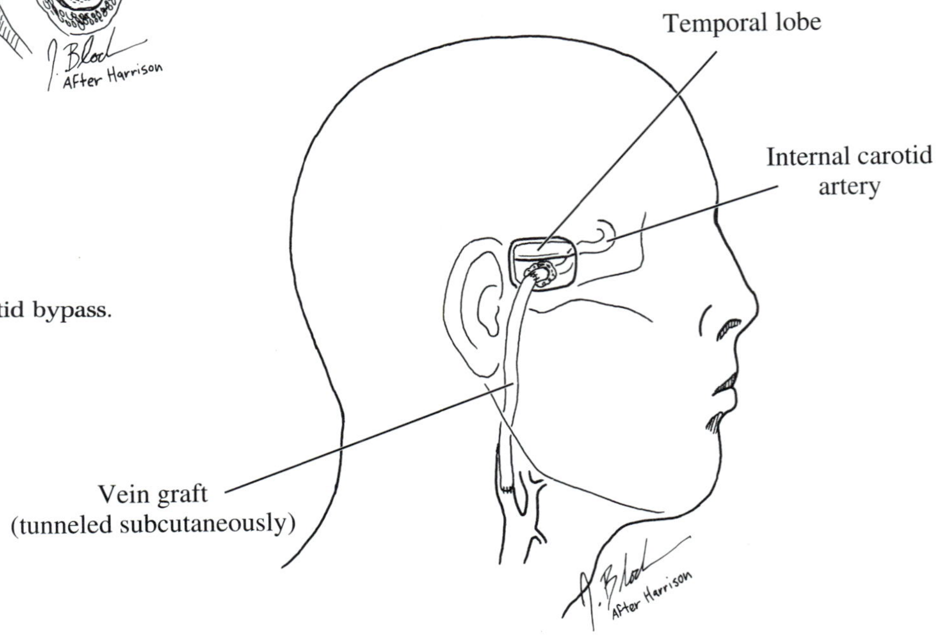

Figure 14. Cervical-to-petrous carotid bypass.

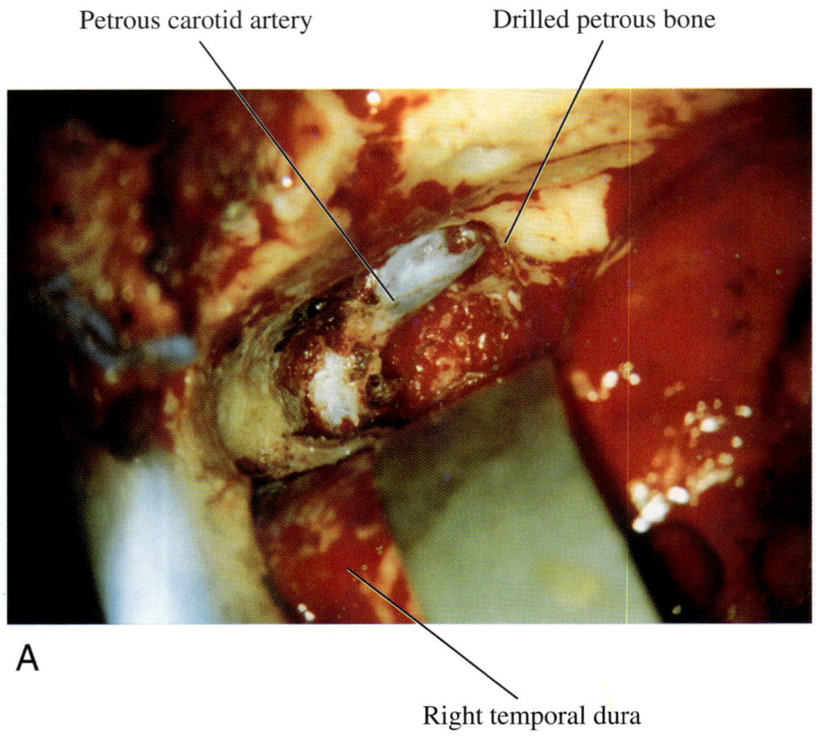

Figure 15. Cervical-to-petrous carotid bypass.

A. Exposure of petrous carotid artery. Note blue discoloration at termination of spontaneous arterial dissection.

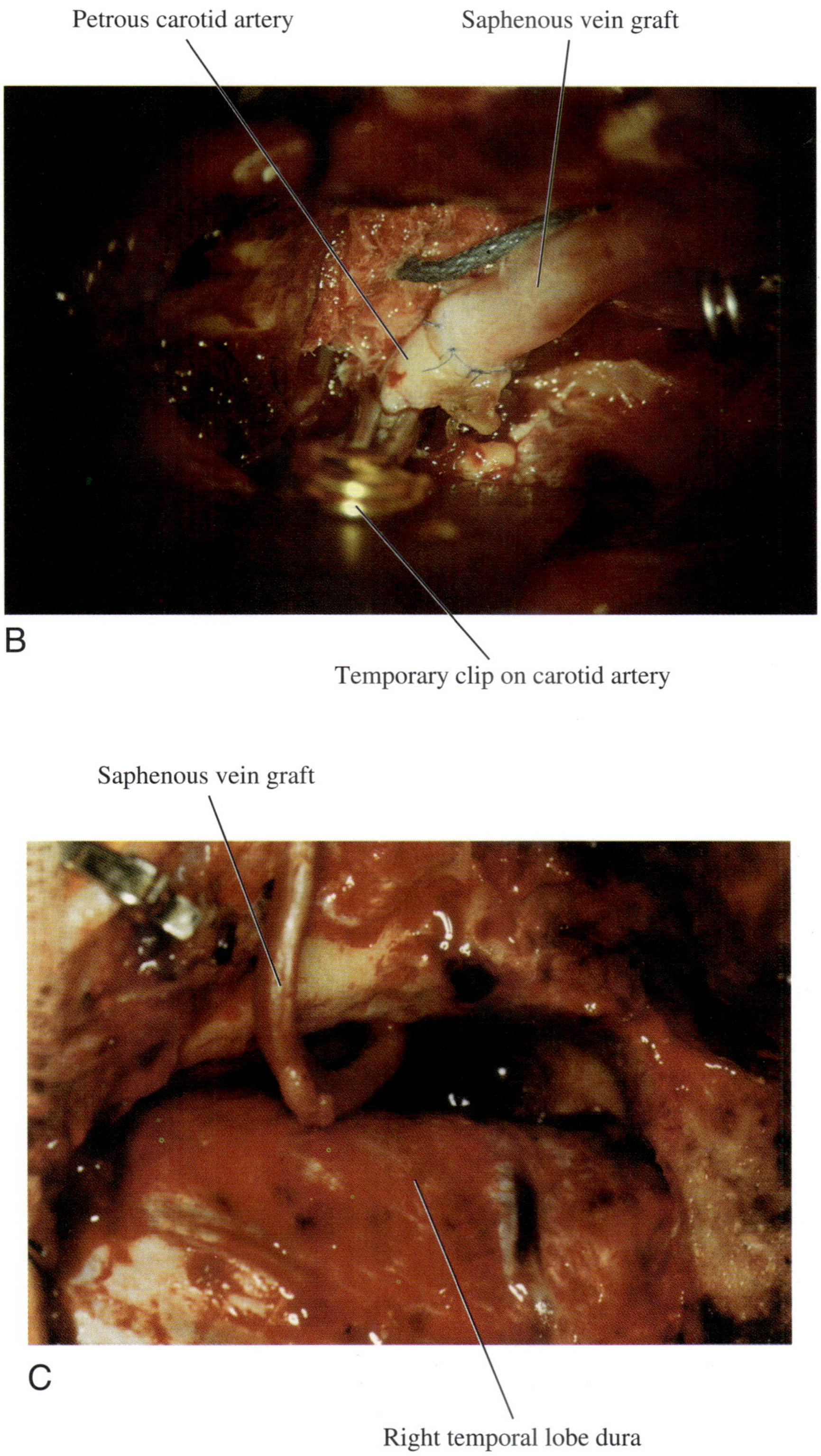

Figure 15. *Continued*

B. Anastomosis of saphenous vein graft to petrous carotid artery (end-to-end).

C. Vein graft in place.

35 Pituitary Tumors

Wesley King

Pituitary tumors represent 10 to 15 per cent of all intracranial neoplasms. With rare exception, these tumors are histologically benign lesions that arise from adenohypophyseal cells. Because of their noninvasive characteristics and the potential for surgical cure in most cases, they are one of the more appealing of the cranial base tumors.

Proper surgical management of patients with pituitary tumors is based on endocrinological and radiological features of the tumor as well as the clinical presentation of the patient and the experience of the surgeon. Because each pituitary adenoma is different, the approach to each tumor should be customized to individual circumstances.

ENDOCRINOLOGICAL CONSIDERATIONS

Collaboration between the neurosurgeon and the endocrinologist is essential preoperatively, perioperatively, and postoperatively. The endocrinological evaluation of pituitary adenomas is well described in the literature and will not be reviewed in detail in this chapter. Broadly speaking, pituitary tumors have been categorized as being hormonally active or inactive. They are also categorized by their immunohistological appearance (Table 1). It has recently become clear that the term *hormonally inactive* may be a misnomer because most of these tumors do produce hormones or fragments of hormones. *Hormonally inapparent* may be a more appropriate categorization. The hormonally active group consists of the prolactin-, growth hormone (GH)-, adrenocorticotropin (ACTH)-, and thyroid-stimulating hormone (TSH)-secreting tumors.

Prolactinomas are the most common of the hormonally active adenomas and account for about 40 per cent of pituitary tumors. The presenting symptoms of these tumors are well known to most clinicians and include amenorrhea with galactorrhea in women and hypogonadism and loss of libido in men. Management in these patients may include medical or surgical measures or a combination of the two.

The mainstay of medical management of prolactinomas remains the dopamine agonist bromocriptine or related drugs. With microadenomas, normalization of hyperprolactinemia can be expected in up to 90 per cent of patients. In the larger tumors, a normal serum prolactin level can be achieved in more than 70 per cent of patients. The role of surgery in the management of these patients remains controversial. With transsphenoidal surgical removal of noninvasive prolactinomas, a "cure" can be achieved in up to 90 per cent of patients, making this a reasonable alternative to lifetime medical management. Surgical treatment of macroadenomas is not as successful; persistent normalization of serum prolactin levels can be expected in less than half the patients.

It is not clear whether or not surgery will improve the medical management by decreasing the requirement for bromocriptine. Several uncontrolled studies have suggested that this may indeed be the case. In our opinion, if a total daily dose of bromocriptine of greater than 7.5 mg is required to normalize the serum prolactin level, surgical treatment should be considered. Surgery is also indicated when a visual deficit does not resolve with bromocriptine treatment or if the tumor is cystic or has produced internal hemorrhage. Surgery should also be considered in pregnant patients and women who are considering pregnancy who have a prolactin-secreting macroadenoma. This is because the volume of tumor can significantly increase during pregnancy and the administration of bromocriptine during pregnancy is not recommended.

Acromegaly is perhaps the least subtle of the hypersecretion syndromes caused by pituitary adenomas. Not only is the disease disfiguring but it is also disabling and has a significant associated morbidity and mortality. Successful management depends on prompt diagnosis and proper integration of surgical and medical therapies. The diagnosis of pituitary acromegaly is based on the identification of acromegalic features in association with elevated levels of GH and somatomedin C (insulin-like growth factor 1, IGF-1) and radiographic evidence of a pituitary mass. Surgery is indicated in most cases, although medical management is rapidly gaining an important

TABLE 1. CLASSIFICATION OF PITUITARY ADENOMAS

PRL-cell adenoma
GH-cell adenoma
Mixed GH-cell/PRL-cell adenoma
ACTH-cell adenoma
FSH/LH-cell adenoma
TSH-cell adenoma
Null cell adenoma
nononcocytic (undifferentiated)
oncocytic

PRL, prolactin; GH, growth hormone; ACTH, adrenocorticotropin; FSH, follicle-stimulating hormone; LH, luteinizing hormone; TSH, thyroid-stimulating hormone.

role in the treatment of these lesions. The criteria for cure in acromegaly has changed over the years. In early reports, a basal GH level of less than 10 ng/mL was evidence of cure. Many of these patients, however, were found to have recurrent disease when followed for a longer period. Later, a more stringent definition required a GH level of no greater than 5 ng/mL. Currently, a patient should not be considered in remission unless the IGF-1 level is normal and the serum GH level suppresses to below 2 ng/mL after oral glucose (100 mg) administration.

Surgery remains the primary mode of treatment for patients with GH-secreting pituitary adenomas. In most cases, transsphenoidal surgery can achieve complete extirpation of the tumor with preservation of normal pituitary function. Only rarely, if the tumor is extraordinarily large, will a craniotomy be required. Surgery is contraindicated in severely debilitated patients or when pituitary hyperplasia from a hypothalamic lesion is suspected. Normalization of basal GH levels is expected to occur in 60 to 90 per cent of patients after surgery and is most frequent when the tumor is a microadenoma and when the preoperative hormone level is less than 40 ng/mL. Relief of acromegalic symptoms and preservation of normal pituitary function are expected in more than 90 per cent of patients.

The medical management of acromegaly is based on the physiological regulation of GH secretion. An analogue of somatostatin, the natural inhibitor of GH release, has been developed and been shown to produce short- and long-term reduction of GH levels when given in 100-μg subcutaneous injections two or three times daily. About 50 per cent of patients with acromegaly normalize their GH and IGF-1 levels after octreotide treatment, and alleviation of the associated signs and symptoms has been observed in 80 per cent. The principal adverse effects of the medication have been gastrointestinal irritability and its association with an increased incidence of gallstones. Although tumor size does decrease in response to octreotide, the effect is not as rapid or as marked as the response of prolactin-secreting macroadenomas to bromocriptine. The indications for octreotide include tumors that are not cured by surgery and patients who are not considered surgical candidates. Octreotide may also play a role as a preoperative adjunct to improve surgical removal of tumor in the future.

ACTH-secreting tumors can be difficult problems. This group of adenomas is characterized by their small size and the morbid systemic manifestations associated with hypercortisolism. Many tumors cannot be visualized with magnetic resonance imaging (MRI). The diagnosis of Cushing's disease is based on information gained from MRI combined with dynamic cortisol and corticotropin testing as well as bilateral inferior petrosal sinus sampling for ACTH. In patients with Cushing's disease, urinary levels of cortisol and 17-hydroxysteroids are increased in 24-hour measurements and are not suppressed with low-dose dexamethasone (0.5 mg orally every 6 hours for 2 days) but are suppressed with high-dose dexamethasone (2 mg every 6 hours for 2 days). A pituitary source for elevated ACTH in a patient with hypercortisolism can be further confirmed by demonstrating a gradient between serum ACTH sampled from the inferior petrosal sinus and that taken simultaneously from a peripheral site. In this test, catheters are placed into both inferior petrosal sinuses by way of the left and right femoral veins. In the case of Cushing's disease, a ratio of central to peripheral corticotropin greater than 2:1 would be expected.

Transsphenoidal surgery for adenomectomy remains the treatment of choice for most patients with Cushing's disease, offering a cure rate as high as 90 per cent when performed by experienced surgeons. If at the time of surgery a tumor cannot be identified, hemihypophysectomy directed by the lateralization of the inferior petrosal sinus study may be performed. Some patients may require complete hypophysectomy if remission is not achieved after the more conservative surgical attempts. Medical therapy is used to control hypercortisolism in the interim before curative surgery in the patient who has failed surgical attempts and is undergoing radiation therapy or to manage patients who are not surgical candidates. Several pharmacological agents that inhibit adrenal steroid metabolism have been tried in the past with limited success. These include metyrapone, aminoglutethimide, and mitotane, all of which have significant adverse effects when administered long term. The antimycotic agent ketoconazole inhibits adrenal and gonadal steroid production, is well tolerated, and should be considered the medical therapy of choice.

So-called hormonally inactive pituitary adenomas are a heterogeneous group of tumors that include true null cell lesions, glycoprotein-producing adenomas, and tumors that immunohistochemically produce pituitary hormones without clinically evident hypersecretion. The majority of this group are the glycoprotein-producing tumors. Because there is not a well-defined associated clinical syndrome, they typically are large lesions at the time of presentation. These adenomas can produce follicle-stimulating hormone, luteinizing hormone, TSH, the alpha subunit that they have in common, or the beta subunit that gives each hormone its specificity. Most tumors cannot be shown to be hormonally active preoperatively and require histochemical examination of the operative specimen to confirm this diagnosis. No adequate medical adjuncts for treating hormonally inactive or inapparent pituitary adenomas exist, and consequently, surgical extirpation remains the primary treatment option for this group of tumors.

GROWTH CHARACTERISTICS

Macroadenomas grow expansively, leaving the sellar region and compressing the optic chiasm and, further, the brain base (Figure 1), whereas microadenomas are restricted to the sella turcica (Figure 2). Hardy proposed a grading system for pituitary adenomas based on the suprasellar extension of the tumor (Figure 3). In type A lesions, the suprasellar expansion bulges into the chiasmatic cistern but does not reach the floor of the anterior third ventricle, whereas type B lesions reach the floor of the third ventricle. In types C and D tumors, the neoplasm is voluminous and bulges into the third ventricle up to the foramen of Monro or has an aberrant expansion into the temporal or frontal fossa, respectively.

It is well known that there is a relation between the invasiveness of a pituitary tumor and its hormone secretory status. Specifically, hormonally active tumors behave in a more invasive manner than hormonally silent adenomas. Previous studies have looked at histological evidence of dural invasion by tumor or the surgeon's observations at the time of surgery. MRI allows preoperative assessment of the relation of the tumor to cranial base structures and determination of the degree of invasiveness.

The normal anatomical relation of the pituitary gland to the cavernous sinuses and carotid arteries is shown in Figure 4. In regard to involvement of the cavernous sinus by pituitary adenomas, we have found two distinct patterns of tumor growth. First, adenomas can truly invade the sinus such that the venous spaces are obliterated and the internal carotid artery is partially or completely surrounded by the tumor (Figure 5). This is frequent with and typical of prolactin-secreting microadenomas or macroadenomas and occasionally is seen in GH-secreting macroadenomas. Second, tumor can compress the cavernous sinus without invading it (Figure 6). On MRI, the internal carotid artery may appear to have tumor partially surrounding it, but in no case is there complete encasement of the artery. This situation is most typical of the nonsecreting, or hormonally inactive, tumors. Frank invasion of the cavernous sinus is exceedingly rare in these tumors, even when they have reached a very large or giant size. At the time of surgery, the surgeon finds an intact capsule adjacent to the cavernous sinus and internal carotid artery, allowing easy removal without bothersome bleeding. The difference in growth characteristics is probably caused by as-yet-undefined biochemical mechanisms.

Vertical expansion of pituitary tumors involves the optic nerves and chiasm, anterior cerebral arteries, and hypothalamus, as shown in Figure 7.

SURGICAL ANATOMY

A complete familiarity with the sellar and lateral parasellar compartment is essential before undertaking surgery by the transsphenoidal or transcranial route. The anatomical relations in this area are well demonstrated in Chapter 9, Figures 9 and 12. As with other approaches, familiarity with the anatomy is best achieved through meticulous cadaveric dissections. The dura of the medial wall of the cavernous sinus is thick like that of the outer layer of the lateral wall. Unlike the lateral wall, an inner layer is absent. The dura of the pituitary fossa, which does have two layers, is contiguous with that of the medial cavernous sinus. Interdural venous channels, in continuity with the cavernous sinus, frequently can be seen passing beneath the pituitary gland and can be the source of bleeding at the time of surgery. Dura separating the gland from the internal carotid artery is drawn in many diagrammatic representations of the parasellar area but typically has not been present in our experience.

The horizontal segment of the internal carotid artery is closely applied to the medial wall of the cavernous sinus, usually separated from it by a thin medial venous space. Along the vertical segment of the internal carotid artery just distal to the foramen lacerum, there are no venous channels medial to the artery. All segments of the intracavernous internal carotid artery can be visualized through the transsphenoidal approach. The posterior vertical segment will be found after it appears distal to the foramen lacerum. After the posterior bend, the artery runs anteriorly as the horizontal segment, which ends at the anterior bend before leaving the cavernous sinus. To enter the subdural space, the artery must pierce the dural ring, which is tenaciously attached to the internal carotid artery. This dural ring actually consists of two fibrous rings that fuse medially where it is continuous with the dura of the diaphragma sellae. Laterally, the dural ring continues as the dura overlying the anterior clinoid process. Several branches of the internal carotid artery can be visualized through the sphenoid sinus. The meningohypophyseal trunk and its branches can be seen arising from the convex portion of the posterior bend, and the artery of the inferior cavernous sinus is seen lateral to the internal carotid artery as it passes above the abducent nerve. Less frequently visualized arteries include the inferior hypophyseal and McConnell's capsular artery.

The neural relations of the medial parasellar area are extraordinarily intricate. The optic nerve exits through the optic canal superomedial to the cavernous sinus with the ophthalmic artery applied to its inferior surface. The ophthalmic artery occasionally arises from the horizontal segment of the internal carotid artery, in which case it enters the orbit through the superior orbital fissure. Cranial nerves III, IV, and VI can be seen lateral to the internal carotid artery in the cadaver dissection shown in Figure 8.

The ophthalmic and maxillary branches of the trigeminal nerve can be exposed transsphenoidally and seldom are injured during surgery on the medial cavernous sinus. Sympathetic nerve fibers run along the internal carotid artery before joining the abducent nerve and ultimately supplying the intraorbital structures.

SURGICAL CONSIDERATIONS

Careful and complete physical and neurological examinations are required before undertaking surgery on the cavernous sinus, regardless of the approach. Because of the risk of vascular and neural injury, patient selection is important. In all cases, an MRI is performed to delineate the extent of the lesion and assess for vascular involvement. The MRI can suggest sellar, clival, or cavernous sinus origin of the lesion. These are critical distinctions when making a differential diagnosis and planning surgery. Figure 9 shows T_1-weighted MRI scan images demonstrating a large pituitary adenoma with suprasellar and intrasellar extension.

Computed tomography supplements MRI by better defining bony destruction in selected cases. MRI usually adequately demonstrates the relation of the neoplasm to the internal carotid artery and documents patency of the artery and cavernous sinus. This is well demonstrated in the MRI scan images in Figure 10, which show an intrasellar pituitary tumor with lateral extension to involve the left cavernous sinus and with lateral displacement of the carotid artery. The MRI scan images in Figure 11 show a large pituitary tumor that is extending far lateral into the cavernous sinus, engulfing the internal carotid artery, with much of the tumor mass lateral to the artery.

With pituitary adenomas, the caliber of the internal carotid artery is invariably normal, even when the artery is completely encased by tumor. This results from the soft consistency of the tumor and the fact that, unlike meningiomas, pituitary adenomas usually do not invade the arterial adventitia. We have not found it necessary to perform routine preoperative cerebral angiography since MRI has been routinely available.

When an invasive pituitary tumor is suspected, preoperative blood studies, including hormonal levels, are essential. These studies may allow a less aggressive surgical approach supplemented postoperatively by medical management or radiation therapy. This is especially true in the case of prolactinomas, for which the role of surgery remains controversial. With prolactinomas, we prefer, when surgery is undertaken, to proceed with the operation shortly after beginning bromocriptine. This medication may promote tumor fibrosis and make resection more difficult. The chance of a hormonal cure in a patient with a prolactinoma invading the cavernous sinus is small with surgery alone, and bromocriptine usually is required postoperatively. Overly aggressive surgery with undue risk of cranial nerve injury is not indicated in this group of pituitary tumors.

Giant pituitary adenomas (Hardy C and D lesions) are worrisome tumors. Symon reported a 19 per cent operative mortality in 16 patients with giant adenomas operated on transcranially. This is in contrast to his group of tumors with suprasellar extension that were not thought to be giant and in which there was an operative mortality of only 1 per cent. We have also seen a significantly higher morbidity rate with larger tumors. The most likely explanation for the increased morbidity is the fact that as the adenomas grow, the subarachnoid space is violated, usually in the region of the cistern of the lamina terminalis. This allows the tumors to engulf and adhere to critical vascular and neural structures. Traction at the time of surgery can thus cause ischemia within the hypothalamus, brain stem, and cerebral hemisphere by compromise of arterial feeders. This would be especially true in the elderly patient, who is more likely to have associated small-vessel cerebrovascular disease. In certain patients, a staged resection, beginning with the transsphenoidal approach, should be considered. An older or a debilitated patient should undergo transsphenoidal biopsy and limited resection followed by irradiation rather than radical resection by way of a craniotomy.

SURGICAL APPROACH

Cavernous sinus involvement should not be a criterion for deciding whether to operate on a pituitary tumor transsphenoidally or transcranially. This decision should be based on the patient's age and health, preoperative symptoms, and direction of tumor growth. The surgeon's experience is also an important consideration. In our opinion, craniotomy should be limited to the patient who is otherwise in good health and whose tumor has grown either eccentrically under the temporal lobe or anteriorly under the frontal lobe. Posterosuperior growth usually can be dealt with satisfactorily through the transsphenoidal route. A craniotomy can also be considered when a transsphenoidal procedure has been unsuccessful at complete tumor removal.

The transcranial and transsphenoidal approaches have been described in Chapters 1 and 9, respectively, and will not be repeated here. Several technical notes regarding the transsphenoidal approach do deserve mention. We prefer to perform this procedure without placing the head in rigid fixation. This allows the surgeon to make subtle changes in the operative view without the need to adjust the operating microscope. We have also found that with experience, the surgeon can perform the entire operation without need for fluoroscopic imaging by paying careful attention to anatomical detail. Specifically, during the initial mucosal dissection along the cartilaginous and bony septum, the surgeon must identify the vomer and sphenoid ostea, which have a constant appearance and relation to the sinus. This should be done before the removal of any bone.

These measures prevent inadvertent exposure of the anterior fossa and keep the surgeon from straying from the midline. Once the sphenoid sinus is entered, the convexity of the sella turcica usually is quite easily identified. There are several circumstances in which we find the image intensifier useful. These include patients with poorly pneumatized sphenoid sinuses that require drilling to expose the sella; patients with acromegaly whose surgical procedures are more frequently difficult because of the mucosal hypertrophy and vascularity; and patients with macroadenomas with large suprasellar extension. In the latter group, fluoroscopic imaging allows one to visualize instruments passed above the sella during tumor removal.

Figure 12 is an intraoperative photograph taken during the removal of a primarily intrasellar adenoma through a transsphenoidal approach. In Figures 13 through 15 the removal of an intrasellar pituitary adenoma is demonstrated using a transnasal paraseptal exposure.

An intraoperative photograph in the case of a giant pituitary adenoma with marked suprasellar extension and compression of the optic nerves and chiasm is shown in Figure 16. This tumor was removed through a subfrontal approach. In Figure 17, the extension of tumor lateral to the carotid artery is demonstrated.

SUMMARY

Pituitary tumors represent a heterogeneous group of tumors characterized by their protean hormonal activity and variable growth patterns. In many cases, the medical and surgical management can be quite challenging. Optimal therapy in these situations requires extensive surgical experience and a comprehensive understanding of the skull base anatomy and neuroendocrine pathophysiological mechanisms.

RECOMMENDED READING

Barkan, A., Kelch, R., Hopwood, N., et al.: Treatment of acromegaly with the long-acting somatostatin analog SMS 201-995. J. Clin. Endocrinol. Metab. 66:16–23, 1988.

Bevan, J., Adams, C., Burke, W., et al.: Factors in the outcome of transsphenoidal surgery for prolactinoma and non-functioning pituitary tumor, including pre-operative bromocriptine therapy. Clin. Endocrinol. 26:541–556, 1987.

Fahlbusch, R., Buchfelder, M., Schrell, U.: Short-term preoperative treatment of macroprolactinomas by dopamine agonists. J. Neurosurg. 67:807–815, 1987.

Hardy, J., Vezina, J.: Transsphenoidal neurosurgery of intracranial neoplasm. *In* Green, R.A., Jr. (ed.): Advances in Neurology. New York: Raven Press, 1976, pp. 261–274.

Hubbard, J., Scheithauer, B., Abboud, C.: Prolactin-secreting adenomas: The preoperative response to bromocriptine treatment and surgical outcome. J. Neurosurg. 67:816–821, 1987.

Klibanski, A., Zervas, N.: Diagnosis and management of hormone-secreting pituitary adenomas. N. Engl. J. Med. 324:822–831, 1991.

Lambets, S., Uitterlinden, P., Vershoor, L., et al.: Long-term treatment of acromegaly with somatostatin analogue SMS 201-995. N. Engl. J. Med. 313:1576–1580, 1985.

Lundin, P., Nyman, R., Burman, P., et al.: MRI of pituitary macroadenomas with reference to hormonal activity. Neuroradiology 34:43–51, 1992.

Scheithauer, B., Kovacs, K., Laws, E., et al.: Pathology of invasive pituitary tumors with special reference to functional classifications. J. Neurosurg. 65:733–744, 1986.

Symon, L., Jakubowski, J.: Transcranial management of pituitary tumors with suprasellar extension. J. Neurol. Neurosurg. Psychiatry 42:123–133, 1979.

Symon, L., Jakubowski, J., Kendall, B.: Surgical treatment of giant pituitary adenomas. J. Neurol. Neurosurg. Psychiatry 42:973–982, 1979.

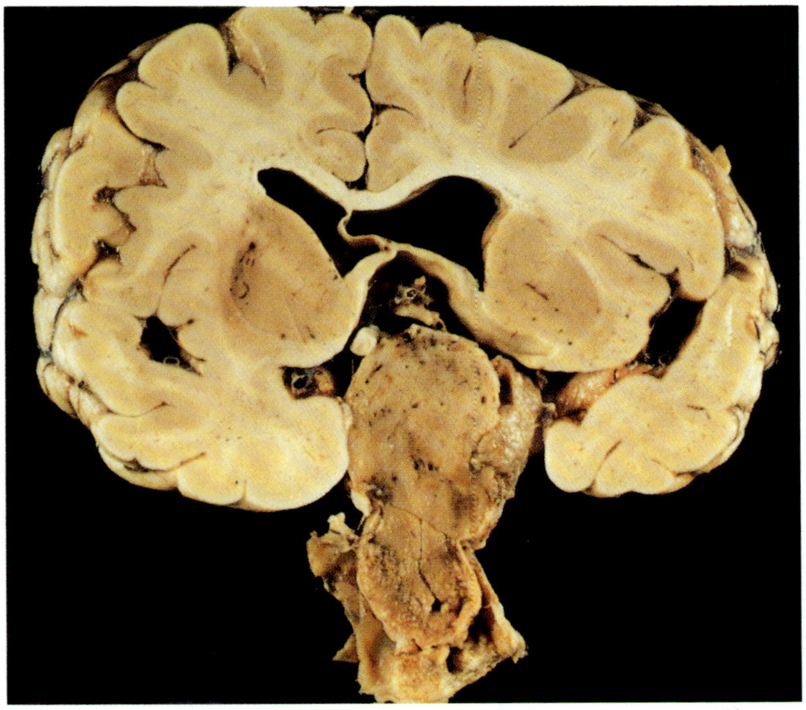

Figure 1. Pituitary macroadenoma widening the sella turcica and compressing brain base structures.

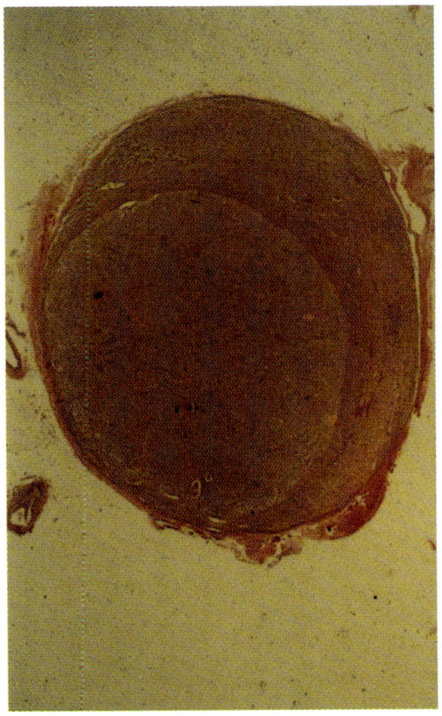

Figure 2. Well-delineated intrasellar pituitary microadenoma compressing surrounding pituitary tissue. Elastica-Van Gieson, overview.

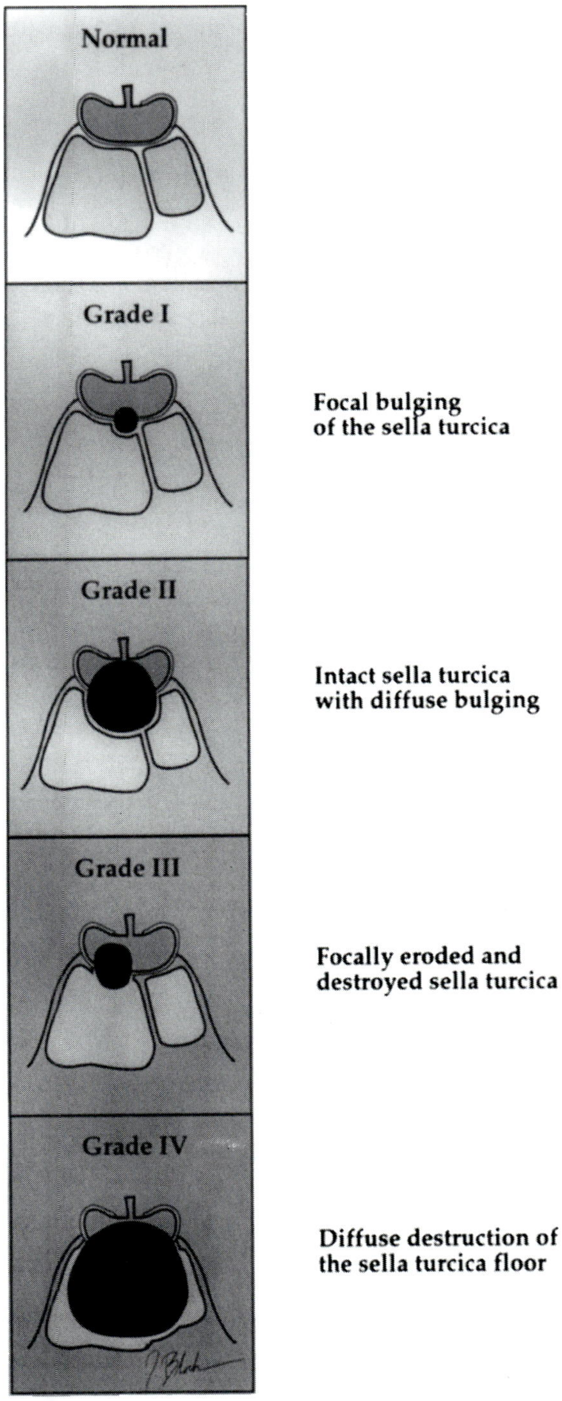

Figure 3. Grading system for pituitary adenomas as proposed by Hardy.

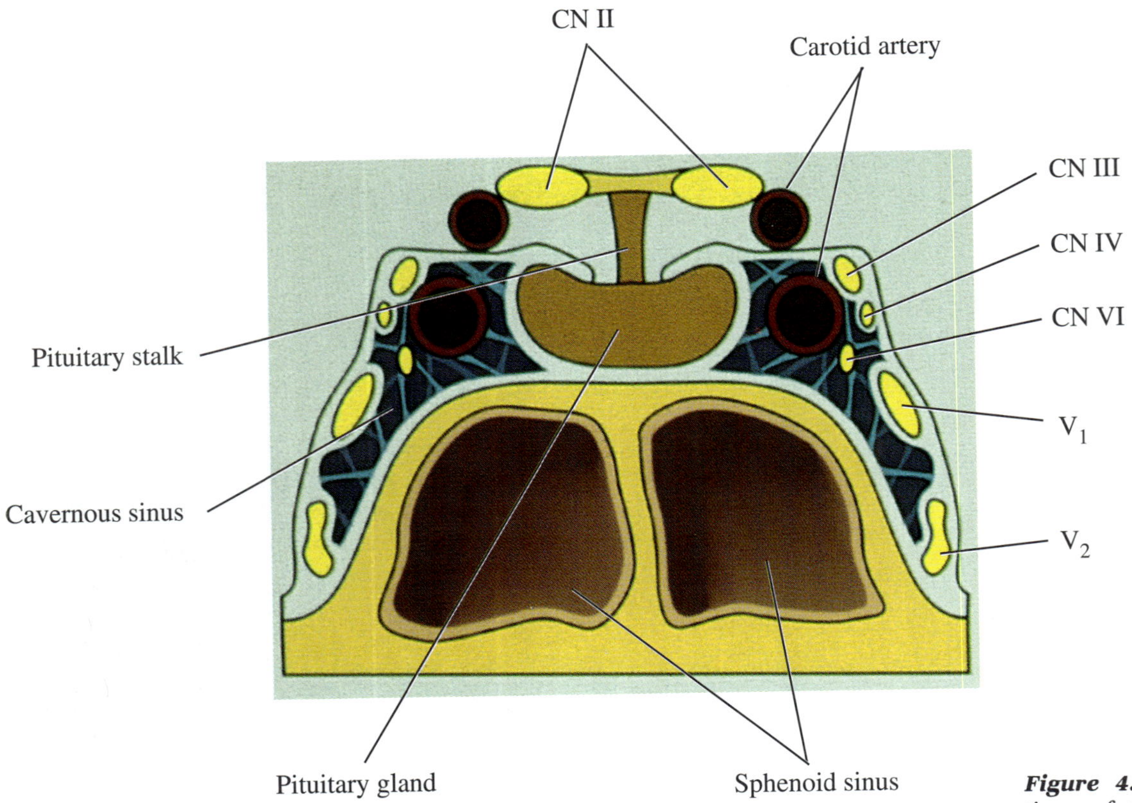

Figure 4. Normal anatomical relations of the pituitary gland to the cavernous sinuses and carotid arteries.

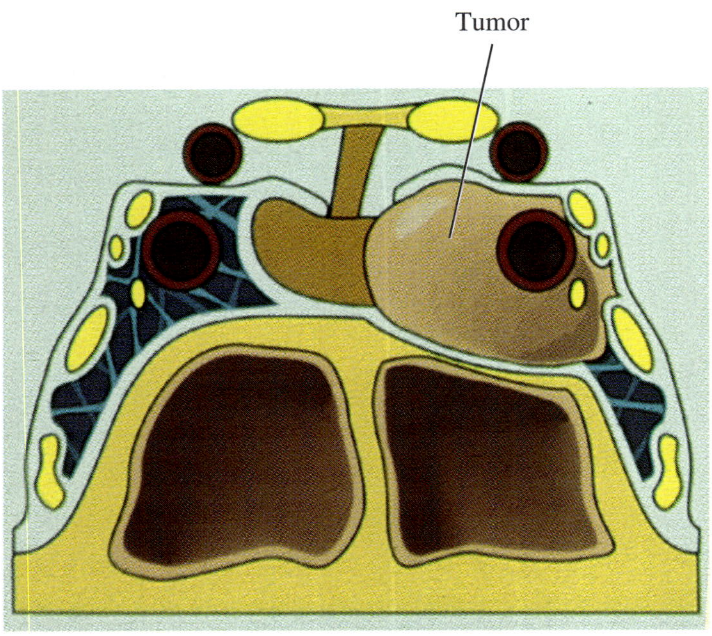

Figure 5. Invasion of the venous spaces of the cavernous sinus, thus completely surrounding the internal carotid artery. This situation is most typical of prolactinomas and GH-secreting lesions.

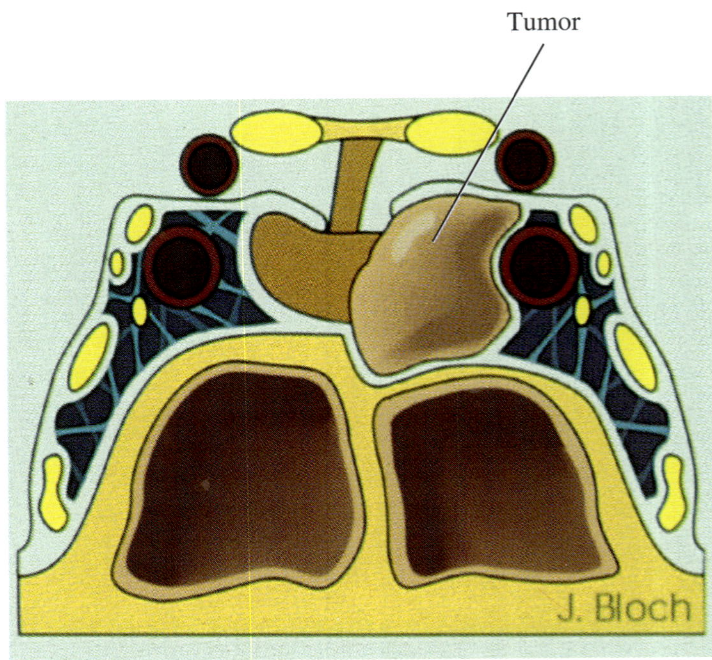

Figure 6. Growth pattern of pituitary adenomas. A tumor can involve the cavernous sinus by displacing the internal carotid artery and venous spaces. In this situation, the tumor is separated from the vascular compartment by dura or a capsule.

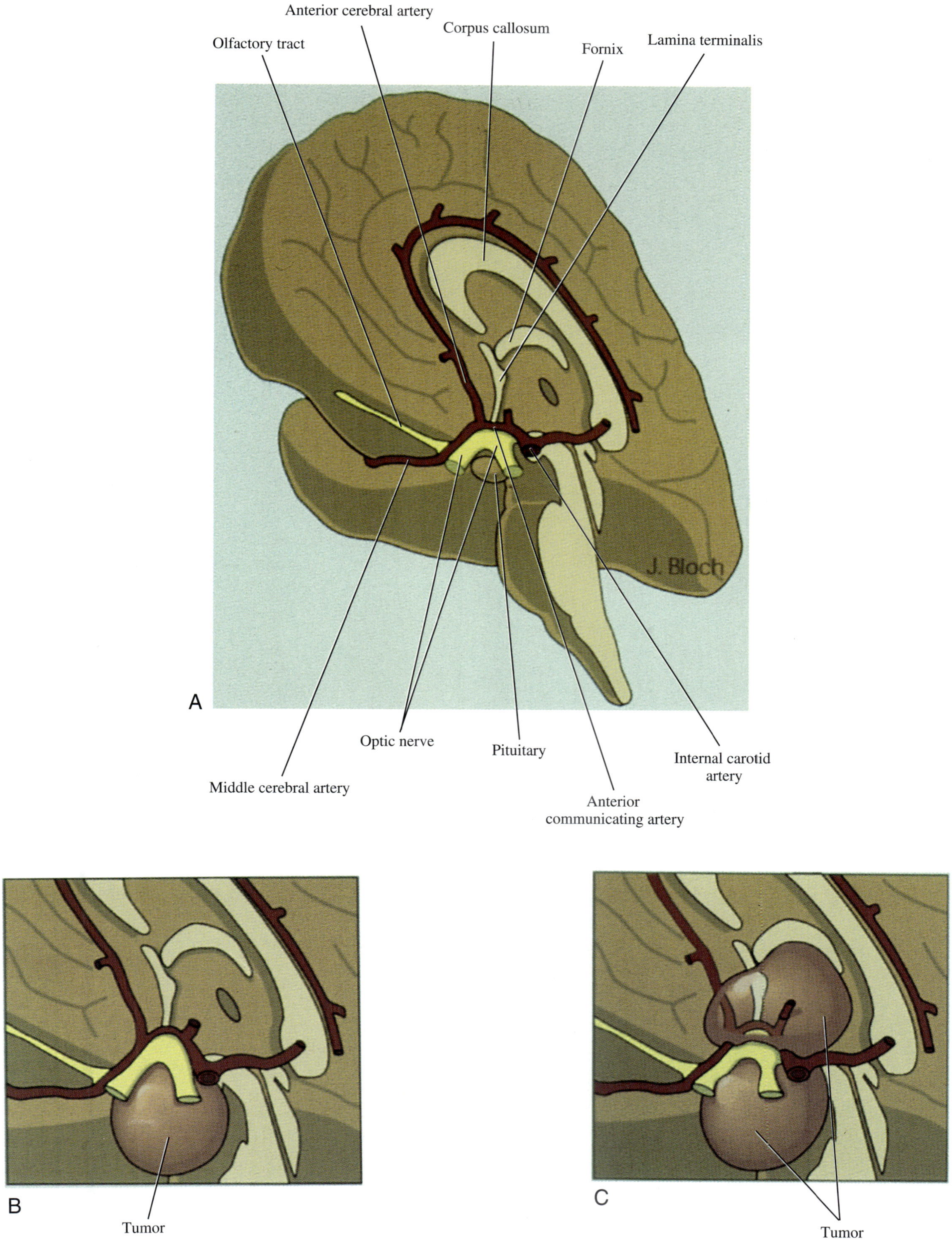

Figure 7. Relation of the pituitary gland to the adjacent neurovascular structures. As the adenoma enlarges, the optic chiasm and anterior cerebral arteries are displaced upward. With further growth, these structures can be engulfed by the tumor.

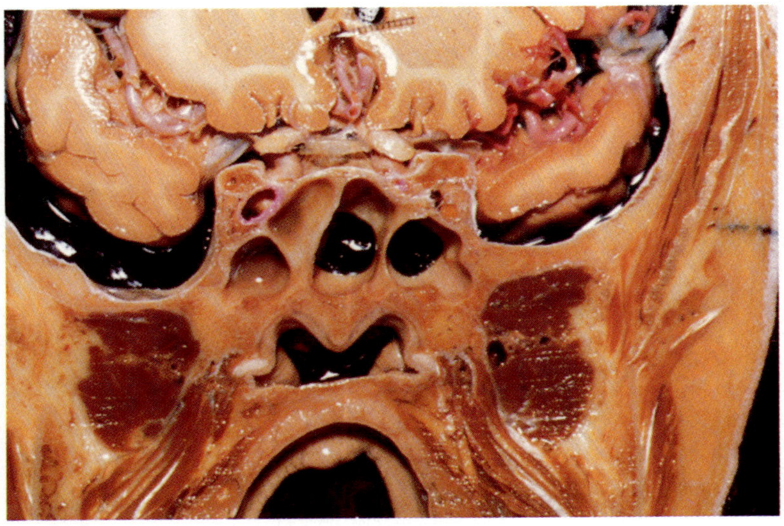

Figure 8. Cadaver dissection showing the anatomical relations in the sellar region with demonstration of cranial nerves III, IV, and VI lateral to the internal carotid arteries.

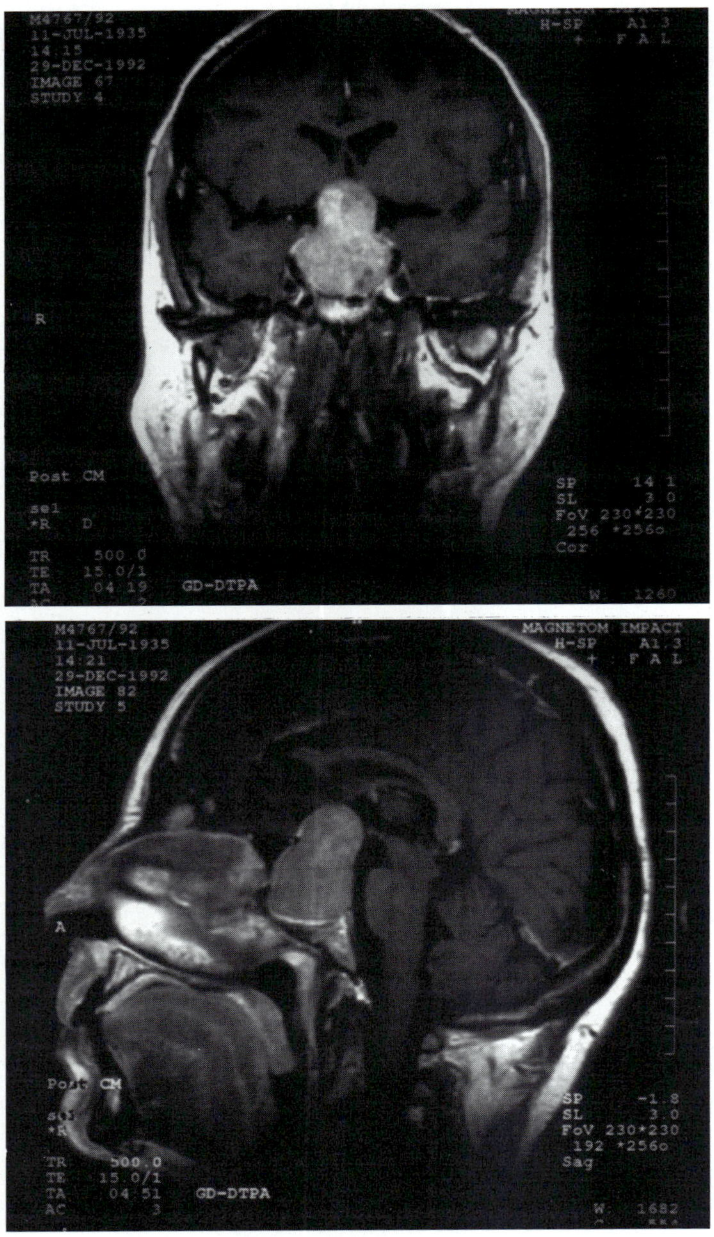

Figure 9. MRI scan images showing suprasellar and intrasellar extension of a large pituitary adenoma.

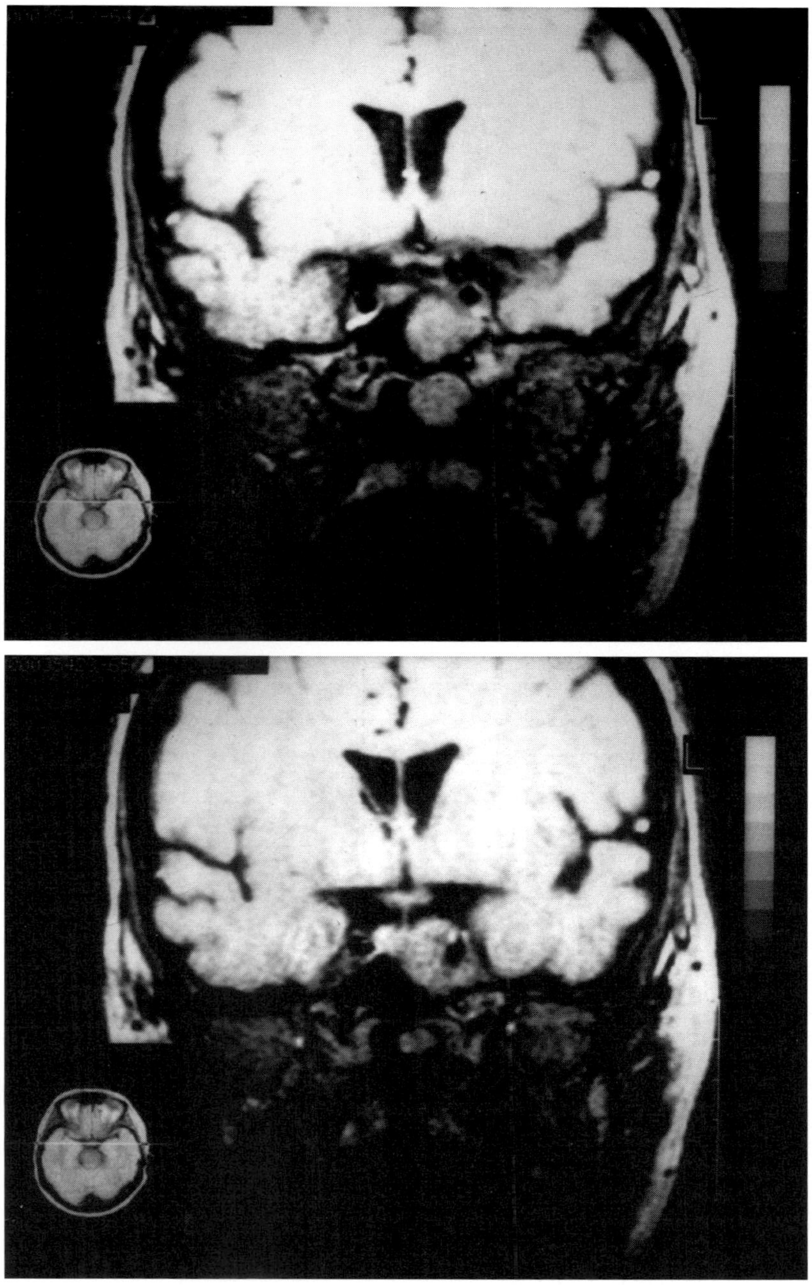

Figure 10. MRI scan images showing an intrasellar pituitary adenoma with lateral extension to involve the left cavernous sinus. The carotid artery is displaced laterally and surrounded by tumor.

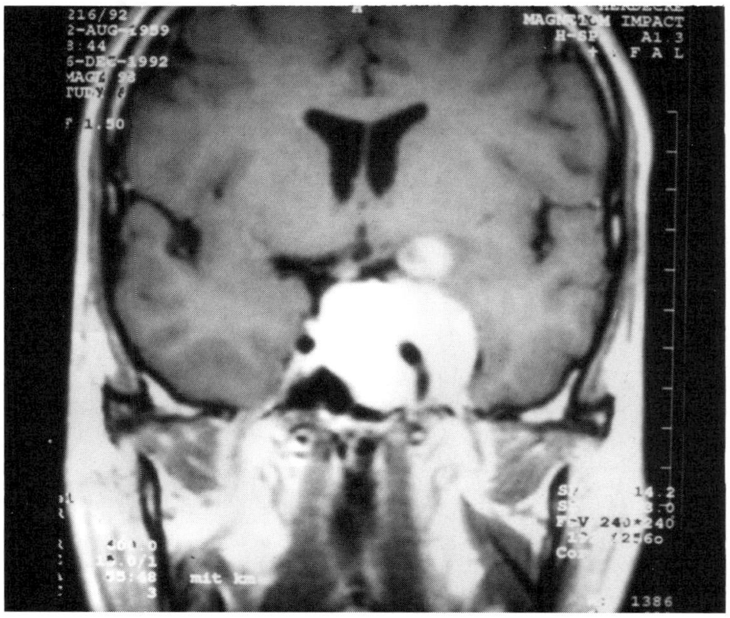

Figure 11. MRI scan image showing a large pituitary adenoma extending far lateral into the cavernous sinus, engulfing the internal carotid artery, with much of the tumor mass lateral to the artery.

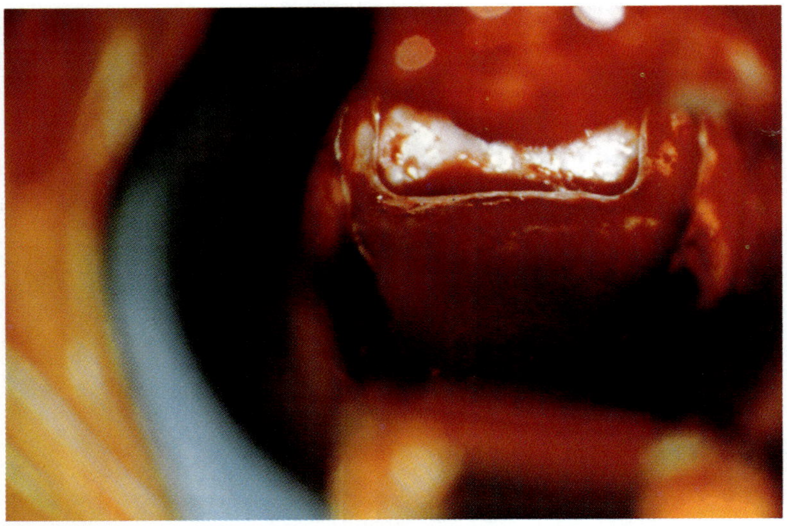

Figure 12. Transsphenoidal approach.

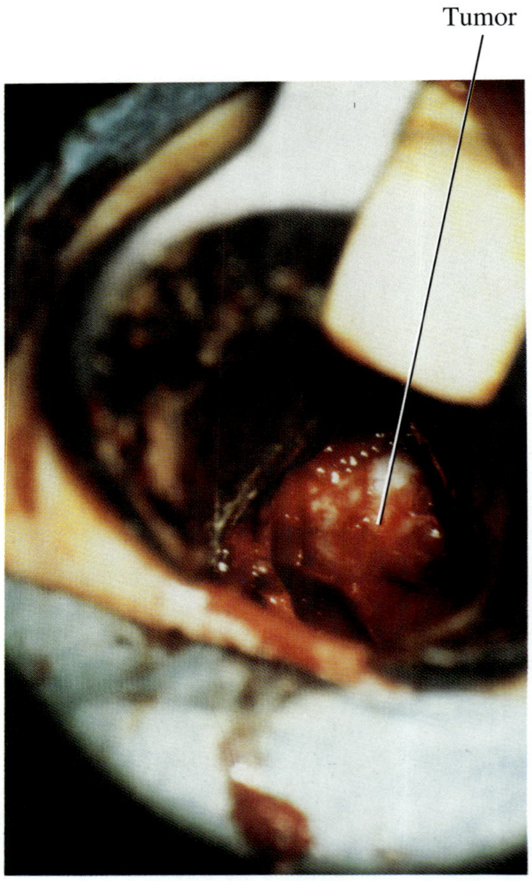

Figure 13. Transnasal paraseptal exposure of an intrasellar pituitary adenoma.

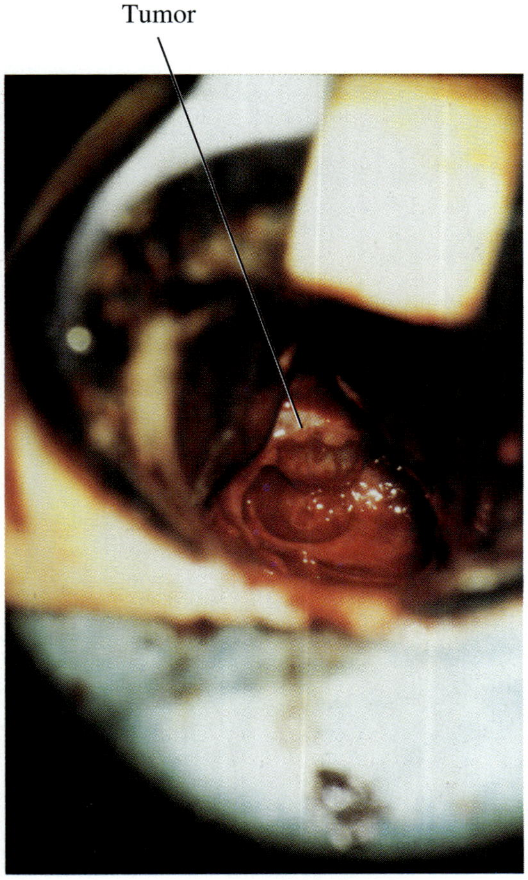

Figure 14. Pituitary tumor.

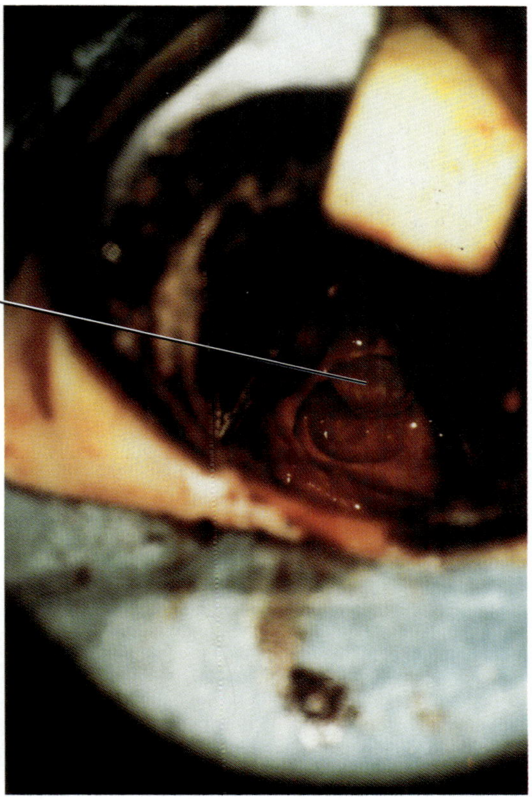

Figure 15. Total removal of tumor.

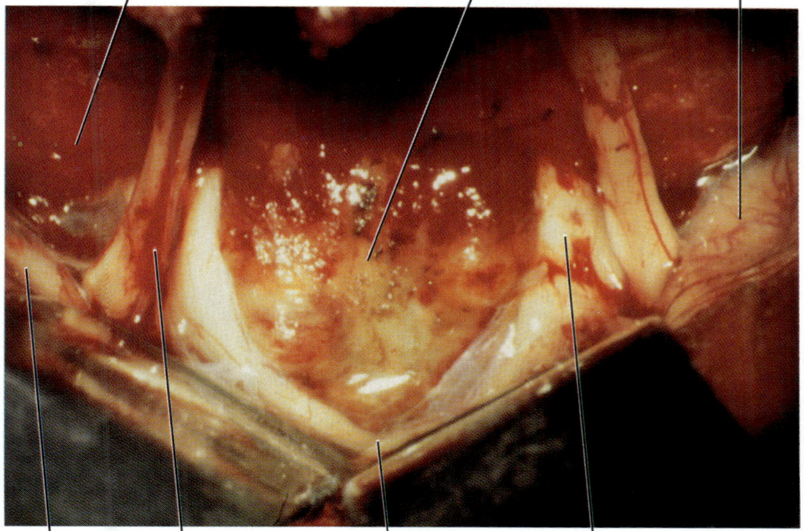

Figure 16. Large pituitary adenoma with compression of the optic nerves and chiasm, with lateral extension of tumor bilaterally to involve the carotid arteries and cavernous sinus.

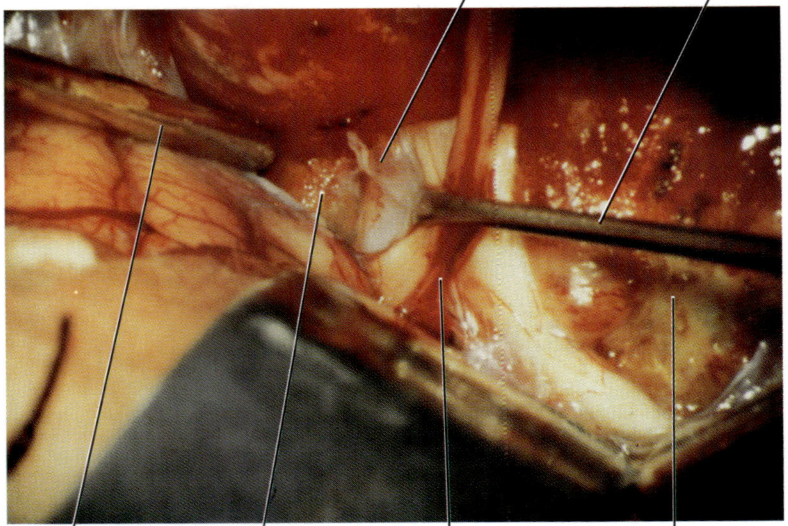

Figure 17. Same case as shown in Figure 16 demonstrating tumor extending lateral to the carotid artery.

36 Optic Glioma

Robert Alan Goldberg *and* Howard R. Krauss

INDICATIONS

Optic gliomas that are isolated to the optic nerve are sometimes an indication for surgical resection. Because this operative procedure obviously causes complete and irreversible loss of ipsilateral vision, surgical decision making in cases in which vision is retained is complex; the biologic capability of the disease process to extend intracranially must be taken into careful consideration.

POSITION

Patient positioning and initial exposure have been described previously in the chapter on transcranial approach to the orbit (Chapter 15).

OPERATIVE PROCEDURE

The bony orbital roof is removed centrally and posteriorly and the entire roof of the optic nerve canal is removed, exposing the superior portion of the optic nerve.

The intracranial optic nerve is then transected posteriorly, taking care to avoid cutting into the fibers of Willebrand's knee, the name given to the axons subtending the supratemporal visual field of the opposite eye that course anteriorly from the chiasm as far as 5 mm.

Dissection of the annulus of Zinn is then performed. The periorbita is opened superiorly over the annulus, and the periosteum is carefully teased off the fibers. CN IV is spared if desired by identifying its insertion on the superior oblique muscle and following this posteriorly as it courses across the superiormost surface of the annulus of Zinn on its way to the superior orbital fissure. It is not always possible to identify and salvage the fourth cranial nerve, and loss of the nerve creates very little cosmetic change in globe position. The optic nerve is exposed within the annulus of Zinn by dissecting through the annulus in the area between the superior rectus and medial rectus muscles. The optic nerve is tightly encased in fibrous tissues in this region, but careful dissection along the surface of the nerve will allow sparing of the cranial nerves running through the superior orbital fissure and intraconal space lateral to the optic nerve.

After the nerve is isolated in the annulus of Zinn, attention is turned to resection of the nerve from the posterior globe. The periorbita is opened anteriorly, and dissection between the superior rectus/levator complex and medial rectus reveals the optic nerve near its insertion to the globe. Malleable retractors protecting neurosurgical cottonoids are used to retract the orbital fat while the optic nerve is dissected from the loose tissues that surround it in the retrobulbar space. The nerve is transected several millimeters posterior to the globe, and traction sutures are placed in the nerve for hemostasis and traction. The nerve is then carefully lifted as it is dissected posteriorly. The ciliary ganglion lies on the lateral aspect of the nerve, and careful dissection can spare the ciliary ganglion, thus preserving sensorimotor innervation to the globe. As the optic nerve is lifted out of the orbital apex, residual inferior fibrous tissues can be lysed, again with care taken to employ meticulous dissection so that the cranial nerves running through the orbital apex may be spared. Bleeding of the ophthalmic artery within the optic canal and apex can be controlled with bipolar cautery. The optic nerve is lifted out of the optic canal and then the intracranial segment can easily be pulled forward, resulting in en bloc resection of the entire segment of intracranial and orbital optic nerve.

CLOSURE

Closure is as described in the previous section on intracranial orbitotomy; if desired, the bony orbital roof can be reconstructed using portions of the inner table of the craniotomy flap, although unless the bony resection has been extensive, reconstruction of the bony roof is generally unnecessary.

RECOMMENDED READING

Alvord, E., Lofton, S.: Gliomas of the optic nerve or chiasm. Outcome by patient's age, tumor site, and treatment. J. Neurosurg. 68:85–98, 1988.

Dutton, J.: Optic nerve gliomas and meningiomas. Neuro. Clin. 9:163–177, 1991.

Housepian, E.: Microsurgical anatomy of the orbital apex and principles of transcranial orbital exploration. Clin. Neurosurg. 25:556–573, 1978.

Hoyt, W., Baghdassarian, S.: Optic glioma of childhood. Br. J. Ophthalmol. 53:793–798, 1969.

Imes, R., Hoyt, W.: Childhood chiasmal gliomas: update on the fate of patients in the 1969 San Francisco study. Br. J. Ophthalmol. 70:179–182, 1986.

Tumor spread in unilateral optic glioma. Study report No. 2. North American Study Group for Optic Glioma. Neurofibromatosis 2:195–203, 1989.

Wright, J., McNab, A., McDonald, W.: Optic nerve glioma and the management of optic nerve tumours in the young. Br. J. Ophthalmol. 73:967–974, 1989.

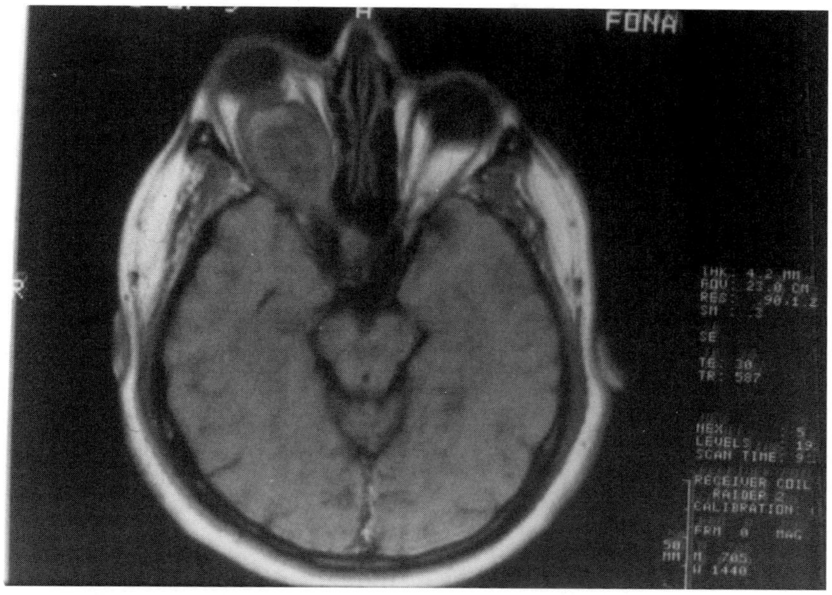

Figure 1. Noncontrast MRI image of a large right optic glioma extending through the optic canal.

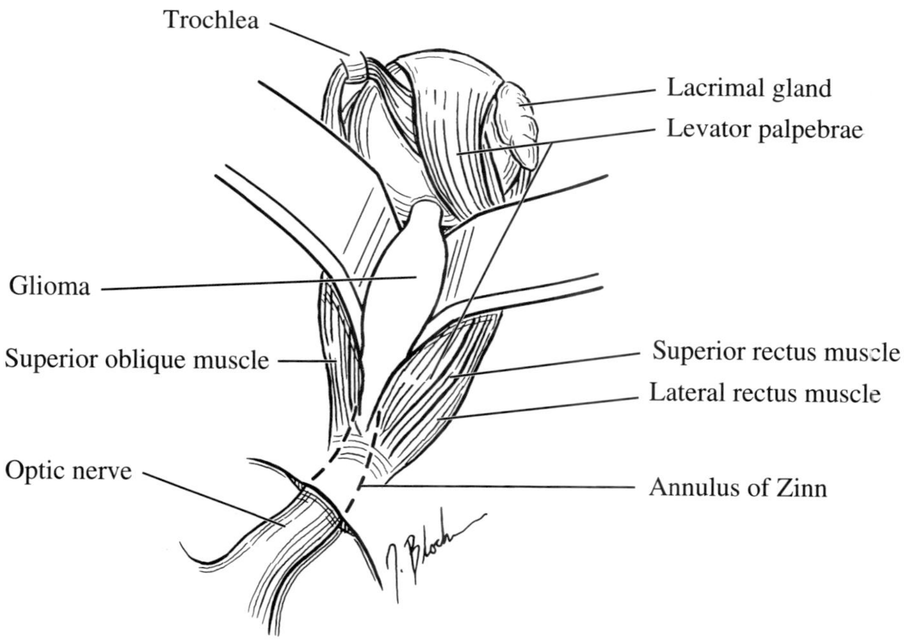

Figure 2. Anatomical relationships in a case of optic nerve glioma.

37 Esthesioneuroblastoma

Esthesioneuroblastomas are rare tumors that arise from the olfactory mucosa. Of primitive neuroectodermal origin, they probably derive from the neuroepithelial sensory cells, although other origins, such as basal or sustentacular cells of the olfactory mucosa, have been suggested. They are malignant tumors which are locally invasive, but distant metastasis (especially to the lungs) has been reported. Local metastasis does occur in as many as 40 per cent of cases. It is the extensive local invasion, histologically characterized by many small tumor nodules (Figure 1), that makes complete removal of these tumors difficult and that leads to the high likelihood of recurrence.

ANATOMICAL CONSIDERATIONS

Because these tumors begin their growth within the nasal cavity and paranasal sinuses, they initially cause nasal obstruction. Recurrent epistaxis and pain are frequent presenting signs. Growth into the orbit produces proptosis and visual signs, sometimes progressing to blindness.

The proximity of the cribriform plate to the point of origin of esthesioneuroblastomas offers the tumor easy access to the floor of the anterior fossa and intracranial expansion. With this extension of tumor, headache is experienced as dural and brain involvement progressively occur.

Esthesioneuroblastomas have been classified by Kadish in terms of anatomical location and extent of growth. Group A relates to those tumors that are confined to the nasal cavity. In group B are those tumors that extend to the paranasal sinuses. Tumors that extend beyond these limits are categorized as group C tumors.

PATHOLOGICAL CONSIDERATIONS

Grossly, these tumors are smooth, soft, and reddish to gray. They are locally invasive and may metastasize regionally or distally, often to the lungs. If not completely removed, they tend to recur.

SURGICAL TREATMENT

Biopsy followed by surgical excision and subsequent radiation therapy is the treatment of choice for these malignant but slow-growing, usually radiosensitive tumors. Some benefit from chemotherapy has been reported in the literature.

For tumors that do not extend intracranially, excision has been carried out by some authors through a transfacial approach only. The tumor mass is exposed through a lateral rhinotomy and ethmoidectomy with a medial maxillectomy, if required. These exposures are outlined in Chapter 19. With intracranial tumor extension, a transfrontal-transbasal approach has sometimes been used. With this approach, the intracranial portion of the tumor can be removed, the cribriform plate and crista gali resected, but the access to the paranasal sinuses is limited. We prefer a combination of a bifrontal craniotomy with a transfacial approach for all types of tumor. Since even small esthesioneuroblastomas frequently show microscopic infiltration of cribriform plate and olfactory nerve, resection of these structures from above must be performed in order to achieve total tumor removal. Similarly, with the transfrontal-transbasal approach only, one cannot visualize the entire paranasal sinuses and thus the risk of remaining tumor may be very high. When both approaches are combined, an en bloc tumor resection is more likely to be carried out; therefore, this should be the procedure of choice.

An example of an esthesioneuroblastoma is demonstrated by magnetic resonance imaging (MRI) scans in Figure 2. This tumor was removed by a combined transfrontal and transfacial approach. Figure 3 shows the planned skin incisions in anteroposterior and lateral projections. The paranasal skin incision and approach to the ethmoid and sphenoid sinuses are seen in Figure 4. Placement of the four burr holes for the transfrontal craniotomy is shown in Figure 5. In Figure 6, the dura is exposed after removal of the craniotomy bone flap.

After opening of the dura, the superior sagittal sinus is doubly ligated and then transected (Figure 7). In Figure 8, both frontal lobes are gently retracted to expose the tumor in the floor of the anterior cranial fossa. After removal of the intracranial portion of the tumor (Figure 9), en bloc resection of the involved bone structures and involved dura is done.

Figure 10 shows complete removal of the tumor, and the paranasal cavity is packed with Xeroform gauze.

The extensive nasal, ethmoidal, anterior fossa skull base defect that remains must be closed in a watertight manner by careful reconstruction. Primary dural closure is attempted, and the remaining dural defect is closed by pericranial flap (Figure 11) or by temporalis fascia or fascia lata graft. Several sutures have been placed (Figure 12), attaching the pericranial flap to the remaining dura at the planum sphenoidale and sphenoid ridge bilaterally. The flap covers the entire anterior skull base and is fixed in place with multiple sutures (Figure 13).

A watertight closure of the dura has been accomplished, as shown in Figure 14. In some cases, a bone graft taken from split cranium, split rib graft, or iliac crest is placed to bridge the bone defect.

As an alternative reconstruction, a three-layer closure consisting of dura followed by a methylmethacrylate cranioplasty plate covering the bone defect and then a flap of pericranium may be used.

Figure 15 shows the craniotomy bone plate replaced. In Figure 16*A*, the transfrontal scalp flap is shown closed, and in Figure 16*B*, the paranasal incision is similarly closed.

In those cases of esthesioneuroblastoma in which intradural growth of tumor is suspected, the operation is done with spinal drainage, and this is continued for 5 days postoperatively.

Patients are placed on antibiotics preoperatively. These are continued for 48 hours postoperatively and then discontinued.

If sacrifice of the nasolacrimal duct becomes necessary during tumor excision, lacrimal drainage can be reestablished by implantation in the buccal soft tissues.

Esthesioneuroblastomas are radiosensitive and are treated with radiation therapy postoperatively. Therapy is started as soon as primary wound healing is assured. Chemotherapy is also used in those tumors that seem to be aggressive in behavior.

COMPLICATIONS

1. Cerebrospinal fluid leak
2. Ascending infection

RECOMMENDED READING

Biller, H.F., Lawson, W., Sachdev, V.P., Som, P.: Esthesioneuroblastoma: Surgical treatment without radiation. Laryngoscope 100:1199–1201, 1990.

Dulguerov, P., Calcaterra, T.: Esthesioneuroblastoma: The UCLA experience 1970–1990. Laryngoscope 102:843–849, 1992.

Meneses, M.S., Thurel, C., Mikol, J., et al.: Esthesioneuroblastoma with intracranial extension. Neurosurgery 27:813–820, 1990.

Sullivan, J.M., Hahn, F.J.: Esthesioneuroblastoma (olfactory neuroblastoma). Nebr. Med. J. 75:176–178, 1990.

Sundaresan, N., Shah, J.P.: Craniofacial resection for anterior skull base tumors. Head Neck Surg. 10:219–224, 1988.

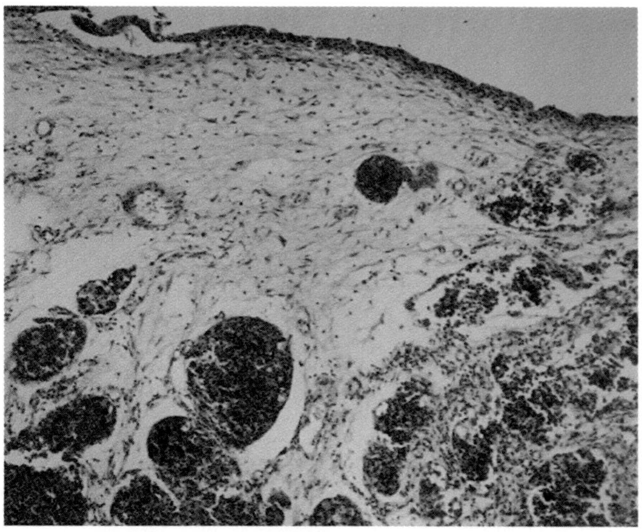

Figure 1. Nodules of esthesioneuroblastoma next to a paranasal sinus. Hematoxylin-eosin, 40×.

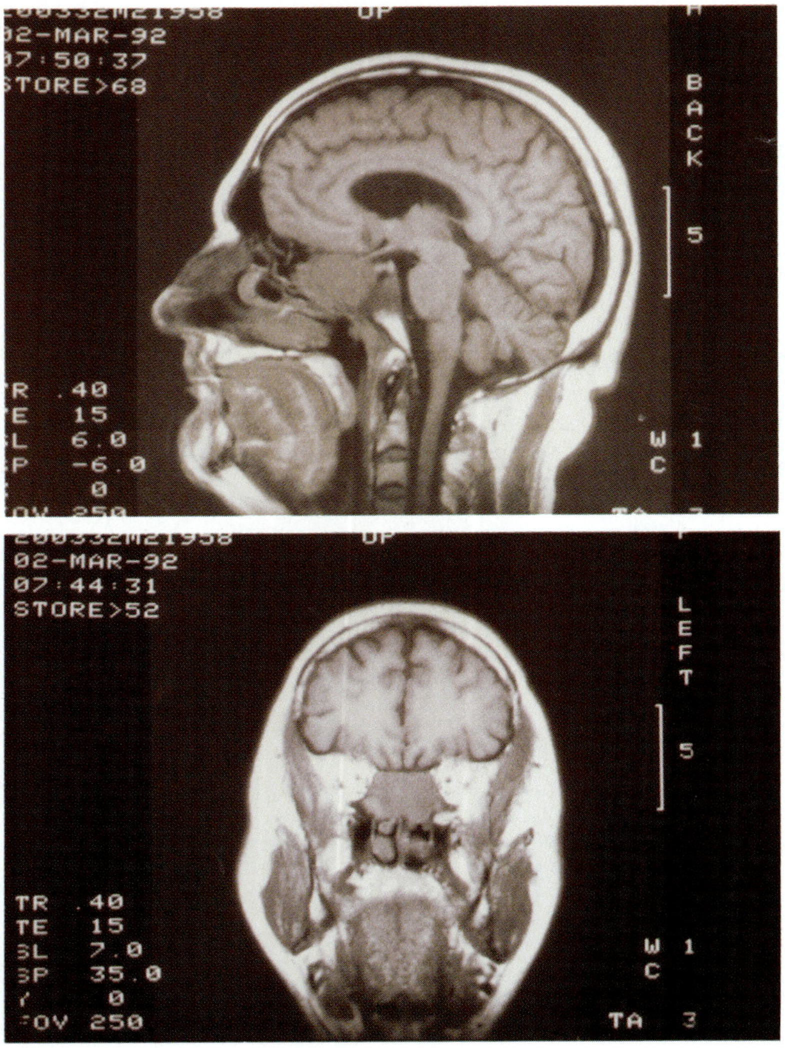

Figure 2. MRI scan images showing an esthesioneuroblastoma.

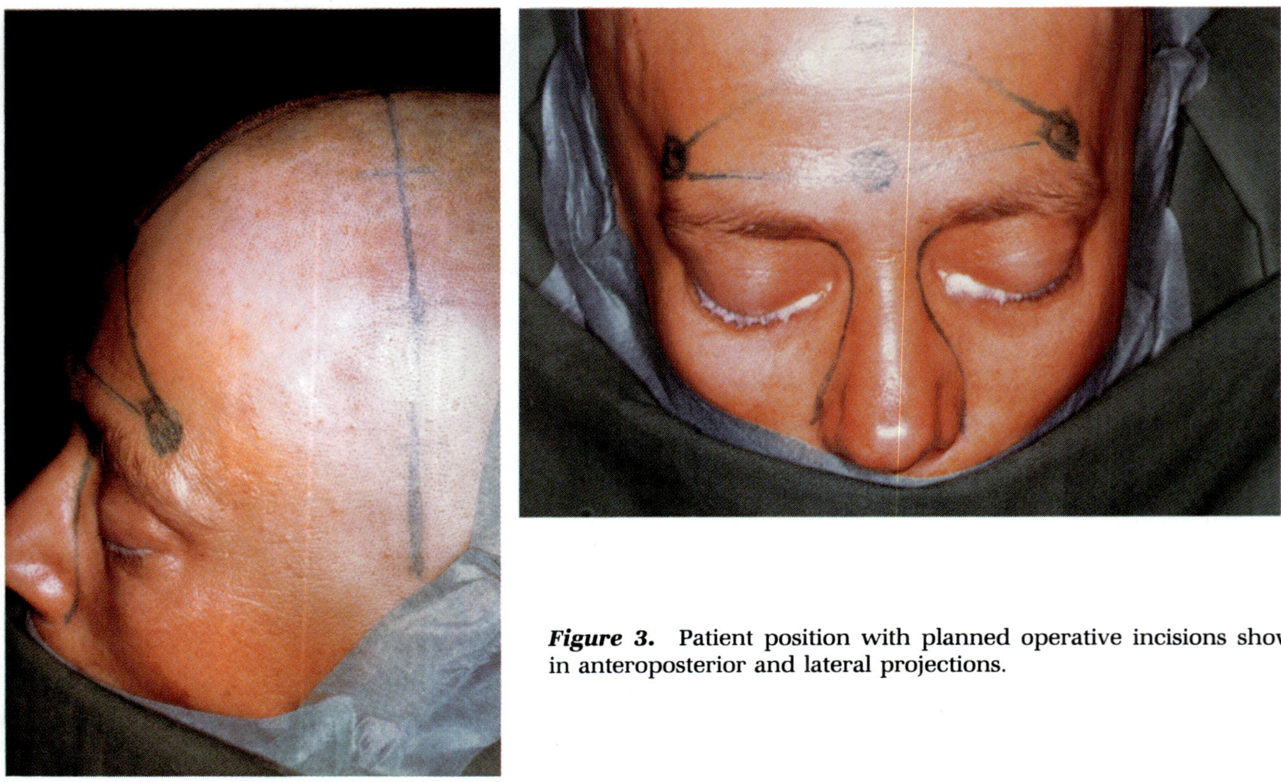

Figure 3. Patient position with planned operative incisions shown in anteroposterior and lateral projections.

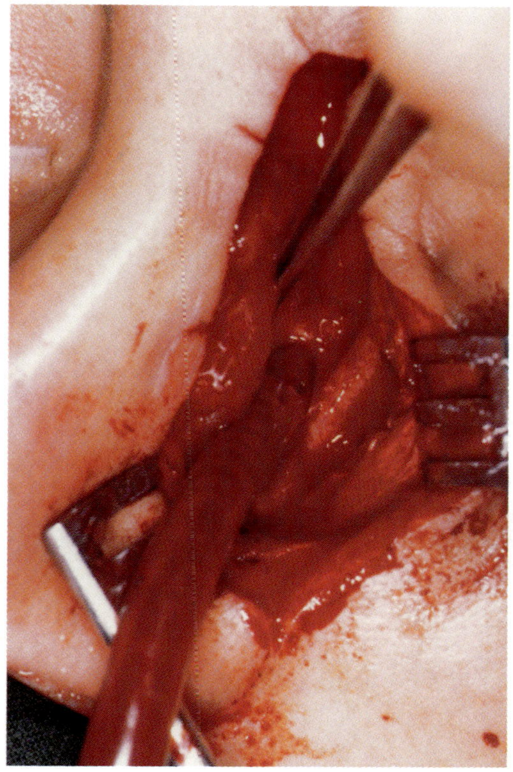

Figure 4. Paranasal skin incision and approach to the ethmoid and sphenoid sinuses for removal of the deep portion of the esthesioneuroblastoma.

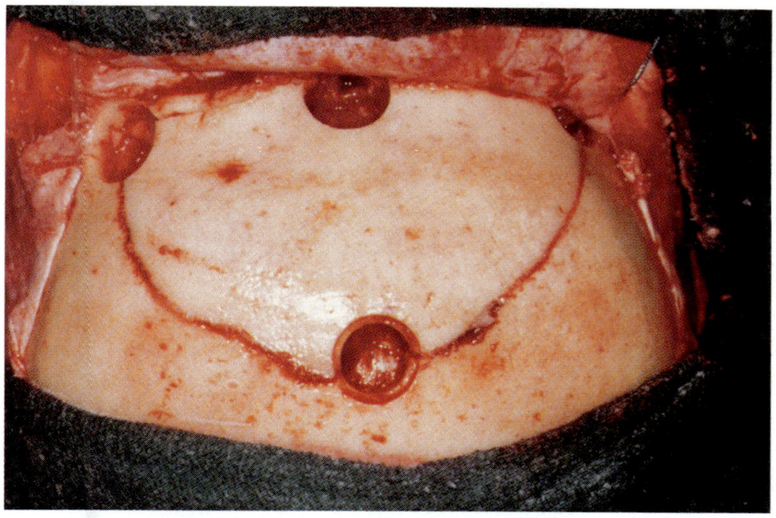

Figure 5. Burr hole placement for transfrontal craniotomy.

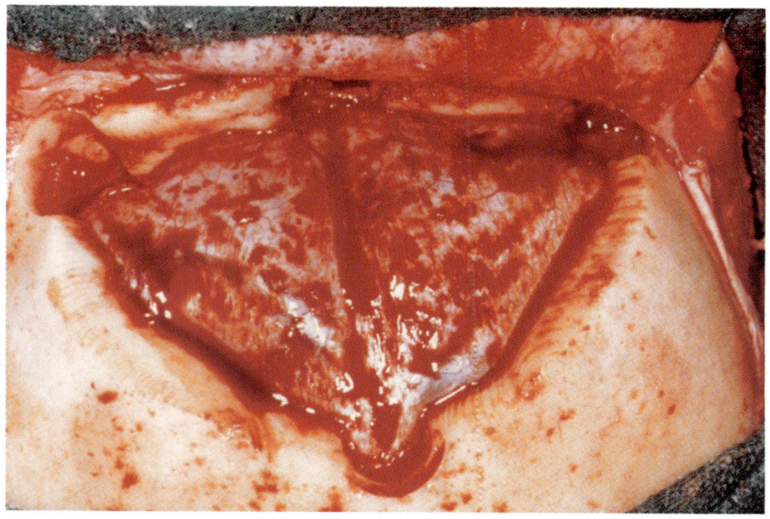

Figure 6. Dura is exposed.

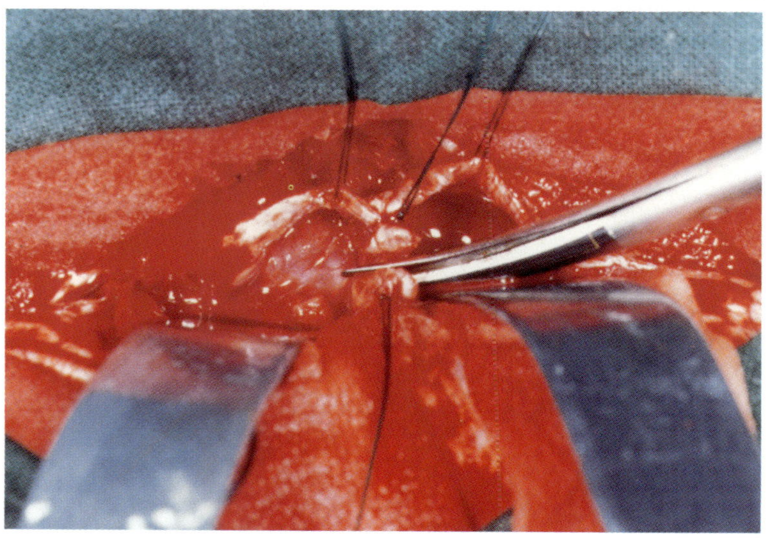

Figure 7. Dura is opened, and the superior sagittal sinus is shown doubly ligated and transected.

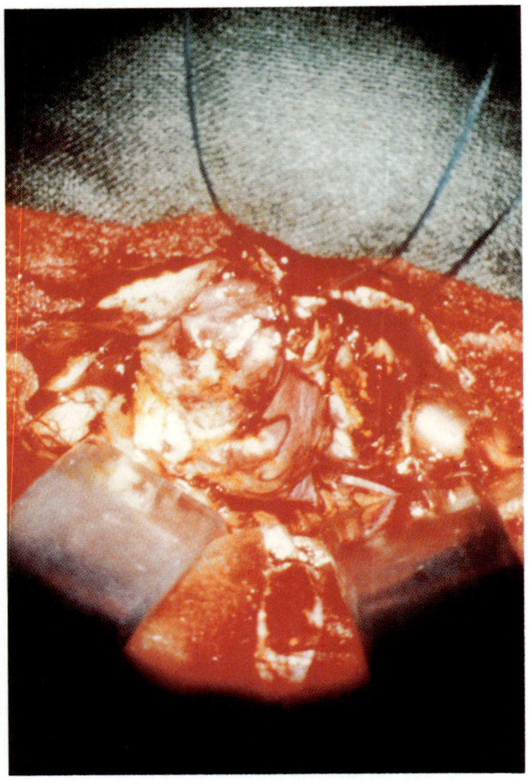

Figure 8. Both frontal lobes are gently retracted to expose the intracranial portion of the esthesioneuroblastoma.

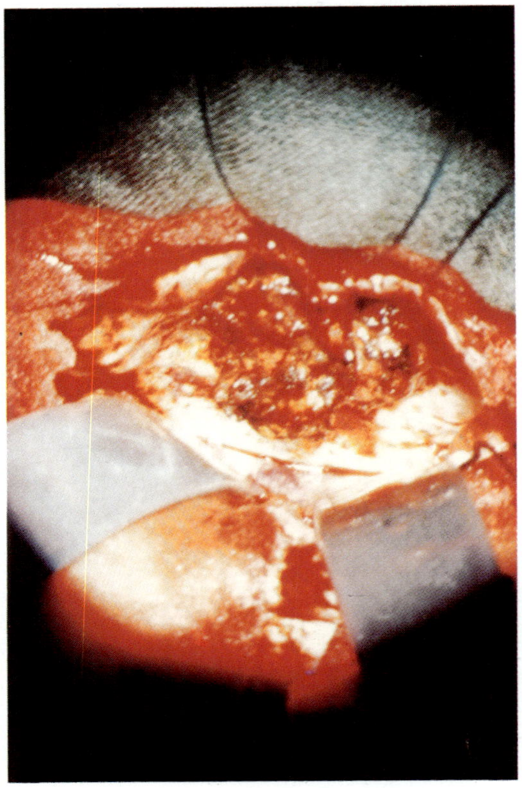

Figure 9. Intracranial tumor removed and en bloc resection of the involved bone structures and involved dura.

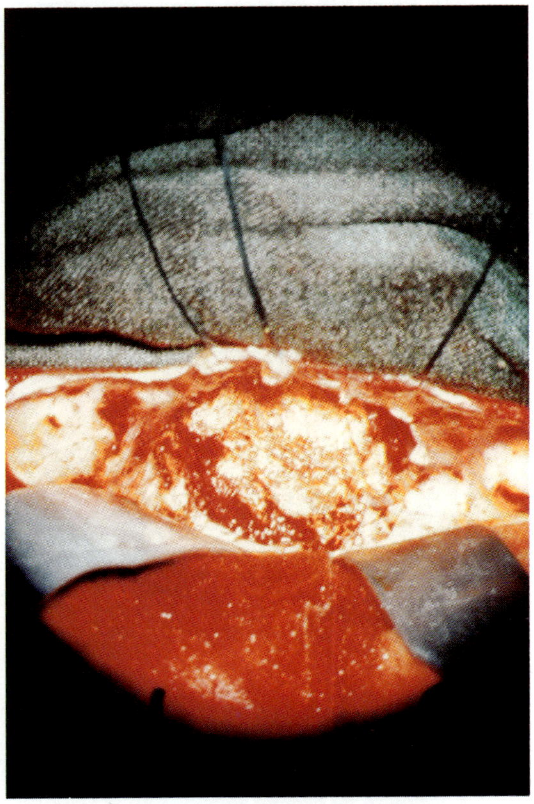

Figure 10. Complete removal of the tumor with packing of paranasal cavity with Xeroform gauze.

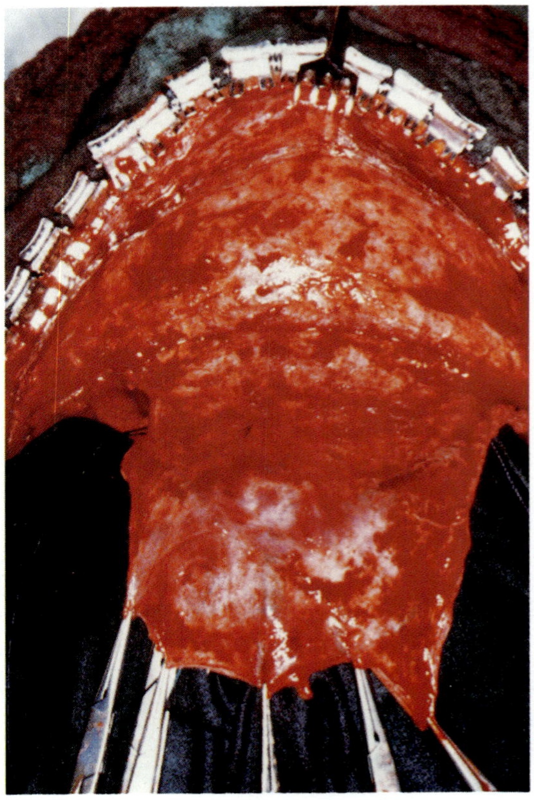

Figure 11. Dural closure with use of pericranial flap.

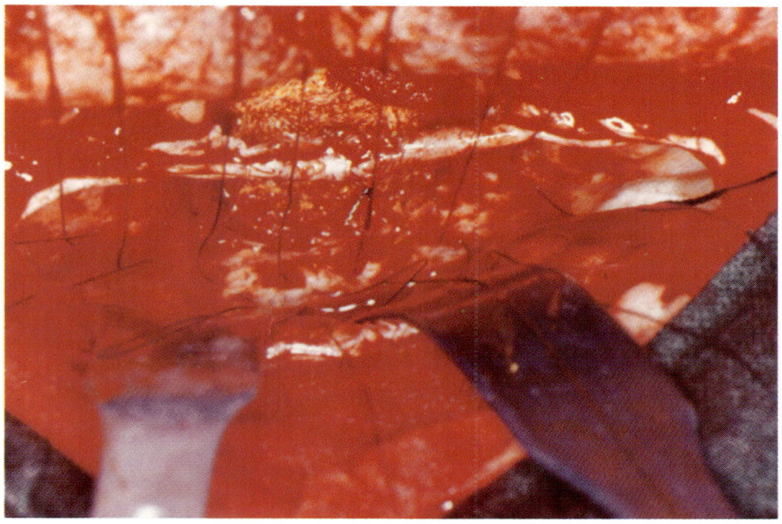

Figure 12. Placement of several sutures to attach the pericranial flap to the remaining dura of the planum sphenoidale and sphenoid ridge bilaterally.

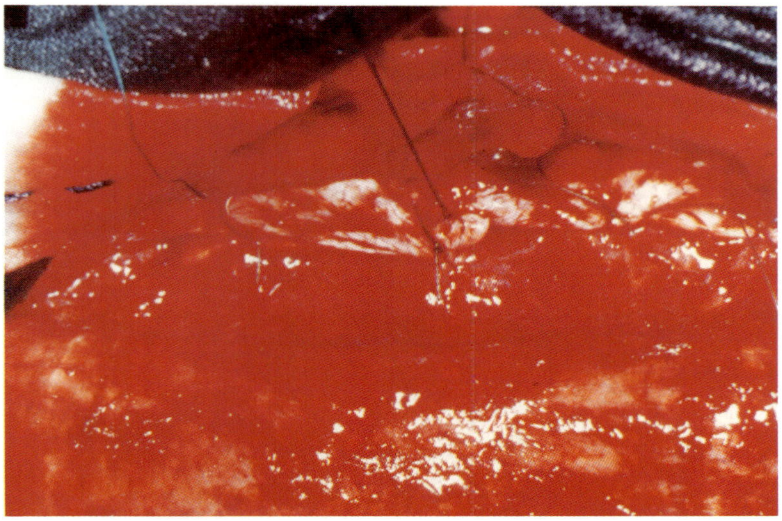

Figure 13. Pericranial flap covering the entire anterior skull base, fixed in place with multiple sutures.

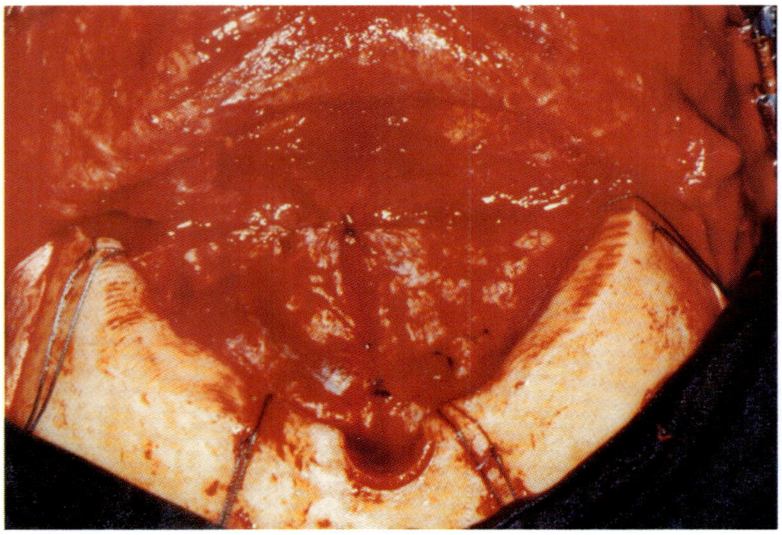

Figure 14. Watertight closure of the dura.

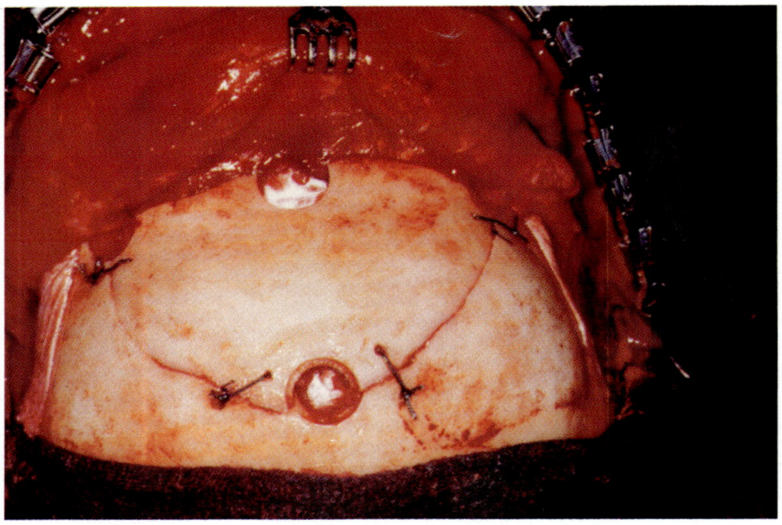

Figure 15. Craniotomy bone plate replaced.

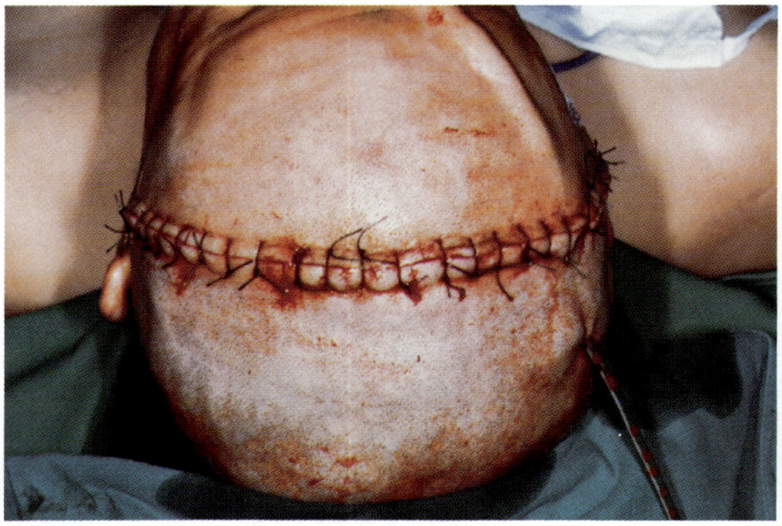

A

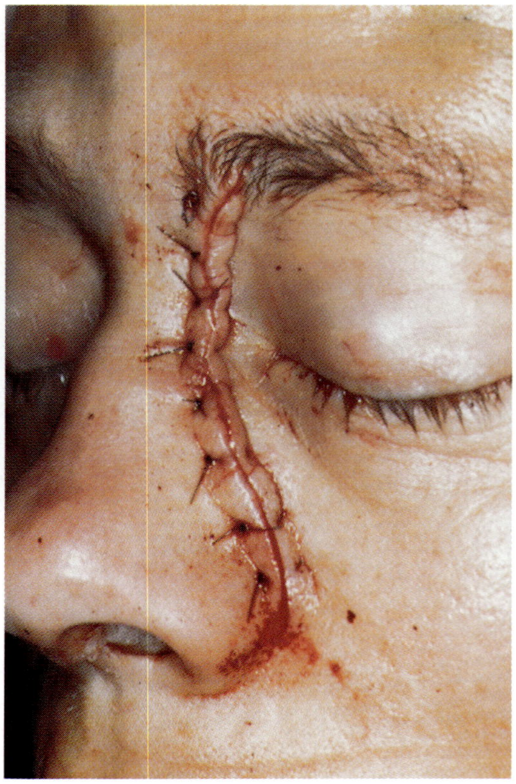

B

Figure 16

A. Transfrontal scalp flap shown closed.

B. Paranasal skin incision shown closed.

38 Juvenile Nasopharyngeal Angiofibroma

INCIDENCE

Juvenile nasopharyngeal angiofibromas are highly vascular fibrous tumors that originate in the region of the sphenopalatine foramen and grow beneath the nasopharyngeal mucosa (Figure 1). In most cases, the tumor extends aggressively into adjoining sinuses with destruction of bone, although it is histologically benign. The tumors are rare and occur exclusively in the nasopharynx. Almost all cases are seen in adolescent boys, who present with symptoms of nasal congestion and recurrent episodes of epistaxis. Cases have been reported in adults, male and female, so that nasopharyngeal angiofibroma without the attribute *juvenile* seems to be a more appropriate term.

ANATOMICAL CONSIDERATIONS

Most juvenile nasopharyngeal angiofibromas arise in the region of the hamulus of the pterygoid process and follow a path of least resistance as they grow. Even though benign, they tend to grow into the nasal cavities and they then extend into the skull base recesses, the infratemporal fossa, the orbit, and the sphenoid sinus. When large, they may cause proptosis or ocular displacement with visual impairment and displace the soft palate downward. They may extend into the cavernous sinus and sphenoid sinus and grow intracranially after eroding the floor of the temporal fossa. Even with such extension, these tumors remain extradural.

DIAGNOSIS

Tumor mass can be visualized by magnetic resonance imaging (MRI) and the extent of bony erosion can be determined by computed tomography (CT). Figure 2 shows axial MRI images of a nasopharyngeal angiofibroma demonstrating typical location of these tumors with remodeling of the walls of the maxillary sinus but also with superior extension into the cavernous sinus and orbital apex. Figure 3*A* shows the same tumor as seen by CT, and Figure 3*B* shows the extensive destruction of the floor of the middle fossa as seen on the bone window CT scan image.

Cerebral arteriography must be relied on to define the blood supply to these highly vascular tumors. Although the internal maxillary artery is the main feeder, tumor supply can be from the internal carotid artery as well as from the external carotid and the vertebral circulations. Preoperative superselective angiography is necessary to evaluate the blood flow, and associated embolization is helpful in reducing bleeding during surgical excision of these tumors.

Figure 4*A* shows a selective external carotid arteriogram that demonstrates the typical intense angiographic stain of an angiofibroma. The tumor is seen to be fed by several branches of the external carotid artery but primarily by the internal maxillary artery. Figure 4*B* shows a selective left internal carotid arteriogram that demonstrates supply to the tumor within the orbital apex and the cavernous sinus region by way of the ophthalmic artery and branches of the cavernous carotid artery. Although the internal maxillary artery and the ascending pharyngeal artery are the main feeders, the meningeal and ophthalmic branches of the internal carotid artery may also supply these tumors.

The treatment of choice for these tumors is surgical removal, although postoperative irradiation may be helpful for residual tumor.

OPERATION

The objective in the removal of these tumors, as in all cranial base tumors, is total excision, if feasible. Further, the objective is to accomplish the surgical procedure with as little blood loss as possible. This is accomplished by extensive preoperative embolization. During surgery, it is important to achieve control of the internal maxillary artery as early in the procedure as possible.

Juvenile angiofibromas of the nasopharyngeal region may be excised through various skull base surgical approaches. For those rare tumors that are primarily displacing the soft palate and presenting into the oral pharynx, a transpalatal approach may be used. This approach is limited in access to the orbits, paranasal sinuses, and skull base.

The transmaxillary-transethmoidal approach offers good access to the nasal cavity, anterior portion of the infratemporal fossa, and inferior orbital fissure (see Chapter 19). For larger tumors that have not eroded through the skull base, a completely extracranial approach is recommended. Use of exposures that enter the cranium is rarely indicated in the excision of nasopharyngeal angiofibromas because intracranial extension so seldom occurs. When it does occur, it is because the tumor has eroded through the skull base but primarily remains extradural.

In Figure 5, the nasopharyngeal angiofibroma that has been demonstrated by diagnostic studies in Figures 2 through 4 is shown intraoperatively. Figure 6 shows partial removal of the tumor, and in Figure 7, the tumor bed is visualized after complete tumor removal. A postoperative CT scan (Figure 8) shows no evidence of residual tumor.

RECOMMENDED READING

Bremer, J.W., Neel, H.B., De Santo, L.W.: Angiofibroma treatment trends in 150 patients during 40 years. Laryngoscope 96:1321–1329, 1986.

Economou, T.S., Abemayor, E., Ward, P.H.: Juvenile angiofibroma. Laryngoscope 98:170–175, 1988.

Piquet, J.J., Chevalier, D.: Surgical treatment of angiofibromas of the nasopharynx—34 cases. Rhinology 27:149–154, 1989.

Samii, M., Draf, W.: Surgery of the Skull Base: An Interdisciplinary Approach. New York: Springer-Verlag, 1989.

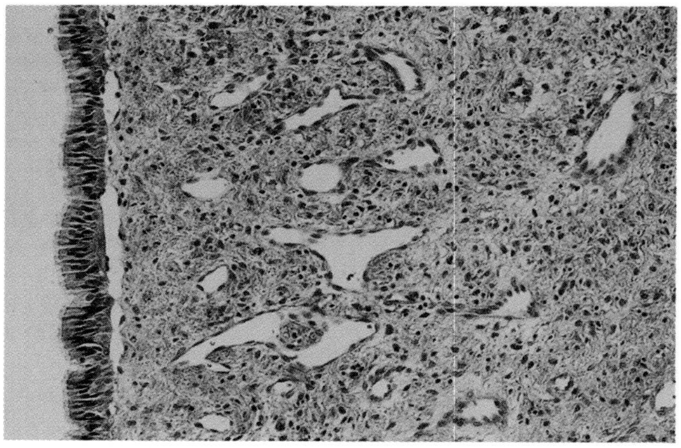

Figure 1. Nasopharyngeal angiofibroma showing a fibromatous tissue with thin-walled vessels of different caliber. Masson-trichrome, 150×.

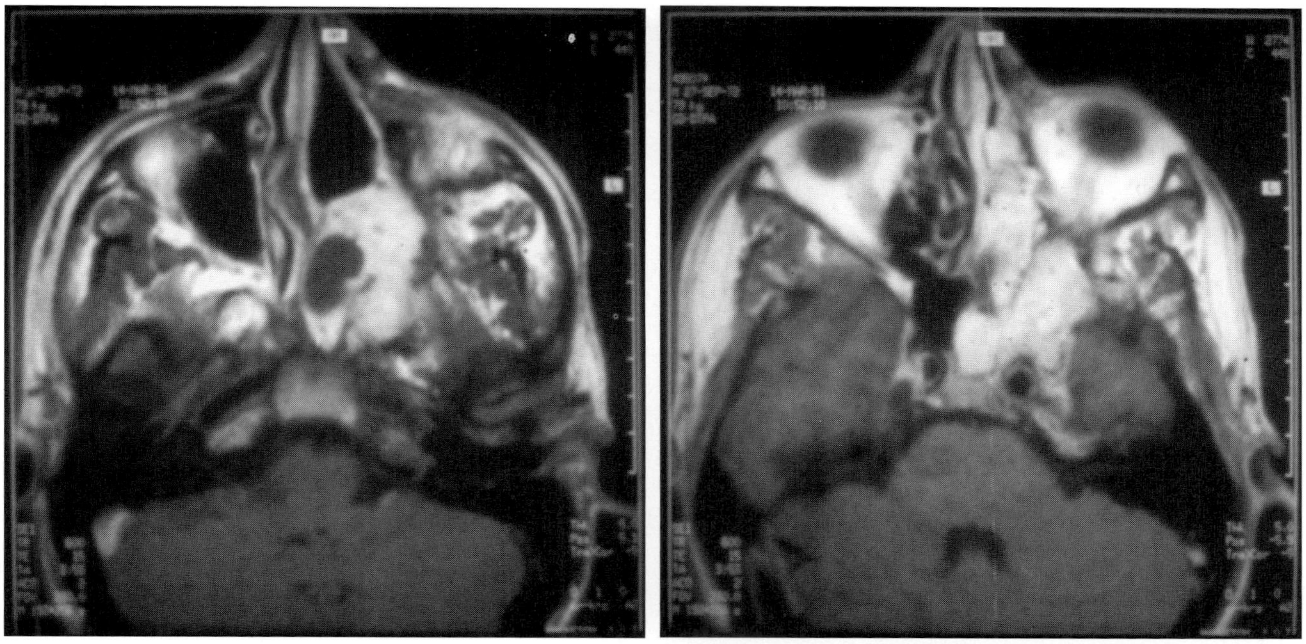

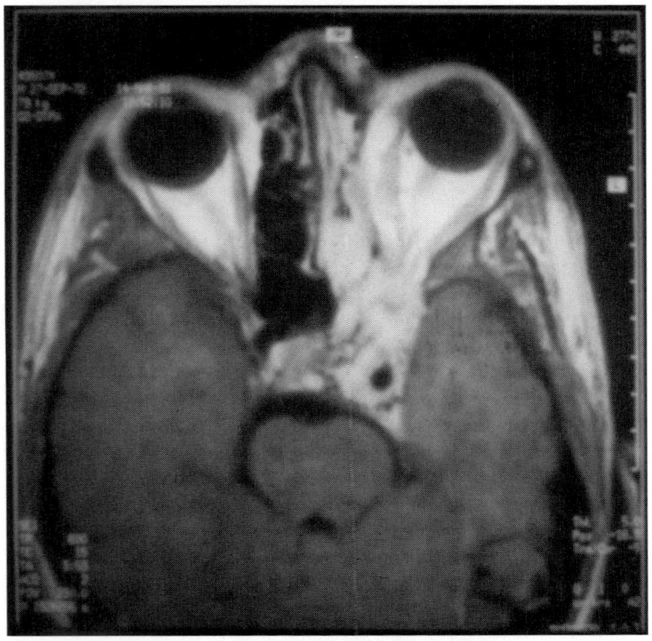

Figure 2. T_1-weighted axial MRI images of a nasopharyngeal angiofibroma showing typical location with remodeling of the walls of the maxillary sinus.

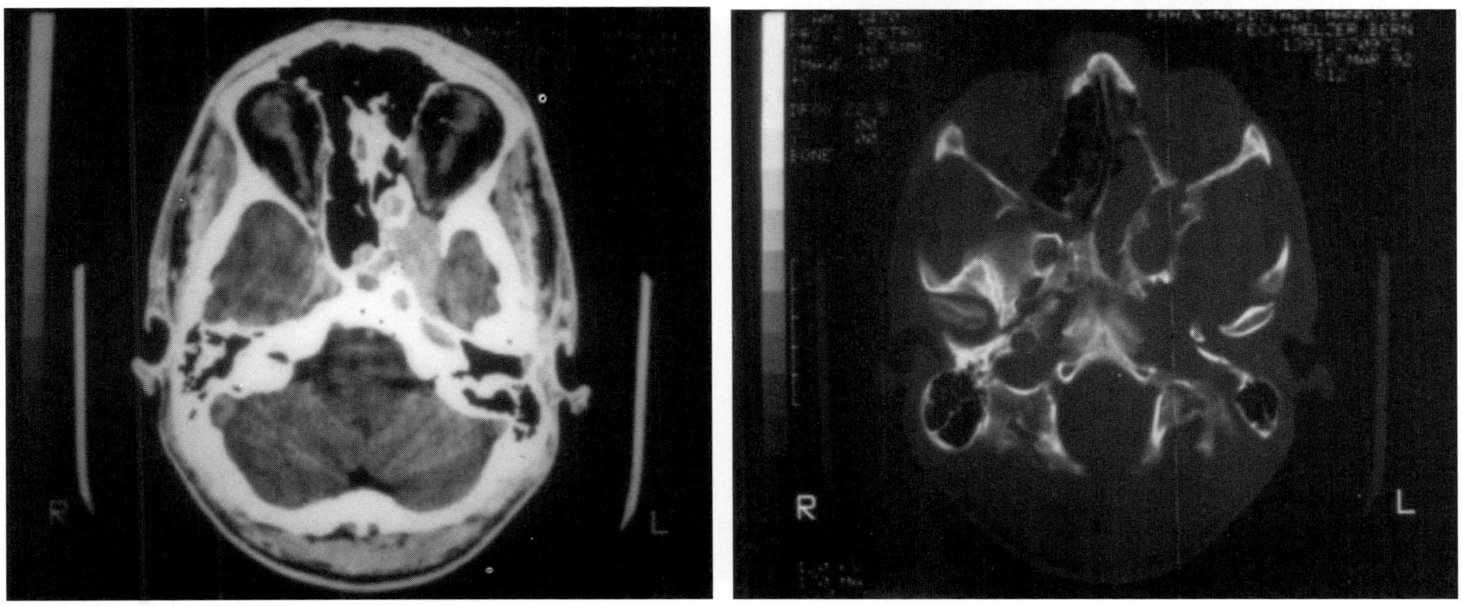

A B

Figure 3.

A. Same tumor as seen on CT scan image.

B. Same tumor with CT bone window image showing extensive bone destruction of the floor of the middle fossa.

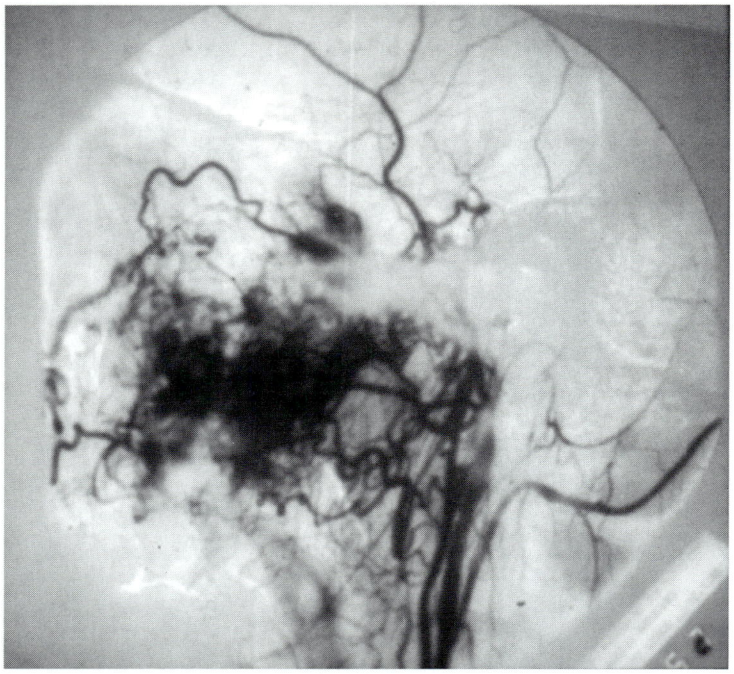

A

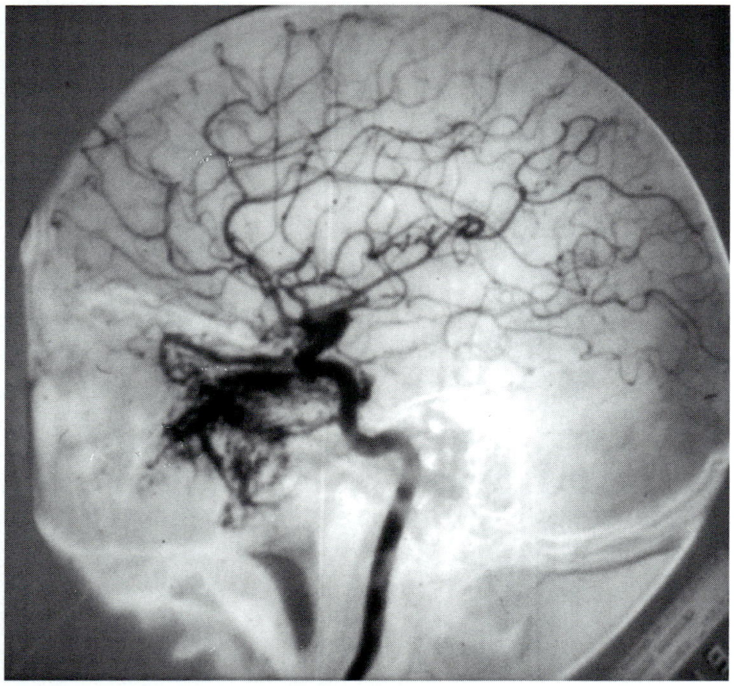

B

Figure 4.

A. Selective external carotid arteriogram demonstrating typical intense angiographic stain of an angiofibroma fed by several branches of the external carotid artery but primarily by the internal maxillary artery.

B. Selective left internal carotid arteriogram demonstrating supply to the tumor within the orbit and the cavernous sinus region by way of the ophthalmic artery and branches of the cavernous carotid artery.

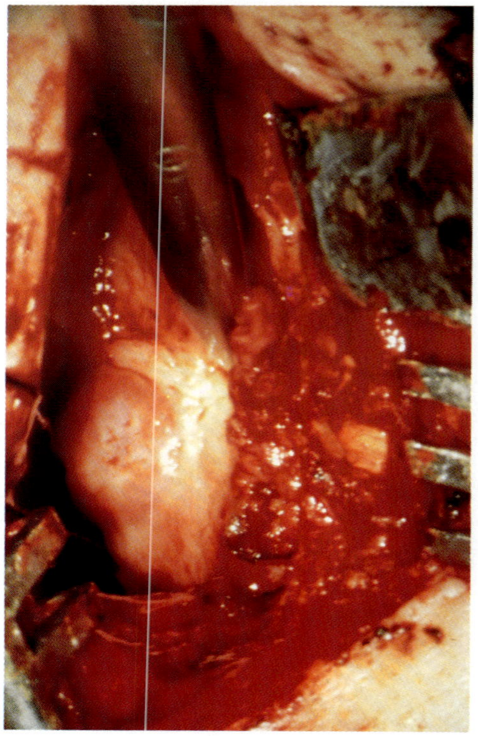

Figure 5. Juvenile nasopharyngeal neurofibroma visualized.

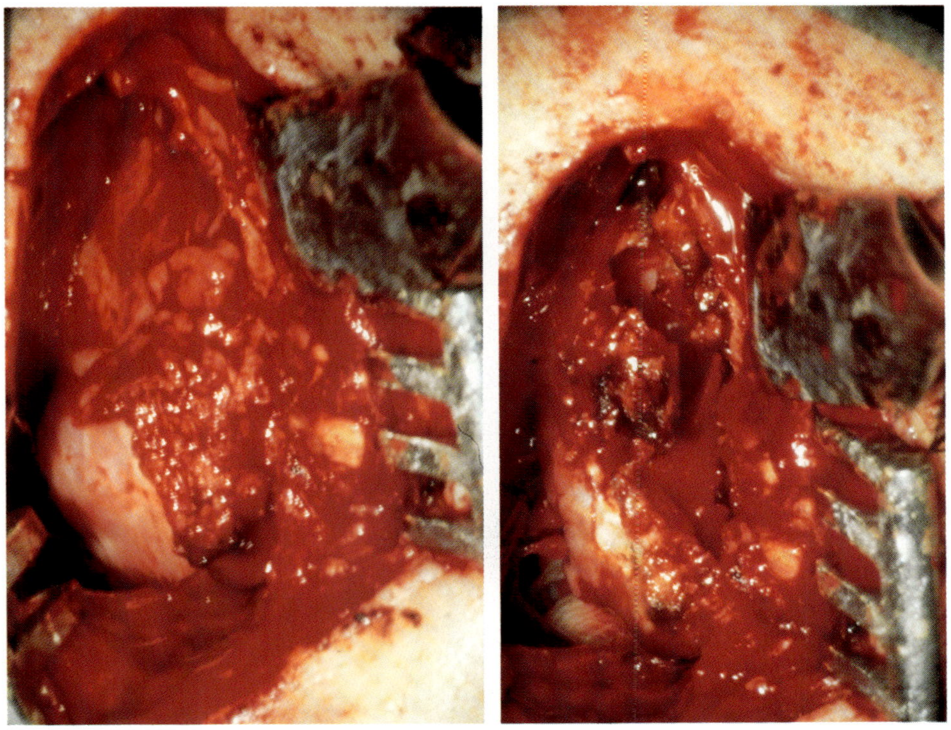

Figure 6. Partial tumor removal.

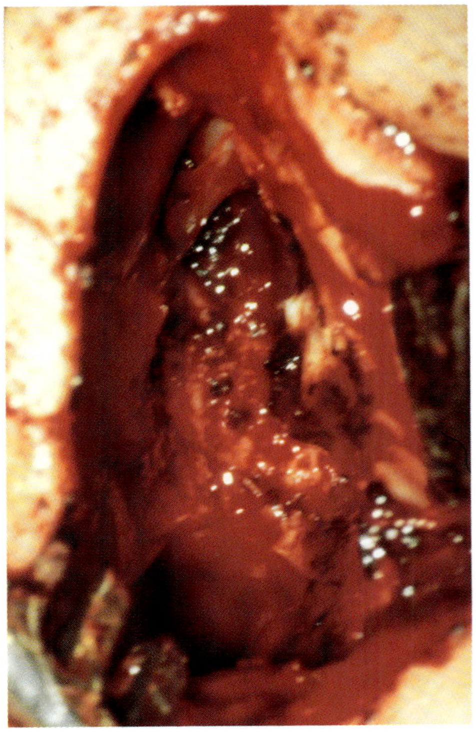

Figure 7. Tumor bed after complete tumor removal.

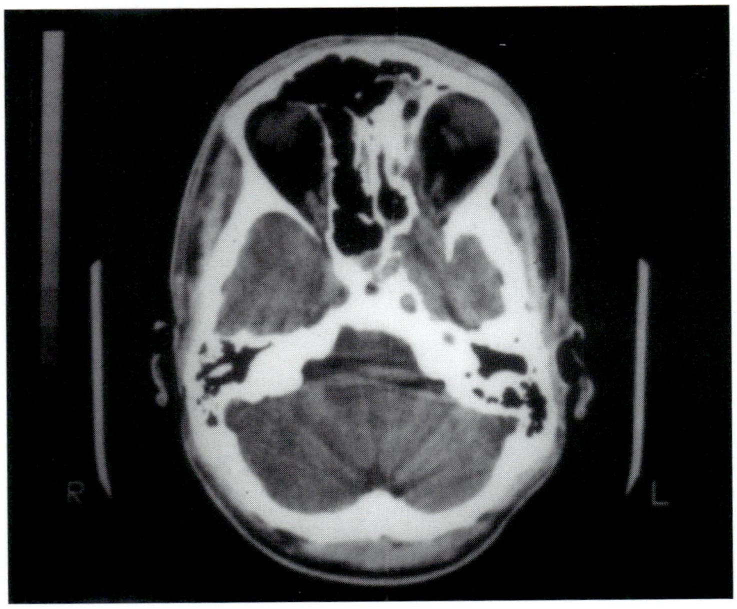

Figure 8. Postoperative CT scan showing no evidence of tumor.

IV

INTERVENTIONAL SKULL BASE NEURORADIOLOGY

Endovascular Therapy 39

Fernando Vinuela *and* Gary Duckwiler

Endovascular therapy has emerged as an important field in the preoperative evaluation and treatment of cranial base tumors and vascular lesions.

ANATOMICAL CONSIDERATIONS: BLOOD SUPPLY OF SKULL BASE

The bone and overlying meninges of the skull base receive a complex blood supply that varies from one region to another. The bone and meninges of the anterior fossa are mainly supplied by the ethmoidal and anterior falcine branches of the ophthalmic artery as well as anterior meningeal branches of the internal maxillary and middle meningeal arteries (Figure 1).

The cavernous sinus and middle fossa share a dual blood supply that originates from external and internal carotid artery circulations. Included are branches of the ophthalmic artery (recurrent meningeal artery) as well as the internal maxillary (artery of the foramen rotundum), middle meningeal, and accessory meningeal arteries (Figures 1–5). Also included are the ascending pharyngeal artery (carotid ramus) and intracavernous branches of the internal carotid artery (inferolateral and meningohypophyseal trunks; Figure 13) (Plate I).

Blood supply of the bone and the dura of the posterior cranial fossa comes from the vertebral artery (anterior and posterior meningeal arteries), ascending pharyngeal artery (hypoglossal and jugular rami; Figure 14), occipital artery (anterior condylar and transmastoid [Figure 19] branches), and the internal carotid artery (lateral and medial clivus branches; Figure 3) (Plate II).

The petrous bone and main contents (auditory apparatus and facial nerve) have a generous plexiform, interconnected blood supply that originates from several arterial sources. Included are the anterior inferior cerebellar artery (artery of the internal auditory canal; Figure 10), middle meningeal and accessory meningeal arteries (petrosal or superior tympanic branches; Figure 11), occipital artery (stylomastoid artery; Figure 12), internal maxillary artery (anterior tympanic artery), internal carotid artery (caroticotympanic artery), and ascending pharyngeal artery (inferior tympanic artery; Figure 4). The dura overlying the petrous bone shares a blood supply similar to that described for the posterior fossa and tentorium (Figure 9) (Plate III).

Blood supply to the tentorium and the tentorial incisura comes from the internal carotid artery (tentorial artery of Bernasconi and Casinari; Figure 15), middle meningeal artery (middle and lateral tentorial arteries), posterior cerebral artery (artery of Davidoff and Schechter; Figure 16), and superior cerebellar artery (Figure 17). Additional arterial supply comes from the vertebral artery (posterior and anterior meningeal arteries; Figure 18), occipital artery (transmastoid artery), and ascending pharyngeal artery (carotid and anterior condyloid rami; Figure 5).

The cranial nerves at the skull base, with the exception of I, II, and VIII, receive substantial blood supply from neuromeningeal branches of the external and internal carotid arteries as they traverse the skull base foramina. This special anatomical disposition needs to be remembered to decrease the untoward complication of cranial nerve palsies that may occur with superselective embolization of skull base vascular lesions.

The internal maxillary artery participates in the blood supply of V_2 (artery of foramen rotundum), V_3, and V_m (accessory meningeal artery) as well as cranial nerve VII (middle meningeal artery). It may also supply cranial nerves III, IV, and VI in the cavernous sinuses through anastomoses with the inferolateral trunk.

The posterior auricular artery supplies the seventh cranial nerve at the stylomastoid foramen (stylomastoid artery). This artery may also arise from the occipital artery.

The ascending pharyngeal artery supplies cranial nerves IX, X, and XI in the jugular foramen (jugular ramus) and cranial nerve XII in the hypoglossal canal (hypoglossal ramus) (Figures 8, 14).

The internal carotid artery supplies all cranial nerves in the cavernous sinus (inferolateral and meningohypophyseal trunks). The vertebral artery may participate through anastomoses in the blood supply of lower cranial nerves (anastomoses with jugular and condyloid branches of the ascending pharyngeal artery).

ENDOVASCULAR THERAPY TECHNICAL CONSIDERATIONS

Magnetic resonance imaging is used to obtain as much preliminary information as possible concerning skull base vascular pathology. The proper angiographic protocol is then selected, depending on the location of the particular skull base lesion to be studied or treated (Table 1).

In evaluating midline skull base vascular lesions or tumors, it is essential to perform bi-

TABLE 1. ANGIOGRAPHIC PROTOCOLS FOR SKULL BASE VASCULAR LESIONS

Lesions in the anterior fossa
Internal carotid angiography (bilateral)
Internal maxillary angiography (bilateral)
Lesions in the middle fossa and cavernous sinus
Internal carotid angiography
Internal maxillary angiography
Middle meningeal angiography
Ascending pharyngeal angiography
Lesions in the posterior fossa
Vertebrobasilar angiography
Occipital angiography
Ascending pharyngeal angiography
Internal carotid angiography
Lesions in the petrous bone
Internal carotid angiography
Internal maxillary angiography
Middle meningeal angiography
Posterior auricular angiography
Ascending pharyngeal angiography
Occipital angiography
Lesions in the tentorium and tentorial edge
Internal carotid angiography
Vertebral angiography
Middle meningeal angiography
Ascending pharyngeal angiography
Occipital angiography

lateral angiography because of the generous dural anastomotic channels. These channels tend to extend across the midline, with contributions from different vascular territories.

SUPERSELECTIVE ANGIOGRAPHY

The development of new generations of microcatheters has dramatically increased the safety of extracranial and intracranial superselective catheterizations of third- and fourth-generation arteries. Microcatheters may be divided into geometry-directed and flow-directed. Their selection is based on the anatomical and dynamic characteristics of the lesion to be embolized. With superselective angiography, the identification of individual feeders to a vascular tumor or malformation is possible. The categorization of the angioarchitecture of the lesion to be embolized can be determined. Finally, the analysis of hemodynamic balance between the lesion and potential anastomotic channels with normal intracranial or extracranial vasculature can be identified.

By injection of amobarbital (Amytal) and lidocaine into arterial feeders, a preembolization functional provocative test can be performed.

PRETHERAPEUTIC FUNCTIONAL TESTING

Temporary Balloon Occlusion of Vessels in the Neck

Presurgical temporary balloon occlusion of internal carotid or vertebral arteries is performed when these arteries appear to be infiltrated by tumor growth at the skull base. Skull base meningiomas and paragangliomas may infiltrate the wall of the internal carotid artery, recruiting blood supply from periadventitial vessels. This is clearly demonstrated on digital angiography (Figure 13*A*). This functional test is performed in the angiography suite with the patient under neuroleptic analgesia and systemic heparinization. Using a transfemoral approach, a non-detachable balloon is inflated in the internal carotid or vertebral artery in the neck, occluding the vessel for 20 to 30 minutes. During this time, permanent electroencephalographic and clinical monitoring is performed by a neurologist. This functional test is complemented by the angiographic documentation of the circle of Willis and, in selected cases, by Xenon-CBF.

Preembolization Superselective Lidocaine and Amytal Injections

The preembolization injection of lidocaine is performed in those feeders of skull base vascular tumors or malformations that potentially may supply cranial nerves. This test appears to be particularly useful before the embolization of stylomastoid and middle meningeal arteries (potential blood supply to the facial nerve). The test elicits a temporary cranial nerve palsy that resolves within a few minutes.

The preembolization injection of Amytal plays a role in those arterial feeders that may be related to the brain or spinal cord. The skull base is an important site of numerous external carotid–internal carotid and vertebral artery anastomoses. These anastomotic channels may be the source of untoward brain or spinal cord strokes during embolization of skull base vascular lesions (dangerous anastomosis; Figures 5*B*, 6). The injection of Amytal into the brain or spinal cord elicits a temporary deficit that warns the endovascular therapist of an untoward clinical complication.

CLINICAL CONSIDERATIONS

Preoperative Embolization of Skull Base Hypervascular Tumors

PARAGANGLIOMAS

Paragangliomas arise from branchiomeric and intravagal paraganglion structures, including the carotid bodies at the bifurcation of the common carotid arteries, the glomus jugulare in the adventitia of the jugular bulb, the glomus tympanicum associated with the glossopharyngeal nerve, the vagal body in the perineurium of the vagus nerve, and the aorticopulmonary ganglia at various levels of the aortic arch.

Most paragangliomas are mainly supplied by the musculospinal branch of the ascending pharyngeal artery and not infrequently from branches of the occipital and posterior auricular arteries (Figures 12, 14). Depending on their extension, paragangliomas may infiltrate the dura, recruiting blood supply from meningeal branches of the internal carotid and vertebral arteries as well as from pial branches of the posterior inferior and anterior inferior cerebellar arteries.

Technique of Endovascular Therapy. The most common embolic agent used for the preoperative occlusion of paragangliomas is polyvinyl alcohol particles (PVA), 200 to 600 microns in diameter.

In cases of tumor infiltration of the internal carotid artery, it may be necessary to perform preoperative temporary or permanent balloon occlusion of this vessel. This maneuver is necessary in paragangliomas that infiltrate the intrapetrous or intracavernous internal carotid artery. The technique drastically reduces intraoperative blood loss, and complications remain rare.

JUVENILE NASOPHARYNGEAL ANGIOFIBROMAS

Juvenile nasopharyngeal angiofibromas are benign, highly vascular tumors that originate in the nasopharynx but may extend into the orbit, infratemporal fossa, and intracranial cavity.

The arterial supply to these tumors arises primarily from branches of the internal maxillary artery, with less frequent involvement of the facial and ascending pharyngeal arteries as well as the ethmoidal branches of the ophthalmic artery. The portion of the tumor that is attached to the skull base may recruit blood supply from the mandibulovidian branch of the internal carotid artery (Figures 7, 13*B*).

Technique of Endovascular Therapy. Embolization is performed immediately before surgery under local anesthesia and in the angiography suite. PVA, 300 to 600 microns in diameter, is the most popular embolic material used, and at the end of the embolization, the trunk of the arterial feeder is occluded with coils or absorbable gelatin sponge (Gelfoam) pellets. The last maneuver avoids early tumor recanalization through local arterial collaterals.

Not infrequently it is necessary to embolize both the internal maxillary and the ascending pharyngeal arteries, if the tumor has extended beyond the midline.

SKULL BASE MENINGIOMAS

Meningiomas represent 15 per cent of all intracranial tumors. When they are in the skull base, they may involve the anterior, middle, or posterior fossa as well as the foramen magnum, cavernous sinus, or tentorium, and they collect their blood supply from regional meningeal vessels (Figures 1, 4, 11, 20). Superselective catheterization of most of these arteries identifies the tumor's blood supply and allows preoperative occlusion of significant portions of the tumor. Before the embolization, it is essential to rule out dangerous external carotid–internal carotid artery anastomosis as well as potential impairment of blood supply to cranial nerves, as they pierce the dura of the skull base.

Technique of Endovascular Therapy. PVA usually is the preferred embolic material. Postembolization steroids may be used to decrease swelling of the tumor and potential compression of cranial nerves and the brain stem. Complications related to embolization of meningiomas are rare.

SCHWANNOMAS (CERVICAL)

The main arterial supply for schwannomas in the neck is from the ascending pharyngeal artery (Figure 21). Selective catheterization of this artery allows preoperative occlusion of the tumor bed with PVA, 300 to 600 microns in diameter. The trunk of the ascending pharyngeal artery is permanently occluded with microcoils after the delivery of PVA. Not unusually, muscular branches of the occipital and ascending cervical arteries are recruited by the tumor and also need to be embolized before surgery.

Embolization of Skull Base Vascular Malformations and Aneurysms

SKULL BASE DURAL ARTERIOVENOUS FISTULAS

Dural arteriovenous fistulas of the skull base may involve the cavernous sinus, transverse/sigmoid sinus, torcula, tentorium, and floor of the middle and anterior fossae (Figures 2, 3, 5, 6, 8–10, 15–19). The clinical presentation is related to the location of the malformation, recruitment of pial venous drainage, intensity of the arteriovenous shunting, and age of presentation.

Technique of Embolization. The endovascular therapy of these lesions may include transarterial, transvenous, or combined endovascular occlusion of the malformation. The therapeutic management of these lesions should be particularly aggressive when they have recruited pial venous drainage (with the potential risk of a serious intracranial hemorrhage). This may involve complete embolization with particles or acrylic material of the external carotid artery feeders as well as transvenous occlusion of the involved dural sinus (e.g., cavernous sinus, transverse sinus). Surgical exposure occasionally is necessary to obliterate the sinus by direct intraoperative embolization.

SPONTANEOUS AND TRAUMATIC INTERNAL CAROTID AND VERTEBRAL FISTULAS

Internal carotid and vertebral arteriovenous fistulas are the most common vascular skull base abnormalities. Posttraumatic intracavernous internal carotid fistulas have been successfully treated by endovascular techniques since 1974.

Technique of Endovascular Therapy. The technique of endovascular balloon occlusion of traumatic carotid cavernous fistulas has been accepted as the method of choice because of its excellent morphological results and low morbidity/mortality. It consists of inflation of a detachable balloon in the cavernous sinus, occluding the fistula and preserving the lumen of the intracavernous internal carotid artery (Figure 22). In cases in which the transarterial approach has failed, the endovascular approach through the inferior petrosal sinus or superior ophthalmic vein or direct surgical exposure of the cavernous sinus may be attempted. In these cases, microcoils, acrylic material, or silk may be used instead of balloons. If the rent in the artery is too large, carotid artery sacrifice may be necessary after balloon test occlusion (see section entitled Pre-Therapeutic Functional Testing).

Intravascular therapy of traumatic carotid cavernous fistulas is successful in 95 per cent of all cases, with an overall morbidity of less than 2 per cent and mortality of less than 0.5 per cent. Spontaneous carotid cavernous fistulas are most often related to dural arteriovenous fistulas of the cavernous sinus or exceptionally to spontaneous rupture of an intracavernous aneurysm.

SKULL BASE VERTEBRAL FISTULAS

Skull base vertebral fistulas may be divided into spontaneous and posttraumatic. Spontaneous vertebrovertebral fistulas may be associated with neurofibromatosis, fibromuscular dysplasia, Ehlers-Danlos syndrome, and other collagen vascular disorders. These lesions are especially difficult to treat because of the generalized mesenchymal vascular disease observed in these patients.

Although nonpenetrating trauma may result in a vertebral arteriovenous fistula, the most common cause for this pathology is penetrating trauma (bullet wounds, stab wounds, needle puncture, or surgery).

Technique of Endovascular Therapy. Endovascular treatment of vertebrovertebral fistulas is primarily transarterial, using detachable balloons or coils to occlude the fistula while preserving the lumen of the vertebral artery (Figure 23). A trapping procedure may need to be performed in those cases in which the vertebral artery cannot be preserved. In those circumstances, a balloon needs to be positioned distal to the fistula site, another at the fistula site, and a third balloon proximal to it to assure fistula closure.

CERVICAL AND INTRACAVERNOUS ANEURYSMS

The most common skull base aneurysms amenable to endovascular therapy are the intrapetrous and intracavernous aneurysms. The vertebral artery aneurysms are relatively rare, although dissecting aneurysms of the distal vertebral artery may be seen and some of them may be treated by the endovascular route.

Skull base aneurysms tend to be large and not infrequently may be partially thrombosed. In their etiology, we must consider trauma (dissecting aneurysms), infection (petrositis), mesenchymal vascular disease (e.g., Ehlers-Danlos syndrome, Takayasu's arteritis), and berry aneurysms. Most of these aneurysms present a wide neck or may be fusiform. Because of this, intra-aneurysmal embolization treatment with either balloons or coils is associated with a high recurrence rate. This is particularly common in intracavernous aneurysms. In these cases, the treatment of choice is transient test occlusion of the involved carotid or vertebral artery followed by permanent occlusion of the parent vessel with detachable balloons (Figure 24).

RECOMMENDED READING

Kuru, Y.: Meningeal branches of the ophthalmic artery. Acta Radiol. (Diagn.) 6:241–251, 1967.

Pollock, J.A., Newton, T.H.: The anterior falcine artery: Normal and pathologic anatomy. Radiology 91:1089–1095, 1968.

Lasjaunias, P., Merland, J.J., Theron, J., et al.: Vascularisation meningée de la fosse cérébrale moyenne. J. Neuroradiol. 4:361–384, 1977.

Lasjaunias, P.: Cranio-Facial and Upper Cervical Arteries. Vol. 1. Baltimore: Williams & Wilkins, 1981.

Lasjaunias, P., Moret, J.: The ascending pharyngeal artery: Normal and pathological radioanatomy. Neuroradiology 11:77–82, 1976.

Theron, J., Lasjaunias, P., Moret, J., et al.: La vascularisation des meninges de la fosse postérieure. J. Neuroradiol. 4:203–224, 1977.

Blunt, M.J.: The blood supply of the facial nerve. J. Anat. 88:520–526, 1954.

Lasjaunias, P., Moret, J.: Normal and nonpathological variations in the angiographic aspects of the arteries of the middle ear. Neuroradiology 15:213–219, 1978.

Bernasconi, V., Casinari, V.: Caratteristiche angiografiche dei meinig iomi del tentorio. Radiol. Med. 43:1015–1026, 1957.

Wollschlaeger, P.B., Wollschaeger, G.: Eine infratentorielle meningeale Arterie. Radiologe 5:451–452, 1965.

Lasjaunias, P., Doyon, D., Edouard, A.: Les paralysies faciales périphériques postembolisation. Ann. Oto-Laryng. (Paris) 95:595–602, 1978.

Lasjaunias, P.: Aspect angiographique de la vascularisation des nerfs craniens. Presented in 4ème Congrès Annuel de la Societé Francaise de Neuroradiologie. Toulouse, May 3–5, 1979.

Dion, J.E.: Principles and methodology. *In* Vinuela, F., Halbach, V.V., Dion, J.E.: Interventional Neuroradiology: Endovascular Therapy of the Central Nervous System. New York: Raven Press, 1992, pp. 17–29.

Horton, J.A., Kerber, C.W.: Lidocaine injection into the external carotid branches: Provocative test to preserve cranial nerve function in therapeutic embolization. AJNR 7:105–108, 1986.

Rauch, R.A., Vinuela, F., Dion, J., et al.: Preembolization functional evaluation in brain arteriovenous malformations: The superselective Amytal test. AJNR 13:303–308, 1992.

Erba, S.M., Horton, J.A., Latchaw, R.E., et al.: Balloon test occlusion of the internal carotid artery with stable Xenon/CT cerebral blood flow imaging. AJNR 9:533–538, 1988.

Peterman, S.B., Taylor, A., Hoffman, J.C.: Improved detection of cerebral hypoperfusion with internal carotid balloon test occlusion and 99mTc-HMPAO cerebral perfusion SPECT imaging. AJNR 12:1035–1041, 1991.

Glenner, G.G., Grimley, P.M.: Tumors of the extra-adrenal paraganglion systems (including chemoreceptors). *In* Atlas of Tumor Pathology, 2nd Ser., Fasc. 9. Washington, D.C.: Armed Forces Institute of Pathology, 1974.

Moret, J., Picard, L.: Vascular architecture of tympanojugular glomus tumors. Its relevance in therapeutic angiography. Semin. Interv. Radiol. 4:291–308, 1987.

Valavanis, A.: Preoperative embolization of the head and neck: indications, patient selection, goals and precautions. AJNR 7:943–952, 1988.

Changani, D.L., Sharma, S.D., Popli, S.P.: Intracranial extensions in nasopharyngeal fibromas. J. Laryngol. Otol. 82:1137–1144, 1969.

Lasjaunias, P., Berenstein, A., Moret, J.: The significance of dural supply of central nervous system lesions. J. Neuroradiol. 10:31–42, 1983.

Lasjaunias, P., Berenstein, A.: Surgical Neuroangiography. Vol. 11: Endovascular Treatment of Craniofacial Lesions. New York: Springer-Verlag, 1987, p. 96.

Russell, D.S., Rubinstein, L.J.: Pathology of Tumors of the Nervous System, 5th ed. Baltimore: Williams & Wilkins, 1989, p. 961.

Abramowitz, J., Dion, J., Jensen, M., et al.: Angiographic diagnosis and management of head and neck schwannomas. AJNR 12:977–984, 1991.

Picard, L., Bracard, S., Mallet, J., et al.: Spontaneous dural arteriovenous fistulas. Semin. Interv. Radiol. 4:219–240, 1987.

Lasjaunias, P., Chiu, M., TerBrugge, K., et al.: Neurological manifestations of intracranial dural arteriovenous malformations. J. Neurosurg. 64:724–730, 1986.

Awad, I.A., Little, J.R., Akrawi, W.P., et al.: Intracranial dural arteriovenous malformations: Factors predisposing to an aggressive neurological course. J. Neurosurg. 72:839–850, 1990.

Halbach, V.V., Higashida, R.T., Heishima, G.B., et al.: Transvenous embolization of dural fistulas involving the transverse and sigmoid sinuses. AJNR 10:385–392, 1989.

Halbach, V.V., Higashida, R.T., Hieshima, G.B., et al.: Treatment of dural fistulas involving the deep cerebral venous system. AJNR 10:393–399, 1989.

Serbinenko, F.A.: Balloon catheterization and occlusion of major cerebral vessels. J. Neurosurg. 41:125–145, 1974.

Debrun, G.M., Vinuela, F., Fox, A.J., et al.: Indications for treatment and classification of 132 CCF's. Neurosurgery 22:285–289, 1988.

Halbach, V.V., Higashida, R.T., Hieshima, G.B., et al.: Transvenous embolization of dural fistulas involving the cavernous sinus. AJNR 10:377–384, 1989.

Teng, M.M., Guo, W.Y., Huang, C.I., et al.: Occlusion of arteriovenous malformations of the cavernous sinus via the superior ophthalmic vein. AJNR 9:539–546, 1988.

Isamat, F., Ferrer, E., Twosw, J.: Direct intracavernous obliteration of high flow CCF's. J. Neurosurg. 65:770–775, 1986.

Higashida, R.T., Halbach, V.V., Tsai, F.Y., et al.: Interventional neurovascular treatment of traumatic carotid and vertebral fistulas: Results in 234 cases. AJR 153:577, 1989.

Beltramello, A., Maschio, A., Piocvan, E., et al.: Spontaneous arteriovenous fistulas of the vertebral artery: Diagnostic and therapeutic considerations. Eur. J Radiol. 8:148, 1988.

Halbach, V.V., Higashida, R.T., Hesihima, G.B., et al.: Treatment of vertebral arterial venous fistulas. AJNR 8:1121, 1987.

Dion, J.: Interventional neuroradiology in head and neck vascular pathology. Categorical course syllabi on interventional neuroradiology. 30th Annual Meeting, ASNR. St. Louis, May 30–June 6, 1992, pp. 373–377.

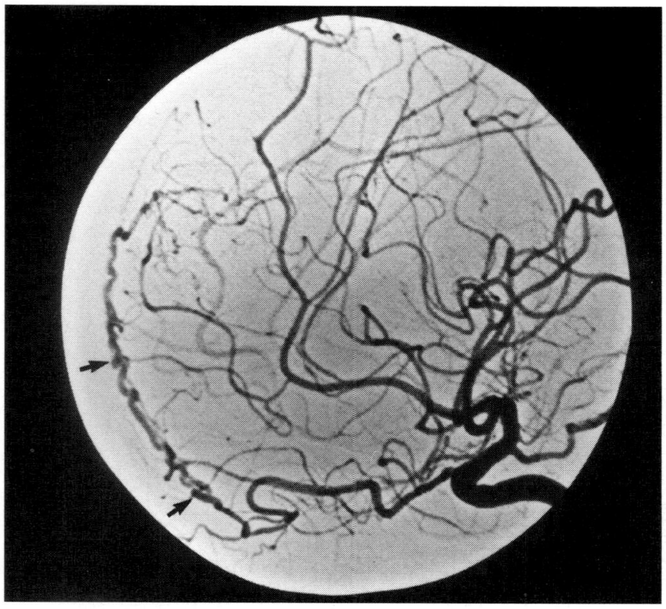

Figure 1. Lateral internal carotid angiogram demonstrates an enlarged anterior falcine artery *(arrows)* that eventually feeds a falcine meningioma. The anterior falcine artery arises from the distal ophthalmic artery.

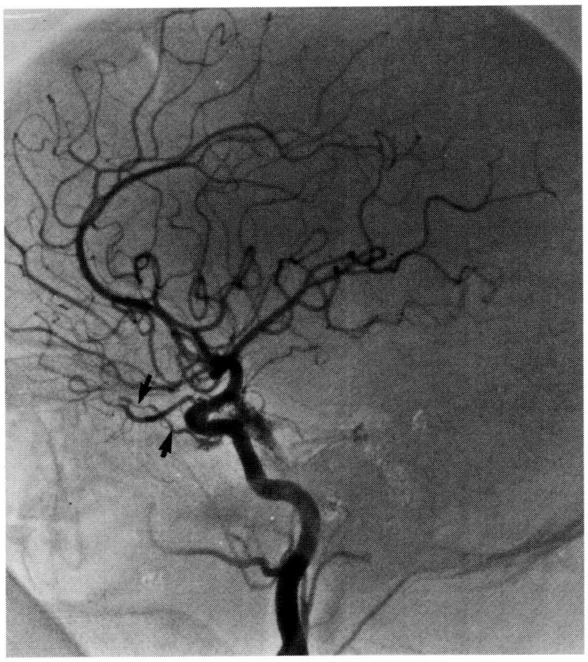

Figure 2. Internal carotid injection, lateral view, shows the recurrent meningeal branch from the ophthalmic artery *(arrows)* feeding a cavernous sinus dural arteriovenous fistula. This artery, along with the ethmoidal branches of the ophthalmic artery, can also supply lesions in the anterior cranial fossa along the tuberculum sella.

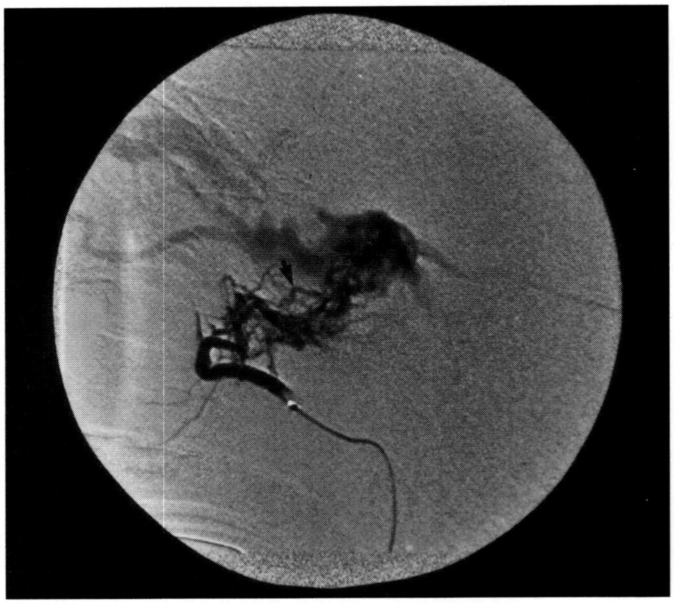

Figure 3. Distal superselective internal maxillary artery injection in lateral projection shows numerous transosseous branches passing through the base of the skull and filling a cavernous sinus dural arteriovenous fistula. Although many of the branches are unnamed, one of the main branches connecting with the inferolateral trunk is the artery of the foramen rotundum *(arrow).*

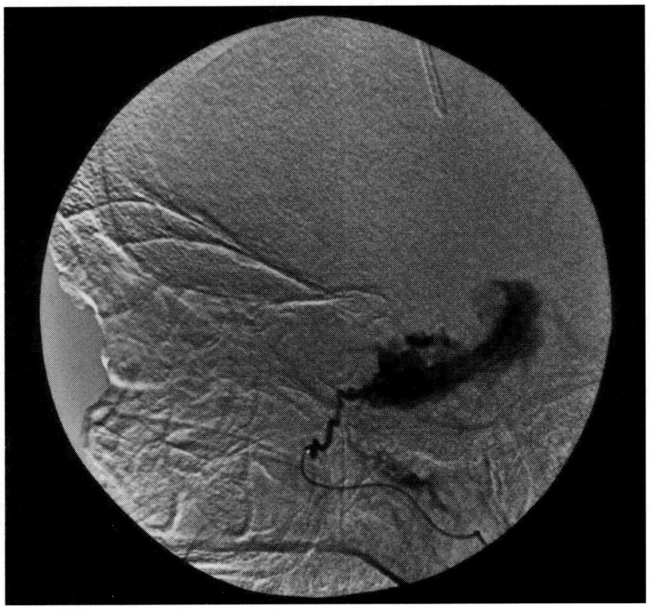

Figure 4. Superselective angiogram of the artery of the foramen rotundum in lateral projection showing filling of a large meningioma in the cavernous sinus. This artery connects the distal internal maxillary with the internal carotid by way of the inferolateral trunk. The second division of the V nerve runs through this canal. This can be a significant collateral when there is carotid occlusion.

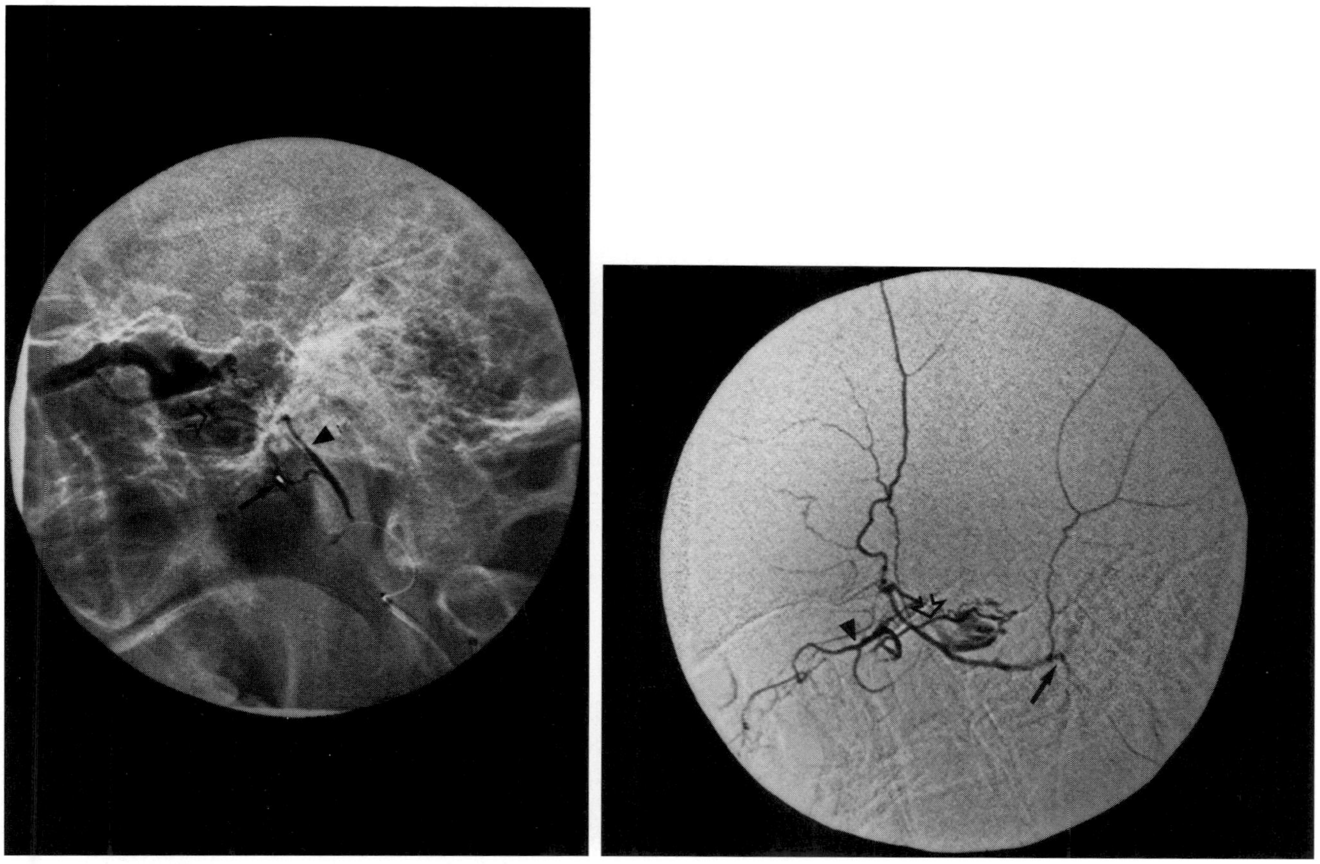

Figure 5.

A. Superselective lateral projection angiogram of the accessory meningeal artery. The microcatheter tip is in the accessory meningeal artery *(arrow)*, and there is reflux into the middle meningeal artery *(arrowhead)*. Note the enlarged artery of the foramen ovale feeding this cavernous sinus dural arteriovenous fistula *(open arrow)*.

B. This is the same patient as in A, but the microcatheter is in the middle meningeal artery *(arrow)*. There is an anatomical variant in this case, with the ophthalmic artery *(arrowhead)* receiving significant supply by way of the middle meningeal. The recurrent meningeal artery of the ophthalmic *(open arrow)* then supplies the dural arteriovenous fistula. The middle meningeal artery, therefore, cannot be embolized because of the high risk of blindness.

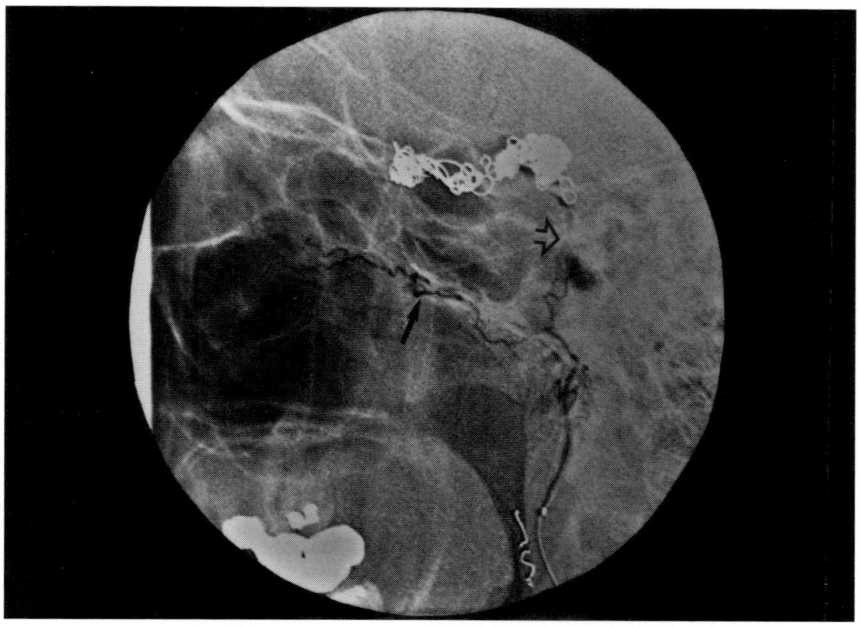

Figure 6. Superselective angiogram of the anterior division of the ascending pharyngeal artery in lateral projection. The superior pharyngeal artery *(arrow)* and carotid ramus *(open arrow)* are well seen. The carotid ramus, which ascends through the foramen lacerum, can anastomose with the internal carotid artery but in this case primarily supplies the cavernous sinus dural arteriovenous fistula (filled with coils from prior transvenous embolization).

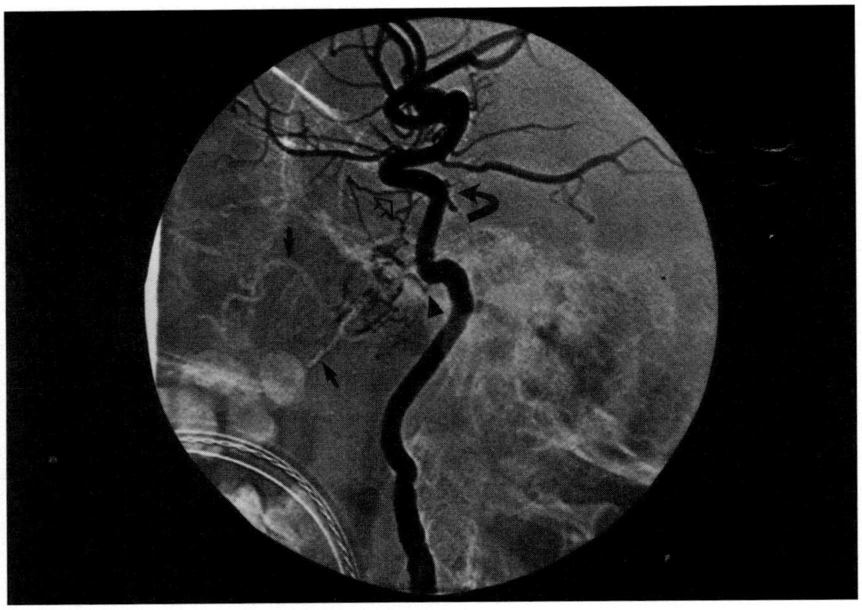

Figure 7. Internal carotid lateral projection. This patient has had prior embolization, as evidenced by the embolic material (glue) *(arrows).* There is also a significant transosseous supply to the juvenile angiofibroma. Residual supply by way of the inferolateral trunk *(open arrow)* and mandibulovidian artery *(arrowhead)* still supplies the residual tumor compartment. Branches of the meningohypophyseal trunk are also identified *(curved arrow).*

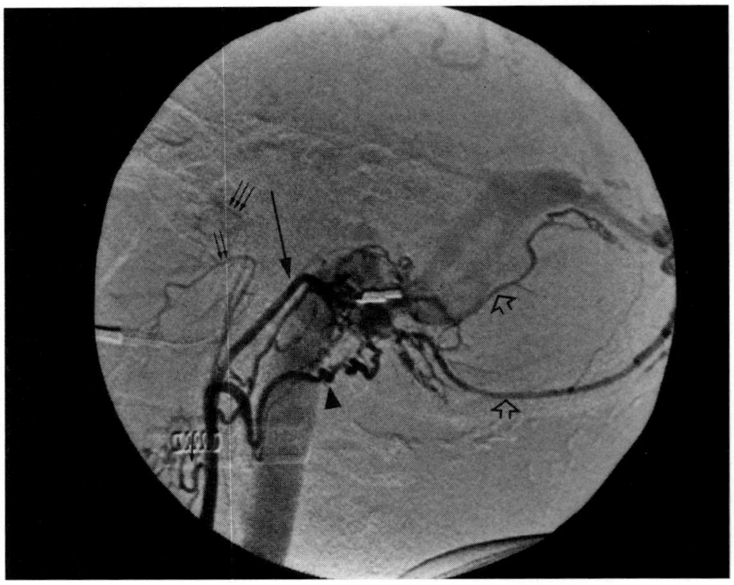

Figure 8. Superselective ascending pharyngeal injection in the lateral projection shows the superior pharyngeal branch *(triple arrow),* neuromeningeal trunk *(long arrow),* middle pharyngeal branch *(double arrow),* and hypoglossal branch *(arrowhead).* This feeds a dural arteriovenous fistula of the tentorium, which subsequently drains into the transverse sinus and eventually the jugular vein. Notice how the branches penetrating the skull base give rise to meningeal branches *(open arrows),* which subsequently serve the fistula.

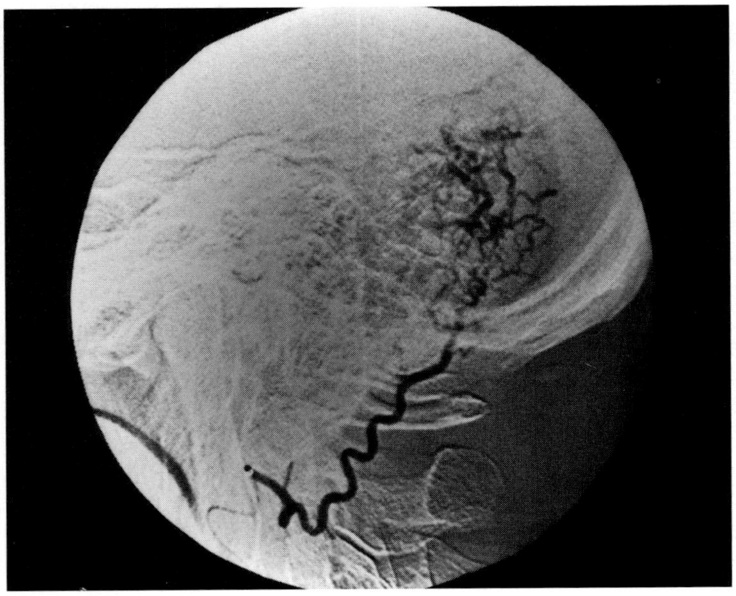

Figure 9. Superselective posterior auricular injection in the lateral projection in a patient with a dural arteriovenous fistula of the transverse sinus shows transosseous branches of the posterior auricular artery. The occipital artery injection *(not shown)* also supplies the fistula through transmastoid branches.

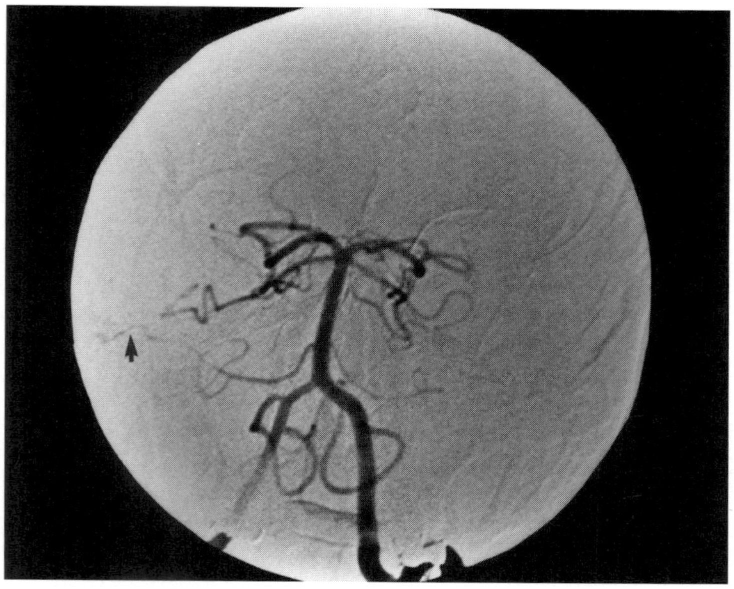

Figure 10. Anteroposterior left vertebral injection shows the distal anterior inferior cerebellar artery on the right serving a dural arteriovenous fistula *(arrow)*. This is in the location of the artery of the internal auditory canal.

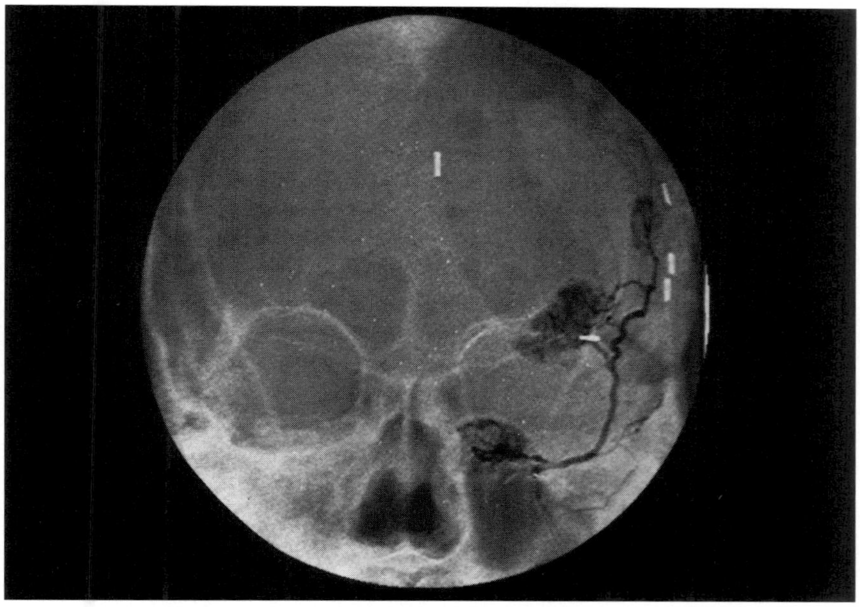

Figure 11. Left middle meningeal artery angiogram in anteroposterior projection shows multiple hemangiopericytomas fed by the middle meningeal artery. After the middle meningeal artery pierces the foramen spinosum, a petrosal branch serves a tumor in the petrous portion of the temporal bone. Additional tumors are seen along the dura more superiorly.

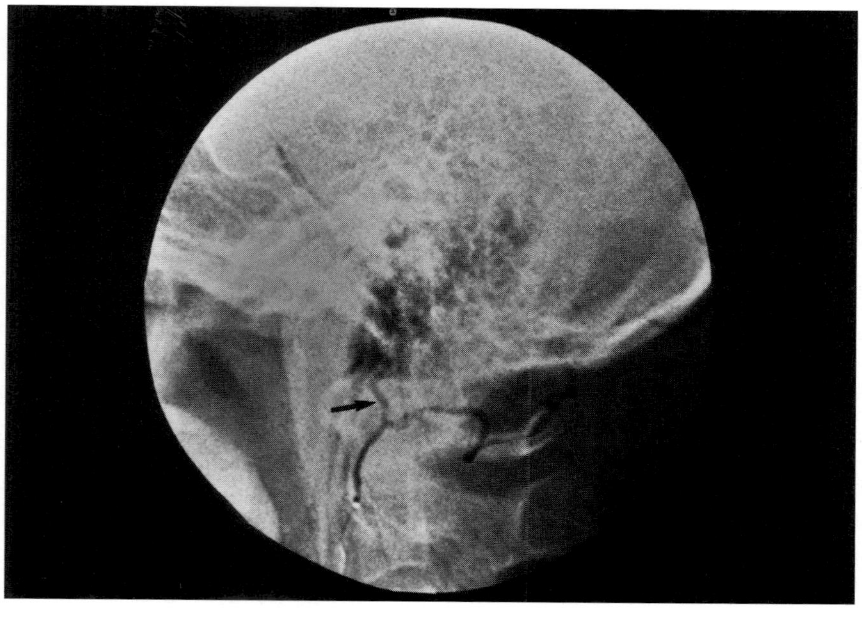

Figure 12. Occipital artery injection, lateral projection, shows the stylomastoid branch of the occipital artery *(arrow)* feeding a vascular tumor at the skull base. This was a paraganglioma (glomus jugulare).

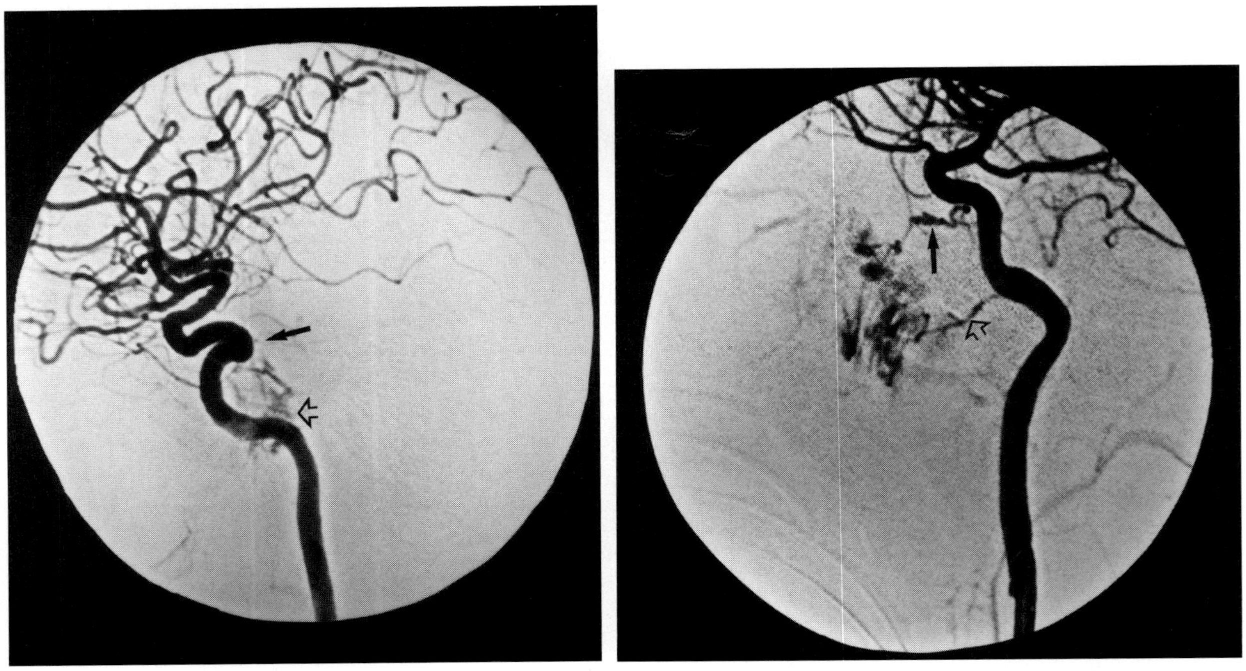

A B

Figure 13.

A. Hemangiopericytoma at the base of the skull shows parasitization of blood flow from the internal carotid artery by way of the meningohypophyseal trunk *(arrow)* and other vessels in the expected location of the caroticotympanic branch *(open arrow)*.

B. Internal carotid injection, lateral view, shows filling of a juvenile angiofibroma from the inferolateral trunk by way of the artery of the foramen rotundum *(arrow)* as well as by way of the mandibulovidian artery *(open arrow)*. Tumors within the petrous portion of the temporal bone may also be fed by these pedicles.

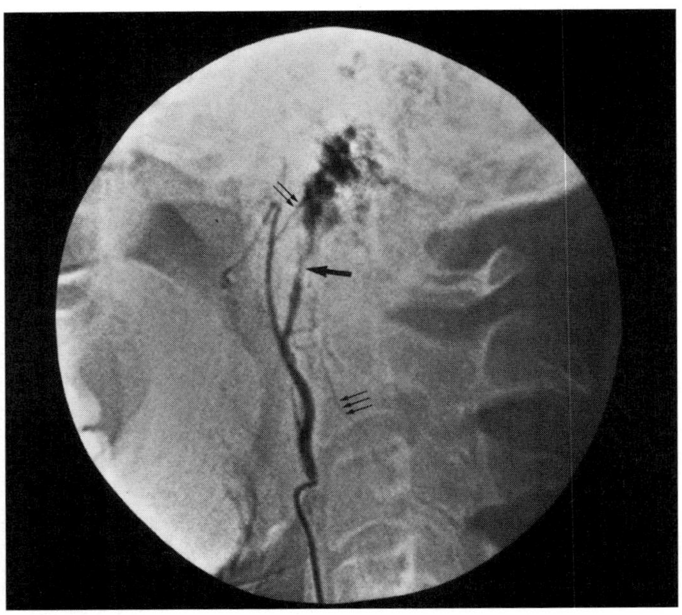

Figure 14. Ascending pharyngeal artery injection, lateral view, shows the neuromeningeal trunk *(arrow)* feeding a paraganglioma at the jugular foramen. The musculospinal division *(triple arrows)* is well seen as well as the inferior tympanic branch of the ascending pharyngeal *(double arrows)*.

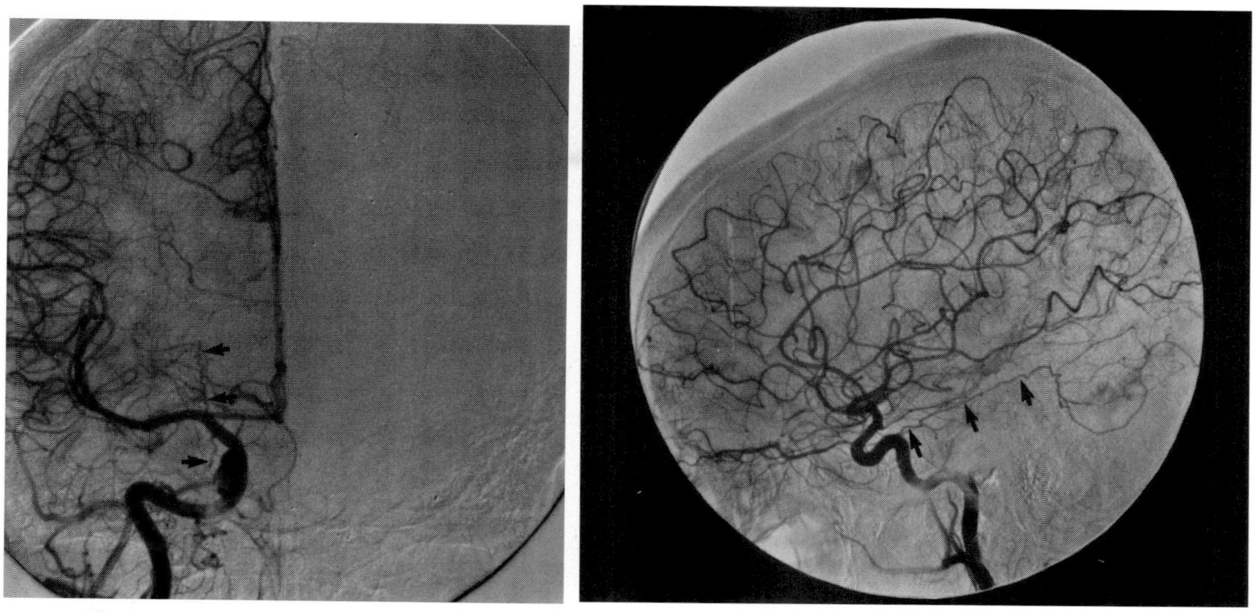

A B

Figure 15.

A. Right common carotid injection, anteroposterior view, shows enlargement of the artery of Bernasconi and Cassinari (marginal tentorial artery) serving a tentorial dural arteriovenous fistula *(arrows)*.

B. Lateral projection in the same patient shows enlargement of the meningohypophyseal trunk, including the artery of the tentorium (Bernasconi and Cassinari) *(arrows)*.

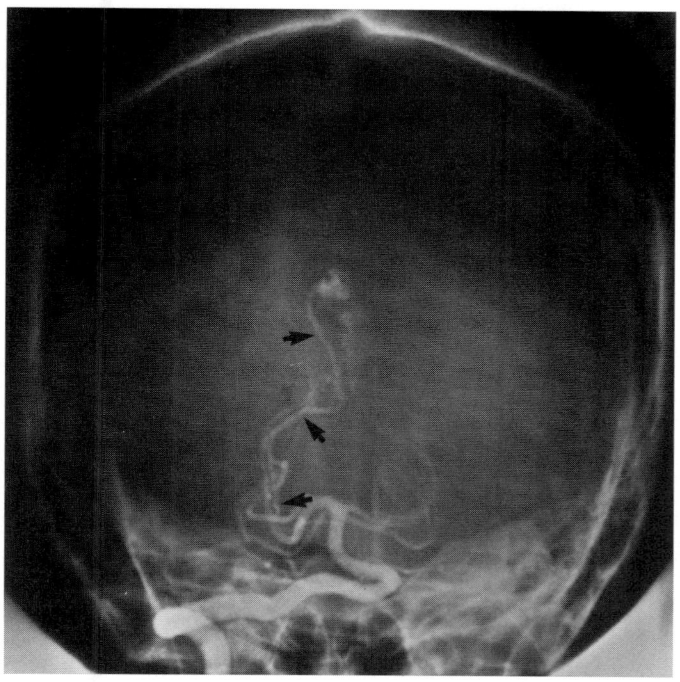

Figure 16. Right vertebral injection in Townes view shows filling of a dural arteriovenous fistula with the primary feeding pedicle from the P1 segment of the posterior cerebral artery. This represents the artery of Davidoff and Schechter *(arrows)*. This is a primary dural branch arising from the posterior cerebral artery. This normally supplies the tentorium and has additional proximal subbranches that can supply a portion of the falx.

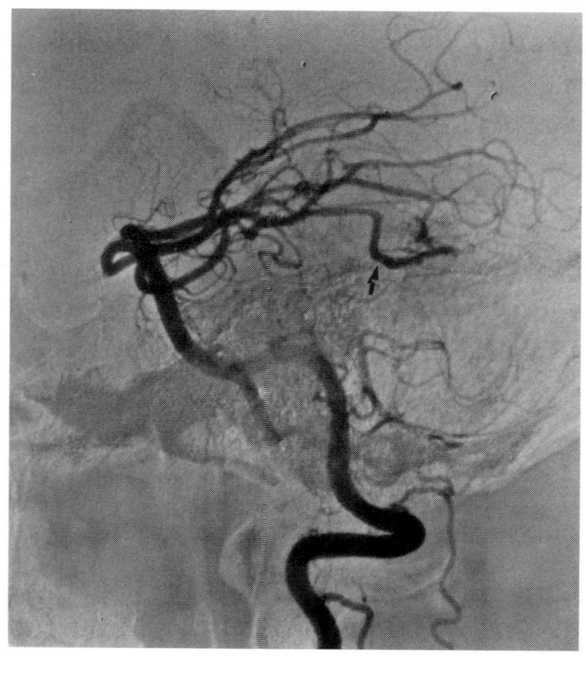

Figure 17. Left vertebral angiogram in lateral projection shows filling of a dural arteriovenous malformation by way of a branch of the superior cerebellar artery *(arrow)*. This may be apparent when there are vascular abnormalities. This artery normally serves the undersurface of the tentorium.

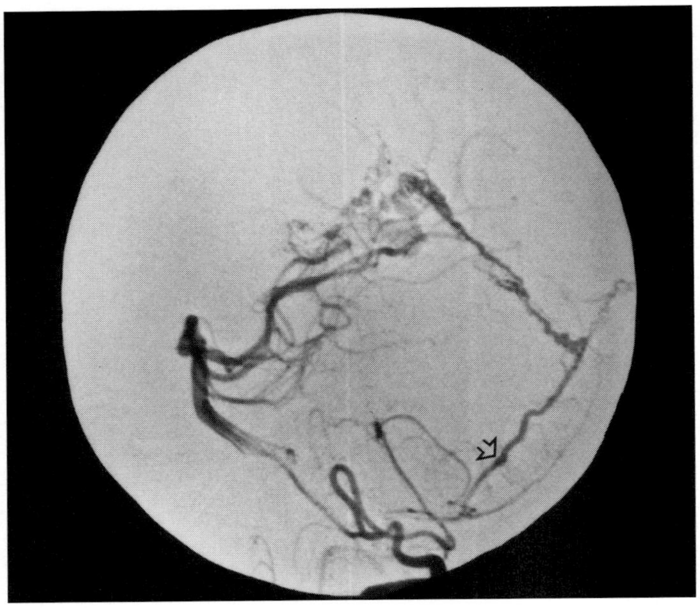

Figure 18. Left vertebral injection, lateral view. There is an arteriovenous malformation of the tentorium fed by a posterior meningeal artery *(open arrow).* This is arising from the distal vertebral artery, and it travels along the dural surface of the inner table and then along the tentorium to reach the fistula site. Anterior meningeal arteries may also arise from the vertebral artery and ascend along the clivus.

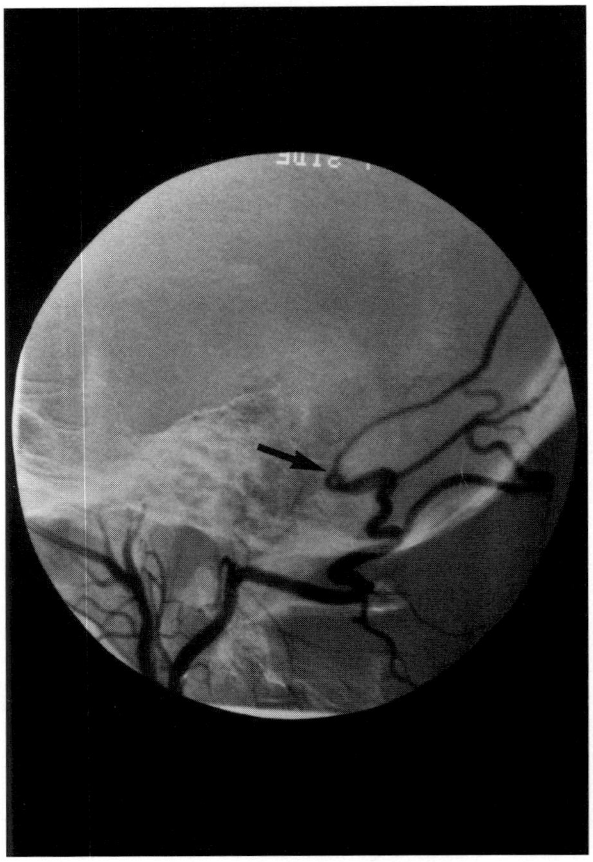

Figure 19. External carotid angiogram, lateral projection, shows marked enlargement of the occipital artery. The patient has a dural arteriovenous malformation of the falx and superior sagittal sinus. The transmastoid branch penetrates to serve the dura. Notice the straight course of the dural vessels as opposed to the sinuous course of the extracranial vessels. The mastoid foramen is the transition point from the exocranial to the intracranial course *(arrow).*

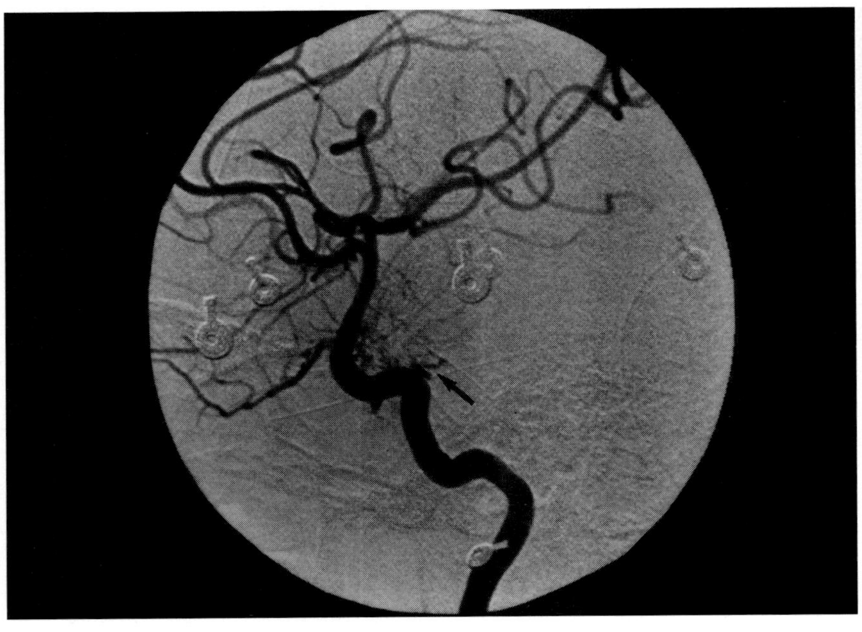

Figure 20. Internal carotid injection, lateral view. There is encasement by a meningioma of the internal carotid artery with parasitization of the adventitial arteries along the wall of the vessel. In addition, there is enlargement of the meningohypophyseal artery *(arrow).*

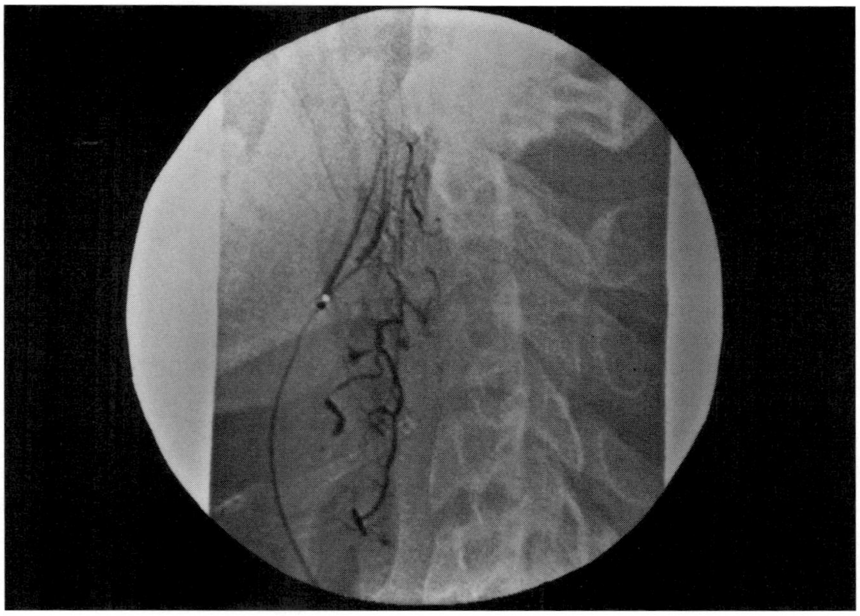

Figure 21. Superselective ascending pharyngeal artery angiogram in a patient with a schwannoma. Notice the "leafless tree" appearance and contrast puddling. This tumor is fed primarily by the musculospinal division of the ascending pharyngeal.

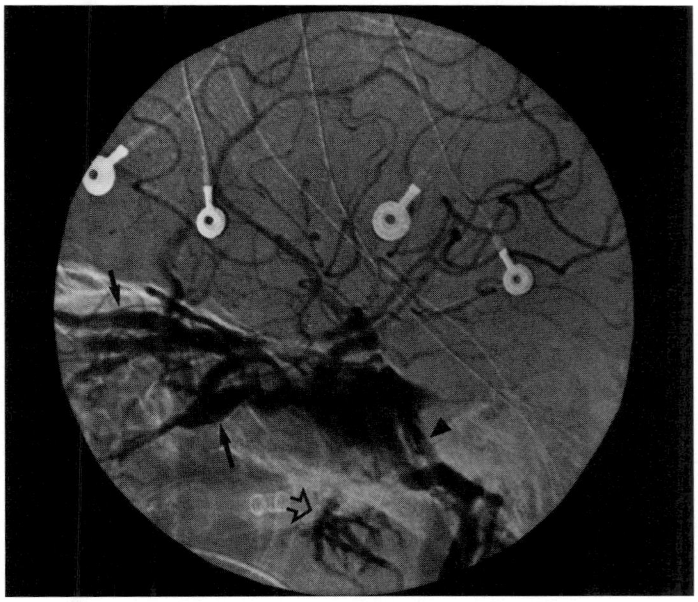

A

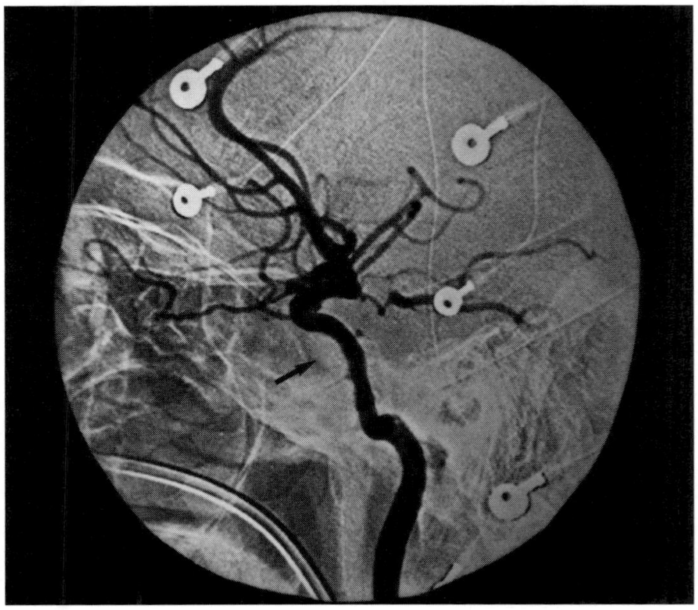

B

Figure 22.

A. Internal carotid injection, lateral view. There is a posttraumatic carotid cavernous fistula, with venous outlet into the orbital veins *(arrows),* inferior petrosal sinus *(arrowhead),* and pterygoid plexus *(open arrow).*

B. After balloon placement *(arrow)* into the venous side of the fistula, the fistula was eliminated with preservation of the internal carotid artery.

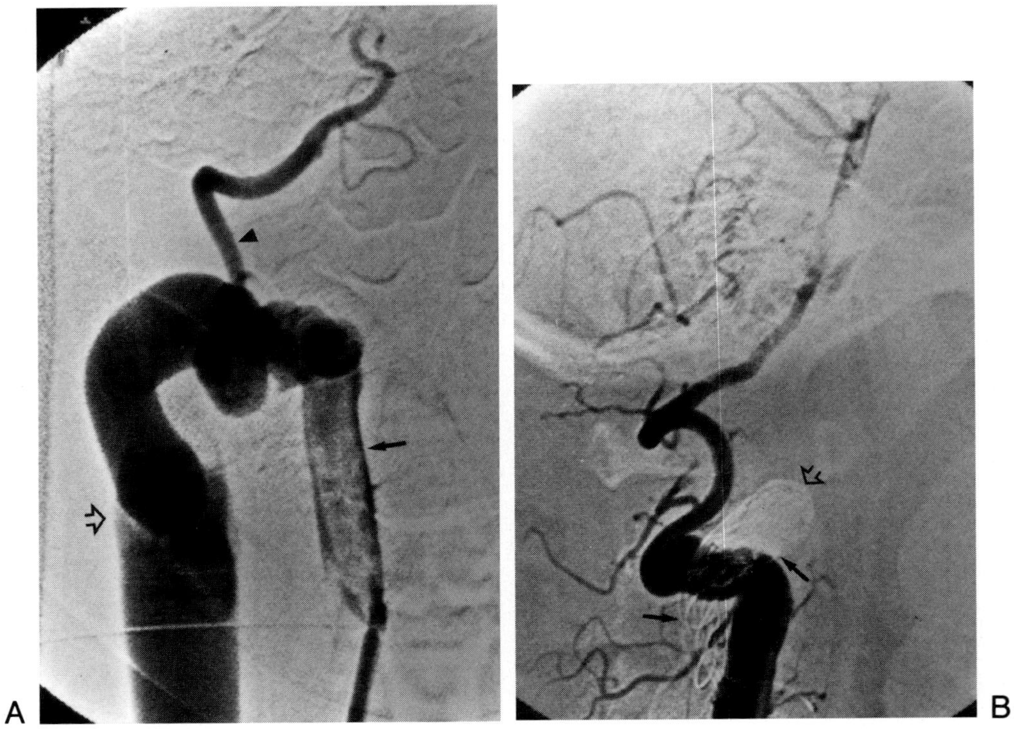

Figure 23.

A. Anteroposterior view, right vertebral artery injection in a 21-year-old woman with a long-standing pulsatile bruit in the neck. This is representative of a congenital arteriovenous fistula. The proximal vertebral artery is very dilated *(arrow)*, and the artery distal to the fistula is normal in caliber *(arrowhead)*. The jugular vein is massively dilated *(open arrow)*.

B. Postembolization lateral view of the vertebral shows elimination of the fistula with preservation of the vertebral artery. In this case, because of the high flow, coils *(arrows)* were placed in the outlet vein before a balloon *(arrowhead)* is placed at the fistula site.

A

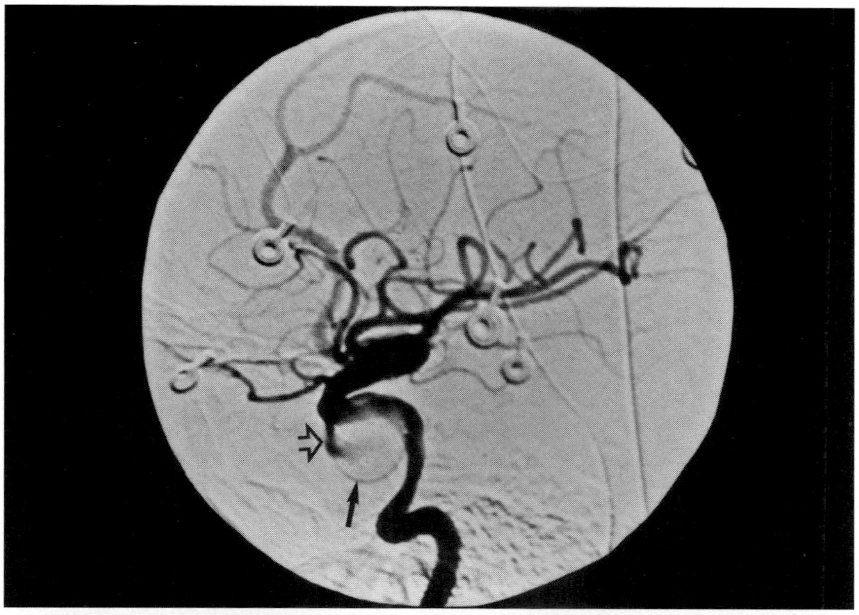

B

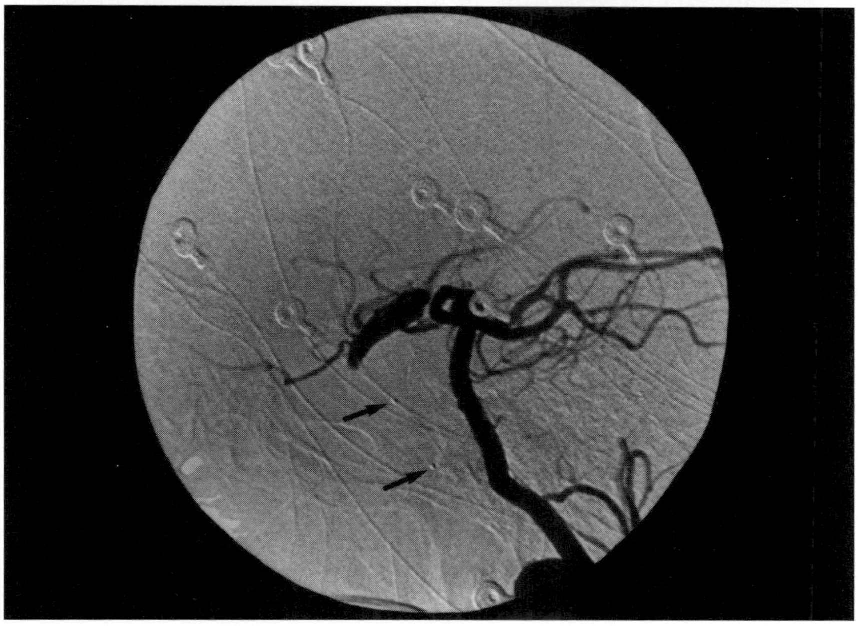

Figure 24.

A. Internal carotid angiogram in lateral projection shows the difficulty in preserving the internal carotid artery when there is a large-necked cavernous aneurysm. There is a balloon within the aneurysm *(arrow)*, but there is also some residual aneurysm filling around the balloon *(open arrow)*.

B. A balloon test occlusion was performed, which the patient tolerated; therefore, the internal carotid artery was sacrificed. This lateral angiogram shows the balloon in place *(arrows show the balloon markers on this subtraction angiogram)* and excellent filling of the carotid territory by way of the posterior communicating artery. The aneurysm no longer fills.

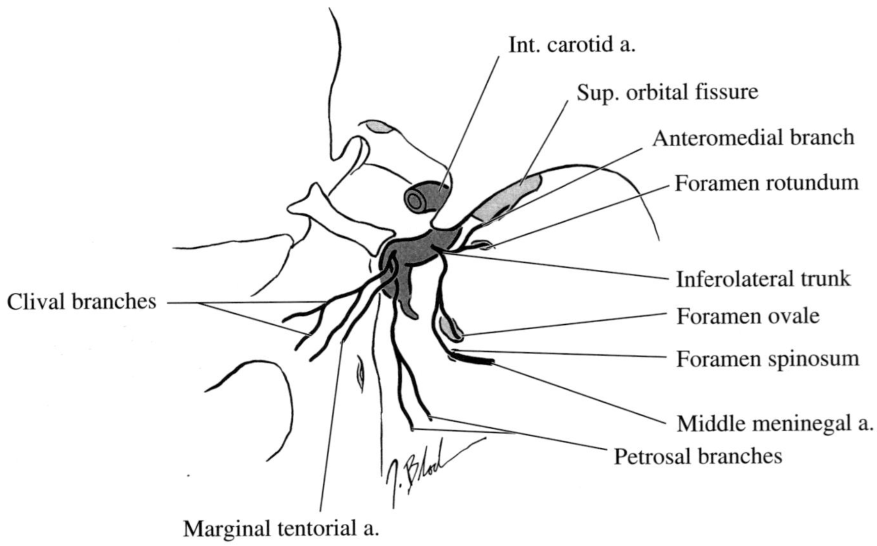

PLATE I

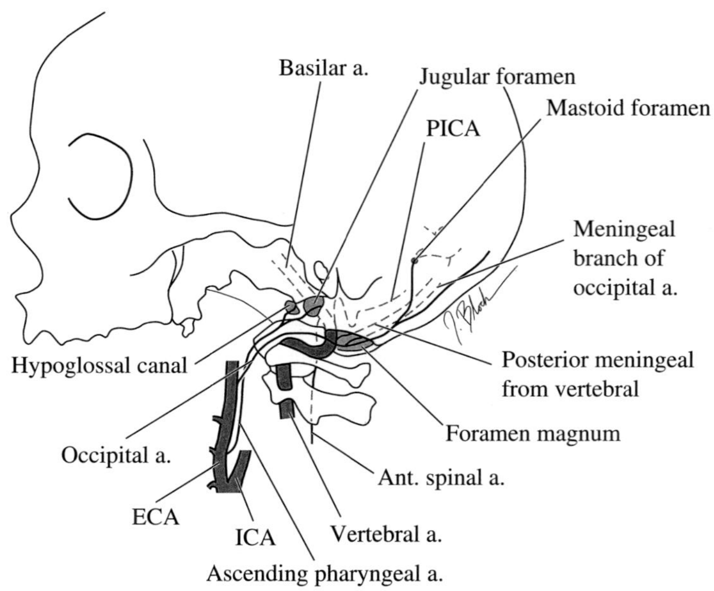

PLATE II

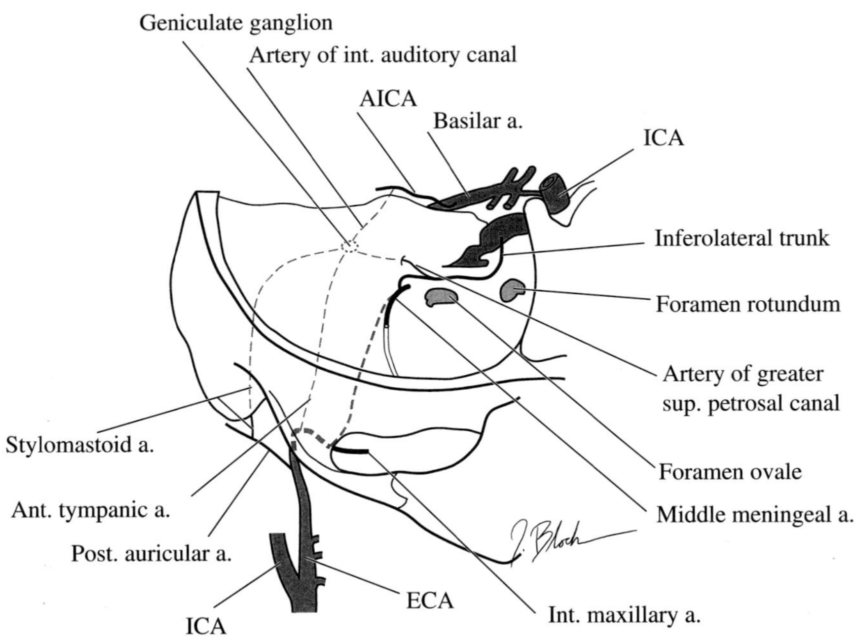

PLATE III

INDEX

Note: Page numbers in *italics* refer to illustrations; page numbers followed by t refer to tables.

Abducent nerve, decompression of, for removal of chordoma, *189*
  preservation of, for removal of petroclival meningioma, 121, *141*
Acoustic neurinoma(s), 152–157, *158–169*
  anatomical considerations in, 152–153, *160–161*
  debulking of, 154, *166*
    cavitron for, 154, *169*
  diagnosis of, 152, *159–160*
  displacement of brain stem from, 152, *159*
  in cerebellopontine angle, 152, *158–160, 163, 168–169*
  in superior vestibular nerve, 153, *162*
  intracanalicular, 152, *160*
    exposure of cerebellopontine angle in, *161*
  middle cranial fossa approach to, 155–156
  origin of, eighth cranial nerve and, 152, *158*
  removal of, complications of, 157
    preservation of vestibular nerve in, *162*
    visualization of fascicles for, 154, *165*
  retrosigmoid lateral suboccipital transmeatal approach to, 153–155, *161–169*
  transcochlear approach to, 157
  translabyrinthine approach to, *21–23*, 156–157
  transotic approach to, 157
Acromegaly, treatment of, 212–213
Adenoma(s), pituitary, 212–216, *217–223*. See also *Pituitary tumor(s).*
Alcohol, polyvinyl, for use in endovascular therapy, 243
Amytal, injection of, during superselective angiography, 242
Aneurysm(s), approaches to, 201–203, *205–209*
  arterial, ruptured, *205*
  embolization of, 243–244, *255*
  paraclinoid, repair of, *206–207*
  paraophthalmic, repair of, *206–207*
Angiofibroma(s), nasopharyngeal, juvenile, 233–234, *234–237*
    blood supply to, *248, 250*
    preoperative embolization of, 243, *248, 250*
Angiography, cerebral, for diagnosis of meningiomas, 117–118
  for diagnosis of vascular lesions of skull base, 242t
  superselective, 242
Angioma, cavernous, pontine, resection of, 63, *65–66*
Angular artery, in orbitotomy with medial approach, *101*
Angular vein, in orbitotomy with medial approach, *101*
Annulus of Zinn, dissection of, in resection of optic gliomas, 224
  in transsphenoidal decompression of optic canal, 112, *113*
Anterior cavernous sinus, exposure of carotid artery in, for repair of aneurysms, 201–202, *205–207*
Anterior cerebral artery. See *Cerebral artery(ies), anterior.*
Anterior choroidal artery, frontal-temporal-orbital approach to, *85*
Anterior clinoid process, meningioma of, removal of, 119–120, *130–134*
  pterional approach to, *8*
  removal of, 201–202, *205–207*
Anterior communicating artery, aneurysm of, ruptured, *205*
  pterional approach to, *8*
Anterior cranial fossa, features of, *77*
Anterior falcine artery, feeding falcine meningioma, *245*
Anterior inferior cerebellar artery. See *Cerebellar artery(ies), inferior, anterior.*
Arachnoid, dissection of, for removal of acoustic neurinoma, 154–155, *166*
  preservation of, with meningioma, 118, *125*
    of cerebellopontine angle, *142*
    petroclival, *140*
Arcuate eminence, middle cranial fossa approach to, *30*
Arterial aneurysm(s), ruptured, *205*. See also *Aneurysm(s).*
Arteriography, carotid, for diagnosis of juvenile nasopharyngeal angiofibroma, 233, *236*
Arteriovenous fistula(s), dural, blood supply to, *246–249, 251–252*
  embolization of, 243–244, *254*
Ascending pharyngeal artery, feeding paraganglioma, *250*
  feeding schwannoma, *253*
  in lateral approach to middle skull base, *46, 47*
Aspirator, ultrasonic, for debulking of cerebellopontine angle meningioma, *143*
Auditory canal, external, in lateral approach to middle skull base, *46*
  internal, anatomic relations in, 153
    cerebellopontine angle acoustic neurinoma in, 152, *158–159*
    cerebellopontine angle meningioma in, removal of, 122, *147–148*
    closure of, after removal of acoustic neurinoma, 154, *165*
    drilling of, for removal of acoustic neurinoma, 154, 155, *163*
    exposure of, for removal of acoustic neurinoma, 153–155, *161–162, 164–165, 169*
    middle cranial fossa approach to, *28, 30*
    translabyrinthine approach to, 18–19, *20–23*
    transotic approach to, 24–25, *25*
Auricular artery, posterior, feeding dural arteriovenous fistula, *248*

Basal approach, transfrontal, 75–76, *76–78*
Basilar artery, aneurysm of, ruptured, *205*
  subtemporal approach to, 202, *208*
  subtemporal transtentorial approach to, *70, 73*
  upper, aneurysms of, approaches to, 202, *208–209*
Basilar trunk, aneurysms of, retrolabyrinthine presigmoid approach to, 202–203, *209*
Bicoronal incision, for subfrontal approach, 3, *4*
Bifrontal craniotomy, for removal of meningioma, 119, *126–127*
Bilateral frontal bone flap(s), for subfrontal approach, 3, *5*
Bill's island, creation of, over sigmoid sinus, *21*
Bone flap(s), for frontal orbital approach, 79, *80–81*
  for frontotemporal approach, 6, *8*
  for middle cranial fossa approach, 27
  for subfrontal approach, 3, *5*
  for subtemporal approach, 9, *10*
  lateral orbitotomy with, 102, *104*
Bone graft(s), for reconstruction of fossa floor, 76, *78*
Bone plate, craniotomy, replacement of, after removal of esthesioneuroblastoma, 227, *232*
Bony optic canal, decompression of, 112, *113*
Brain, compression of, from chordoma, *188*
Brain base, compression of, from pituitary macroadenoma, 214, *217*
Brain stem, after transoral exposure, *97*
  decompression of, for removal of chordoma, *189*
  displacement of, from acoustic neurinoma, 152, *159*
    from meningioma of craniocervical junction, *149*
    from petroclival meningioma, *137*
  dissection of, for removal of meningioma of cerebellopontine angle, *144*
  epidermoid cyst on, *173*
Bromocriptine, for management of prolactinomas, 212
Burr hole(s), placement of, for frontotemporal approach, 6, *7*
    for removal of esthesioneuroblastoma, *229*
    for subfrontal approach, 3, *4–5*
    for suboccipital lateral retrosigmoid approach, *14*
    for subtemporal approach, *10*
Bypass procedure(s), for skull base, 203–204, *210–211*

C1, arch of, drilling of, for oral approach to clivus and C1–C2, 95, *97*
C2 spinal nerve, anterior branch of, in lateral approach to craniocervical junction, *57*
Calcification, in craniopharyngioma, 176, *180, 183*
Caldwell-Luc sinusotomy, 86, *89*
Canthal ligament(s), medial, in orbitotomy with medial approach, *101*
Canthotomy, lateral, 102, *103*
Capitis inferior muscle, oblique, in lateral approach to craniocervical junction, *57*
Carotid arteriography, for diagnosis of juvenile nasopharyngeal angiofibroma, 233, *236*

Carotid arteriovenous fistula(s), embolization of, 243–244
Carotid artery, anatomical relations of, to pituitary gland, *218*
bifurcation of, 82, *84*
displacement of, from chemodectoma, 191, *193*
exposure of, in anterior cavernous sinus, for repair of aneurysms, 201–202, *205–207*
in carotid cave, for repair of aneurysms, 201–202, *205–207*
in frontal-temporal-orbital approach, *85*
extension of pituitary tumor to, *218, 223*
identification of, in transsphenoidal decompression of optic canal, *113*
infraclinoid, exposure of, for repair of aneurysms, *205–206*
internal, cholesterol granuloma at, *199*
displacement of, by pituitary tumor, *221*
dissection of chemodectoma from, *195*
exposure of, for removal of meningioma of anterior clinoid, *133*
in frontal-temporal-orbital approach, *84*
feeding hemangiopericytoma, *250*
feeding juvenile nasopharyngeal angiofibroma, *248, 250*
feeding meningioma, *252*
globular meningioma surrounding, 117, *123*
in approach to pituitary tumors, 214, *220*
in lateral approach to middle skull base, *46–47*
in subtemporal-transzygomatic approach, *42*
neurinoma near, *52*
petrous, subtemporal transtentorial approach to, *70*
preservation of, in removal of petroclival meningioma, *141*
reconstruction of, after repair of paraclinoid aneurysm, *207*
relation to jugular bulb, at skull base, *50*
subtemporal transtentorial approach to, *70–71, 73*
transsphenoidal approach to, *36*
intracavernous, violation of, complications of, 83
lateral approach to, 43–45, *46–53*
anatomical considerations in, 43, *46–47*
Carotid bypass, cervical-to-petrous, 204, *210–211*
petrous-to-supraclinoid, 203–204, *210*
Carotid cave, exposure of carotid artery in, for repair of aneurysms, 201–202, *205–207*
Carotid cavernous fistula, blood supply to, *253*
Carotid dural ring, dissection of, for repair of aneurysms, *205*
Carotid prominence, transsphenoidal approach to, *35*
Carotid ramus, feeding cavernous sinus dural arteriovenous fistula, *247*
Carotid trunk, external, in lateral approach to middle skull base, *46–47*
Caudal cranial nerve(s), exposure of, lateral approach to, *53*
Caudal orbitotomy, 107, *108*
Cavernous angioma, pontine, resection of, 63, *65–66*
Cavernous fistula, carotid, blood supply to, *253*
Cavernous sinus(es), anatomical relations of, to pituitary gland, *218*
anterior, exposure of carotid artery in, for repair of aneurysms, 201–202, *205–207*
blood supply to, 241, *246*
dural arteriovenous fistula of, blood supply to, *246–247*
Cavernous sinus(es) *(Continued)*
extension of tumors into, transsphenoidal approach to, 33, *37*
inferior, artery of, transsphenoidal approach to, *36*
invasion of, by pituitary tumor, *218*
meningioma of, blood supply to, *246*
removal of, 120, 121, *134–135, 138–141*
subtotal, 121, *136–138*
pituitary tumor in, *221*
structures surrounding, 82, *85*
subtemporal transtentorial approach to, *73*
Cavitron, for debulking of acoustic neurinoma, 154, *169*
C1–C2 joint, oral approach to, 95–96, *96–97*
removal of, in lateral approach to craniocervical junction, *57*
Cerebellar artery(ies), inferior, anterior, aneurysms of, retrolabyrinthine presigmoid approach to, 202–203, *209*
dissection of, for removal of epidermoid cyst, 171, *173*
for removal of meningioma of cerebellopontine angle, *143*
feeding dural arteriovenous fistula, *249*
preservation of, for removal of acoustic neurinoma, 152–153, 156–157
for removal of chordoma, *189*
suboccipital lateral retrosigmoid approach to, *15*
posterior, in lateral approach to craniocervical junction, *58*
pre–sigmoid sinus approach to, *65*
suboccipital lateral retrosigmoid approach to, *15*
superior, feeding dural arteriovenous fistula, *251*
in subtemporal-transzygomatic approach, *42*
pre–sigmoid sinus approach to, *64–65*
subtemporal transtentorial approach to, *70, 73*
Cerebellar tonsil, suboccipital medial approach to, *17*
Cerebellopontine angle, acoustic neurinoma in, 152, *158–160, 163, 168–169*
anatomical relations in, 45, *51, 97*
epidermoid cyst in, 170, *172–173*
exposure of, in intracanalicular acoustic neurinoma, *161*
in suboccipital lateral retrosigmoid approach, 12, *15*
meningiomas of, removal of, 120–122, *142–148*
middle cranial fossa approach to, *28*
neurinoma near, *52*
pre–sigmoid sinus approach to, 63, *64–65*
transotic approach to, 24–25, *25*
Cerebellum, in subtemporal-transzygomatic approach, *42*
pre–sigmoid sinus approach to, *64*
Cerebral angiography, for diagnosis of meningiomas, 117–118
Cerebral artery(ies), anterior, displacement of, by pituitary tumor, *219*
frontal-temporal-orbital approach to, *84–85*
pterional approach to, *8*
transsphenoidal approach to, *35*
middle, frontal-temporal-orbital approach to, *84–85*
pterional approach to, *8*
posterior, feeding dural arteriovenous fistula, *251*
pterional approach to, *8*
subtemporal transtentorial approach to, *70, 73*
subtemporal-transzygomatic approach to, *42*
Cerebral monitoring, during petrous-to-supraclinoid carotid bypass, 204
Cervical aneurysm(s), embolization of, 244
Cervical schwannoma(s), preoperative embolization of, 243, *253*
Cervical spinal cord, suboccipital medial approach to, *17*
Cervical-to-petrous carotid bypass, 204, *210–211*
Chemical meningitis, after removal of epidermoid cysts, 171
Chemodectoma(s), 190–191, *192–196*
anatomic considerations in, 190
approach to, 190–191, *193–196*
blood supply to, *249–250*
diagnosis of, 190
histologic features of, 190, *192*
preoperative embolization of, *193*, 242–243, *249–250*
resection of, 45
Chiasmatic groove, subtemporal transtentorial approach to, *69*
Cholesterol granuloma(s), 170–171, *172–173*, 197–198, *198–200*
anatomic considerations in, 197
clinical presentation of, 197
histologic features of, 197, *198*
pre–sigmoid sinus approach to, 198, *200*
treatment of, 197–198, *200*
Chondroma(s), 186–187
Chondrosarcoma(s), 186–187
Chordoma(s), 186–187, *188–189*
of upper clivus, *88*
Choroidal artery, anterior, frontal-temporal-orbital approach to, *85*
Ciliary artery, posterior, lateral orbital approach to, *104*
Ciliary ganglion, lateral orbital approach to, *104*
Ciliary nerve, posterior, lateral orbital approach to, *104*
Cisterna magna, exposure of, in suboccipital medial approach, *17*
Clinoid process, anterior, meningioma of, removal of, 119–120, *130–134*
pterional approach to, *8*
removal of, 201–202, *205–207*
posterior, subtemporal transtentorial approach to, *69*
Clivus, chordoma of, extradural, *188*
with displacement of pons, *188*
ethmoidal sphenoidal approach to, 93, *94*
exposure of, for midface degloving, 87, *91–92*
in lateral approach to middle skull base, *49*
in transfrontal basal approach, *77*
meningiomas of, removal of, 122
oral approach to, 95–96, *96–97*
posterior, anatomical relations in, *97*
sublabial paraseptal sphenoidal approach to, 86–87, *88–92*
subtemporal transtentorial approach to, *69*
upper, chordoma of, *88*
Closure, for caudal orbitotomy, 107
for cranial orbitotomy, 105
for ethmoidal sphenoidal approach to sella and clivus, 93
for frontal orbital approach, 79, *81*
for frontal-temporal-orbital approach, 83
for frontotemporal approach, 6–7, *8*
for lateral approach to craniocervical junction, 55
for lateral approach to middle skull base, 45, *53*
for lateral orbitotomy with bone flap, 102
for middle cranial fossa approach, 28, *31*
to acoustic neurinoma, 156
for midface degloving, 87, *92*
for oral approach to clivus and C1–C2, 95–96
for pre–sigmoid sinus approach, 63
for removal of esthesioneuroblastoma, 227–228, *230–232*

Closure *(Continued)*
for resection of optic gliomas, 224
for retrosigmoid lateral suboccipital transmeatal approach to acoustic neurinoma, 155
for subfrontal approach, 3–4, *5*
for suboccipital lateral retrosigmoid approach, 13
for suboccipital medial approach, 16
for subtemporal approach, 9
for subtemporal transtentorial approach, 69
for subtemporal-transzygomatic approach, 41, *42*
for transconjunctival medial orbitotomy, 98
for transfrontal basal approach, 75–76, *78*
for translabyrinthine approach, 19
to acoustic neurinoma, 157
for transotic approach, 25
for transsphenoidal decompression of optic canal, 112
Cochlea, middle cranial fossa approach to, *28*
subtemporal transtentorial approach to, *70*
Cochlear nerve, anatomic relations of, *161*
dissection from acoustic neurinoma, 154, *166–167*
middle cranial fossa approach to, *28*
preservation of, for removal of acoustic neurinoma, *162, 164*
Communicating artery(ies), anterior, aneurysm of, ruptured, *205*
pterional approach to, *8*
posterior, frontal-temporal-orbital approach to, *85*
pterional approach to, *8*
subtemporal transtentorial approach to, *70*
Computed tomography (CT), for diagnosis of acoustic neurinomas, 152, *159–160*
for diagnosis of epidermoid cysts, 170
for diagnosis of meningiomas, 117
Cranial base, meningiomas of, common locations of, 118, *124*
Cranial fossa. See *Fossa.*
Cranial nerve(s), blood supply to, 241
caudal, exposure of, lateral approach to, *53*
compression of, from petroclival meningioma, *137*
dissection of, in removal of meningioma of cerebellopontine angle, *144*
eighth, and origin of acoustic neurinomas, 152, *158*
exposure of, for removal of acoustic neurinoma, 154, 156–157, *169*
in frontal-temporal-orbital approach, *84–85*
in approach to pituitary tumors, 214–215, *220*
in lateral approach to craniocervical junction, *58*
in lateral approach to middle skull base, *46–47*
in transoral approach to clivus, *97*
involvement of, with meningioma of cerebellopontine angle, *142*
lower, visualization of, for removal of acoustic neurinoma, *165*
preservation of, for removal of meningioma of cerebellopontine angle, *146–147*
for removal of meningioma of craniocervical junction, *150*
pre-sigmoid sinus approach to, *64*
suboccipital lateral retrosigmoid approach to, *15*
subtemporal transtentorial approach to, *70, 73*
transsphenoidal approach to, *36–37*
Cranial nerve IV, approach to, for cranial orbitotomy, 105, *106*
Craniectomy, for removal of chemodectoma, *194*
Craniectomy *(Continued)*
for suboccipital lateral retrosigmoid approach, 12, *14*
for suboccipital medial approach, 16, *17*
rectosigmoid, *20*
suboccipital, for lateral approach to craniocervical junction, 54–55, *57*
Craniocervical junction, course of vertebral artery at, 54, *57*
exposure of, *58*
lateral aproach to, 54–55, *55–61*
meningioma of, removal of, 122, *148–151*
Craniopharyngioma(s), 176–179, *180–185*
approaches to, choice of, 177
calcification in, 176, *180, 183*
classification of, 176, *180*
cystic, 176, *180*
frontotemporal approach to, 178–179
growth patterns of, 176, *182*
histologic features of, 176, *180*
incidence of, 176
infiltrative, 176, *180*
origin of, sites of, 176, *181*
postoperative complications from, 179
preoperative management of, 177
pterional approach to, 178–179
anatomic relations in, 177, *183*
resection of, 176
anatomic considerations in, 177
subfrontal approach to, 178, *183–185*
anatomic relations in, 177, *183*
subtemporal approach to, 179
suprasellar, displacement of optic nerves by, *182*
removal of, *184–185*
transcallosal approach to, 179
transsphenoidal approach to, 177–178
Craniotomy, bifrontal, for removal of meningioma, 119, *126–127*
for frontal orbital approach, 79, *80–81*
for frontal-temporal-orbital approach, 82–83, *84–85*
for frontotemporal approach, 6, *7–8*
for middle cranial fossa approach, 27–28, *30–31*
for pre-sigmoid sinus approach, 62–63, *64–65*
for removal of petroclival meningioma in cavernous sinus, *139*
for suboccipital medial approach, 16, *17*
for subtemporal approach, 9, *10*
for subtemporal transtentorial approach, 67
for subtemporal-transzygomatic approach, 40, *42*
for transfrontal basal approach, 75, *76–78*
for translabyrinthine approach, 18–19, *20–23*
for transotic approach, 24, *25*
Craniotomy bone plate, replacement of, after removal of esthesioneuroblastoma, 227, *232*
Craniotomy flap, frontotemporal, placement of, for removal of meningioma of anterior clinoid, *131*
Cribriform plate, transfrontal basal approach to, *76*
transsphenoidal approach to, *35*
Crista galli, transfrontal basal approach to, *76*
Crockard transoral retractor, placement of, 95, *96*
Cushing's disease, treatment of, 213
Cyst(s), dermoid, 170–171, *172, 174–175*
epidermoid, 170–171, *172–173*
Cystic craniopharyngioma(s), 176, *180*
Cytokeratin staining, for identification of chordoma, 186, *188*

Degloving, midface, 86–87, *88–92*
use of Gelpi retractors for, 86, *90*
Dermoid cyst(s), 170–171, *172, 174–175*
Desmarres retractor, for transcutaneous orbitotomy, 98 *100*
Diaphragma sellae, transsphenoidal approach to, *37*
Digastric muscle, posterior belly of, in lateral approach to middle skull base, *46*
transection of, for removal of chemodectoma, *194*
Drainage fistula, creation of, for treatment of cholesterol granuloma, 197, *200*
Dura, frontal, cranial orbital approach to, *106*
exposure of, in frontal orbital approach, *81*
in lateral approach to middle skull base, *47*
pre-sigmoid sinus approach to, *64–65*
resection of, for removal of esthesioneuroblastoma, *230*
for removal of meningioma of cerebellopontine angle, *145*
Dura graft(s), lyophilized, for closure of dural defects, 45, *53*
Dural arteriovenous fistula(s), blood supply to, *246–249, 251–252*
embolization of, 243–244, *254*
Dural defect(s), closure of, after removal of esthesioneuroblastoma, *230–231*
with lyophilized dura grafts, 45, *53*
covering of, by pericranial flap, for removal of meningioma of anterior clinoid process, *134*
Dural opening, for frontotemporal approach, 6, *8*
for lateral approach to craniocervical junction, 54–55, *58*
for pre-sigmoid sinus approach, *65*
for removal of esthesioneuroblastoma, *229*
for removal of meningioma of anterior clinoid, *132*
for retrosigmoid lateral suboccipital transmeatal approach, to acoustic neurinomas, 153
for subfrontal approach, 3, *5*
for suboccipital lateral retrosigmoid approach, 12, *15*
for suboccipital medial approach, 16, *17*
for subtemporal approach, 9, *10*
for subtemporal transtentorial approach, 68, *73*
for subtemporal-transzygomatic approach, 40, *42*
for transfrontal basal approach, 75
for transsphenoidal approach, 32, *35*
Dural reconstruction, after removal of chemodectoma, *196*
after removal of chordoma, 187, *189*
after removal of esthesioneuroblastoma, *230–231*
Dural ring, carotid, dissection of, for repair of aneurysms, *205*

Eighth cranial nerve, and origin of acoustic neurinomas, 152, *158*
Embolization, of aneurysms, 243–244, *255*
Endovascular therapy, 241–244, *245–255*
anatomical considerations in, 241, *245–247*
pretherapeutic functional testing in, 242
superselective angiography for, 242
technical considerations in, 241–242
use of polyvinyl alcohol in, 243
Epidermoid cyst(s), 170–171, *172–173*
Esthesioneuroblastoma(s), 226–227, *227–232*
Ethmoid sinus, exposure of, for ethmoidal sphenoidal approach to sella and clivus, 93, *94*
Ethmoidal artery(ies), identification of, for transcutaneous orbitotomy, 98, *101*
severing of, for transsphenoidal decompression of optic canal, *113*
Ethmoidal sphenoidal approach, to sella and clivus, 93, *94*

Extended maxillotomy, 87, *91–92*
External auditory canal, in lateral approach to middle skull base, *46*
External carotid trunk, in lateral approach to middle skull base, *46–47*
Extradural chordoma, of clivus, *188*
Eyelid(s), tarsi of, in orbitotomy with medial approach, *101*

Facial approach(es), 86–113. See also specific approaches, e.g., *Clivus, sublabial paraseptal sphenoidal approach to.*
Facial artery, in lateral approach to middle skull base, *46*
Facial nerve, anatomic relations of, 153, *161*
  dissection of, for removal of chemodectoma, *194*
    from acoustic neurinoma, 154, *166–167*
  preservation of, in middle cranial fossa approach, 26–28, *30–31*
    in removal of acoustic neurinoma, 155, 156, *162, 164, 169*
    in translabyrinthine approach, 18–19, *20–23*, 156
    in transotic approach, 24–25, *25*
  reconstruction of, after removal of acoustic neurinoma, 155
Falcine artery, anterior, enlarged, feeding falcine meningioma, *245*
Falx, dural arteriovenous fistula of, blood supply to, *252*
Fistula(s), arteriovenous, dural, blood supply to, *246–249, 251–252*
    embolization of, 243–244, *254*
  cavernous, carotid, blood supply to, *253*
  fistula drainage, creation of, for treatment of cholesterol granulomas, 197, *200*
  vertebrovertebral, blood supply to, *254*
    embolization of, 244, *254*
Flocculus, pre-sigmoid sinus approach to, *64*
Foramen lacerum, subtemporal transtentorial approach to, *69*
Foramen magnum, exposure of, for midface degloving, *92*
  lateral rim of, removal of, in lateral approach to craniocervical junction, *57*
  meningioma in, resection of, through lateral approach to craniocervical junction, 55, *61*
  narrowing of, from extradural chordoma, *188*
  subtemporal transtentorial approach to, *69*
Foramen ovale, artery of, feeding cavernous sinus dural arteriovenous fistula, *247*
  subtemporal transtentorial approach to, *69*
Foramen rotundum, artery of, feeding dural arteriovenous fistula of cavernous sinus, *246*
    feeding juvenile nasopharyngeal angiofibroma, *250*
    feeding meningioma of cavernous sinus, *246*
Foramen spinosum, subtemporal transtentorial approach to, *70*
Fossa, interpeduncular, exposure of, intradural transtentorial, 68, *72*
  middle, blood supply to, 241
    bony destruction in, from nasopharyngeal angiofibroma, *235*
    exposure of, in panoramic orbitotomy, *111*
    floor of, See *Fossa floor.*
  temporal-infratemporal, lateral approach to, 43, *46–53*
Fossa dura, subtemporal transtentorial approach to, *73*
Fossa floor, anatomical relations in, *69, 71–72*
  reconstruction of, with bone grafts, 76, *78*
  transfrontal basal approach to, *76*
Fovea ethmoidalis, caudal orbital approach to, 107, *108*
Frontal approach(es), 75–85. See also specific approaches, e.g., *Transfrontal basal approach.*
Frontal bone flap(s), for subfrontal approach, 3, *5*
Frontal dura, cranial orbital approach to, *106*
  exposure of, in frontal orbital approach, *81*
Frontal lobe(s), retraction of, for removal of esthesioneuroblastoma, *230*
Frontal nerve, cranial orbital approach to, *106*
Frontal orbital approach, 79, *80–81*
Frontal sinus(es), cranial orbital approach to, *106*
  transfrontal basal approach to, *76*
  transsphenoidal approach to, *35*
Frontal-temporal-orbital approach, 82–83, *83–85*
Frontotemporal approach, 6–7, *7–8*
  to craniopharyngiomas, 178–179
Frontotemporal craniotomy flap, placement of, for removal of meningioma of anterior clinoid, *131*

Gelpi retractor(s), use of, for midface degloving, 86, *90*
Geniculate ganglion, subtemporal transtentorial approach to, *70*
Giant pituitary tumor(s), management of, 215
Gingival margin, transsphenoidal approach to, *35*
Glasscock-Jackson classification, of glomus tumors, 190, 191t
Glenoid fossa, exposure of, for lateral approach to middle skull base, *47, 48*
Glioma(s), optic, 224, *225*
Globe, displacement of, retraction suture for, 98, *99*
  lateral orbital approach to, *104*
Globular meningioma, surrounding internal carotid artery, 117, *123*
Glomus jugulare tumor(s), 190, *193*
  blood supply to, *249*
  preoperative embolization of, 242–243, *249–250*
Glomus tympanicum tumor(s), 190
Glomus tumor(s), classification of, 190, 191t
Granuloma(s), cholesterol, 197–198, *198–200*. See also *Cholesterol granuloma(s).*
Greater occipital nerve, in lateral approach to craniocervical junction, 54, *56–57*
Greater superficial petrosal nerve, middle cranial fossa approach to, *30*
  subtemporal transtentorial approach to, *70*
Growth hormone, levels of, in acromegaly, 213

Hard palate, mucosa of, elevation of, for midface degloving, 87, *91*
Hearing, preservation of, 18
Hemangioblastoma, exposure of, through lateral approach to craniocervical junction, 55, *59–60*
Hemangiopericytoma(s), blood supply to, *249–250*
Hypervascular tumor(s), of skull base, preoperative embolization of, 242–243, *248–250, 253*
Hypoglossal schwannoma, resection of, through lateral approach to craniocervical junction, 55, *60*

Incision(s), bicoronal, for subfrontal approach, 3, *4*
  for caudal orbitotomy, 107
Incision(s) *(Continued)*
  for ethmoidal sphenoidal approach to sella and clivus, 93, *94*
  for frontal orbital approach, 79
  for frontal-temporal-orbital approach, 82, *83–84*
  for frontotemporal approach, 6, *7*
  for lateral approach to craniocervical junction, 54
  for lateral approach to middle skull base, 44, *50*
  for lateral orbitotomy with bone flap, 102, *103*
  for middle cranial fossa approach, 27, *29*
  for midface degloving, 86–87, *88*
  for oral approach to clivus and C1–C2, 95, *96*
  for pre-sigmoid sinus approach, 62, *63*
  for removal of chemodectoma, *194*
  for removal of esthesioneuroblastomas, *228–229*
  for subfrontal approach, 3, *4*
  for suboccipital lateral retrosigmoid approach, 12, *14*
  for suboccipital medial approach, 16, *17*
  for subtemporal approach, 9, *10*
  for subtemporal transtentorial approach, 67, *70*
  for subtemporal-transzygomatic approach, 40, *41–42*
  for transcutaneous orbitotomy, 98, *100*
  for transfrontal basal approach, 75
  for translabyrinthine approach, 18, *20*
  for transotic approach, 24, *25*
  for transsphenoidal approach, 32, *34*
  for transsphenoidal decompression of optic canal, 112, *113*
  Kronlein, for lateral orbitotomy with bone flap, 102, *103*
  lid crease, for transcutaneous orbitotomy, 98–99, *100*
  Lynch, for transcutaneous orbitotomy, 98–99, *100*
    for transsphenoidal decompression of optic canal, 112, *113*
  midline occipital, for suboccipital medial approach, 16, *17*
  modified Wright, for lateral orbitotomy with bone flap, 102, *103*
  paramedian, for oral approach to clivus and C1–C2, 95, *96*
  preauricular, for subtemporal approach, 9, *10*
    for subtemporal-transzygomatic approach, 40, *41*
  retroauricular, for lateral approach to middle skull base, 44, *50*
  scalp, for subtemporal-transzygomatic approach, 40, *41*
  subbrow, for transcutaneous orbitotomy, 99, *100*
  sublabial, for transsphenoidal approach, 32, *34*
  trap-door, for middle cranial fossa approach, 27, *29*
Inferior cavernous sinus, artery of, transsphenoidal approach to, *36*
Inferior cerebellar artery, anterior. See *Cerebellar artery(ies), inferior, anterior.*
  posterior. See *Cerebellar artery(ies), posterior, inferior.*
Inferior oblique muscle, lateral orbital approach to, *104*
Inferior pharyngeal constrictor muscle, in lateral approach to middle skull base, *46*
Infiltrative craniopharyngioma(s), 176, *180*
Infiltrative meningioma(s), debulking of, 118
  partial removal of, 121, *136–138*
Infraclinoid carotid artery, exposure of, for repair of aneurysms, *205–206*
Infraorbital foramen, exposure of, for midface degloving, *88*

Infratentorial dura, exposure of, in presigmoid sinus approach, *65*
Infundibular stalk, transsphenoidal approach to, *35*
Internal auditory canal. See *Auditory canal, internal.*
Internal carotid arteriovenous fistula(s), embolization of, 243–244
Internal carotid artery. See *Carotid artery, internal.*
Internal jugular vein, in lateral approach to middle skull base, *46–47*
Internal maxillary artery, exposure of, for midface degloving, 87, *91*
Interpeduncular fossa, exposure of, intradural transtentorial, 68, *72*
Interventional neuroradiology, 239–244, *245–255*
Intracanalicular acoustic neurinoma, 152, *160*
  exposure of cerebellopontine angle in, *161*
Intracavernous aneurysm(s), embolization of, 244, *255*
Intracavernous carotid artery, violation of, complications of, 83
Intraventricular meningioma, 117, *123*

Jugular bulb, lateral approach to, 44–45, *47*
  preservation of, for removal of acoustic neurinoma, 153–154
  relation to internal carotid artery, at skull base, *50*
Jugular foramen, chemodectoma in, *192*
  lateral approach to, 43–44, *46–53*
  neurinomas of, resection of, lateral approach to, 45, *51–53*
Jugular vein, lateral approach to, anatomical considerations in, 43, *46–47*
Juvenile nasopharyngeal angiofibroma(s), 233–234, *234–237*
  blood supply to, *248, 250*
  preoperative embolization of, 243, *248, 250*

Keyhole burr hole(s), placement of, for frontotemporal approach, 6, *7*
  for subfrontal approach, 3, *4*
Kronlein incision, for lateral orbitotomy with bone flap, 102, *103*

Lacrimal duct(s), in orbitotomy with medial approach, *101*
Lacrimal nerve, cranial orbital approach to, *106*
Lacrimal sac(s), in orbitotomy with medial approach, *101*
Lamina papyracea, removal of, for transsphenoidal decompression of optic canal, 112, *113*
Lateral approach, to middle skull base, 43–46, *46–53*
Lateral canthotomy, 102, *103*
Lateral orbitotomy, 102, *103–104*
  transconjunctival, 102, *103*
  with bone flap, 102, *104*
Lateral parasellar area, transsphenoidal approach to, *37*
Lateral position, for suboccipital lateral retrosigmoid approach, 12, *13*
Lateral retrosigmoid approach, suboccipital, 12–13, *13–15*
Lateral semicircular canal, in lateral approach to middle skull base, *47*
Lateral transcondylar approach, to vertebral artery aneurysms, 203, *209*
Levator palpebrae muscle, cranial orbital approach to, *106*
Levator-superior rectus complex, cranial orbital approach to, *106*
Lid crease incision, for transcutaneous orbitotomy, 98, *100*
Lidocaine, injection of, during superselective angiography, 242
Limbus sphenoidale, subtemporal transtentorial approach to, *69*
Lingual artery, in lateral approach to middle skull base, *46*
Longissimus capitis muscle, in lateral approach to middle skull base, *46*
Longus capitis muscle, retraction of, for midface degloving, *92*
Lower cranial nerve(s), visualization of, for removal of acoustic neurinoma, *165*
Lynch incision, for transcutaneous orbitotomy, 98–99, *100*
  for transsphenoidal decompression of optic canal, 112, *113*
Lyophilized dura graft, for closure of dural defects, 45, *53*

MacCarty burr hole, placement of, for subfrontal approach, 3, *4*
Macroadenoma(s), pituitary, compression of brain base from, 214, *217*
Magnetic resonance imaging (MRI), for diagnosis of acoustic neurinoma, 152, *159–160*
  for diagnosis of epidermoid cysts, 170
  for diagnosis of meningiomas, 117, *124*
Major septum, transsphenoidal approach to, *35*
Mandible, inferior margin of, in lateral approach to middle skull base, *47*
Mandibulovidian artery, feeding juvenile nasopharyngeal angiofibroma, *248, 250*
Marginal tentorial artery, feeding dural arteriovenous fistula, *251*
Masseter muscle, in lateral approach to middle skull base, *46–47*
Mastoid, middle cranial fossa approach to, *28*
Mastoid tip, exposure of, for removal of chemodectoma, *194*
  in lateral approach to middle skull base, *46*
Mastoidectomy, translabyrinthine approach to, 18–19, *20–23*
Maxilla(e), anterior walls of, exposure of, for midface degloving, *88*
Maxillary arch, exposure of, for midface degloving, *88*
Maxillary artery, internal, exposure of, for midface degloving, 87, *91*
Maxillary buttress, attachments of, removal of, for midface degloving, *90*
Maxillary sinus, exposure of, in lateral approach to middle skull base, *49*
  panoramic orbital approach to, *110*
  walls of, remodeling of, from nasopharyngeal angiofibroma, *235*
Maxillary wall(s), removal of, for midface degloving, *89*
Maxillotomy, extended, 87, *91–92*
Meckel's cave, meningioma of, removal of, 120, *134–135*
  trigeminal neuroma in, *11*
Medial approach, suboccipital, 16, *17*
Medial canthal ligament, in orbitotomy with medial approach, *101*
Medial orbitotomy, transconjunctival, 98, *99–100*
Meningeal artery(ies), feeding hemangiopericytomas, *249*
  middle, subtemporal transtentorial approach to, *71*
  posterior, feeding dural arteriovenous fistula, *252*
  superselective angiography of, *247*
Meningioma(s), 117–122, *123–151*
  blood supply to, *252*
  clinical presentation of, 117
Meningioma(s) *(Continued)*
  cranial base, common locations of, 118, *124*
  diagnosis of, 117–118, *124*
  extension of, into sphenoid sinus, *126–127*
  falcine, blood supply to, *245*
  globular, surrounding internal carotid artery, 117, *123*
  histologic features of, 117
  incidence of, 117
  infiltrative, debulking of, 118
    partial removal of, 121, *136–138*
  intraventricular, 117, *123*
  of anterior clinoid, removal of, 119–120, *130–134*
  of cavernous sinus, blood supply to, *246*
    removal of, 120, *134–135*
      subtotal, 121, *136–138*
  of cerebellopontine angle, removal of, 120–122, *142–148*
  of clivus, removal of, 122
  of craniocervical junction, removal of, 122, *148–151*
  of foramen magnum, resection of, through lateral approach to craniocervical junction, 55, *61*
  of Meckel's cave, removal of, 120, *134–135*
  of olfactory groove, removal of, 119, *125–128*
    postoperative computed tomographic findings after, *128*
  of orbital sphenoidal area, removal of, 120, *134–135*
  of paranasal sinuses, removal of, 119, *127–128*
  of parasellar area, removal of, 120, *134–135*
  of planum sphenoidale, removal of, 119, *125–128*
  of sphenoid ridge, removal of, 119–120, *130–134*
  of tuberculum sellae, removal of, 119, *125–130*
    with compression of optic nerve, *129*
  petroclival, removal of, 120–122, *136–141*
  preoperative embolization of, 243
  removal of, bifrontal craniotomy for, 119, *126–127*
    principles of, 118–119, *124–125*
  tentorial, removal of, 120–122, *136–148*
  with preservation of arachnoid sheath, 118, *125*
Meningioma en plaque, compressing optic chiasm, 117, *123*
Meningitis, chemical, after removal of epidermoid cysts, 171
Microadenoma(s), pituitary, in sella turcica, 214, *217*
Midbrain, pterional approach to, *8*
Middle cerebral artery, frontal-temporal-orbital approach to, *84–85*
  pterional approach to, *8*
Middle ear, middle cranial fossa approach to, *28*
Middle fossa. See *Fossa, middle.*
Middle fossa approach, 26–28, *28–31*
  to acoustic neurinomas, 155–156
Middle meningeal artery, subtemporal transtentorial approach to, *71*
Middle skull base, lateral approach to, 43–46, *46–53*
Midface degloving, 86–87, *88–92*
  use of Gelpi retractors for, 86, *90*
Midline occipital incision, for suboccipital medial approach, 16, *17*
Modified Wright incision, for lateral orbitotomy with bone flap, 102, *103*
MRI (magnetic resonance imaging). See *Magnetic resonance imaging (MRI).*
Muscle flap, temporalis, in middle cranial fossa approach, *29*
  retraction of, for subtemporal-transzygomatic approach, 40, *42*

Muscle layer(s), exposure of, in lateral approach to craniocervical junction, 54, *56*

Nasal cavity, exposure of, in lateral approach to middle skull base, *50*
Nasal concha(e), in orbitotomy with medial approach, *101*
Nasal paraseptal sphenoidal approach, to sella and clivus, 86–87, *88–92*
Nasal septum, transsphenoidal approach to, *37*
Nasal turbinate(s), transsphenoidal approach to, *35, 37*
Nasopharyngeal angiofibroma(s), juvenile, 233–234, *234–237*
  blood supply to, *248, 250*
  preoperative embolization of, 243, *248, 250*
Nasopharynx, exposure of, in lateral approach to middle skull base, *50*
Neck, vessels in, temporary balloon occlusion of, 242
Nerve(s). See specific names, e.g., *Cranial nerve(s).*
Neurinoma(s), acoustic, 152–157, *158–169*. See also *Acoustic neurinoma(s).*
  near cerebellopontine angle, *52*
  of jugular foramen, resection of, lateral approach to, 45, *51–53*
  trigeminal, in Meckel's cave, *11*
Neuroradiology, interventional, 239–244, *245–255*

Oblique capitis inferior muscle, in lateral approach to craniocervical junction, *57*
Oblique muscle(s), inferior, lateral orbital approach to, *104*
  superior, cranial orbital approach to, *106*
    lateral orbital approach to, *104*
Occipital artery, feeding dural arteriovenous fistula, *252*
  feeding paraganglioma, *249*
  in lateral approach to middle skull base, *46*
Occipital incision, midline, for suboccipital medial approach, 16, *17*
Occipital nerve, greater, in lateral approach to craniocervical junction, 54, *56–57*
Octreotide, for treatment of acromegaly, 213
Oculomotor nerve, in subtemporal-transzygomatic approach, *42*
  preservation of, for removal of petroclival meningioma, *141*
Odontoid, drilling of, for oral approach to clivus and C1–C2, 95, *97*
Olfactory fiber(s), transfrontal basal approach to, *76*
Olfactory groove, meningioma of, removal of, 119, *125–128*
    postoperative computed tomographic findings after, *128*
Olfactory nerve, exposure of, for removal of meningioma of anterior clinoid, *133*
Operative procedure, for transsphenoidal approach, 32–33, *33–37*
Ophthalmic artery, exposure of, for repair of paraclinoid aneurysm, *206*
  feeding dural arteriovenous fistula of cavernous sinus, *246*
  transsphenoidal approach to, *36*
Optic canal, panoramic orbital approach to, *110*
  transsphenoidal approach to, *35*
    for decompression, 112, *113*
Optic chiasm, compression of, by meningioma en plaque, 117, *123*
    by pituitary tumor, *223*
  displacement of, by pituitary tumor, *219*
  frontal-temporal-orbital approach to, *84*
  pterional approach to, *8*
Optic foramen, exposure of, for repair of aneurysms, *205*
  subtemporal transtentorial approach to, *69*
Optic glioma(s), 224, *225*
Optic nerve, compression of, by pituitary tumor, *223*
    from meningioma of tuberculum sellae, *129*
  decompression of, for removal of craniopharyngioma, *184*
  displacement of, by suprasellar craniopharyngioma, *182*
  dissection of, in resection of optic gliomas, 224
  exposure of, for bifrontal craniotomy for removal of meningiomas, 119, *126–127*
    for orbitotomy with medial approach, *100*
    for removal of meningioma of anterior clinoid, *133*
  frontal-temporal-orbital approach to, *84*
  lateral orbital approach to, *104*
  pterional approach to, *8*
  subtemporal transtentorial approach to, *70*
  transsphenoidal approach to, *36–37*
Oral approach, to C1–C2, 95–96, *96–97*
  to clivus, 95–96, *96–97*
Orbit(s), anatomical structures in, *110*
  bony decompression of, for removal of meningioma of orbital sphenoidal area, 120, *135*
  exposure of, for panoramic orbitotomy, *110–111*
    for transconjunctival lateral orbitotomy, *103*
    in frontal-temporal-orbital approach, *84*
    in transfrontal basal approach, *75, 78*
  removal of bone from, for caudal orbitotomy, 107, *108*
Orbital apex, anatomical structures at, *110*
  exposure of, in panoramic orbitotomy, *111*
Orbital approach, frontal, 79, *80–81*
Orbital fissure(s), superior, exposure of, in panoramic orbitotomy, *111*
Orbital floor, exposure of, for transconjunctival lateral orbitotomy, 102, *103*
Orbital septum, in orbitotomy with medial approach, *101*
Orbital sphenoidal area, meningioma of, removal of, 120, *134–135*
Orbitotomy, caudal approach for, 107, *108*
  cranial approach for, 105, *106*
  frontal-orbital approach for, 105, *106*
  lateral approach for, 102, *103–104*
    transconjunctival, 102, *103*
    with bone flap, 102, *104*
  medial approach for, 98–99, *99–101*
    transconjunctival, 98, *99–100*
    transcutaneous, 98–99, *100–101*
    transethmoidal, 99
  panoramic, 109, *110–111*
  paranasal-ethmoidal approach for, 98–99, *99–101*
Otic capsule, dissection of, *21–22*

Panoramic orbitotomy, 109, *110–111*
Paraclinoid aneurysm(s), repair of, *206–207*
Paraganglioma(s), 190–191, *192–196*. See also *Chemodectoma(s).*
Paramedian incision, for oral approach to clivus and C1–C2, 95, *96*
Paranasal cavity, packing of, after removal of esthesioneuroblastoma, *230*
Paranasal sinus(es), exposure of, in transfrontal basal approach, 75, *77*
  meningiomas of, removal of, 119, *127–128*
Paranasal-ethmoidal approach, for orbitotomy, 98–99, *99–101*
Paraophthalmic aneurysm(s), repair of, *206–207*
Parasellar area, lateral, transsphenoidal approach to, *37*
  meningioma of, removal of, 120, *134–135*
Paraseptal approach, transnasal, to pituitary tumors, 216, *222–223*
Paraseptal sphenoidal approach, to sella and clivus, 86–87, *88–92*
Park bench position, for suboccipital lateral retrosigmoid approach, 12, *13*
  modified, for lateral approach to craniocervical junction, *56*
Parotid duct, in lateral approach to middle skull base, *46*
Parotid gland, dissection of, for removal of chemodectoma, *194*
  in lateral approach to middle skull base, *46–47*
Pars nervosa, transsphenoidal approach to, *35*
Pearly tumor(s), 170–171, *172–173*
Pericranial flap, for covering dural defect, after removal of esthesioneuroblastoma, *230–231*
    after removal of meningioma of anterior clinoid, *134*
Periorbital landmark(s), *101*
Periosteum, elevation of, from orbit, for lateral orbitotomy with bone flap, *104*
Petroclinoid ligament, in subtemporal-transzygomatic approach, *42*
Petroclival area, exposure of, intradural transtentorial, 68, *72*
Petroclivus, meningiomas of, removal of, 120–122, *136–141*
Petrosal nerve(s), subtemporal transtentorial approach to, *70, 71*
  superficial, greater, middle cranial fossa approach to, *30*
Petrosal sinus(es), superior, exposure of, in pre-sigmoid sinus approach, 62, *64*
    subtemporal transtentorial approach to, *70*
Petrosal vein, pre-sigmoid sinus approach to, *64*
Petrosectomy, partial, anatomical considerations in, *47*
Petrous apex, cholesterol granulomas of, 197–198, *198–200*
Petrous bone, anatomical relations in, *69–70, 74*
  blood supply to, 241
  chemodectoma in, *192*
  nerves in, anatomic relations of, *161*
Petrous internal carotid artery, subtemporal transtentorial approach to, *70*
Petrous pyramid, subtemporal transtentorial approach to, *69*
Petrous-to-supraclinoid carotid bypass, 203–204, *210*
Pharyngeal artery, ascending, feeding paraganglioma, *250*
    feeding schwannoma, *253*
    in lateral approach to middle skull base, *46, 47*
Pharyngeal constrictor muscle, inferior, in lateral approach to middle skull base, *46*
Pharyngeal retractor, placement of, 95, *96*
Pituitary adenoma(s), 212–216, *217–223*. See also *Pituitary tumor(s).*
Pituitary gland, anatomical relations of, to cavernous sinuses and carotid arteries, *218*
  transsphenoidal approach to, *35–36*
Pituitary macroadenoma(s), compression of brain base from, 214, *217*
Pituitary microadenoma(s), in sella turcica, 214, *217*
Pituitary tumor(s), 212–216, *217–223*
  classification of, 212, 212t
  endocrinological considerations in, 212–214
  extension of, intrasellar, *220*
    to carotid artery, *218*, 223
  giant, management of, 215
  grading system for, 214, *217*
  growth characteristics of, 214, *217–219*
  preoperative management of, 215, *220–221*

Pituitary tumor(s) *(Continued)*
structures affecting, *218, 220, 223*
suprasellar extension of, *220*
surgical anatomy in, 214–215, *220*
surgical approach to, 215–216, *222–223*
Planum sphenoidale, meningiomas of, removal of, 119, *125–128*
subtemporal transtentorial approach to, *69*
Polyvinyl alcohol (PVA), for use in endovascular therapy, 243
Pons, displacement of, from chordoma of clivus, *188*
subtemporal transtentorial approach to, *73*
Pontine cavernous angioma, resection of, 63, *65–66*
Position, for caudal orbitotomy, 107, *108*
for ethmoidal sphenoidal approach to sella and clivus, 93
for frontal orbital approach, 79
for frontal-temporal-orbital approach, 82, *83*
for frontotemporal approach, 6, *7*
for lateral approach to craniocervical junction, 54, *55–56*
for lateral approach to middle skull base, 44
for middle cranial fossa approach, 26–27, *29*
for midface degloving, 86
for oral approach to clivus and C1–C2, 95
for petrous-to-supraclinoid carotid bypass, 203
for pre-sigmoid sinus approach, 62
for subfrontal approach, 3, *4*
for suboccipital lateral retrosigmoid approach, 12, *13*
for suboccipital medial approach, 16
for subtemporal approach, 9
for subtemporal transtentorial approach, 67, *70*
for subtemporal-transzygomatic approach, 40, *41*
for transfrontal basal approach, 75
for translabyrinthine approach, 18
for transotic approach, 24
for transsphenoidal approach, 32, *33*
for transsphenoidal decompression of optic canal, 112
lateral, for suboccipital retrosigmoid approach, 12, *13*
park bench, for suboccipital lateral retrosigmoid approach, 12, *13*
modified, for lateral approach to craniocervical junction, *56*
prone, for suboccipital lateral retrosigmoid approach, 12, *13*
semisitting, for lateral approach to craniocervical junction, *56*
for suboccipital lateral retrosigmoid approach, 12, *13*
Posterior auricular artery, feeding dural arteriovenous fistula, *248*
Posterior cerebral artery. See *Cerebral artery(ies), posterior.*
Posterior ciliary artery, lateral orbital approach to, *104*
Posterior ciliary nerve, lateral orbital approach to, *104*
Posterior clinoid process, subtemporal transtentorial approach to, *69*
Posterior clivus, anatomical relations in, *97*
Posterior communicating artery, frontal-temporal-orbital approach to, *85*
pterional approach to, *8*
subtemporal transtentorial approach to, *70*
Posterior inferior cerebellar artery. See *Cerebellar artery(ies), inferior, posterior.*
Posterior meningeal artery, feeding dural arteriovenous fistula, *252*
Preauricular incision, for subtemporal approach, 9, *10*
for subtemporal-transzygomatic approach, 40, *41*
Presigmoid approach, 62–63, *63–66*
retrolabyrinthine, to anterior inferior cerebellar artery aneurysms, 202–203, *209*
to basilar trunk aneurysms, 202–203, *209*
to cholesterol granulomas, 198, *200*
to meningiomas of petroclivus, 120–121, *136–141*
Presigmoid-transtentorial approach, to petroclival meningioma in cavernous sinus, 121, *138–141*
Prolactinoma(s), 212, 215
Prone position, for suboccipital lateral retrosigmoid approach, 12, *14*
Pterional approach, 6–7, *7–8*
for removal of meningiomas of orbital sphenoidal area, 120, *134–135*
for removal of meningiomas of sphenoid ridge and anterior clinoid, 119–120, *130–134*
to basilar artery aneurysm, 202, *208*
to craniopharyngiomas, 178–179
anatomic relations in, 177, *183*
Pterygoid plate, exposure of, for midface degloving, 87, *92*
Pterygoid process, exposure of, in lateral approach to middle skull base, *49*
Pterygopalatine fossa, exposure of, in panoramic orbitotomy, *110–111, 111*
PVA (polyvinyl alcohol), for use in endovascular therapy, 243
Pyriform apertures, enlargement of, in transsphenoidal approach, 32, *34*

Radiation therapy, for treatment of chemodectomas, 191
for treatment of chordomas, 187
Rectus muscle(s), cranial orbital approach to, *106*
Retraction suture(s), for displacement of globe, 98, *99*
Retractor(s), Desmarres, for transcutaneous orbitotomy, 98, *100*
Gelpi, use of, for midface degloving, 86, *90*
pharyngeal, placement of, 95, *96*
transoral, Crockard, placement of, 95, *96*
Retroauricular incision, for lateral approach to middle skull base, 44, *50*
Retrolabyrinthine presigmoid approach, to anterior inferior cerebellar artery aneurysms, 202–203, *209*
to basilar trunk aneurysms, 202–203, *209*
Retrosigmoid approach, lateral, suboccipital, 12–13, *13–15*
to acoustic neurinomas, 153–155, *161–169*
to meningioma of cerebellopontine angle, 122, *142–148*
to tentorial meningioma, 121
Retrosigmoid craniectomy, *20*
Retrosigmoid lateral suboccipital transmeatal approach, to acoustic neurinomas, 153–155, *161–169*
Rule of 50s, 18

Sagittal sinus(es), superior, dural arteriovenous fistula of, blood supply to, *252*
transection of, for removal of esthesioneuroblastoma, *229*
Saphenous vein graft, placement of, for cervical-to-petrous carotid bypass, 204, *211*
Scalp incision, for subtemporal-transzygomatic approach, 40, *41*
Schwannoma(s), blood supply to, *253*
cervical, preoperative embolization of, 243, *253*
hypoglossal, resection of, through lateral approach to craniocervical junction, *55, 60*
resection of, middle cranial fossa approach to, *30*
Schwannoma(s) *(Continued)*
vestibular, 152–157, *158–169*. See also *Acoustic neurinoma(s).*
Sella turcica, anatomical relations of, *35*
ethmoidal sphenoidal approach to, 93, *94*
exposure of, in transfrontal basal approach, *77*
floor of, removal of, for midface degloving, *90*
transsphenoidal approach to, *35*
pituitary microadenoma in, 214, *217*
sublabial paraseptal sphenoidal approach to, 86–87, *88–92*
Semicircular canal(s), fenestration of, *21*
lateral, in lateral approach to middle skull base, *47*
superior, identification of, in middle cranial fossa approach, 27, *30–31*
subtemporal transtentorial approach to, *70*
Semisitting position, for lateral approach to craniocervical junction, *56*
for suboccipital lateral retrosigmoid approach, 12, *13*
Semispinalis muscle, penetration of, by greater occipital nerve, *56*
Septum, major, transsphenoidal approach to, *35*
orbital, in orbitotomy with medial approach, *101*
Sigmoid sinus, creation of Bill's island over, *21*
exposure of, for removal of chemodectoma, *194–195*
in pre-sigmoid sinus approach, 62, *64*
in lateral approach to middle skull base, *47*
Sinus(es). See specific types, e.g., *Paranasal sinus(es).*
Sinusotomy, Caldwell-Luc, 86, *89*
Skin flap, for frontotemporal approach, 6, *7*
Skull base, blood supply to, 241, *245–247*
bypass procedures for, 203–204, *210–211*
exposure of, in panoramic orbitotomy, *110–111*
hypervascular tumors of, preoperative embolization of, 242–243, *248–250, 253*
middle, lateral approach to, 43–46, *46–53*
relation of internal carotid artery to jugular bulb at, *50*
removal of dermoid cyst from, *174*
vascular lesions of, angiographic protocols for, 242t
Sphenoid ridge, meningioma of, removal of, 119–120, *130–134*
Sphenoid sinus, exposure of, for ethmoidal sphenoidal approach to sella and clivus, 93, *94*
for removal of meningioma of anterior clinoid, *133*
in lateral approach to middle skull base, *49*
extension of meningioma into, *126–127*
floor of, removal of, 32, *34*
in transsphenoidal decompression of optic canal, *113*
keel of, 32, *34*
transsphenoidal approach to, *35, 37*
Spinal cord, cervical, suboccipital medial approach to, *17*
Spinal nerve(s), C2, anterior branch of, in lateral approach to craniocervical junction, *57*
Splenius capitis muscle, in lateral approach to middle skull base, *46*
Stapes, middle cranial fossa approach to, *28*
Stenver's-projection radiograph, for identification of superior semicircular canal, 27, *31*
Sternocleidomastoid muscle, dissection of, for removal of chemodectoma, *194*
in lateral approach to middle skull base, *46*
Styloglossus muscle, in lateral approach to middle skull base, *47*
Stylohyoid muscle, in lateral approach to middle skull base, *46–47*

Stylopharyngeus muscle, in lateral approach to middle skull base, *47*
Subbrow incision, for transcutaneous orbitotomy, 99, *100*
Subfrontal approach, 3–4, *4–5*
  to craniopharyngiomas, 178, *183–185*
    anatomic relations in, 177, *183*
Sublabial incision, for transsphenoidal approach, 32, *34*
Sublabial paraseptal sphenoidal approach, to sella and clivus, 86–87, *88–92*
Submandibular gland, in lateral approach to middle skull base, *46*
Suboccipital craniectomy, for lateral approach to craniocervical junction, 54–55, *57*
Suboccipital lateral retrosigmoid approach, 12–13, *13–15*
  to meningiomas of cerebellopontine angle, 122, *142–148*
  to tentorial meningiomas, 121
Suboccipital medial approach, 16, *17*
Subtemporal approach, 9, *10*
  for removal of meningiomas of Meckel's cave, 120
  to basilar artery aneurysms, 202, *208*
  to craniopharyngiomas, 179
Subtemporal transtentorial approach, 66–69, *69–74*
Subtemporal-transzygomatic approach, 40–41, *41–42*
Superficial petrosal nerve, greater, middle cranial fossa approach to, *30*
    subtemporal transtentorial approach to, *70*
Superficial temporal artery, in lateral approach to middle skull base, *46*
Superior cerebellar artery. See *Cerebellar artery(ies), superior.*
Superior oblique muscle, cranial orbital approach to, *106*
  lateral orbital approach to, *104*
Superior orbital fissure, exposure of, in panoramic orbitotomy, *111*
Superior petrosal sinus, exposure of, in pre-sigmoid sinus approach, 62, *64*
  subtemporal transtentorial approach to, *70*
Superior sagittal sinus, dural arteriovenous fistula of, blood supply to, *252*
  transection of, for removal of esthesioneuroblastoma, *229*
Superior semicircular canal(s), identification of, in middle cranial fossa approach, 27, *30–31*
  subtemporal transtentorial approach to, *70*
Superior thyroid artery, in lateral approach to middle skull base, *46*
Superselective angiography, 242
Supraclinoid internal carotid artery, subtemporal transtentorial approach to, *70*
Supraorbital nerve, cranial orbital approach to, *106*
  in orbitotomy with medial approach, *101*
  transfrontal basal approach to, *76*
Supraorbital rim, exposure of, in frontal-temporal-orbital approach, *84*
Suprasellar craniopharyngioma(s), displacement of optic nerves by, *182*
  removal of, *184–185*
Suprasellar epidermoid cyst, *172*
Supratentorial dura, exposure of, in presigmoid approach, *65*
Supratrochlear nerve, cranial orbital approach to, *106*
  in orbitotomy with medial approach, *101*
Suture(s), retraction, for displacement of globe, 98, *99*
Sylvian fissure, dissection of, for removal of meningioma of anterior clinoid, *132*
Sympathetic nerve, transsphenoidal approach to, *36*
Tarsus (tarsi), of eyelids, in orbitotomy with medial approach, *101*
Temporal area, dermoid cyst in, *174*
Temporal artery, superficial, in lateral approach to middle skull base, *46*
Temporal lobe, pterional approach to, *8*
Temporal-infratemporal fossa, lateral approach to, 43, *46–53*
Temporalis muscle flap, in middle cranial fossa approach, *29*
  retraction of, for subtemporal-transzygomatic approach, 40, *42*
Temporomandibular joint, lateral approach to, *48*
Temporo-occipital-petrosal approach(es), 40–74. See also specific approaches, e.g., *Subtemporal-transzygomatic approach.*
Tentorial artery, marginal, feeding dural arteriovenous fistula, *251*
Tentorial flap, retraction of, 68
Tentorial notch, anatomical relations in, *42*, *71–72*
Tentorium, blood supply to, 241
  dural arteriovenous fistula of, blood supply to, *248*, *251–252*
  excision of, in subtemporal transtentorial approach, 68, *73–74*
  meningiomas of, removal of, 120–122, *136–148*
  transection of, in pre-sigmoid sinus approach, 63, *64*
Third ventricle, obliteration of, by craniopharyngioma, *183*
Thyrohyoid muscle, in lateral approach to middle skull base, *46*
Thyroid artery, superior, in lateral approach to middle skull base, *46*
Tonsil(s), cerebellar, suboccipital medial approach to, *17*
Transcallosal approach, to craniopharyngiomas, 179
Transcochlear approach, 24–25, *25*
  to acoustic neurinomas, 157
Transcondylar approach, lateral, to vertebral artery aneurysms, 203, *209*
Transconjunctival lateral orbitotomy, 102, *103*
Transconjunctival medial orbitotomy, 98, *99–100*
Transcutaneous medial orbitotomy, 98–99, *100–101*
Transethmoidal medial orbitotomy, 99
Transethmoidal-transsphenoidal approach, to chordomas, 187, *188–189*
Transfacial approach, to esthesioneuroblastomas, 226
Transfrontal basal approach, 75–76, *76–78*
Transfrontal-transbasal approach, to esthesioneuroblastomas, 226, *228–229*
Translabyrinthine approach, 18–19, *20–23*
  to acoustic neurinomas, *21–23*, 156–157
Transnasal paraseptal approach, to pituitary tumors, 216, *222–223*
Transoral retractor, Crockard, placement of, 95, *96*
Transotic approach, 24–25, *25*
  to acoustic neurinomas, 157
Transsphenoidal approach, 32–33, *33–37*
  to craniopharyngiomas, 177–178
  to decompression of optic canal, 112, *113*
  to nasal septum, *37*
  to pituitary tumors, 215–216, *222*
Transtentorial, transcavernous, transpetrous approach, to basilar artery aneurysms, 202, *208*
Transverse sinus, exposure of, in pre-sigmoid sinus approach, 62, *64*
Trap-door incision, for middle cranial fossa approach, 27, *29*
Trigeminal nerve, compression of, from petroclival meningioma, *137*
Trigeminal nerve *(Continued)*
  decompression of, for removal of epidermoid cyst, *173*
  dissection of, from epidermoid cyst, *173*
Trigeminal neuroma, in Meckel's cave, *11*
Trochlea, in orbitotomy with medial approach, *101*
Trochlear nerve, in subtemporal-transzygomatic approach, *42*
Tuberculum sellae, meningioma of, removal of, 119, *125–130*
    with compression of optic nerve, *129*
  subtemporal transtentorial approach to, *69*
Tumor(s). See specific types, e.g., *Pituitary tumor(s).*
Tumor blush, from chemodectoma, *193*
Turbinate(s), nasal, transsphenoidal approach to, *35*, *37*

Ultrasonic aspirator, for debulking of cerebellopontine angle meningioma, *143*
Unilateral frontal bone flap(s), for subfrontal approach, 3, *5*
Upper basilar artery, approaches to, for repair of aneurysms, 202, *208–209*
Upper clivus, chordoma of, *88*

V2, exposure of, in lateral approach to middle skull base, *49*
Vascular lesion(s), 201–204, *205–211*
  of skull base, angiographic protocols for, 242t
Vascular malformation(s), embolization of, 243–244
Vein of Labbé, pre-sigmoid sinus approach to, *64*
Ventricle(s), third, obliteration of, by craniopharyngioma, *183*
Vertebral arteriovenous fistula(s), embolization of, 243–244
Vertebral artery, aneurysms of, lateral transcondylar approach to, 203, *209*
  course of, at craniocervical junction, 54, *57*
  feeding vertebrovertebral fistula, *254*
  in lateral approach to craniocervical junction, *58*
  suboccipital medial approach to, *17*
Vertebrobasilar artery(ies), after transoral exposure, *97*
Vertebrovertebral fistula, blood supply to, *254*
  embolization of, 244, *254*
Vestibular function, preservation of, 18
Vestibular nerve(s), anatomic relations of, *161*
  fascicles of, visualization of, for removal of acoustic neurinoma, 154, *165*
  inferior, preservation of, in removal of acoustic neurinoma, *162*
  superior, acoustic neurinoma arising in, 153, *162*
Vestibular schwannoma(s), 152–157, *158–169*. See also *Acoustic neurinoma(s).*
Vestibule, middle cranial fossa approach to, *28*
Vomer, exposure of, in lateral approach to middle skull base, *49*

Wright incision, modified, for lateral orbitotomy with bone flap, 102, *103*

Zygoma, in lateral approach to middle skull base, *46*, *48*